Dent

Disclaimer

The material contained in the book (some of which) has been provided by contributing authors. The publisher and editors disclaim any responsibility about the originality of contents

Jaypee's Dental Dictionary

Priya Verma Gupta MDS (Pedodontics)
MA Rangoonwala College of Dental Sciences and
Research Center
Pune, India

LC Gupta MD (Rad) DMRE, MD (PSM), FAMS, DSC (Hon)
Retd Director Medical, Border Security Force
India

Sujata Sarabahi MS, MCh, DNB, MNAMS
Maxillofacial and Plastic Surgeon
Associate Professor
Vardhman Mahavir Medical College and
Safdarjung Hospital, New Delhi, India

 Jaypee Brothers

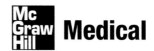 **Mc Graw Hill Medical**

© 2011, Jaypee Brothers Medical Publishers
First published in India in 2009 by

 Jaypee Brothers Medical Publishers (P) Ltd.

Corporate Office
4838/24 Ansari Road, Daryaganj, **New Delhi** - 110002, India, +91-11-43574357

Registered Office
B-3 EMCA House, 23/23B Ansari Road, Daryaganj,
New Delhi 110 002, India
Phones: +91-11-23272143, +91-11-23272703, +91-11-23282021, +91-11-23245672, Rel: +91-11-32558559 Fax: +91-11-23276490, +91-11-23245683
e-mail: jaypee@jaypeebrothers.com
Website: www.jaypeebrothers.com

First published in USA by The McGraw-Hill Companies, 2 Penn Plaza, New York, NY 10121. Exclusively worldwide distributor except South Asia (India, Nepal, Sri Lanka, Bhutan, Pakistan, Bangladesh, Malaysia).

ISBN-13: 978-0-07-175998-4
ISBN-10: 0-07-175998-0

Dedicated to
dynamic, indefatigable spirit of
Padma Shri Dr LK Gandhi
who has been a significant milestone of dental care
for his kind guidance
and wholehearted support

Contributors

Harsh Mohan, MBBS, MD, FIC (Path), FUICC
Prof and Head, Department of Pathology
Government Medical College
Chandigarh, India

Vikram Gandhi, MDS, MNAMS
Reader, Department of Orthodontics
Institute of Dental Sciences of Technologies
Modinagar, Uttar Pradesh, India

Ajay Vidhyarthi, MS, FICS, Fellow (Surgical Oncology)
Senior consultant oncosurgery
Ranchi, Jharkhand, India

Sugandha Mohan, BDS
Government Medical College
Rohtak, Haryana, India

Anurag Singh, MDS (Oral and Maxillofacial Surgery)
Senior Resident
Safdarjung hospital
New Delhi, India

Nikhil Das, BDS
Roma Dental Clinic
Aligarh, Uttar Pradesh, India

Amitha Hegde, MDS
Prof and Head, Department of Pedodontics and
Preventive Dentistry
AB Shetty Memorial Institute of Dental Sciences
Deralakatte, Manglore, Karnataka, India

Vivek Hegde, MDS (Endodontics)
Prof and Head, Department of Endodontics and
Operative Dentistry
MA Rangoonwala College of Dental Sciences and
Research Center, Pune, Maharashtra, India

Pooja Ahmad, BDS
Dental Institute of Guy's, King's and St Thomas's
Kings College
London, United Kingdom

Subhadra H N, MDS (Pedodontics)
DY Patil Dental College
Mumbai, Maharashtra, India

Jyoti Gupta, MDS
Prof and HOD, Department of
Oral Medicine and Radiology
Krishna Medical University and
School of Dental Sciences
Karad, Maharashtra, India

Sachin Dangay, MDS
Senior Consultant Prosthodontics
Delhi Dental Care
New Delhi, India

Ritu Sharma, MDS (Endodontics)
Associate Professor
Department of Endodontics and Operative Dentistry
Hindustan Institute of Dental Science
Uttar Pradesh , India

Anjula Bhagat, MBBS
USA

IS Mehta, BDS
Dental Surgeon
New Delhi, India

Preface

The world of dental sciences has changed dramatically over the last two decades and simultaneously so has the public awareness about dental health increased many folds. To provide qualified health managers new dental colleges and superspecialities are developing fast.

All learning in science is based on education in vocabulary. Mostly dictionaries are concerned with words while encyclopedias explain the object which describes the word to be understood and used correctly. It is a balanced product of both. We have catered to the needs of postgraduate students by including definitions and diseases which they ought to know.

Editors have made special efforts to include maximum words not only related to dentistry but also all other related medical specialities which have a bearing on dental care. The dictionary has been made pictorial to make the reading more interesting and to give a visual impact to the readers.

Appendices have been added. The main objective was to collect useful and frequently used information from various other sources to make it easily available between the two covers of the book.

We are grateful to Prof Dr Harsh Mohan, a man of pathology and his daughter Dr Sugandha who have provided many of the histological slides to make the dictionary more pictorial and useful. Similarly Dr KD Tripathi who is a milestone in the field of pharmacology has been a source of constant academic encouragement to us.

We are also happy to include some line sketches by master Rohan Gupta for better elaboration of certain terms.

Lastly and most importantly we must express our debt and enduring gratitude to our publisher/family friend and guide Shri Jitendar P Vij, Shrimati Raman Vij and young commander Mr Ankit Vij who have published this book of words in four colors and on art paper at a reasonable price.

We would like to express our thanks in advance to anybody who will spare his valuable time to take the trouble to inform us of any shortcomings in this dictionary and we will surely make the necessary amendments in the next edition.

Priya Verma Gupta
LC Gupta
Sujata Sarabahi

Contents

PLATE 1

CRANIAL NERVE

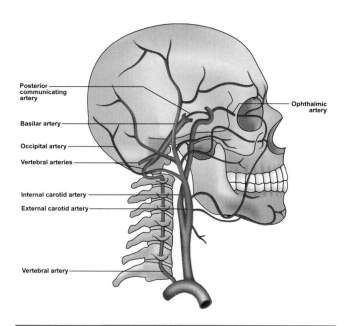

Posterior communicating artery

Ophthalmic artery

Basilar artery

Occipital artery

Vertebral arteries

Internal carotid artery

External carotid artery

Vertebral artery

Arterial blood supply

PLATE 2

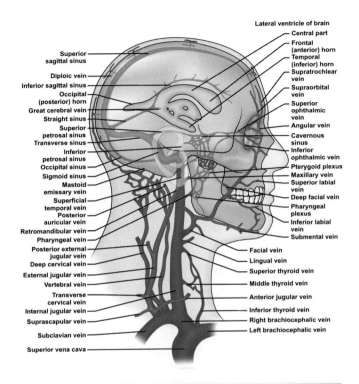

Lateral ventricle of brain
Central part
Frontal (anterior) horn
Temporal (inferior) horn
Supratrochlear vein
Supraorbital vein
Superior ophthalmic vein
Angular vein
Cavernous sinus
Inferior ophthalmic vein
Pterygoid plexus
Maxillary vein
Superior labial vein
Deep facial vein
Pharyngeal plexus
Inferior labial vein
Submental vein
Facial vein
Lingual vein
Superior thyroid vein
Middle thyroid vein
Anterior jugular vein
Inferior thyroid vein
Right brachiocephalic vein
Left brachiocephalic vein

Superior sagittal sinus
Diploic vein
Inferior sagittal sinus
Occipital (posterior) horn
Great cerebral vein
Straight sinus
Superior petrosal sinus
Transverse sinus
Inferior petrosal sinus
Occipital sinus
Sigmoid sinus
Mastoid emissary vein
Superficial temporal vein
Posterior auricular vein
Retromandibular vein
Pharyngeal vein
Posterior external jugular vein
Deep cervical vein
External jugular vein
Vertebral vein
Transverse cervical vein
Internal jugular vein
Suprascapular vein
Subclavian vein
Superior vena cava

Venous supply

PLATE 3

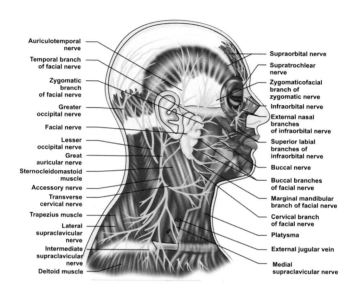

Auriculotemporal nerve

Temporal branch of facial nerve

Zygomatic branch of facial nerve

Greater occipital nerve

Facial nerve

Lesser occipital nerve

Great auricular nerve

Sternocleidomastoid muscle

Accessory nerve

Transverse cervical nerve

Trapezius muscle

Lateral supraclavicular nerve

Intermediate supraclavicular nerve

Deltoid muscle

Supraorbital nerve

Supratrochlear nerve

Zygomaticofacial branch of zygomatic nerve

Infraorbital nerve

External nasal branches of infraorbital nerve

Superior labial branches of infraorbital nerve

Buccal nerve

Buccal branches of facial nerve

Marginal mandibular branch of facial nerve

Cervical branch of facial nerve

Platysma

External jugular vein

Medial supraclavicular nerve

Nerve supply of head and neck

PLATE 4

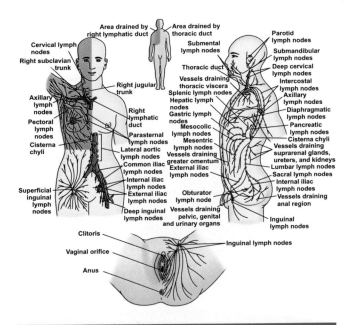

Area drained by right lymphatic duct
Area drained by thoracic duct

Cervical lymph nodes
Right subclavian trunk
Axillary lymph nodes
Pectoral lymph nodes
Cisterna chyli
Superficial inguinal lymph nodes

Right jugular trunk
Right lymphatic duct
Parasternal lymph nodes
Lateral aortic lymph nodes
Common iliac lymph nodes
Internal iliac lymph nodes
External iliac lymph nodes
Deep inguinal lymph nodes

Submental lymph nodes
Thoracic duct
Vessels draining thoracic viscera
Splenic lymph nodes
Hepatic lymph nodes
Gastric lymph nodes
Mesocolic lymph nodes
Mesentric lymph nodes
Vessels draining greater omentum
External iliac lymph nodes
Obturator lymph node
Vessels draining pelvic, genital and urinary organs

Parotid lymph nodes
Submandibular lymph nodes
Deep cervical lymph nodes
Intercostal lymph nodes
Axillary lymph nodes
Diaphragmatic lymph nodes
Pancreatic lymph nodes
Cisterna chyli
Vessels draining suprarenal glands, ureters, and kidneys
Lumbar lymph nodes
Sacral lymph nodes
Internal iliac lymph nodes
Vessels draining anal region
Inguinal lymph nodes

Clitoris
Vaginal orifice
Anus
Inguinal lymph nodes

Lymph nodes

PLATE 5

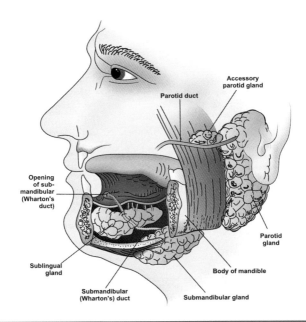

Accessory
parotid gland

Parotid duct

Opening
of sub-
mandibular
(Wharton's
duct)

Parotid
gland

Sublingual
gland

Body of mandible

Submandibular
(Wharton's) duct

Submandibular gland

Salivary glands

PLATE 6

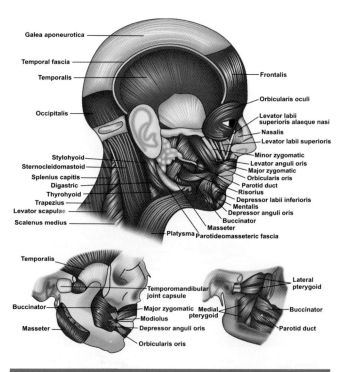

Muscles of facial expression

PLATE 7

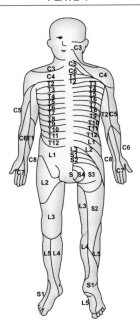

Anterior and posterior view of dermatomes

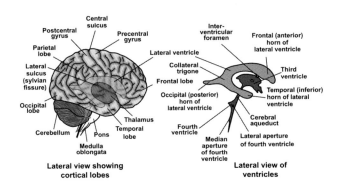

Lateral view showing cortical lobes

Lateral view of ventricles

Lateral view of corticle lobes and ventricles

PLATE 8

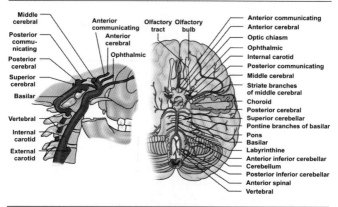

Arteries of head, neck, base of brain

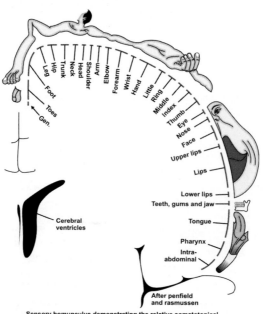

Sensory homunculus demonstrating the relative somatotopical
representation in the somesthetic cortex of the brain

Motor-sensory homunculus

PLATE 9

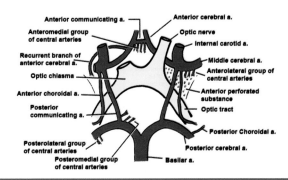

Circle of Willis

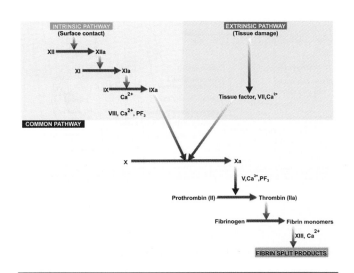

Intrinsic and extrinsic pathways of blood coagulation

PLATE 10

CRANIAL NERVES

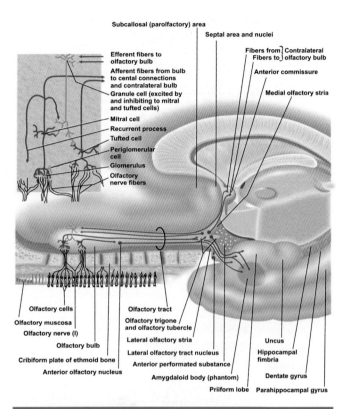

Subcallosal (parolfactory) area

Septal area and nuclei

Fibers from ⎤ Contralateral
Fibers to ⎦ olfactory bulb

Anterior commissure

Medial olfactory stria

Efferent fibers to
olfactory bulb

Afferent fibers from bulb
to cental connections
and contralateral bulb

Granule cell (excited by
and inhibiting to mitral
and tufted cells)

Mitral cell

Recurrent process

Tufted cell

Periglomerular
cell

Glomerulus

Olfactory
nerve fibers

Olfactory cells

Olfactory muscosa

Olfactory nerve (I)

Olfactory bulb

Cribiform plate of ethmoid bone

Anterior olfactory nucleus

Olfactory tract

Olfactory trigone
and olfactory tubercle

Lateral olfactory stria

Lateral olfactory tract nucleus

Anterior performated substance

Amygdaloid body (phantom)

Priiform lobe

Uncus

Hippocampal
fimbria

Dentate gyrus

Parahippocampal gyrus

Olfactory nerve (I)

PLATE 11

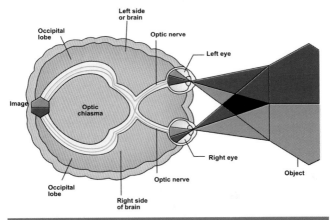

Optic nerve (II)

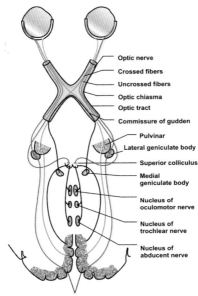

Occulomotor nerve (III), Trochlear nerve (IV), Abducent nerve (VI)

PLATE 12

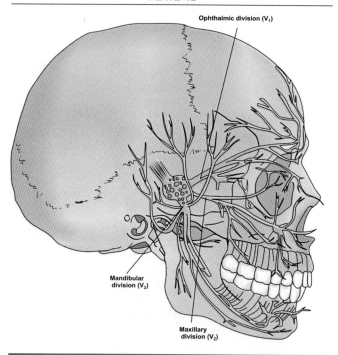

Ophthalmic division (V₁)

Mandibular division (V₃)

Maxillary division (V₂)

Trigeminal nerve (V)

PLATE 13

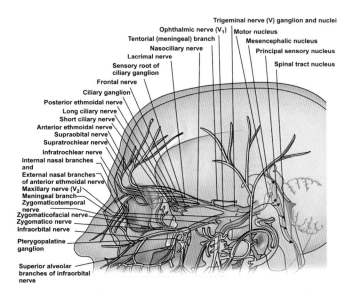

Trigeminal nerve (V) ganglion and nuclei
Ophthalmic nerve (V₁)
Tentorial (meningeal) branch
Nasociliary nerve
Lacrimal nerve
Sensory root of ciliary ganglion
Frontal nerve
Ciliary ganglion
Posterior ethmoidal nerve
Long ciliary nerve
Short ciliary nerve
Anterior ethmoidal nerve
Supraobital nerve
Supratrochlear nerve
Infratrochlear nerve
Internal nasal branches and
External nasal branches of anterior ethmoidal nerve
Maxillary nerve (V₂)
Meningeal branch
Zygomaticotemporal nerve
Zygomaticofacial nerve
Zygomatico nerve
Infraorbital nerve
Pterygopalatine ganglion
Superior alveolar branches of infraorbital nerve

Motor nucleus
Mesencephalic nucleus
Principal sensory nucleus
Spinal tract nucleus

Trigeminal ophthalmic nerve (V₁)

PLATE 14

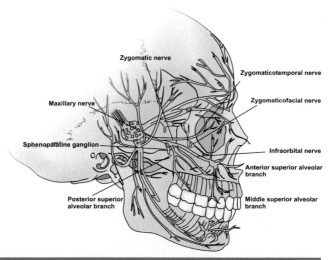

Zygomatic nerve

Zygomaticotemporal nerve

Zygomaticofacial nerve

Maxillary nerve

Sphenopalatine ganglion

Infraorbital nerve

Anterior superior alveolar branch

Posterior superior alveolar branch

Middle superior alveolar branch

Trigeminal maxillary nerve (V₂)

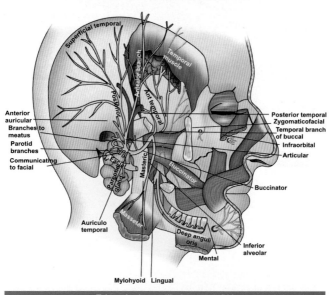

Superficial temporal

Temporal muscle

Posterior

Anterior branch

Ant temporal

Posterior temporal

Zygomaticofacial

Temporal branch of buccal

Infraorbital

Articular

Anterior auricular

Branches to meatus

Parotid branches

Communicating to facial

Parotid gland

Masseteric

Buccinator

Buccinator

Auriculo temporal

Masseter

Deep anguli oris

Mental

Inferior alveolar

Mylohyoid   Lingual

Trigeminal mandibular nerve (V₃)

PLATE 15

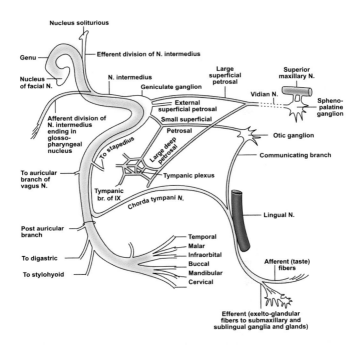

Facial nerve (VII)

PLATE 16

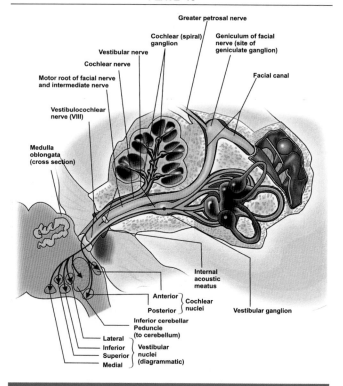

Greater petrosal nerve

Cochlear (spiral) ganglion

Geniculum of facial nerve (site of geniculate ganglion)

Vestibular nerve

Cochlear nerve

Facial canal

Motor root of facial nerve and intermediate nerve

Vestibulocochlear nerve (VIII)

Medulla oblongata (cross section)

Internal acoustic meatus

Anterior } Cochlear
Posterior } nuclei

Vestibular ganglion

Inferior cerebellar Peduncle (to cerebellum)

Lateral
Inferior
Superior
Medial

Vestibular nuclei (diagrammatic)

Vestibulocochlear nerve (VIII)

PLATE 17

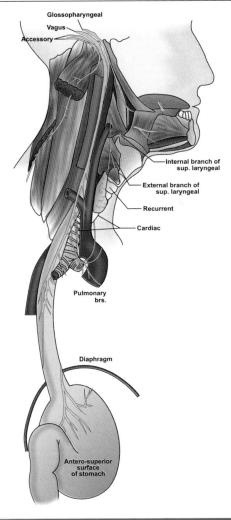

Glossopharyngeal
Vagus
Accessory

Internal branch of
sup. laryngeal

External branch of
sup. laryngeal

Recurrent

Cardiac

Pulmonary
brs.

Diaphragm

Antero-superior
surface
of stomach

Glossopharyngeal nerve (IX)

PLATE 18

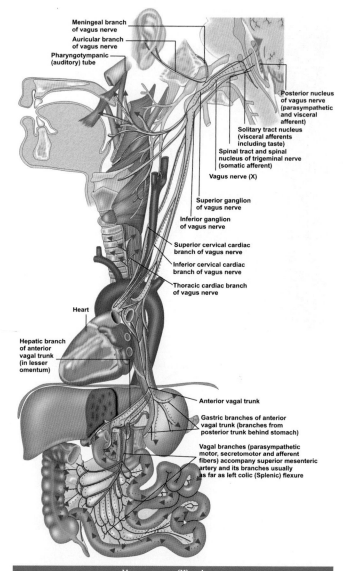

Meningeal branch
of vagus nerve

Auricular branch
of vagus nerve

Pharyngotympanic
(auditory) tube

Posterior nucleus
of vagus nerve
(parasympathetic
and visceral
afferent)

Solitary tract nucleus
(visceral afferents
including taste)

Spinal tract and spinal
nucleus of trigeminal nerve
(somatic afferent)

Vagus nerve (X)

Superior ganglion
of vagus nerve

Inferior ganglion
of vagus nerve

Superior cervical cardiac
branch of vagus nerve

Inferior cervical cardiac
branch of vagus nerve

Thoracic cardiac branch
of vagus nerve

Heart

Hepatic branch
of anterior
vagal trunk
(in lesser
omentum)

Anterior vagal trunk

Gastric branches of anterior
vagal trunk (branches from
posterior trunk behind stomach)

Vagal branches (parasympathetic
motor, secretomotor and afferent
fibers) accompany superior mesenteric
artery and its branches usually
as far as left colic (Splenic) flexure

Vagus nerve (X) schema

PLATE 19

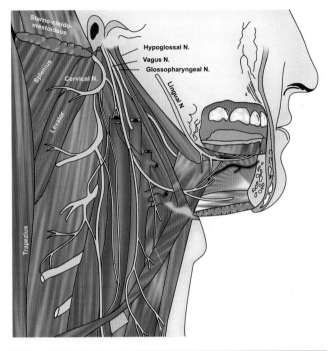

Sterno-cleido-mastoideus

Splenius

Cervical N.

Levator

Hypoglossal N.

Vagus N.

Glossopharyngeal N.

Lingual N

Trapezius

Accessory nerve (XI)

PLATE 20

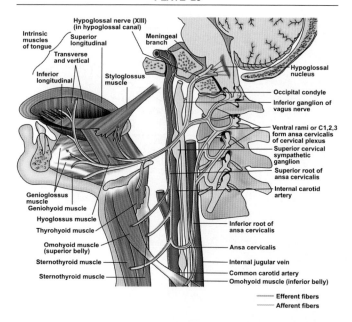

Intrinsic muscles of tongue

Superior longitudinal

Hypoglossal nerve (XIII) (in hypoglossal canal)

Meningeal branch

Transverse and vertical

Inferior longitudinal

Styloglossus muscle

Hypoglossal nucleus

Occipital condyle

Inferior ganglion of vagus nerve

Ventral rami or C1,2,3 form ansa cervicalis of cervical plexus

Superior cervical sympathetic ganglion

Superior root of ansa cervicalis

Internal carotid artery

Genioglossus muscle

Geniohyoid muscle

Hyoglossus muscle

Thyrohyoid muscle

Omohyoid muscle (superior belly)

Sternothyroid muscle

Sternothyroid muscle

Inferior root of ansa cervicalis

Ansa cervicalis

Internal jugular vein

Common carotid artery

Omohyoid muscle (inferior belly)

------- Efferent fibers
——— Afferent fibers

Hypoglossal nerve (XII)

PLATE 21

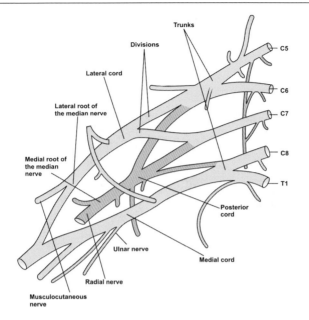

Trunks

Divisions

Lateral cord

Lateral root of
the median nerve

Medial root of
the median
nerve

C5

C6

C7

C8

T1

Posterior
cord

Ulnar nerve

Medial cord

Radial nerve

Musculocutaneous
nerve

Branchial plexus

PLATE 22

OSTEOLOGY

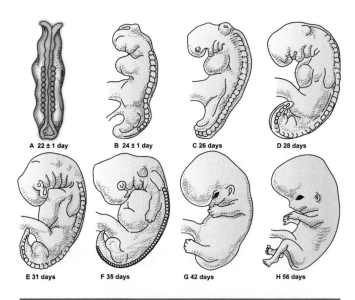

A 22 ± 1 day

B 24 ± 1 day

C 26 days

D 28 days

E 31 days

F 35 days

G 42 days

H 56 days

Human embryo at various stages of development. The relative size has been distorted to emphasize cooorespondence of parts

PLATE 23

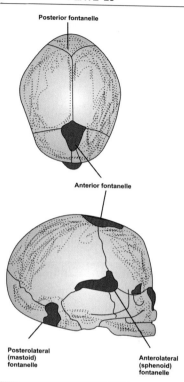

Posterior fontanelle

Anterior fontanelle

Posterolateral
(mastoid)
fontanelle

Anterolateral
(sphenoid)
fontanelle

The fontanelles

PLATE 24

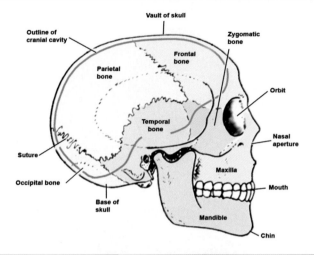

(A) Skull

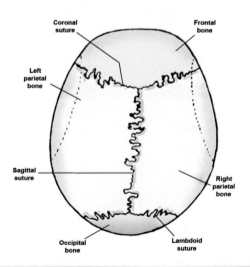

(B) Skull

PLATE 25

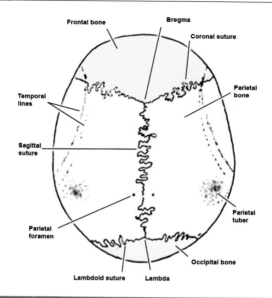

Frontal bone

Bregma

Coronal suture

Temporal lines

Parietal bone

Sagittal suture

Parietal foramen

Parietal tuber

Occipital bone

Lambdoid suture

Lambda

Bregma

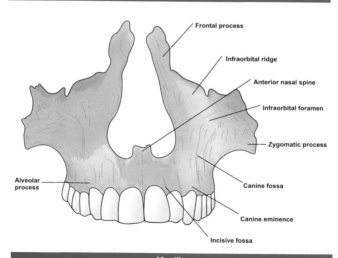

Frontal process

Infraorbital ridge

Anterior nasal spine

Infraorbital foramen

Zygomatic process

Alveolar process

Canine fossa

Canine eminence

Incisive fossa

Maxilla

PLATE 26

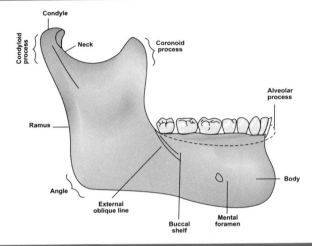

Mandible(D)

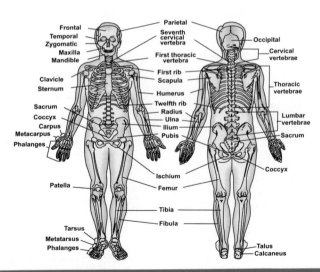

Anterior and posterior view of the human skeleton

A (in reference to cephalometrics) is the deepest midline point in curved bony outline from base to alveolar process of the maxilla.

A beta are the type of fibers which carry sensations like touch, pressure and position.

A delta are the type of fibers which carry sharp pain with a speed of 12-20 m/sec.

Abdominal region refers to abdominopelvic cavity that is divided into '9' regions. The central regions are epigastric, umbilical and hypogastric. Epigastric literally means upon stomach. Umbilical is centremost region surrounding umbilicus and hypogastric region is just below umbilical region. Six regions are on either side, i.e. three to the left and three to the right. These are known as hypochondriac, lumbar and iliac region. Iliac regions are also known as inguinal regions.

Abdominopelvic cavity is a region that is located below diaphragm. Upper portion is called abdominal cavity and contains liver, gallbladder, pancreas, spleen and kidney. Lower portion is known as pelvic cavity. It extends down from the level of hip and contains rectum urinary bladder and internal parts of reproductive system.

Abducent nerve is a sixth cranial nerve. It supplies lateral rectus muscle and turns eye ball laterally.

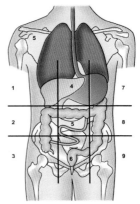

Abdominal quadrants

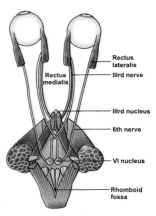

Abducent nerve

Aberrant salivary glands are those salivary gland tissue that develops at a site where it is not found usually. These are frequently seen in cervical region near the parotid gland. Most aberrant glands in neck occur in upper portion of neck.

A

Abfraction is said to have occurred when minute stresses develop around the cervical margins of teeth as a result of the flexure of the root and the crown of the tooth. The cracks propagate from occlusal forces established along the tooth and from abrasion and erosion.

Abortion means spontaneous or induced termination of pregnancy before the fetus is independently viable or the expulsion of an embryo or fetus before it has reached to the stage of viability prior to about 20 weeks of gestation. Therapeutic abortion is done to save woman's life. Complication includes shock and sepsis.

Abrasion is a wearing away of tooth structure due to friction of a foreign object. Most commonly it is caused by tooth brushing and is seen at the cervical margin of teeth. It is more common on left side than right one. It can also be confused with root surface caries. Radiographically it is seen as well-defined horizontal radiolucency along the cervical margin of a tooth. Habitual cigar holder may cause abrading of an incisal edge. Harder materials tend to be more abrasion resistant than soften ones.

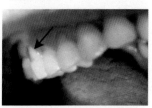
Abrasion cavities with gingival recession

Abrasive index is a method of rating the abrasiveness of dentifrices.

Abrasive refers to the material which causes wear or abrasion of another material.

Abscess refers to a local infection which can be caused due to severe decay, periodontal disease, or trauma. It is characterized by swelling and pain. If an abscess ruptures, it will be accompanied by sudden relief from pain due to a reduction in pressure. A foul taste may also be noticed.

Absent bowel sounds refers to an inability to hear any bowel sounds in any abdominal quadrant. Abdomen distends and risk of perforation or peritonitis develops. It may require immediate attention.

Absentmindedness can be described as habitual inattention marked by preoccupation with thoughts. There is no attention to external stimuli.

Absolute humidity is the weight of water vapour in a unit volume of air. It is expressed as gramms per kg or gramms per cubic meter of air.

Absolute reliability is quantified by standard error of measurement. It is an extent to which a score varies on repeated measurement.

Absorption can be described as penetration of one material into another. Absorption (in reference to radiology) is a process through which X-ray imparts some or all of its energy to the material through which it passes; it depends on the atomic structure of matter and wavelength of the X-ray beam. Absorption also refers to the accumulation of substance at an interface in a concentration different from concentration of substance in bulk.

Absurdity is an idea or expression which is nonsensical, incoherent or meaningless.

Abuse means misuse.

Abutment is a teeth adjacent to an empty space in mouth which will be used to support the prosthetic device which will the space.

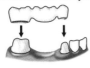

Abutment tooth

Academic refers to formal education.

Acanthesthesia refers to the skin sensation in which there is feeling of pinprick.

Acanthosis nigricans may be benign, malignant and pseudo-acanthosis nigricans. Benign form seems to be genetic. Malignant form is associated with internal malignancy. It develops after 40 years of age. Pseudoacanthosis is a most common form. Tongue and lips appear to be involved more. Lips may be enlarged and covered by papillomatous growths, specially the angle of mouth. Buccal mucosa shows a velvety white appearance with papillary lesions. Gingival papillomatosis with periorofacial mucosal and skin lesions is seen. Gastric adenocarcinoma may develop. There is no treatment for disease.

Acatalepsia refers to the inability to comprehend or reason.

Acataphasia refers to the inability to correctly form a sentence.

Access opening is a procedure done to obtain access to the pulp chamber of the tooth in order to do root canal therapy.

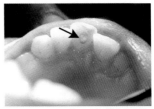

Access opening of an incisor

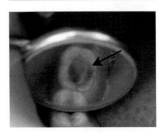

Access opening of a molar

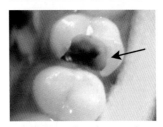

Access opening of a premolar

Accessory gland is a gland that assists organs in doing their function.

Accessory muscle refers to the muscle that participates and assists a major muscle.

Accessory nerve is a motor cranial nerve number eleven. Cranial motor root supplies muscles of soft palate, pharynx and larynx and the spinal root supplies sternocleido-mastoid and trapezius muscles.

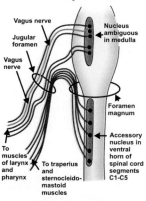

Accessory nerve

Acesulfame refers to the non-cariogenic sweetener about 200 times sweeter than sucrose with a pleasant taste and no aftertaste.

Acetabulum is the large cup shaped cavity on the innominate bone in which femur fits in.

Acetic acid is a chemical found in fixed solution that stops the action of developer.

Acircular refers to the slender needle like.

Acid attack refers to the action of acids that is released from plaque upon enamel.

Acid-base balance refers to the balance of body fluids that is maintained at pH 7.3–7.45 on the alkaline side. Acidic products of the body's metabolism are excreted in urine in combination with bases such as sodium and potassium. These bases are thereby lost to the body and acid-base balance is maintained.

Acid etching is an interim procedure where selective etching of the portions of enamel rods with 37% of phosphoric acid is done in order to increase the surface area and surface energy thereby improving adhesion.

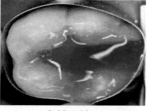

Acid etching

Acid-etch technique is a treatment of tooth enamel with an acid to produce a roughening by dissolving the top layer of enamel to expose the enamel rods and prisms.

Acid is a substance that releases hydrogen ions to a solution. The higher the hydrogen ion concentration of a solution the greater its acidity.

Acidophilic adenoma refers to the small benign lesion of salivary gland. It is more common in woman. The tumor usually measures 3 to 5 in cms above the age of 60. It is composed of large cells with eosinophilic cytoplasm. Lymphoid tissue is commonly present. Malignant transformation is rare and it has to be excised.

Acidulated phosphate fluoride (APF) is a therapeutic agent usually supplied as a gel to increase the fluoride content of dental tissue.

Acinar cells are those cells that are commonly found in salivary glands. The acinar cells are of two types when stained by optical microscopy, i.e. basophilic serous cells and eosinophilic mucous cells. On the basis of their acinar secretary cell composition, the secretions of the parotid and von Ebner's gland are classified as serous. The secretions of submandibular and sublingual glands are mixed. The serous and mucous cells also play on important role in protein glycoprotein secretion.

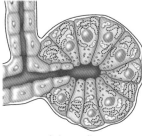

Acinar cells

Acini are pancreatic cells that secrete serous fluid with digestive enzyme.

Acinic cell tumor refers to the pleomorphic adenoma; these are not common neoplasm of salivary gland. Parotid is affected and is not frequently seen in intraoral sites. Clinical features include, size of lesion is about 3 cm, overlying skin is intact, lesion is well defined and slow growing, cystic spaces makes it fluctuant, rarely lip or cheek may be involved. Surgical excision is the solution.

Acne fulminous is an acute onset of extreme severity. It develops abruptly. Numerous large painful papules, nodules and cysts tends to develop. There may be painful arthropathy. Systemic and local steroids may be required.

Acne vulgaris refers to the condition where acne develops over face during teenage. Lesions consist of papules and pustules with black and white heads. Face, back and chest are generally affected. Acne with virilization is due to androgen secreting tumor of adrenal, ovary and testis. Treatment is long and response is slow and uncertain.

Aconite poisoning is mainly used for homicidal purpose. Arrows are poisoned by pastes of aconite by hilly tribes to kill their enemies. Powdered aconite is sprinkled in water of tanks and wells so that who so ever drinks may die. It is extremely unstable hence is difficult to detect if after death.

Acousticophobia refers to the morbid fear of sound or noise.

Acquired congenital reflex is a reflex that develops after the eruption of the posterior primary teeth, from 18 months of age onwards, the child tends to swallow with the teeth brought together by the masticatory muscles action without tongue thrust.

Acquired immunity refers to the immunity that is acquired after birth. It can be described as resistance that is weak or absent in the first exposure but then increases dramatically with subsequent exposures to the same specific pathogen.

Acquity is a sharpness of visual perception.

Acrocinesia refers to the excessive movement.

Acrodermatitis enteropathica is a rare disease affecting childhood and transmitted as an autosomal recessive character. It may be due to zinc deficiency. Patient develops skin lesions, hair loss, nail changes along with diarrhea. Retarded body growth and mental changes also occur. Buccal mucosa, palate, gingiva and tonsils may show red and white spots. Erosions and ulcers are seen along with severe halitosis zinc supplements will be the treatment of choice.

Acrodynia occurs in young infants. There are many cutaneous manifestations. Ear, nose, cheeks become pink. Patient has cold, clammy feeling and the skin over affected area peels off easily. Photophobia, lacrimation, muscular weakness, hypertension and stomatitis is also seen. Drooling of saliva is there, gingiva becomes sensitive to pain, exhibiting ulcer. Mastication becomes difficult. Administration of BAL is helpful.

Acromegaly develops due to excessive growth hormone from anterior pituitary gland. Hands, fingers and feet are enlarged. Face becomes longer. Voice becomes husky. Visual disturbance develops.

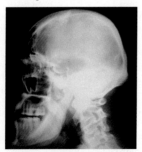

Acromegaly

Acrosoma is a specialized structure of the sperm containing enzymes.

Acrylic is a family of organic molecules carbon-carbon double bond which form polymers useful in making dentures.

Acrylic faced cast metal crown refers to the crown that can be used as long-term provisional crown during the intermediate stage in a large scale oral reconstruction. However it has its own disadvantages as it gets detoriated in the oral cavity by being worn away, discoloring and due to marginal leakage.

Acrylic is a dental material used for prosthesis and various types of appliances. It consists of powder called polymer and a liquid called monomer, when mixed it sets into a hard acrylic by a process called curing. Heat cured acrylic is used for dentures and orthodontic appliances. While cold cured acrylic is used for denture repairs, impression trays and temporary crowns.

Acrylic jacket crowns are used as provisional crowns since they are more permanent than the usual simple temporary procedures and less costly than cast metal crowns. These types of crowns are usually used where other form of treatment such as periodontal or orthodontic treatment is to be done before the final placement of crown.

Actatic speech refers to the unco-ordinated verbal communication.

Actin refers to the muscle protein used in contraction.

Actinomyces is a gram-positive, non-motile, non-spore-forming organisms occurring as rods and filaments that vary considering in length. Filaments are usually long and slender and are branching.

Actinomycosis is caused by gram-positive, non-acid fast branched filamentous bacteria. It is a chronic granulomatous fibrosing disease. Organism may enter the tissues through the oral mucous membrane and may remain localized or spread to the adjacent soft tissue. Skin overlying the abscess is purplish red and indurated or often fluctuant. Mandible is generally involved.

Protein (immunoglobulin) globules
Granule   Filamentous bacteria

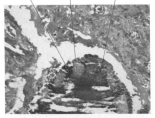

Actinomycosis

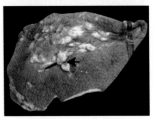

Actinomycosis skin

Action potential is the rapid change in the membrane potential of excitable nerve and muscle cells associated with the conduction of impulses along the cell membrane.

Action tremors range in speed between 7 to 11 Hz and more distally than proximally. Such tremors can easily be suppressed by beta blockers. Alcohol may abolish but withdrawal tremors may appear again.

Activation phase is the activation phase of endothelial binding triggers by factors binding to receptors on neutrophils surface. They include fragments of collagen, soluble factors, by products of complement cascade, Chemokines, PAF, Leukotriene B4, and PGD2. Each leukocyte chemotactic factor is recognized by a specific receptor on the leukocyte surface of the transmembrane receptor family. Contact with even minute amount of such a factor either dissolved in the blood or bound to the endothelial surface triggers diameter changes in the surface adhesion properties of neutrophils. It also induces changes in the conformation of integrins on leukocyte surfaces enabling them to bind specific glycoprotein ligands on endothelium. Chemokines unmasks the binding activities of integrins called MAC–1 Leukocyte Functional Ag (LFA), which can then bind to ICAM-1 on activated endothelial cell.

Active eruption refers to the emergence of the tooth in the oral cavity from its position in the jaw (*see* Figure on page 8).

Active exercises are movements of body due to voluntary contraction and relaxation of muscle.

Active immunity is of 2 types natural or acquired. It occurs naturally when disease is caused by micro-organism and protection against further attack by that micro-organism is conferred to the individual if the body recovers from the disease.

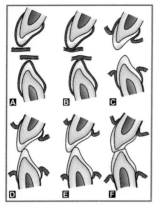
Active eruption

Active memory refers to the short-term memory.

Acupressure is a type of therapy where physician puts light and medium pressure on certain specific points. Their aim is to stimulate the body's electro-magnetic energy to help body's own recuperative powers to remove energy blockage. Block-age is due to production of lactic acid and carbon monoxide in muscle tissue resulting in stiff musculature. Removal of block-age relaxes the whole body.

Acupuncture is a system of science where the needles are inserted into patient's skin to treat diseases. Chinese thought that life force flows through the meri-dians. Flow of force when blocked results in disease. Needles are inserted at specific sites. Acupun-cture releases endorphins which act as natural analgesics. Acupun-cture has shown successful results in dental surgery and in process of delivery.

Acute abdomen is a persistent, severe abdominal pain of sudden onset. There may be fever. Abdominal wall may be tense due to appendicitis, salpingitis and peritonitis.

Acute adenitis is a simple inflammation of lymph gland. Glands are body guard of specific area and these enlarge when infection develops in their area. In different type of diseases pattern of gland involvement is different. In infection these enlarge but may remain mobile, in TB, these may be matted, in malignancy these may be enlarged and fixed.

Acute atrophic candidiasis is red patch of atrophic raw, painful mucosa which develops with minimal evidence of pseudo-membrane. Depapillation of tongue and antibiotic sore throat may be seen.

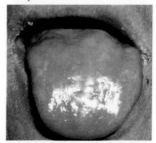
Depapillated tongue

Acute bacterial sialadenitis is caused by streptococcus pyogenes and staphylococcus aureus. Bacteria reach the gland through Stensen's duct. Diabetes, Sjögren's syndrome are the causative factors. Clinical features include sudden onset of painful swelling in the preauricular region. Parotid glands may be involved unilaterally or bilaterally. Fever, weakness and redness of skin over parotid are seen. There may be difficulty in swallowing. Antibiotics are helpful.

Acute cholecystitis is an inflammation of gallbladder always associated with gallstones. There is peritoneal pain with overlying skin tenderness and muscle rigidity in right hypochondrium. Referred pain may be radiating to back on right shoulder. Nausea and vomiting may be present. Tenderness and muscle guarding develops in right upper quadrant. In some cases palpable mass of globular shape below right costal palpable margin moving with respiration may be feet. Serum bilirubin will be raised. There may be area of hyperesthesia over right subcapsular region.

Acute cold exposure is said to have occurred when body temperature is less than 35°C. Vasodilatation increases the risk of hypothermia. It may result in dizziness, dyspnea, confusion and inco-ordination. Signs include shivering, dysarthria and altered mental status. Person may suffer from hypotension and respiratory depression.

Acute cystitis is an infection of the bladder most commonly due to coliform bacteria and enterococci. Route of infection is ascending from urethra. Frequency, urgency, dysuria with suprapubic discomfort is common. Ladies may develop hematuria especially after intercourse. Urine shows pyuria and bacteriuria. Uroflox responds well.

Acute dacrocystis refers to the condition where patient presents with pain and swelling near the medial canthus of the eye associated with epiphora. Nose appears red, hot, ill defined and very tender. On pressure over the swelling there is no regurgitation through the puncta. Edema and redness may extend to lower eyelid. Submandibular lymph node may be enlarged and tender.

Acute epididymitis occurs when the route of infection is via urethra to the ejaculatory duct and then down the vas deferens to the epididymis. Symptoms of uretheritis, pain at tip of urethera or cystitis may develop. Pain develops in scrotum radiating to spermatic cord or flank. Prostate may be tender.

Acute gingivitis refers to the inflammation of gingiva, it is the disease of sudden onset and short duration; the condition may be painful in nature

Acute hepatitis refer to the inflammation of lever due to bacteria present within hours or 1-2 days after symptoms. While patients with chronic hepatitis present less acutely with a history of months that could be mostly tuberculous in origin.

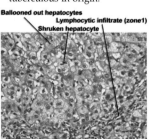
Ballooned out hepatocytes
Lymphocytic infiltrate (zone1)
Shruken hepatocyte

Acute hepatitis

Acute herpes' zoster is due to the neurotropic virus travelling along the involved nerve. It causes neuritis and vesicular disease of skin and mucous membrane. Eruption is located to a single dermatome. High dose antiviral therapy in acute phase of herpes zoster improves the rate of healing. Intensity of pain is also reduced. Post-herpetic neuralgia may continue in old persons.

Acute herpetic stomatitis is an acute viral infectious disease. In 1939 Dodd isolated virus from gingivostomatitis. Patient develops fever, irritability, headache, pain and regional lymphadenopathy. Lips, tongue and buccal mucosa are also involved. Painful gingival swelling develops with yellowish fluid filled vesicles, ulcers develop in varying size. These heal automatically within 7-14 days and leave no scar. Isolation can be detected in tissue culture.

Acute illness is the one that comes on suddenly and for a short period.

Acute inflammation is characterized by signs of acute inflammation, i.e. redness, heat, swelling, pain and loss of function. In early stage acute inflammation, edema fluid, fibrin and neutrophils accumulate in the extracellular space of damaged tissue (*see* Figure).

Acute intolerance is a strong negative reaction to a minimal amount of anoxing object.

Acute iritis refers to conjuctival infection around cornea. There may be severe pain, blurred vision, photophobia and constricted pupil.

Acute leukemia may be lymphoblastic and myeloblastic. It may be acute or chronic depending

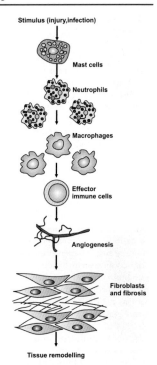

Stimulus (injury,infection)

Mast cells

Neutrophils

Macrophages

Effector immune cells

Angiogenesis

Fibroblasts and fibrosis

Tissue remodelling

Acute inflammation

upon the nature and progression of disease. Development is sudden with fever, sore throat, headache, swelling of lymph glands, petechial hemorrhage in skin and mucous membrane. Spleen, kidney and liver become enlarged. Decrease in platelet may lead to hemorrhage. Terminal infection is frequent (*see* Figure on page 11).

Acute lingual tonsillitis gives rise to unilateral dysphagia and feeling of lump in throat. Lingual tonsil may appear enlarged and congested. It may be studded

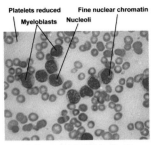

Platelets reduced   Fine nuclear chromatin
  Myeloblasts   Nucleoli

Acute myeloblastic leukemia

with follicles. Cervical lymph nodes may be enlarged. Treatment is by antibiotics.

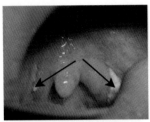

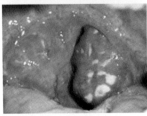

Acute tonsillitis

Acute lymphonodular pharyngitis is an acute febrile disease of children. Sore throat, fever and loss of appetite develop. Symptoms last from 4 to 14 days. Oral manifestation consists of white to yellowish solid papules surrounded by a narrow erythema. It contains packed nodules of lymphocytes.

Acute maxillary sinusitis refers to the periapical infection and may involve maxillary sinus. Patient develops pain and swelling over sinus. Pressure over maxillary sinus will increase pain. Fever and pain may be radiated to the ear. Antibiotics and anti-inflammatory drugs help.

Acute melancholia can be characterized by constant headache, insomnia, irritability and gastric upsets. Onset is gradual. Hallucinations and delusions are very common. Suicidal and homicidal impulses may be seen. Patient may get excited over a minor incident. It may be followed by mania and lucid interval cyclically.

Acute myocardial infarction (AMI) is a clinical syndrome caused by a deficient coronary arterial blood supply to a region of myocardium that results in cellular death and necrosis. This syndrome is usually characterized by severe and prolonged substernal pain but more intense and longer duration than angina pectoris. Cause of acute myocardial infarction in more than 90% of cases is coronary artery disease. Other risk factors include obesity and undue stress, also elevated blood pressure and/or elevated blood cholesterol. Immediate predisposing failures for AMI include a significant decrease in blood flow through the coronary arteries, as in coronary thrombosis (*see* Figure on page 12).

Acute necrotizing ulcerative gingivitis (ANUG) is an endogenous oral infection having necrosis of gingiva. Blood diseases and

A

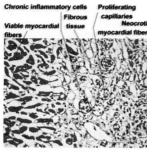

Chronic inflammatory cells / Proliferating capillaries
Fibrous tissue / Neocrotic myocardial fibers
Viable myocardial fibers

Myocardial infarct

severe nutritional deficiencies may also result in it. It develops sudden pain, tenderness, profuse salivation and spontaneous bleeding. Typical fetid odor develops. Lesion consist of painful, punched out, necrotic ulcers developing on interdental papillae and gingival margin but lips, tongue and palate may also be involved. Gingiva bleeds on touch and is covered by a gray, necrotic pseudomembrane. Patient is not able to eat. Pain is a superficial pressure type. Trench mouth was the term given during World War I when in trenches soldiers suffered from acute necrotizing of ulcerative gingivitis. It is an overgrowth of organisms prevalent in normal flora. Disease is not transmissible. Organisms work symbiotically named fusiform bacillus and spirochetes.

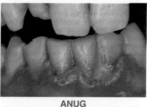

ANUG

Acute otitis media is a condition where patient is a young child and complaints of pain in ear. There may be hear loss, fever, vomiting, and diarrhea. Tympanic membrane is bulging. Bloody then serosanguinous and finally purulent otorrhea may follow. Spontaneous perforation of tympanic membrane gives relief.

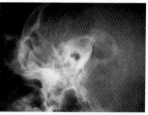

Otitis media

Acute pain is associated with the pain of sudden onset and short duration.

Acute pancreatitis is an idiopathic condition. Sudden onset of acute excruciating epigastric pain with radiation to back is the main complaint. Pain is more in supine position and there is some relief when patient sits up. Low grade fever, tachycardia and hypotension are common. Bowel sounds are depressed. Green coloration of flanks indicates severe necrotizing pancreatitis. Ultrasound is a good modality to diagnose it.

Acute pericoronitis an infection or abscess associated with a partially erupted tooth or fully erupted tooth that is covered completely or partially by a flap of tissue.

Acute phase response is most soluble mediators of innate immunity found in relatively small amount in the serum under normal conditions. Concentration of these proteins can increase 1000 fold during serious injury as part of co-ordinated protective response called *"Hepatic acute phase response'.* Liver temporarily increases its synthesis of more than a dozen serum proteins that participate in antimicrobial defense. Response occurs when hepatocytes are exposed to certain cytokines like 1L-6, 1L-1, TNF, LPS of bacteria.

Acute proliferative glomerulo-nephritis is a renal condition where the renal symptoms develop after a period of 10 days. Fifty percent of patient develops hypertension. Urine is of high specific gravity of smoky color. Urinary rudiments contain red cells casts and granular casts. Transient elevation in BUN and serum creatinine may be seen. There may be frank hematuria with periorbital hematoma. Hematuria may be gross or microscopic with oliguria. Both kidneys are swollen. External surface can be smooth with petechiae.

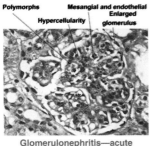

Polymorphs   **Mesangial and endothelial Enlarged**
Hypercellularity   **glomerulus**

Glomerulonephritis—acute

Acute pulpalgia refers to the development of pulpal inflam-mation or pulpitis. Increased intra-pulpal pressure is the stimulus that is applied to the sensory nerves of the pulp and leads to severe toothache. It occurs with a large carious lesion or with restoration. Severe pain is elicited with thermal changes especially cold. Pain is of lancinating type. Intensity of pain increases when patient lies down, when entrance to the diseased pulp is not wide pain becomes severe. Pulp contains large number of bacteria. There is no specific treatment and once pulpitis occurs, the damage is irreparable. Tooth involved with acute pulpitis may be treated by pulp therapy.

Acute pyelonephritis this condition is uncommon in contrast to acute cystitis. Vesicoureteric infection, pregnancy and instrumentation may predispose to it. Diabetes predisposes to infection. Person develops loin pain, high fever and often rigors. There may be much destruction of cortex sparing of glomeruli and blood vessels.

Acute renal failure is a sudden onset of renal failure generally associated with Liguria. In a few weeks renal function is restored. There are two mechanisms ischemia and nephrotoxicity.

Acute retroviral syndrome is a non-specific viral syndrome occurring 1-6 weeks following HIV exposure. Many of the clinical features may go unrecognized. Symptoms include fever, sweats, malaise, truncal rash, mouth pain and neck stiffness. Liver and spleen are enlarged. Fever with lymphadenopathy develops.

Acute suppurative osteomyelitis is a squeale of periapical infection. Dental infection is the commonest

A

cause. Staphylococcus aureus and staphylococcus albus are the commonest one. Maxilla or mandible may be involved. There will be severe pain, enlargement of lymph glands. WBC count is elevated. Once periostitis develops there is no swelling or reddening of skin. On X-ray lytic lesion is noted. Individual trabeculae becomes fuzzy and indistinct. Separated fragment of dead bone is called sequestrum. For large sequestrum surgical removal is to be done.

Adaptation refers to the manner in which working end of an instrument is placed against the surface of the tooth to get maximum adaptability or proximity to the tooth surface and avoid soft tissue trauma.

Adaptive immune system is said to have occurred when innate system is breached, a specific response is mounted to each infectious agent and the infectious agent is remembered to prevent it causing infection later.

Addicted is the one who is dependent and has a strong psychological reliance on a specific drug.

Addiction is a habit forming and has a compulsive physiological need for it.

Addition polymerization is a polymerization process involving free radicles in which no byproduct is formed as the chain grows.

Addition silicone is a silicone polymer resulting from free radical polymerization of vinyl group of platinum catalysts.

Adduction is a movement of body part toward the middle of the body.

Adenoameloblastoma arises from residual odontogenic epithelium. In early stage tumor is completely radiolucent. It may be solid or may contain large cystic areas. It forms duct like structures. Site of occurrence is more in maxilla. Vast majority measure 1.5 to 3 cm. Minute calcifications are also seen under microscope. In advanced stage, sufficient calcification occurs to produce clusters of radiopaque foci with the radiolucency. Majority occurs in unerupted tooth or in the walls of dentigerous cyst. Mostly involved teeth are maxillary canine, lateral incisors, mandibular premolar. Slow growth expands the cortical plates and produces a clinical signs of swelling and asymmetry is seen. Radiographs shows destructive lesions of jaw which may or may not be well circumscribed. Soft tissues are not involved.

Adenocarcinoma occurs more commonly in relation to minor salivary glands. The tumor is slow growing with no surface ulceration. It is a painless mass. Later on tumor grows faster. Swelling becomes painful. Ulceration and loss of sensation develops. Under microscope one can see numerous proliferating malignant ductal epithelial cells. There will be areas of hemorrhage and necrosis (*see* Figure on page 15).

Adenocystic carcinoma is a malignant neoplasm arising from glandular epithelium. It is a most common malignant tumor of submandibular salivary gland. Glands of palate and tongue can also be involved. Parotid tumor

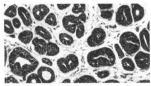
Adenocarcinoma

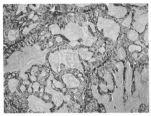
Adenocarcinoma high power

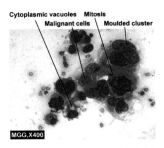
Cytoplasmic vacuoles   Mitosis
   Malignant cells   Moulded cluster
MGG, X400
Adenocarcinoma and ascitic fluid

produces a subcutaneous mass anterior to or below the external ear. Pain is a very common feature in this tumor. There is fixation and induration of tumor. Submandibular gland tumors become quite large. While palatal lesions are often accompanied by delayed healing of socket once tooth has been extracted. If greater palatine nerve is involved palatal parasthesia will develop. Treatment involves excision followed by radiotherapy because tumor cells are radiosensitive.

Adenofibroma is a frequent neoplasm of youth occurring below the age of 25 years. These are usually small, painless tumors discovered incidently. Adenofibroma occasionally undergoes spontaneous infarction and necrosis during pregnancy. Necrosis usually produces no symptoms.

Adenoids are gland like, known as pharyngeal tonsils. These are paired lymphoid structures in the nasopharynx.

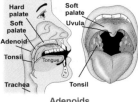
Location of tonsils and adenoids
Hard palate   Soft palate
Soft palate   Uvula
Adenoid
Tonsil   Tongue
Trachea   Tonsil
Adenoids

Adenoid squamous cell carcinoma develops in younger age. Lesion appears as elevated nodule. It shows scaling, crusting and ulceration. There is a proliferation of surface dysplastic epithelium. Surgical excision helps.

Adenolymphoma is a benign salivary gland neoplasm. It is also known as *Warthin's tumor* and develops in parotid gland tumor is superficially lying just beneath the parotid capsule. It is firm but not palpable. It consists of cystic spaces with intraluminar projections. It contains lot of lymphoid tissue. It may develop due to proliferation of ectopic salivary gland tissue. Some think that it is a hemartous growth than a true neoplastic lesion. It comprises 20% of all parotid tumors. It is well encapsulated and movable. It is a slow growing well circumscribed soft and painless, and can grow up to 2-4 cm in diameter. It gives a compressible and doughy feeling on palpation, on cut surface confluent cystic spaces are seen and chocolate colored fluid comes out. Dense fibrous capsule surrounds it. Malignant transformation is rare. Surgical excision is to be done.

Adenoma thyroid is a solitary discrete nodule. These arise from follicular epithelium known as follicular adenomas. It is well circumscribed solitary, round, rubbery, firm and well capsulated. Cut surface is brown and translucent.

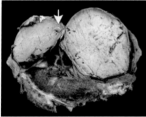

Capsule   Compressed follicles   Fetal follicles

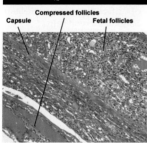

Adenoma thyroid

Adenomatoid odontogenic tumor is well encapsulated lesion having preference for maxilla than mandible. Often it presents as a cystic lesion with a missing tooth.

It has several masses of mural nodules composed of duct like structures. Amorphous calcification is seen radiographically.

Adhesion refers to the force of attraction between the molecules or atoms on two different surfaces as they are brought into contact with one another or it can be described as the surface attachment of two materials. In simple words it refers to the sticking together of unlike substances.

Adjuvant therapy is the treatment given after the primary treatment such as radiation therapy or hormonal therapy.

Admissed alloy is an amalgam alloy containing particles of different composition, i.e. silver tin or silver copper particles.

Adolescence is the period of transition from childhood to adulthood. It can also be described as period of 3 to 4 years after puberty; extending from the earlier signs of sexual maturity until the attainment of physical and emotional maturity.

Adolescent caries are lesions in teeth and surfaces those are relatively immune to caries. There is relatively small opening in enamel with extensive undermining of enamel. Rapid penetration of enamel and extensive involvement of dentin is seen. The rapid progression of the lesion does not permit an effective pulpal response with little or no secondary dentin.

Adrenal gland is an endocrine gland composed of cortex and medulla. These are two organs situated at upper poles of kidneys and are embedded in perirenal fat. Size of these is 1½ x ¾ x ½ an inch. Right is pyramidal in shape while left one is crescent shaped. Adrenal cortex produces and secretes more than 30 steroid hormones, of which cortisol, a glucocorticoids, is widely considered the most important. Cortisol helps the body adapt to stress.

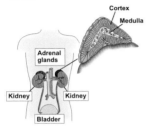

Adrenal glands

Adrenaline is a hormone secreted by medulla of adrenal glands. It is first hormone to be discovered. Under emotional stress; BP rises due to its liberation. Blood sugar and BMR also rises. Chemically it is hydroxyl, dihydroxy phenyl ethylemethyline.

Adulteration of milk is a process where the milk is adulterated by addition of skimmed milk powder, gelatine or starch with maida or arrow root after extraction of fat to make it thick. Common methods of adulteration of milk are adding water to increase the quantity. Second most common is extraction of cream from milk partially or completely.

Adulthood refers to the stage of growth and development where ossification and growth are virtually completed during early adulthood, i.e. upto 18 to 25 years of age. There after developmental changes occur very slowly.

Advanced acute pulpalgia is a stage of pulpal pathology where the pain is very severe the most excruciating acute pain known to man. Patient may even become hysterical due to pain. Relief from this pain is embarrassingly by simple cold water. The history is self-incriminating. Symptoms are violent. The involved tooth usually can be pointed out by patient and is tender to percussion too. Because the inflamed pulp reacts so violently to heat, the most decisive test is the heat test. As soon as not gutta-percha touches the involved tooth, the patient develops subgluteal vacuum and patient rises up in the chair as if stabbed. Cold water is instantly applied and pain subsides. Local anesthesia gives blessed relief.

Advanced interproximal lesion refers to the carious lesion that extends to the dentino-noenamel junction (DEJ) or through the DEJ and into the dentin, but does not extend through the dentin greater than half the distance toward the pulp. An advanced lesion affects both enamel and dentin.

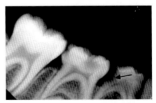

Advanced proximal caries

Adypsia is an abnormal absence of thirst. It occurs in hypothalamic

A

injury/tumor, head injury, cirrhosis and bronchial tumor.

Aerobic bacteria are micro organism that require oxygen to live or aerobic bacteria are the bacteria which grow in oxygen rich environment; in the oral cavity the bacteria are found outside the sulcus.

Aerobic is a physiological process in which oxygen is required.

Aerobic training is a process of training when consumption of oxygen develops muscles ability to sustain activity.

Aerosol refers to mist.

Afebrile is absence of fever.

Afferent is nerve that carry sensory messages toward the brain.

Afferent impulse is an impulse travelling toward the central nervous system.

Aflatoxin is a toxic metabolite of mould Aspergillus flavus discovered in 1960. Infected groundnuts result it. Other nuts may also contain it. Aflatoxin B1 is acutely toxic and carcinogenic. If it is consumed by cows, aflatoxin M1 may be found in milk and cheese.

Agar hydrocolloids are the impression materials that are compounded from reversible agar gels. When heated they liquefy or go into solution state and on cooling they return to gel state. It is usually extracted from seaweed. It is a polysaccharide in nature. Agar impressions are unstable on standing so model should be made at earliest by origin Agar is a gelatine like substance obtained from seaweed.

Age of abrasion describes the likelihood as to when the abrasion occurred, e.g. fresh abrasion is bright red and oozing. In 24 hours bright red scab forms which becomes reddish grows and covers the defect under scab. In 7-10 days scab dries up, shrinks and falls leading to discoloration. For complete healing it takes 14 days.

Age of bruise describes the likelihood of the forniation of bruise, e.g. a bruise is red just after infliction and it becomes blue on 3rd day. On 4th day it becomes brown due to hemosiderin. On 5th and 6th color becomes green. 7th to 11th day color is yellow due to bilirubin and after 2 weeks color becomes normal.

Age refers to the chronological or date of birth.

Agglutination is the clumping together of cells distributed in a fluid, generally a result of antigen antibody reaction.

Aglycogeusia refers to the condition where the affected individual is not able to distinguish sugar solution from water.

Agnosia refers to the condition where there is the loss of ability to recognize objects by one sense organ while other sense organs may recognize it. Auditory agnosia is the inability to recognize familiar sounds. Lesions in left angular gyrus produce finger agnosia. Anonsognosia is a denial of disease in the affected body part.

Agranulocytopenia refers to the marked reduction in granular leukocytosis. Toxic effect of certain drugs like chloramphenicol, phenyl butazone may result in it. Long-term administration of analgesics, diuretics and anticoagulants may cause it. Ionizing radiation, TB, malaria and typhoid may also induce agranulocytosis.

Fever, generally starts with chills and sore throat. Skin becomes pale. Even jaundice may develop, Regional lymphadenitis may develop, Urinary tract infection may develop, Rectal ulcerations are common, Severe leukopenia develops, Neutrophils count comes down to 0-2%. Agranulocytic angina develops showing necrotizing ulceration over gingival, soft palate and cheeks. Excessive salivation is noted. Ulcers develop which are covered by yellow/ gray membrane. Ulcers may start bleeding. Halitosis develops. Opportunistic fungal infections may develop.

Agranulocytosis is a condition where there is marked decrease in the number of circulating neutrophils. In primary Agranulocytosis cause is not known while in secondary one cause can be traced out. Reaction may be allergic one. It can occur at any age. Disease starts as high fever with chill and sore throat. Patient suffers from weakness and prostration. Development a necrotizing ulceration of oral mucosa. Salivation increases. Necrosis of gingiva may develop. Rapid destruction of supporting tissues follows. Granular white blood cells disappear from circulation due to idiosyncrasy towards certain drugs like sulphonamides, phenylbutazone and phenothiazines. Person will develop fever, rigor and extreme weakness. Throat shows brownish gray or white exudates and there may be an ulceration of tonsils and buccal mucosa. Lymph glands are enlarged.

Agraphia is an inability to express thoughts in writing. It generally occurs due to cerebrovascular accidents.

AIDS is a disabling or life threatening disease caused by human immunodeficiency virus. Major signs include 10% weight loss. Chronic diarrhea and fever of one month may occur. Minor signs include persistent cough of one month, recurrent herpes zoster, and generalized lymphadenopathy. Most common oral manifestations are hairy leukoplakia, oral candidiasis and Kaposi's sarcoma. Other infections associated with it are orolabial herpes, aggressive pathological periodontal disease and dryness of mouth. Acute infection occurs 3 to 6 weeks after initial contact with HIV. Nonspecific syndrome occurs during which joints pain, gastrointestinal symptoms and a macular rash predominate. These self-limiting symptoms persist for 2-3 weeks. Eights to twelve weeks after infection, antibody to HIV can be detected in serum. After acute infection person enters the symptomatic phase of the disease. The average time from infection to development of disease is 8 to 10 years. During this period T4 lymphocytes comes down from 800 mm^3 to 50 mm^3. Oral manifestations in HIV infected patients are Oral candidiasis occurring in 30% to 90% cases. Persistent ulcers of mouth in AIDS should be biopsied for deep fungal infections. Hairy leukoplakia has been noted in HIV positive homosexuals. Recurrent herpes simplex virus progresses to large chronic oral lesions. Ulcers are surrounded by raised white border. Lesions may co-exist with genital and anal lesions. Painful oral ulcers caused by cytomegalovirus may be seen. Kaposi's sarcoma is the most common oral neoplasm in AIDS. Early lesions look like hemangiomas, flat or raised discolorations. Generalized gingivitis and periodontitis develop.

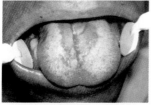
Oral candidias in HIV patient

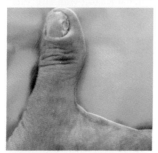
Herpes infection in HIV patient

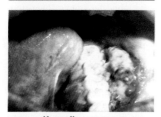
Kaposi's sarcoma

AIDS of CNS has phases of primary infection, asymptomatic infection and established phase. In primary phase 10% patients have aseptic encephalitis and virus can be isolated from CSF. During asymptomatic phase there is also aseptic meningitis but virus is not recoverable from CSF. Prednisolone may give relief. In established disease neurological features are very common when peripheral T4 cell count falls below 500/c mm. Dementia is a well known feature of HIV disease. These patients have neuronal atrophy and gliosis. There will be slowness of thought, loss of interest and withdrawal from society.

Air powder abrasive polisher is a polishing device that sprays a solution of sodium bicarbonate and water to remove stain and plaque from the surface of tooth.

Air velocity is measured by aremometer. At a height of 10 meters velocity is measured. It is measured in meters per second.

Air-water syringe is a device which delivers a stream of water or air and can also deliver a forceful spray of air and water. It is generally used to rinse the patient's mouth.

Airway obstruction is a condition where partial or complete airway obstruction may occur either due to trauma or any underlying pathology. Dyspnea and cyanosis may occur in seconds and death may occur due to asphyxia or reflex cardiovascular collapse.

ALARA is a concept of radiation protection where radiation is to be kept at minimum. It stands for AS LOW AS REASONABLY ACHIEVABLE.

Albinism is the absence of pigment in skin, hair and eyes of an animal. Absence of chlorophyll in plants.

Albright's syndrome is like fibrous dysplasia of bone. There is replacement of spongy bone by a peculiar fibrous tissue. Radiographs will show radiopacity and radiolucency, some like compact bone other like cystic bone. The cause of endocrine manifestation in Albright's syndrome is not known. Transformation to malignancy occurs. Radiotherapy is not advised.

Albumin is a plasma protein which helps in regulation of the osmotic concentration of the blood.

Albuminuria refers to the presence of albumin in urine usually due to kidney disorder.

Alcohol toxicity refers to the condition where skin becomes cold and clammy. Body temperature is lowered. Respiration is slow, shallow and noisy. Pulse is weak and accelerated. Pupils become sluggish and various reflexes are generally depressed.

Alcoholic hepatitis consists of alcoholic hyaline, hepatic infiltration with polymorphonuclear cell and intralobular connective tissue proliferation. Person may be asymptomatic to mild illness. Hepatomegaly with splenomegaly is common. Fever and jaundice are common. Testicular atrophy, parotid enlargement and loss of body hair are often seen. In severe form ascites, edema and encephalopathy are seen. Treatment includes high calorie diet and vitamin supplement. Proteins are restricted and corticosteroids 20-40 mg may be tried.

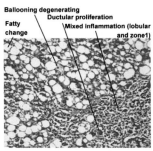
Alcoholic hepatitis

Alcoholic ketoacidosis occurs after drinking binge by a malnourished, chronic alcoholic resulting in elevated anion gap acidosis. Symptoms include anorexia, nausea abdominal pain and orthostatic dizziness. There may be odor of ketone on breath, tachycardia and tachypnea.

Aldrich syndrome is a rare hereditary disease transmitted as an X-linked recessive trait. It generally develops in infancy. It develops thrombocytopenic purpura and eczema over face. Eczema is of allergic origin. Spontaneous bleeding of gingiva is frequently seen. There is an abnormality of platelets. There is no specific treatment.

Alginate is an impression material used for recording impressions dentures. It gives an accurate impression, without distortion. It is mixed by powder and water at room temperature. This sets within a few minutes. Material is an elastic one but the disadvantage is if kept for long. It undergoes dimensional changes. So it should be repeatedly rinse in cold running water and dip in sodium hypochloride.

A

Alimentary canal is a digestive tract consisting of mouth, esophagus, stomach duodenum and large intestine (*see* Figure).

Alitame is an artificial sweetener that is 2000 times sweeter than sucrose. It is formed from Laspartic acid and D-alanine having a clean taste and is stable.

Alkaptonuria or ochronosis which is a recessively inherited inborn error of metabolism, is characterized by deposition of dark pigments in bones, joints and nasal cartilages. Occasionally brownish discoloration of the permanent dentition can also be observed.

All and none phenomenon is said to have occurred where nerve or muscle cell either will respond or not respond at all. It responds maximally every time. It is not related with the intensity of stimulus.

Allergic sialadenitis is a non-neoplastic, non-inflammatory enlargement of salivary gland. Enlargement is bilateral and painless. Periauricular portion of enlargement is noted. Salivary potassium content is enlarged and salivary sodium content is reduced. Some may occur due to toxic reaction to drugs. Allergic sialadenitis is a self-limiting disease.

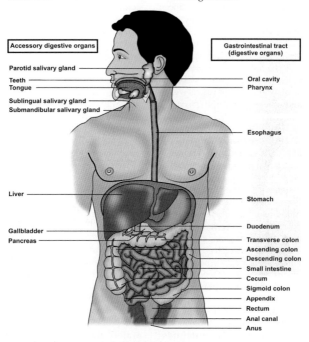

| Accessory digestive organs | | Gastrointestinal tract (digestive organs) |

Parotid salivary gland
Teeth
Tongue
Sublingual salivary gland
Submandibular salivary gland

Oral cavity
Pharynx

Esophagus

Liver

Stomach

Gallbladder
Pancreas

Duodenum
Transverse colon
Ascending colon
Descending colon
Small intestine
Cecum
Sigmoid colon
Appendix
Rectum
Anal canal
Anus

Alimentary canal

Allergic stomatitis refers to the condition where allergic reactions may cause acute multiple vesicles and ulcers of oral mucosa or a lichenoid reaction. Oral drugs may also cause the condition. The fixed drug eruption is characterized by localized area of erythema, edema and vesiculation at the site of drug contact. Contact allergy is caused by a delayed type hypersensitivity reaction to topical antigen. Contact allergy to dental amalgam is usually caused by mercury. Tooth paste allergy is rare but occurs. It results in fissuring of lips, perioral esquamation, edema, angular cheilitis and swelling of gingiva.

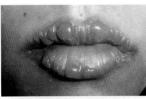

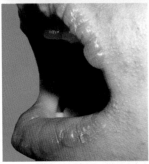

Allergic stomatitis

Allergy is abnormal tissue reactivity after exposure to a foreign antigen resulting in release of histamine.

Allograft refers to the graft of tissues between individuals of same species but of disparate genotype.

Allopurinol is the xanthine oxidase inhibitor which quickly lowers plasma urate and urinary uric acid concentration. It facilitates topus mobilization.

Alloxan is a pyrimidine derivative that can induce diabetes by destroying islets of Langerhan's.

Alloy for dental amalgam is a silver tin alloy containing other metals generally copper and zinc which will be mixed with mercury to form dental amalgam.

Alloy is a mixture of two or more metals. It exhibits metallic properties and is composed of one or more elements, i.e. brass is an alloy of copper and zinc.

Alopecia areata develops well circumscribed patches of nonscarring scalp alopecia without skin changes. Patches may develop on beared, pubic areas and axilla. This disorder is recurrent.

Alopecia refers to baldness, loss of hair.

Alpha-fetoprotein is a normal fetal protein which passes from fetus into the amniotic fluid and maternal serum. At 16 weeks gestation increased levels suggest fetal spina bifida with Down's syndrome.

Alternate current is a current in which electron flows in opposite direction.

Alternative medical therapy is the treatment outside the main stream of traditional therapy.

Althesin is a steroid anesthetic agent. It is injected slowly IV in a dose of 0.05 to 0.075 ml/kg body weight, rapid induction of anesthesia occurs. It has a very short duration of anesthesia and recovery is rapid. Extravenous injection does not produce tissue damage.

Alumina slips casting is a process for forming alumina cores that gives very high strength values of around 500 MPa. Advantage of it is high strength and good fitting. Disadvantages include high initial cost, long processing time and lack of bonding to the tooth structure.

Aluminium is a metal that occurs in rock and clay. It is found in animal and plants. Aluminium cooking vessels are not harmful at all.

Aluminous porcelain is a strong dental porcelain. It is 40 to 50 percent by weight alumina, a crystalline made of aluminum oxide (Al_2O_3).

Alveolar bone is the bone surrounding the root of the tooth; loss of this bone is typically associated with severe periodontal disease.

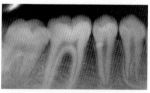

Alveolar bone

Alveolar bone loss refers to the loss of bone that surrounds and supports the teeth in mandible or maxilla. Alveolar bone loss could be horizontal or vertical bone loss (*see* Figure again).

Alveolar cavitational osteopathosis refers to the cavity

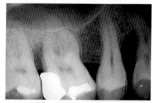

Alveolar bony defect

which is not demonstrable on X-ray but is able to locate clinically on surgical procedure.

Alveolar crest fibers refer to the fibres that extend obliquely from the cementum to the alveolar crest. These fibers prevent extrusion and prevent the lateral movements of the tooth.

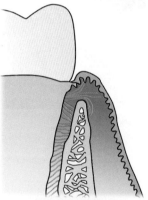

Alveolar crest fibers

Alveolar crest is the highest portion of alveolar bone or it is the most coronal portion of alveolar bone found between the teeth, composed of dense cortical bone appearing radiopaque.

Alveolar eminence is the outline of the root on the facet portion of the bone.

Alveolar mucosa is a nonkeratinized epithelium characterized by a smooth and shiny surface. The absence of keratin makes the alveolar mucosa redder than the pink gingival tissue. This tissue has abundance of elastic fibers and is readily movable. Mucosa covers the vestibule and floor of mouth and becomes buccal and labial mucosa. Its width increases with age and eruption of teeth.

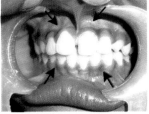

Alveolar mucosa

Alveolar osteitis is unpredictable and can be mistaken for osteomyelitis. Pain starts a few days after extraction of tooth. Pain is deep seated, severe and throbbing. There is no clot in the socket. Also known as Dry Socket.

Alveolar process is that portion of the mandible or maxilla which surrounds the root of a tooth.

Alveolar soft part sarcoma is a rare tumor. Lesions in tongue and floor of mouth have been reported. Tumor is composed of large cells with fine granular cytoplasm. Lesions are slow growing, well circumscribed masses with no gross features. Radical surgical excision is an accepted treatment.

Alveolectomy is a surgical procedure that is performed to produce a smooth alveolar ridge, either by removing the sharp bony spicules, postsurgical procedure or by augmenting the ridge.

Alveolus is the bony socket in which the root of the tooth sits.

Alveoplasty is a surgical reduction and reshaping of alveolar ridge.

Alzheimer's disease is a degenerative disease of an old age. There is neuronal loss in cerebral cortex with convolution atrophy, especially over frontal and temporal lobe. Some amount of ventricular enlargement takes place. There develops thickened neuritic process. Number of plaque in one field is directly correlated with degree of memory loss. Disturbance of speech function takes place. CSF (cerebrospinal fluid) is normal and EEG shows generalized slowing. CT (computed tomography) and MRI (magnetic resonance imaging) shows dilatation of lateral ventricles and widening of cortical sulci.

Amalgam carrier refers to the dental hand instrument that is used to carry and dispense freshly mixed amalgam into a cavity preparation. The lever forces a plunger to push contained amalgam from the cylinder.

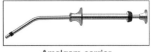

Amalgam carrier

Amalgam is a silver alloy and the most commonly used restorative material. It's one of the metal is mercury which gives silver color to the filling thus commonly it is also known as silver filling. In average deep cavities, the pulp is affected mainly by the cold and hot stimuli that result from the thermal conductive properties of amalgam. In such cavities pain is

A

due to unlined cavities resulting in an inflammatory response after 3 days to 5 weeks. Marginal leakage that occurs due to improper condensation of amalgam into the cavity has been shown to cause damage to pulp restorations. Pulpal response to silver amalgam restoration may occurs shortly after placement. Delayed expansion is one of the most common complication.

Amalgam carver is a hand instrument used to carve the anatomical features on the occlusal aspect of an amalgam restoration.

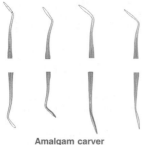

Amalgam carver

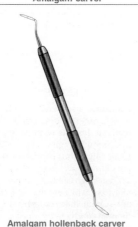

Amalgam hollenback carver

Amalgam tattoo is a flat, bluish grey lesion of oral mucosa resulting due to the introduction of amalgam particles into the tissue. The metallic particles disperse in tissue resulting in permanent area of pigmentation. It is mostly seen on gingiva or edentulous ridge.

Amalgam well refers to a small metal disk to hold the mixed amalgam.

Amalgamation is a process of mechanically mixing the dental amalgam alloy with mercury.

Amalgamator is a device used to mix mercury with amalgam alloy.

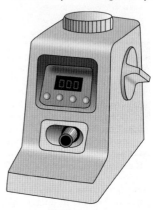

Amalgamator

Ambisexuality refers to the erotic interest toward both males and females.

Amblyopia is a functional loss of vision without any organic defect. There is blurring and inability to focus generally found in alcoholics.

Ameloblastic fibrodontoma is a well circumscribed lesion. Lesion is small measuring 1 to 2 cm in diameter. Occasionally these lesions will become huge. It does not evade bone hence curettage serves the purpose.

Ameloblastic fibroma is an uncommon neoplasm of odontogenic origin. It is a true mixed odontogenic tumor, containing nests and strands of ameloblastic epithelium. Calcified dental structures are not seen. X-ray features are of simple ameloblastoma. There will be a well defined unilocular radiolucency. Multilocular lesions may occur. Vast majority occurs in mandible and highest incidence is in premolar region. Tumor is often associated with unerupted teeth. Mitotic activity is not common. There may be a paucity of blood.

Ameloblastic odontome is an odontogenic neoplasm characterized by simultaneous presence of ameloblastoma and composite odontoma. Mild pain with delayed eruption of teeth is a presenting feature. On radiograph central destruction of cortical plates are seen.

Ameloblastoma is a true neoplasm. It originates in 80% cases from mandible. It develops insidiously as a central lesion of bone which is slowly destructive. It may ulcerate or fungate disfiguring the patients face. Radiographically it shows multilocular cyst like lesion of bone. After surgery recurrence is rare (*see* Figure under).

Ameloblasts are the epithelial cell of the enamel organ. It is responsible for the formation of enamel (*see* Figure on page 28).

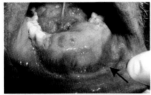

Ameloblastoma mid line

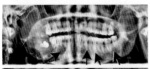

Multilocular-ameloblastoma

Unilocular ameloblastoma

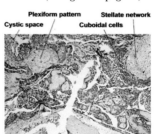

Plexiform pattern   Stellate network
Cystic space   Cuboidal cells

Ameloblastoma (Histological section)

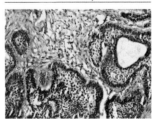

Ameloblastoma-high power

A

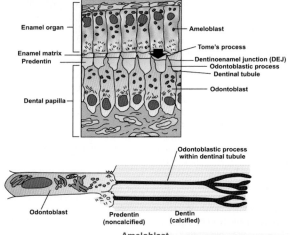

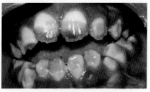

Ameloblast

Amelogenesis imperfecta is defined as a spectrum of hereditary defects in the function of ameloblasts and mineralization of enamel matrix that results in teeth with multiple generalized abnormalities affecting the enamel layer only. It is entirely an ectodermal disturbance, since the mesodermal components of the tooth are basically normal. The anomaly occurs in the general population in the range of 1 in 14,000. Three basic type of amelogenesis imperfecta are hypoplastic: Type in which there is defective formation of matrix, hypocalcification type in which there is defective mineralization of the formed matrix, Hypomaturation type in which enamel crystallites remain immature (*see* Figure).

Amelo-onychohypohidrotic syndrome is characterized by defective nails with subungual

Amelogenesis imperfecta

hyperkeratosis seen with sweat gland hypofunction and severe hypoplastic-hypocalcified crowns.

Amino acids are basically proteins in nature. Twenty-two amino acids are known of which 8 cannot be synthesised in our body in sufficient quantity and hence are to be supplied from outside. Essential amino acid includes isoleucine, leucine, lysine, methionine, phenylalanine, theonine, tryptophan and valine. Growing children needs histidine.

Aminoglycosides are bactericidal. They cause misreading of mRNA by the ribosome, leading to abnormal protein production. To enter the bacterium, aminoglycosides need to be actively transported across the cell membrane. This does not occur in anaerobic organisms, which are therefore, resistant.

Amniocentesis is the removal of amniotic fluid for analysis. It is a procedure to detect birth defects.

Amoebiasis entemoeba histolytica exists in two forms the trophozoite form and the cystic form. Later is involved in transmission by food, fingers and flies. In intestine it results in amoebiasis. Hepatic amoebiasis is the commonest manifestation of extra-intestinal amoebiasis. Large liver abscesses contain reddish brown fluid and cellular necrotic tissue.

Amoebic liver abscess is a condition where *E. histolytica* invades colonic mucosa and carried to liver by portal circulation to form microabscess. Microabscesses confluent to make larger one. Posterior lobe is the commonest site to form abscess. There will be abdominal pain, fever, rigor and sweating. In pleural irritation one will develop intercostals tenderness and cough. As complication it may rupture into pleural, pericardial sac or into peritoneal cavity. Radiograph will show elevated right dome with restricted mobility. Metronidazole and Ampicillin in high doses is effective (*see* Figure).

Amoebic lung abscess develops by spreading across the diaphragm from liver. It is more common in liver. Prior to rupture of amoebic abscess there is generally a non-suppurative effusion. It is known

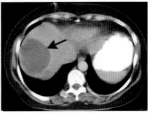
Liver abcess

as sympathetic effusion. Amoebic abscess may show tropozites of E. *histolytica* along the margins of healthy and necrotic tissue.

Amorphous is without any long range order of atoms or groups of atoms.

Amperage is the number of electrons that pass through a conductor, the strength of electric current.

Amplitude is defined as the total height of the wave oscillation from the top of the peak to the bottom. A measurement of the amount of energy in the wave, larger the amplitude, greater the amount of energy that can do useful work.

Amylase is an enzyme that converts starch into sugar.

Amyloid spleen follicles appears as small granules on gross inspection known as sago spleen. In another variety follicles are spared and amyloid is deposited in the wall of sinuside.

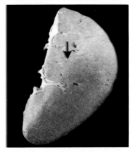

A

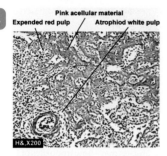

Expended red pulp / Pink acellular material / Atrophiod white pulp

H&,X200

Apple-green birefringence   Arteriole

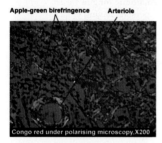

Congo red under polarising microscopy.X200

Pink acellular material
Expanded red pulp   Atrophied white pulp

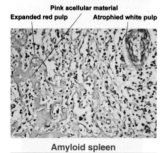

Amyloid spleen

Amyloidosis kidney can result in enlargement of kidney. Pathologically glomeruli are filled with amorphous deposits staining with congo red. Primary amyloidosis results in end stage of renal disease with in 2-3 years. Renal transplantation is an option.

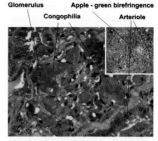

Glomerulus   Apple - green birefringence
Congophilia   Arteriole

Amyloidosis kidney

Anabolic therapy is the use of testosterone or analogs to building lean body mass.

Anacrotic pulse refers slow rising pulse.

Anaerobic bacteria are those bacteria's that do not need oxygen to grow. They are generally associated with periodontal disease.

Analgesia is the absence of sensitivity to pain. It indicates a specific type of spinal cord lesion. It always occurs with loss of temperature. These fibers travel together in spinal cord. It can occur with paresthesia. It can be classified partial or total below the level of lesion. When develops abruptly it is due to trauma.

Analgesics are drugs used to eliminate or reduce sensation of pain. These drugs are used to alter the central perception of pain. Site of action is cortex. These can be narcotic or non-narcotics.

Analog image is a radiographic image produced by a conventional film.

Analysis of variance is a group of statistical tests used to analyse differences between two or more groups based on positioning the sum of squares into that attributable to between group differences and that attributable to within group differences.

Anaphylactoid/ Pseudo-allergic reactions are non-immunologic release of mediators from mast cells and basophils.

Anaphylaxis is Type I hypersensitivity reaction or an acute, severe, allergic reaction characterized by sudden collapse, shock or respiratory/circulatory failure following an injection of an allergen where there is exaggerated immunologic reaction that results from release of vasoactive substances such as histamine. There is an increased susceptibility to an allergen resulting from previous exposure to it.

Anaplasia is a growth of abnormal cells.

Anatomic crown refers to the entire crown, extending from cusp tip to the cementoenamel (CE) junction.

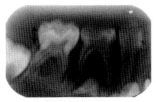

Anatomic crown

Anatomic mouth breather is one whose lip morphology does not permit complete closure of mouth. Such as patient having short lower lip. Removal of any nasopharyngeal obstruction, rapid maxillary expansion, vestibular screen may be the treatment of choice.

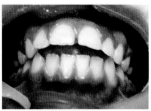

Mouth breathing and
tongue thrust

Anatomic tongue thrust occurs in persons having enlarged tongue and can have an anterior tongue posture.

Anchor suture are the type of suture that are used to close the facial and lingual flaps and adapts them tightly against the tooth. The needle is placed at the line angle area of the facial or lingual flap adjacent the tooth, anchored around the tooth, passed beneath the opposite flap and tied.

Anergy refer to non-responsiveness to antigen T cells may become anergic when exposed to antigen in the absence of activation signal.

Anesthesia is a medication which relieves the sensation of pain.

Aneurysmal bone cyst is a solitary lesion of young adults below 20 years of age. Radiographically bone is extended. Lesion is cystic and may show soap bubble appearance. Bone is eccentrically ballooned. It consists of fibrous connective tissue stroma with blood filled spaces. Numerous young fibroblasts are seen. Surgical curettage and excision is treatment of choice.

Aneurysm is a localized dilatation of blood vessel due to weakening, thinning and stretching of wall. It is more common in aorta. It may

A

be saccular, fusiform, mycotic and dissecting aneurysm.

Angina pectoris classification includes stable angina / classic angina which is usually the result of coronary artery disease. Stable angina is triggered by strenuous activity, emotional stress or cold weather. The 'pain' of stable angina lasts from 1-15 minutes and builds gradually. The pain of stable angina is relieved by rest or administration of nitroglycerin. Variant angina /Prinzmetal's angina — more likely to occur when patient is at rest than during physical exertion or emotional stress. Coronary artery spasm is the cause of variant angina. Variant angina is more common in women under the age of 50 years. Signs apart from chest pain, syncope, dyspnea and palpitation. Nitroglycerin usually provides prompt relief of pain. Unstable angina— Lies intermediate between stable angina and acute myocardial infarction. Unstable angina is the result of progression of atherosclerosis. Episodes of pain associated with unstable angina may persist for up to 30 minutes. Three characteristics used to define unstable angina, i.e. angina of recent onset, caused by minimal exertion, increasingly severe, prolonged or frequent angina, angina both at rest and with minimal exertion.

Angina pectoris: Angina a Latin word describing a spasmodic, cramp like, choking feeling or suffocating pain, pectoris is Latin for chest. Angina is defined as a characteristic thoracic pain usually substernal, precipitated chiefly by exercise, emotion or a heavy meal; relieved by vasodilator drugs and a few minutes rest and result of a moderate inadequacy of coronary circulation.

Angioedema collections is the collection of fluid in the skin, mucous membrane or viscera due to over production of anaphylotoxin.

Angioedema is an occasional manifestation of hypersensitivity in man. It presents as an intense edema of face, pharynx and larynx. It may cause respiratory obstruction needing tracheostomy. It is due to release of histamine from sensitized most cells in face and buccal cavity.

Angio-neurotic edema is a nonhereditary form and is due to food allergy. It manifests itself as a smooth diffuse edematous swelling involving face, lips, chin and eyes. Feeling of itching or pricky sensation is there. Skin is of normal color. Hereditary form has visceral involvement and is serious. Edema develops due to vascular swelling.

Angioplasty is a medical procedure in which vessels occluded by arteriosclerosis are opened. This technique was developed in 1977. This is done in patients who don't respond to medical treatment as well as don't require by pass surgery also.

Angiosarcoma is the malignant vascular neoplasm and not HIV related; oral cavity is the rare site. These are rapidly proliferative and present as nodular tumors. These can arise from lymph or blood vessel. Even after radical excision they have a poor prognosis (*see* Figure on page 33).

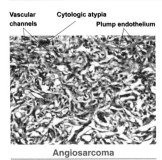

Vascular channels — Cytologic atypia — Plump endothelium

Angiosarcoma

Angle A is a figure formed by two lines diverging from common.

Angle of facial convexity is formed by the intersection of glabella – subnasale line and subnasale – soft tissue pogonion line. Mean value is 12° and SD is ± 4°. A smaller positive or negative value suggests a class III relationship. A high positive value reflects a class II relationship. The value of this angle, however, does not reveal the localization of the deformity.

Angle of mandible is an area of mandible where body meets the ramus.

Anglo-Saxon system is a method used for diagnosing pit and fissure caries, which consists of certain "liberal" criteria's, described by Horowitz, HS, in 1972. Description of the system: The pits and fissures on the occlusal, vestibular and lingual surfaces are carious when the explorer "catches" after insertion with moderate to firm pressure and when the "catch" is accompanied by one or more of the following signs of decay: Softness is noted at the base of the area. Opacity adjacent to the area provides evidence of undermining or demineralization. Softened enamel adjacent to the area may be scraped away by the explorer. These areas should be diagnosed as sound when there is apparent evidence of demineralization, but no evidence of softness.

Angular chelitis is also known as angular cheliosis. It may be caused by *Candida Albicans*, streptococci or staphylococci. Riboflavin folate and iron deficiency may also result in it. General protein deficiency can also result it. Recurrent trauma from dental flossing may also be implicated.

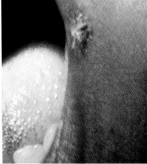

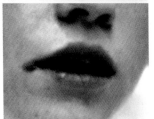

Angular chelitis

Angulation refers to the angle formed between the blade of the instrument and the tooth surface.

A

Anhidrosis is an abnormal deficiency of sweat. It can be localized or generalized. Localized anhidrosis being limited to a part rarely affects thermo-regulation. Anhidrosis may develop due to neurological or skin disorders.

Ankyloglossia is the fusion between tongue and floor of mouth. Partial ankyloglossia is known as tongue tie. Restricted movement of tongue results in difficulty in speech. Clipping of the lingual frenum is part of treatment.

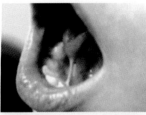

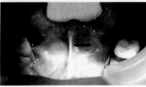

Ankyloglossia

Ankylosing spondylitis is a chronic inflammatory disease affecting joints of axial system. Disease starts insidiously in sacroiliac joints with pain and stiffness. There is progressive limitation of back motion. Eventually the entire spine becomes fused. Chest expansion becomes limited. ESR is high. Erosion and sclerosis of sacroiliac joints are first to be noticed. Peripheral joints when involved don't show any demineralization or erosion. Non-steroid anti inflammatory drugs are used.

Ankylosis is the term given to the fusion between cementum of teeth and the underlying bone. Generally the deciduous teeth are affected in which bone has fused to cementum and dentin preventing exfoliation of tooth and eruption of underlying permanent tooth. Tooth erupts into oral cavity but does not reach the occlusal plane. In addition adjacent permanent teeth are taller occlusocervically. Anky-losed tooth sounds solid on percussion.

Annealing refers to a low temperature heat treatment for removing residual stress, e.g. heating of a direct gold filling to remove gaseous impurities from the surface.

Anode is the positive electrode in the X-ray tube. It converts electrons into X-ray photons.

Anodontia refers to the congenital absence of teeth. It may be total or partial. This term cannot be applied to teeth that have developed, but have failed to erupt. It may involve dental or permanent dentition. False anodontia develops due to extraction of all teeth. Etiology of single missing tooth is unknown. It may have family history too.

Anomaly is a deviation from the normal or expected outcome.

Anorexia nervosa is an eating disorder or an abnormal psychic condition in which person looses all desire for food and even develops nausea due to self-starvation. Girls think that they are overweight and will do excessive exercise and cut their consumption of food. Patient has low esteem.

Anosmia refers to a loss of smell is called anosmia and perverted smell as persomia. Anosmia is due to common cold and nasal conjestion, unilateral anosmia occurs due to brain tumors. Olfactory hallucination occurs in lesions of uncus, hippocampus and psychosis.

Antagonists refers to the teeth in opposing arches that usually contact each other in occlusion.

Anterior - situated in front of.

Anterior cerebral artery occlusion – affects motor and sensory cortices representing contralateral leg causing motor weakness and sensory loss. Anterior cerebral artery is a branch of internal carotid and supplies medial surface of frontal and parietal lobes and corpus callosum.

Anterior cord syndrome includes analgesia and thermo-anesthesia which occur bilaterally below the level of lesion. There is flaccid paralysis.

Anterior cranial base length (Se-N) is the measurement of the anterior cranial base performed using the center of the superior entrance to the sella turcica as a set point. The correlation of this criterion with the length of the jaw bases enables the assessment of the proportional averages of these bases.

Anterior cross bite is a condition characterized by reverse over jet where one or more maxillary anterior teeth are in lingual relation to the mandibular teeth. Anterior cross bites should be intercepted and treated at an early

stage so as to prevent a minor orthodontic problem from progressing into a major dentofacial anomaly. An old orthodontic maximum states "The best time to treat a cross bite is the first time it is seen".

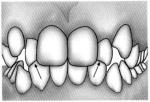
Anterior cross bite

Anterior partial crown in the earlier days before the use of metal ceramic crowns, when there was no satisfactory facing material, partial crowns were the only alternative to restore individual teeth.

Anterior teeth refers to the front teeth, i.e. incisors and canines.

Anterograde amnesia refers to the loss of memory following the accident.

Anthropometry is a study of various landmarks established on dry skull are measured viewing individuals by using soft tissue points overlying the bony landmarks.

Anti-embolic stockings refers to elastic stockings.

Antibiotics are the substances that are produced by or derived from bacteria that may either kill the microorganism (bactericidal) or may retard their growth (bacteriostatic) so that the body's own immune system can overcome the infection.

Antigen is "any foreign substance that elicits an immune response (e.g. the production of specific antibody molecules) when introduced into the tissues of a susceptible animal and is capable of combining with the specific antibodies formed.

Antimicrobial is a chemo-therapeutic agent that works by destroying or reducing the number of bacteria present.

Antiseptics are antimicrobial agents that are applied topically or subgingivally to destroy microorganisms and inhibit their reproduction. These inhibit the growth and multiplication of bacteria. Generally it does not kill bacteria.

Antisialagogue refers to substance that prevents salivation.

Antitoxin is a specific type of antibody produced by body in response to a toxin.

Antivitamins are substances known as vitamin antagonists, which block the synthesis or metabolism of vitamins. Drug methotrexate is antagonist of folic acid; antibiotics interfere with vitamin K synthesis. These are known to be present in natural foods, e.g. thiaminase in raw fish. Some synthetic antagonists of vitamins are used as drugs in the therapy of neoplasm, e.g. methotrexate infections, e.g. pyrimethamine. Neoplastic cells and microorganisms are much more sensitive than normal cells but high doses of antivitamins can cause vitamin deficiency.

Anxiety disorder is a condition where patient shows excessive anxiety and worry about a number of events and activities for at least 6 months. Symptoms include restlessness, fatigability, difficulty with concentration, irritability and sleep disturbances. Person may develop hyper-tension.

Anxiety tremors are fine and rapid. It is seen in thyrotoxicosis.

Anxiolytics are anxiety reducing drugs.

Aortic dissection is an entrance of blood into aortic media. Underlying conditions associated with it include, hypertension and atherosclerosis. Person will develop abrupt severe pain. Pain is sharp and tearing. Systolic BP is higher than > 150 ++. One may hear aortic insufficiency murmur. Pulse deficit is increased.

Aortic regurgitation is usually asymptomatic until middle age. It persists with left side failure or chest pain. There will be wide pulse pressure with left sided failure or chest pain. There will also be hyperactive enlarged pulse pressure, hyperactive enlarged left ventricle. Diastolic murmur along left sternal border will be heard. ECG shows left ventricular hypertrophy.

Aortic stenosis causes delayed and diminished carotid pulse with soft, absent or paradoxically split S2. Harash systolic murmur with thrill along left sternal border often radiating to neck is heard ECG shows left ventricular hypertrophy. Angina pectoris frequently occurs.

Apathy is an absence or suppres-sion of interest in the external environment and personal affair. It may be caused by alcohol, drug abuse, neurological or psycholo-gical disorder.

Apex is the pointed extremity of a structure.

Apexification is a root induction procedure of a nonvital tooth where a medicament is applied within a root canal which allows a calcified barrier to form across the open apex.

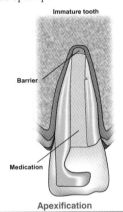

Apexification

Apexogenesis is a root induction procedure in a vital tooth where the normal development of the apex of a root is expected by placing a medicament within the pulp chamber of tooth. Treatment of a vital pulp is by pulp capping or pulpotomy.

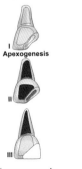

Apexogenesis

Aphasia is a defect of language function secondary to brain damage. Dysphagia is a failure of language to develop normally.

Aphrodisiac is a substance that stimulates the sexual desire and activity but claims have not been proved scientifically.

Aphthous stomatitis is an idiopathic, noninfectious inflammatory disease. Ulcers develop recurrently on nonkeratinized oral mucosa. There are 3 types of ulcers. Minor aphthous stomatitis produces small ulcers which heal within 10 days. Major aphthous ulcers produce larger ulcers and takes longer time to heal. It heals by scarring and at least one ulcer is always present. Herpetiform aphthae present multiple painful ulcers of 1 to 20 mm affecting nonkeratinized area. Ulcers are superficial with an erythematous halo. These are non-indurated and painful. Reiter's syndrome is a immune mediated disease. It produces lesions like oral aphthous ulcers, polyarthritis, uretheritis and conjunctivitis.

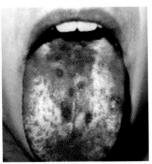

Stomatitis affecting tongue

A

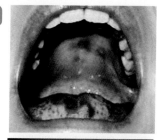

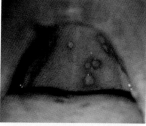

Stomatitis affecting palate

Apical curettage is the surgical removal of infectious material surrounding the apex of a tooth root.

Apical fibers are the periodontal fibers that radiate in the apical portion from the cementum to the bone and keep the tooth intact within the socket.

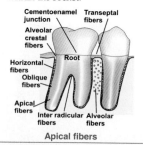

Apical fibers

Apical foramen is the opening at the end of the root of a tooth through which the tooth receives its nerve and blood supply.

Apical heart rate is the number of ventricular contractions per minute.

Apical periodontal cyst is a true cyst because cavity is lined by epithelium. It is asymptomatic. Tooth is rarely painful or even sensitive to percussion. Apical periodontal cyst is a lesion due to chronic inflammatory process. On X-ray cyst may be of greater size, occasionally apical periodontal cyst exhibits a thin radiopaque line around radiolucent area.

Apicectomy is a surgical procedure done to remove the infected apical portion of tooth. Main purpose is to save the tooth where root filling is not feasible. It is the final alternative to extraction.

Aplasia of mandibular condyle is the abnormality associated with other abnormalities also. In one side facial abnormality shift of mandible towards affected side occurs during opening. In bilateral cases shift is not there. Osteoplasty is the treatment.

Aplasia of salivary glands refers to any one of the gland that may be missing. Cause is not known. It may result in dry mouth. Oral mucosa looks dry and pebbly. Cracking of lips and fissuring of corners of mouth is seen. Food debris may accumulate around tooth. There is no particular treatment.

Aplastic anemia is a dramatic decrease in all circulating blood cells because of depression of bone marrow activity. Primary is congenital while secondary may be due to ionizing radiation, benzene, cyclophosphamide and viral hepatitis. Higher doses of chemotheraphy destroy stem cells which are not recovered. Lymphadenopathy is not seen. Platelet count falls gradually. Skin rashes, nose bleed and gum bleeding are common.

Apocrine sweat glands are associated with hair follicles and are found in axillary and genital areas. These respond to emotions and become active when person is frightened, upset in pain or is sexually excited. It does not have a strong odor.

Apparent density is a mass of sample divided by volume it occupies.

Appendicitis is an inflammation of appendix which lies one inch below the ileocaecal valve. All the taeniae of colon converge at the base of appendix. As appendicitis progresses the organs swells up due to accumulated pus within the lumen. It leads to compromise in blood supply, gangrene and perforation.

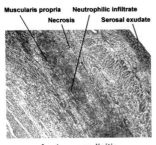

Muscularis propria · Neutrophilic infiltrate · Necrosis · Serosal exudate

Acute appendicitis

Appendicular skeleton is a part of skeleton that includes the bones of upper extremities, the lower extremities, the pelvic girdle and pectoral girdle.

Appetite center is a cluster of neurons in the lateral hypothalamus whose impulses cause an increase in appetite.

Apposition is the laying down of, or addition of.

Apraxia is an inability to carry out an organised voluntary movement despite the fact that motor and sensory pathways are normally intact. There is no paralysis. It is due to loss of acquired motor skills.

Apthous ulcer lesions are confined to oral mucosa and burning sensations starts 2 to 48 hours earlier. Initially localised area of erythema develops. With in hours a small white papule develops which ulcerates and enlarges. Ulcers are round, symmetrical and shallow. Multiple lesions are present. Lesions are very painful and interfere with speech and eating. Lesions heal slowly leaving scars. Use of tropical corticosteroids are helpful.

Aqueous humor is a watery fluid that fills anterior chamber of the eye in front of lens.

Arch is a curvature; both the maxillary and mandibular ridge form a horseshoe shaped arch.

Arch bars are the prefabricated form of metal bars which are used for mandibular fixation particularly when the patient has an insufficient number of suitably shaped teeth to enable other effective wiring to be carried out. After reduction, the teeth on the main fragments are tied together to a metal bar which has been bent to conform to dental arch.

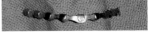

Arch bar

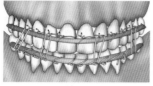

Arch bar

Argon lasers are those lasers that have an active medium of argon gas that is fiber optically delivered in continuous-wave and gated-pulse modes. Two emission wavelengths, and both are visible to the human eye 488 nm (blue in color) and 514 nm (blue-green). Both wavelengths are not well absorbed in dental hard tissues and are poorly absorbed in water. It can be used as an aid in caries detection. The diseased, carious area appears as dark orange-red color and is easily discernible from the healthy structures.

Ariboflavinosis is a deficiency of vitamin B_2 showing swollen, cracked, bright-red lips, enlarged tender magenta red tongue, cracking at the corners of mouth and congested conjunctiva.

Armamentarium includes equipment, books, materials and instruments essential to professional practice.

Arsenic is colorless, tasteless and odorless. Small quantity is required to kill a man, i.e. 0.2 gm. A pinch of white arsenic about 20 grams. Fatal period is 12-48 hours. It is tastelss so easily mixed with sweets. It has cumulative properties. But it can be detected with absolute certainty from each of burial place, burnt ashes and hair/teeth for a long period even after death.

Arterial hemorrhage bleed profusely and lost blood is bright red in color and blood comes out in jet. The rise and fall of which synchronise with the pulse of the patient.

Arterio-venous malformations develop due to a mesh of abnormally thin vessels. Larger ones are seen in posterior half of hemispheres forming a wedge like lesion. Bleeding of AVM is principally intraparenchymal patient may develop seizure, focal neurological deficits, impaired higher functions and headache. X-ray skull will show calcification in AVM while MRI will show pattern of blood flow in lesion and will spot the thrombus too.

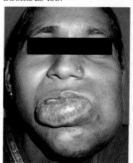

Arterio-venous **malformation**

Arthenocoria means slow dilation or constriction of the pupils in response to light changes. Photophobia may be present.

Arthralgia is the pain in a joint without swelling or other sign of arthritis.

Articular angle is a constructed angle between the upper and lower parts of posterior contours of the facial skeleton. Its size depends on the position of the mandible, it is larger if the mandible is retrognathic but small if the mandible is prognathic. It decreases with anterior positioning of the mandible, closing of the bite, and mesial migration of the posterior segment teeth and increases with posterior relocation of the mandible, opening of the bite and distal driving of the posterior teeth.

Articular cartilage is a layer of hyaline covering the joint surface of epiphysis.

Articular prominence is a rounded projection of temporal bone located anterior to glenoid process.

Articulate to come together.

Articulating head rest is a head rest that can be moved in multiple directions.

Articulating paper is a fairly heavy weight paper impregnated with ink like carbon paper. When paper is inserted in patients mouth and teeth are closed together paper leaves marks at higher points.

Articulation is the point where two or more adjacent bones create a joint.

Articulator is a mechanical device used to replicate functional movements of the jaw to casts.

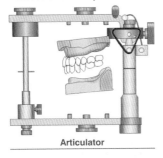

Articulator

Artifacts are physical evidence within a qualitative research design which contributes to the understanding of research question.

Artificial insemination is an artificial introduction of semen into vagina, cervix or uterus. In artificial insemination homologus is the process in which husband's semen is only used. In artificial insemination donor – semen of donor other than husband is used while in pooled donor semen of husband is added.

Aryl acetic acid derivative has a pharmacological effects similar to other NSAIDS, i.e. inhibition of synthesis of prostaglandins. Its potency is greater than indomethacin. It is rapidly absorbed. In joint fluid it is 8 times to that of plasma concentration.

Aseptic meningitis is common and is not generally fatal in children. It is caused by one of enterovirus like poliovirus. Next common cause is virus infection. CSF shows lymphocytosis.

Aseptic technique includes measures that reduce or eliminate microorganisms.

Aspartame is better known as nutrasweet and appears to be non-cariogenic. It is devoid of an after taste but is contraindicated in phenylketonuria as it contains phenylalanine. It is derived from protein.

Aspirate refers to draw back.

Aspirator refers to an apparatus employing suction or the tube-like straw which the dentist place in your mouth for suction.

Assistant's stool is the chair used by assistant to provide dental treatment to the patient.

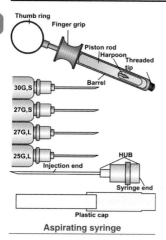

Aspiring syringe

Assistant's zone is the part of work circle where the dental assistant is positioned during the delivery of dental treatment. Best position is 2 to 4 O'clock position.

Asthma is defined as a disease characterized by an increased responsiveness of the trachea and bronchi to various stimuli and manifested by wide spread narrowing of the airways that changes either spontaneously or as a result of therapy. Acute asthmatic episodes are usually self-limiting, however clinical entity termed "status asthmaticus" characterized by a persistent exacerbation of asthma. Individuals who suffer from status asthmaticus experience wheezing, dyspnea, hypoxia and other symptoms that are refractory to two or three doses of adrenergic agents. Asthma can be manifested by a coughing spell, with or without sputum production and wheezing. Breathing during an asthmatic attack is labored. Blood pressure may rise in acute episode attacks, also heart rate increases rate of more than 120 beats/minute. If left untreated, acute asthmatic episode may last minutes or hours. Termination of attack is usually heralded by a period of intense coughing with expectoration of a thick, tenacious mucus plug. This is followed immediately by a sensation of relief and a clearing of the air passages.

Asymmetric Tonic Neck Reflex shows that when the body is at rest and not crying, the patient keeps his head on one side, the arms and the legs on the same side extend, while the opposite limbs go into flexion. The reflex is prominent between 2nd and 4th month. Persistence of the reflex beyond the age of 6 to 9 months or a constant neck posture is abnormal and usually indicates spastic cerebral palsy or poor control over the motor functions.

Asymmetry is to be occurred when aesthetic, tooth size, shape and gum contour are not as close to identical from one side of the mouth to the other. Ideally, the incisal edges of your teeth should follow the contour of the upper lip.

Asynergy is an impaired coordination of muscles or organs that normally function harmoniously. It may develop due to disorder of basal ganglion and cerebellum.

Atherogenesis is the formation of atherosclerotic lesion on the walls of arteries.

Atherosclerosis is a generalized and slowly progressive disorder of aorta and large and medium sized muscular arteries. It is the main cause of arteriosclerosis. Lesion develops slowly over years. Atherosclerosis is known to undergo ulceration, hemorrhage, calcification and thrombosis. Hypertension accelerate atherosclerosis which in turn increases chances of ischemic heart disease.

Athetosis is a slow, purposeless writhing movement of limbs, face or tongue. These movements increase when patient carries out voluntary movements. Posthemiplegic athetosis is unilateral. Some amount of rigidity brings slowness. Discrete individual movements of lips, tongue and hand are abnormal.

Athletes' foot is a fungal infection characterized by vesicles, fissures, ulcers and itching. It commonly affects toes.

Atomic weight is the total number of protons and neutrons in nucleus of an atom.

Atopic dermatitis is a chronic, itching superficial inflammation of skin. There may be family history too. Exact cause is unknown. Patients have high serum levels of lgE antibodies; child may develop red, weeping, crusted lesions on the face, scalp and extremities. Itching is a constant feature. Later dermatitis may become generalized. Secondary bacterial infections and regional lymphadenitis are common. Diagnosis is entirely clinical.

Atresia is a closure or absence of a usual opening.

Atrial fibrillation is an irregularity in ventricular beats created by inconsistent impulses through AV node transmitted to the ventricles at irregular intervals.

Atrial septal defects are small and moderate defects that may be asymptomatic. With large shunts exertional dyspnea or cardiac failure may develop. Right ventricular and pulmonary artery pulsations are palpable and visible. S2 is widely split.

Atropine is named after one of leading fates called 'atropos'. It is well absorbed from body surface. It reduces all secretions except milk. Smooth muscles are relaxed. Its side effects include dry mouth, tachycardia, urinary retention and constipation.

Attached gingiva is the part of gingiva which is in continuation with the marginal gingiva. It is firm and resilient and tightly bound to the underlying periosteum of the alveolar bone. In children, it appears less dense and redder than in adults due to less keratinized epithelium with its greater vascularity. The attached gingiva is more black because of lesser connective tissue density and its texture is less stippled. The two unique characteristics of the attached gingiva in children are the interdental clefts and the retrocuspid papilla. The interdental clefts are normal anatomic feature found in the interradicular zones underlying the saddle areas. The retrocuspid papilla is found approximately 1mm below the free gingival groove on the attached gingiva lingual to the mandibular canine. It occurs in 85% of children and apparently decreases with age.

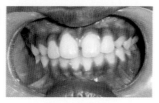

Attached gingiva

Attached subgingival plaque is a bacterial plaque located below the gingival margin that is attached to tooth.

Attenuated live vaccine: Live vaccine contains organism of reduced virulence due to culturing under unfavorable conditions.

Attrition is a physiological or mechanical wearing down of a tooth due to contact of another tooth as in during mastication in old age. There develops flattening of an incisal edge. There is slight mobility of teeth in their sockets. Man shows severe attrition than woman.

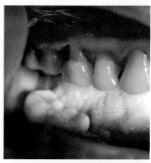

Attrition and abrasion

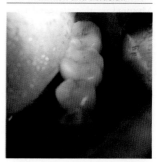

Attrition on posterior teeth

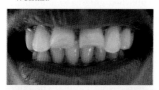

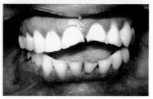

Attrition

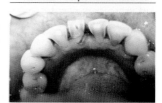

Severe attrition

Atypical facial neuralgia is a dull, aching and throbbing pain due to vascular component. It is accompanied by muscle pain. Pain is diffusely located even though persistent and variable. Quality of pain being acute, sudden, intense exacerbations gives it a neuralgic quality.

Atypical odontalgia is a persistent pain in tooth with no abnormality found in tooth on any type of examination. Odontalgia word comes from Greek word odont means tooth and algo means pain. Cavity and exposure of nerve causes pain. But tooth pain which occurs when there is no dental disease is called atypical odontalgia. It generally occurs after root canal treatment or tooth extraction.

Atypical orofacial pain is a condition where patient is not able to locate and identify the quality of pain. Emotional breakdown, tears and hysteria are not uncommon. On account of pain person does not leave work place. Referred pain also may be poorly localized and pain of vascular origin in head becomes difficult to separate from atypical facial pain. Atypical facial pain is not associated with trigger zones.

Augmentation material includes three primary augmentation materials in dentistry intramucosal, endodontic and bone substitute materials. Material should be easy to fabricate, biocompatible, sterilize and should shape intraoperatively.

Auricle is the portion of external ear.

Auricle

Auricular lymph nodes can be palpated bilaterally in front and behind of ears.

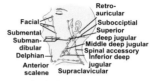
Auricular lymph nodes

Autistic behavior is the exaggerated self centered behavior marked by a lack of responsiveness to other people. It develops in schizophrenic children.

Autograft is the graft taken from patient's own skin which is best used to cover the wounds. The best donor site is the patient's thighs or upper arm. But in case of extensive burns these areas can be reused to obtain grafts again after 2 weeks because usually thin grafts are taken. In case the area is extensive, scalp is a good donor site because it can be reused many times as a donor area.

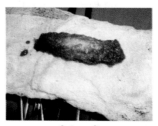
Autograft

Autoimmune disease is a disease that is characterized by tissue injury caused by a cell mediated immune response against constituents of body's own tissues.

Autoimmunity is caused by pathogenic immune reactions against self-antigens.

Autotransformer is a voltage compensator that corrects for minor fluctuations in current flowing throughout the X-ray machine.

Autogeneous refers to self-generated, self-propagated. It originates within an organism.

Automatic processing is the method used to process films in which all film processing steps are automated.

Autonomic nervous system is a part of nervous system that controls involuntary body functions, such as salivation, sweat and heart beat.

Autopsy is a postmortem examination.

Autotransplant refers to the procedure where transfer of a tissue or organ to another place in same person.

Avascular refers to the absence of blood supply.

Avidin is a protein present in white of an egg which combines with vitamin H and makes it available to the body. It is inactivated in cooked eggs.

Avitaminosis means without vitamins.

Avulsion is the tearing away of a tendon or ligament attachment from bone.

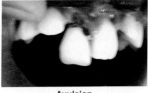
Avulsion

Axial is opposite of appendicular. It is pertaining to the central portion of body.

Axial wall is the vertical axis of a tooth.

Axon the process that carries impulses away from the cell body of a nerve.

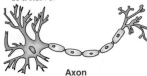
Axon

B **Babinski's reflex** refers to the stroking of the lateral surfaces of the planter surface of the foot from the head to the toe that results in flexion of the toe.

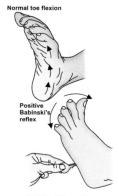

Normal toe flexion

Positive Babinski's reflex

Babinski's reflex

Backache refers to the pain occurring in the back due to any reason. Malignant tumors will have night rest pain. Mechanical pain is worse with activity. There will be weight loss, malaise and loss of appetite.

Backward decay or caries refers to the kind of carious progress where caries process in dentin progresses much further than it does in enamel, i.e. when the spread of caries along the DEJ exceeds the caries in the contagious enamel, from the junction and is termed as backward caries.

Bacteremia refers to the presence of bacteria in blood stream.

Bacterias are classified as plants but without chlorophyll. These can cause dental decay, periodontal disease, TB, typhoid, tetanus, diphtheria etc. In presence of unfavorable conditions these develop a protective mucoid coating which helps them to survive. In favorable condition these become virulent again. Killing of spores is difficult.

Bacterial plaque is a dense, organized matrix of micro-organism that forms on the teeth, gingiva and restorations. It is a cause of poor oral hygiene, dental caries and periodontal diseases. In a recently cleaned mouth, it contains leukocytes, epithelial cells and a few gram positive cocci. 2-14 days old plaque will contain leukocytes, rods, gram negative bacteria, white cells and gram positive cocci.

Bacterial sialadenitis can be unilateral/bilateral swelling of parotid gland. Swelling may involve pre and post auricular areas. Trismus results, from pain and swelling. Occasionally fever, chill and leucocytosis may be seen. In chronic infection recurrent bouts of acute exacerbation may be seen. Antibiotic helps.

Bacterial spore is a resistant form of bacteria encapsulated by a thick wall which enables the cell to survive in unfavorable environment of growth.

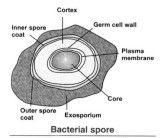

Cortex

Germ cell wall

Inner spore coat

Plasma membrane

Core

Outer spore coat

Exosporium

Bacterial spore

Bactericide is an agent that is capable of destroying bacteria.

Bacteriocins are proteins produced by certain bacteria that can kill other bacteria.

Bacteriophage is a virus that infects a bacterium or simply inhibits the growth of bacteria.

Bacterium is a microorganism capable of causing disease, a primitive single celled organism without membranous organelles.

Baking powder is a mixture which liberates CO_2 when moistened/heated. Sodium bicarbonate is the source of CO_2 and an acidic substance is required such as tartric acid. Quick acting powders contain tartrate and liberate CO_2.

Ball scaler number b2-b3 is a popular heavy sickle with wider and heavier blades used for removing granulation tissue, fibrous interdental tissue and tenacious subgingival deposits.

Bar over denture is a male portion of appliance that provides stability and is attached to another tooth in the same dental arch.

Barbed broaches are disposable hand instruments for removing the pulp. It is made of fine wire with multiple barbs when broach is inserted in a root canal and rotated it engage the pulp which can be taken out with broach. After use these are thrown out.

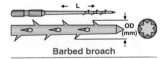

Barbed broach

Barbiturates are the drugs that are widely used in treatment of mild anxiety. These produce sedation and drowsiness and reduced concentration.

Barbiturates-antidotes best antidotes are bemegride or megimide and daptazol. They are given with IV 5% glucose drip in a dose of 15 mg of daptazol and 50 mg of bemegride every 5 minutes until pharyngeal and laryngeal reflexes return to normal.

Barlow's sign is an indicator of congenital dislocation of hip detected during first 6 weeks of life.

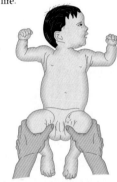

Barlow's sign

Baroreceptor reflex is a nervous reflex which senses sudden change in blood pressure and then stimulates heart and blood vessels to bring hypertension in normal range.

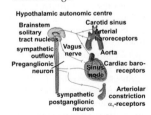

Baroreceptor reflex

Barré's pyramidal sign is an inability to hold the lower legs still with the knees flexed. Place the patient prone and his knees at 90°. Then ask him to hold his lower legs still. If he cannot maintain this position, you have observed the cause of pyramidal tract disease.

Barré's sign is a delayed contraction of iris seen in mental deterioration.

Basal cell adenoma is a tumor that develops in major salivary glands especially parotid gland. These are painless and grow slowly. It has a well defined connective tissue capsule. Cells are isomorphic. Cytoplasm is scanty and ill defined. Tumor has to be removed.

Basal cell carcinoma is a locally aggressive malignant neoplasm that develops on the sun exposed surface over skin. It does not metastasize. It generally involves middle one third of face in 4th decade of life. It arises from basal layer of epidermis or from hair follicle. Direct strong sun light is the causative factor. It starts as a small, elevated papule which ulcerates, heals over and then breaks down. Untreated lesion grows on. Common site involved includes upper lip, nasolabial folds, cheek, forehead etc. It does not arise from oral mucus membrane. It starts as a slow growing small nodule. It develops into central crusted ulcer with an elevated but smooth rolled border. It develops as a sole lesion. If not treated it invades adjacent structures There is basaloid cell's proliferation but cells don't show any mitosis. In some cases squamous cell may occur in tumor. Surgical treatment followed by radiotherapy gives good results.

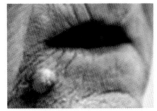
Basal cell carcinoma

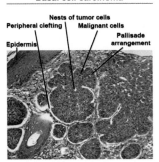
Basal cell carcinoma skin

Basal metabolic rate refers to the process when body is at complete rest, 12 hours after meal energy is needed to maintain the heart beat, respiration etc. But largely to maintain body temperature and tension of muscle, is known as BMR. It is related to muscle mass and surface area of body. For infants BMR is 50-70 k cal per square meter per hour. Average BMR is about 1500 k cal per day. It is under control of thyroid gland and is increased in fever and hyperthyroidism.

Base metal refers to the metal that oxidized readily. It is an alloy composed of metals that are neither precious nor noble. It was developed in 1970 based on nickel and chromium. A thin invisible chromium oxide layer provides a

B

complete and impervious film. It does not dull the surface finish. They are low in cost but their hardness makes occlusal adjustment, polishing and crown removal very difficult.

Base plane angle is the angle between the maxillary and mandibular jaw bases also is used to determine the inclination of the mandibular plane. In horizontal growth pattern this angle is small (23.4° at 9 years and 20.5° at 15 years), whereas is vertical growth pattern it is larger (329° at 9 year and 30.9° at 15 years).

Basic research is the systemic application of scientific method leading to the establishment of new knowledge or theory.

Basilar migraine is a headache of occipital region and is very severe. Aura includes disturbance of vision. Numbness, tingling of lips, hands and feet occurs. Some may have vertigo, diplopia, dysarthria and aggressive outbursts. Basilary artery spasm is responsible of it.

Basophils are white blood cell that stains the basic dyes. It consists of coarse granules in the cytoplasm.

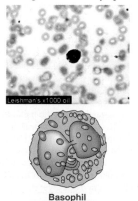

Basophil

Bass method is a method of tooth brushing where the tooth brush is oriented in a 45° angle to the long axis of the tooth and a vibratory motion is used to remove debris or plaque.

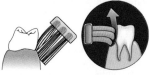

Bass technique

B-cell is a b-lymphocyte that produces and secrets antibodies.

B-cell lineage is ability to synthesize protein called immunoglobulin. Mature B-cells can express Ig in two different forms.

BCG Vaccination came in 1948 that is when it was accepted universally. It is given intradermally and protects for 20 years. After about 230 subautmes over a period of 13 years were able to evolve a strain known as Calmette-Guerin or BCG.

Beau's lines are transverse white linear depression on the finger nails. These lines may develop after severe illness or due to toxicity. It may also be seen in malnutrition, nail bed trauma and coronary artery disease.

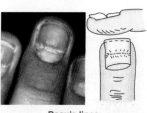

Beau's lines

Bed bath includes washing with water at the bedside only.

Bed sore is a type of ulcer that is situated over a pressure point. Size and shapes of ulcers are variable. It may extend up to the bone. It is covered by pale dirty slough. Edge is clean cut and sloping. There may be sero purulent fluid.

Beer is an alcoholic beverage produced by fermentation of cereals. First step is malting of barley. On sprouting, enzyme amylase develops which hydrolyses starch into dextrin's and maltose. Sprouted barley is dried and extracted with hot water to produce wort. Then hops are added to ferment. A slow fermentation is continuously increasing the alcoholic content and forming the CO_2. Beer contains 3-7% alcohol and 30-60 k cal per 100 ml.

Behavior learning theory is a learned behavior and confirm to the laws of learning theory with no underlying causes and no more emotional or psychologic problems. The learning theory advocates that nonnutritive sucking stems from adaptive response. According to this theory since habit behavior is learned, it can presumably be unlearned. For instance an infant associates sucking with pleasurable feelings such as hunger, satiety and being held. These events will be replaced in later life by transferring the sucking action to the most suitable objects available namely, the thumb or fingers. Learning theorists say that conditioning results in the development of habit (Pavlov 1928). A conditioned reflex is a reflex response, acquired by repeated pairing the stimulus with another stimulus that normally does produce the response. This is an example of one stimulus to another. Conditioning and stimulus generalization can intimate a habit, which if continuously repeated or reinforced will become a learned pattern.

Behavior therapy is an application of interventions based on an understanding of learning principles.

Beliefs are the concepts that a person holds to be true.

Bell's palsy pain behind ear may precede the paralysis for a day or two. MRI may show swelling with enhancement of geniculate ganglion and facial nerve. Exposure to cold may cause it. Person is not able to close one eye. Food collects between the teeth and lips and saliva may dribble from corner of mouth. There is no sensory loss and recovery takes place soon.

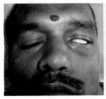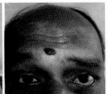

Bell's palsy

Benign cementoblastoma is a true neoplasm of functional cement blasts. These develop in younger age group. Mandible is affected more. Radiographically tumor mass is attached to the tooth root and appears as a well circumscribed dense mass. It is outlined by thin radiolucent line.

Benign chondroblastoma develops between the age group of 5-25 years of age. It is composed of closely packed, polyhedral cells with occasional foci of chondroid matrix. Surgical excision is advised, recurrence is common.

Benign cystic teratoma of ovary contains several types of tissue representing two or three embryonic layers. Tumors are unilateral with cystic spaces.

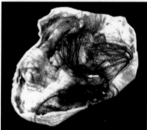

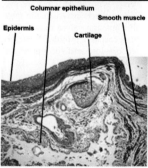

Columnar epithelium

Smooth muscle

Epidermis

Cartilage

Benign cystic teratoma ovary

Benign fibrous histiocytoma lesion develops in skin over breast. They may develop on a previous scar of the skin and appear as lesion in which firm nodule is covered by shiny pink epithelium. Wide local excision is required.

Benign neonatal convulsions refers to the familial benign neonatal convulsions which are dominantly inherited. Most cases are mapping to chromosome 20q and some to 8q. The onset is on 3rd day of life. Short duration attacks with tonic syndromes and ocular symptoms. Ocular remissions occur. Between seizures infants are well.

Benign osteoblastoma was first described in 1954 by Dublin and Johnson. Vertebral column is mostly involved. Lesion is well circumscribed. Actively proliferating osteoblasts pave the irregular trabaculae of new bone. Conservative surgical excision is the treatment.

Benjamin theory (1960) says, "Thumb sucking arises from the rooting or placing reflex seen in all mammalian infants. Rooting reflex is the movement of the infant's head and tongue towards an object touching his cheek. The object is usually the mother's breast but may also be a finger or a pacifier. This rooting reflex disappears in normal infants around 7-8 months.

Beri beri is a condition that occurs due to severe persistent deficiency of thiamine (vitamin B_1). Heart is enlarged due to dilatation and hypertrophy of all chambers especially right ventricle occurs. Muscle fibers show varying degrees of degeneration.

Beta-titanium orthodontic wires – the composition of titanium-molybdenum is 77.8% titanium, 11.3% molybdenum, 6.6% zirconium and 4.3% tin. Molybdenum results in excellent formability or capability for permanent deformation. These wires have true ability to weld.

Bezold's sign is a swelling and tenderness of the mastoid area. It indicates mastoiditis.

Bhang is a combination of dried leaves and small stalks of cannabis. Bhang is taken in sweets, sharbat, ice creams and kulfi. Bhang contains 15% cannabrinol. Fatal dose is 10 mg/kg body weight. It results in mood of elevation. In excitement patient starts laughing loudly. In severe poisoning sensation of tingling and numbness of skin will result. Patient may go to sleep.

Bicuspids refers a type of tooth that has two cusps, i.e. premolars. The first and second bicuspids; they are the 4th and 5th teeth from the midline of the oral covity respectively. These are the posterior teeth that are used for chewing.

Bifid means cleft into two parts and branches.

Bifurcation means having two branches, or dividing into two parts.

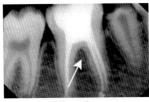

Bifurcation

Bilateral refers to both sides.

Bilateral condylar neck fractures refer to the bilateral bony injury to the condylar neck of the mandible. In such fractures usually there is considerable displacement of one side or the other.

Bilateral extracapsular fractures refer to the condylar neck fractures occurring on both the sides and are of two types: low condylar neck fractures and high condylar neck fractures. Operative reduction of atleast one side of fracture to restore ramus height is desirable. In case of high condylar neck fracture inter-maxillary fixation (IMF) is done for up to 6 weeks and maintained until bony union has occurred

Bilateral fracture occurs on both sides of the body due to combination of direct and indirect violence. Condylar neck and canine regions are the most common sites

Bilateral intracapsular fractures are the fractures occurring in the condyle. The occlusion is slightly deranged in these cases and immobilization of 3-4 weeks may be required to achieve stable union.

Bilateral renal artery occlusion produces anuria or severe oliguria. Person may develop low back pain, fever, flank tenderness and hematuria.

Bile pigments are produced by liver and is stored in gallbladder. It consists of bile salts sodium glycocholate and sodium taurocholate. Bile pigments are bilirubin and biliverdin. *Bile salts* are used in digestion of fats and bile pigments being waste are excreted in feces.

Bimanually is the physical examination using both hands.

Binangle refers to an instrument having two off setting angles in its shank.

Binary alloy is an alloy that is composed of two elements.

Bioavailability it is the amount of drug reaching the systemic circulation in the unmetabolized form and absorption through bodily surfaces.

Bioburden refers to any visible organic debris in dentistry.

Bioengineer is a person who has knowledge of engineering along with biology and functions as a scientist in health care field.

Biofilm is a community of bacteria embedded in exopolysaccharide that adhere out an inert or living surface.

Biofilm is a well organized, cooperating community of microorganisms. The slim layer that forms on rocks in streams is a classic example of a biofilm. So is the plaque that forms in the oral cavity. Biofilms are everywhere in nature. They form under fluid conditions. It is estimated over 95 percent of bacteria existing in nature are in biofilms. Sometimes biofilms are seen as positive source used for detoxification of waste water and sewage. More often biofilms provide a challenge for humans. Human biofilm infections include dental cavities, gum diseases, ear infections and some infections of the prostate gland and heart. When bacteria in a biofilm aggregate on surfaces, they produce copious amounts of a sugary, mucus coating. In case of our mouth, teeming bacteria can in just a few hours erect the microscopic equivalent of a coral reef on our teeth. Biofilm refers to a polysaccharide layer containing colony forming bacteria.

Biologic pocket depth/ Histologic pocket depth is the distance measured between the gingival margin and the base of the pocket.

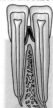

Biologic pocket depth

Biological indicator is also known as spore test to know whether sterilization has been done or not.

Biological therapy is a treatment to stimulate or restore the ability of the immune system to fight infection.

Biometrics is defined as the science of statistical biology, the collection and statistical analysis of data regarding a living organism.

Biopsy is the removal of tissue from the living organism for the purpose of examination at microscopic level. It not only helps in diagnosis but determines the nature of any unusual lesion. Total excision of a small lesion for study is known as Excisional biopsy. While in biopsy only a small part is removed for diagnostic biopsy.

Bio-stimulation is a photo chemical interaction which describes the stimulatory effects of laser light on biochemical and molecular processes that normally occur in tissues such as healing and repair.

Biotin was obtained from egg yolk in 1936. It is known as vitamin 'H' also. Its daily requirement is one microgram. Its deficiency rarely develops. Use of antibiotics destroys the vitamin. Raw white egg prevents its absorption. It is required in synthesis of hemoglobin and manufacture of glycogen. Raw egg contains avidin which binds with biotin preventing its absorption.

Bipolar refers to two poles.

Birth history is the history of new born during birth that includes the type of delivery, occurrence of any complication during birth such as Rh incompatibility or neonatal jaundice.

Bisferiens pulse is a combination of collapsing pulse and low rising pulse.

Bite block is a device used to hold the mouth open during mouth surgery.

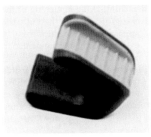

Bite block

Bite plane a fixed appliance made of acrylic used to correct cross bite.

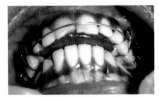

Anterior bite plane

Bite registration is a procedure used to orient upper and lower models of the teeth in proper bite relationship during fabrication of crown.

Bitewing film is an intraoral radiograph used to examine crowns of both maxillary and mandibular teeth biting surface on the same film.

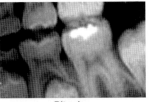

Bitewing

Bitewing vertical is an intraoral film used to examine the level of alveolar bone in mouth. It is placed with long portion of a film in a vertical direction.

Biting habits refers to the self inflicting habits such as nail biting, pencil biting and lip biting.

Bitot's spot are triangular, foamy, rough and raised patches seen on bulbar conjunctiva in vitamin A deficiency. These don't interfere with vision. These are generally bilateral. If more than 2% children between 0-5 years show Bitot's spot in community. It is known as community X-erosis.

B

Black lesions are the lesions that occur due to foreign body deposition. It may be developed due to altered blood pigment and necrosis. If an alteration in blood pigment occurs with oxidation and drying black color may appear in crust. Gangrene gives a black color. As dead tissue sloughs a depressed lesion with a black periphery develops.

Black's cavity classification is the classification system given by Dr GV Black who has coded the cavities according to location on the tooth.

Black stain develops when a black deposit takes the form of thin line or band just above the free gingiva. Black stain is dominated by Actinomyces. These are highly retentive calculus like stain, black or dark brown in color, occurring on the gingival third along the gingival margin also known as brown stain. The stain appears as a continuous or interrupted line following the gingival margin. This line may be 1 mm wide with no appreciable thickness or it may also appear as heavy deposits which will be slightly elevated from the tooth surface and is easily detectable. The teeth frequently appear clean and shiny with a lower tendency to bleed. Black stain has a calculus like appearance and is generally composed of microorganisms embedded deep in a matrix. These stains can occur at any age but are more common in child-hood, females and frequently found in clean mouth. These stains tend to recur despite maintenance of personal hygiene but the severity may reduce with meticulous plaque control methods.

Blastocyst is a stage in embryology following morula.

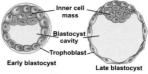

Blastocyst

Blastomycosis is a fungal infection caused by *blastomyces dermatitidis*. It is a normal habitant of soil. In chronic form, low grade fever and mild cough may develop. Oral lesions are rarely the primary lesions but if occurs, it is of nonspecific painless verrucous ulcer with undurated borders. Patients will show pulmonary lesions on X–ray. It may cause shortness of breathing, weight loss and blood tinged sputum. There will be development of painless ulcer with indurated borders. In some cases hard nodules and radiolucent jaw lesions can be seen. Diagnosis is made on biopsy.

Bleaching is the lightening of the color of a tooth through the application of a chemical agent to oxidize the organic pigmentation of the tooth.

Bleeding index is an index that is used to score the status of gingiva where presence or absence of bleeding is recorded by inserting a periodontal probe into the sulcus.

Bleeding time is a diagnostic test that provides an assessment of adequacy of platelet function not the number. It means how much it takes a standardized skin incision to stop bleeding by formation of clot. It is 1-6 minutes.

Blepharoclonus is an excessive blinking of eyes. This extra pyramidal sign occurs with disorders of basal ganglia and cerebellum.

Blind spot is the area on retina that has no rods or cones. So any image that focuses on blind spot cannot be seen.

Blink reflex occurs when we gently tap the glabella (junction between the nose and forehead), both eyelids of the neonate blink.

Blocking is a cognitive disturbance resulting in interruption of a stream of speech or thoughts. Blocking may occur in normal individuals but most commonly occurs in schizophrenia.

Blood borne pathogens are the microorganisms present in blood that cause disease.

Blood brain barrier is a structural and functional barrier formed by astrocytes and blood vessel walls in the brain. It prevents some products diffusing from the blood into brain tissue.

Blood pressure is a measurement of two blood vessels. The first is the pressure of the blood against the arterial blood vessels and second is the pressure against the blood vessels as the heart relaxes between contractions. It is known as diastole.

Blood sugar is a test used to assess the level of sugar in blood. Fasting blood sugar is 80-100 mg/100 ml. The level rises after meals 140 mg/100 ml but rapidly returns to normal unless person is suffering from diabetes. Glucose provides energy and is stored in liver as glycogen.

Blue color weakness develops from diminished or absent blue receptors.

Blue grass appliance (1991) was introduced by Haskell, this is a habit breaking appliance for children with a continued thumb sucking habit, which is affecting the mixed or permanent dentition. It consists of a modified six sided roller machined from teflon to permit purchase of the tongue. This is slipped over a 0.045 stainless steel wire soldered to molar orthodontic bands. This appliance is placed for 3-6 months. Instructions are given to turn the roller instead of sucking the digit. Digit sucking is often seen to stop immediately.

Blue lesions there is no biological blue pigment. Some cystic lesions containing clear fluid appear blue and some vascular lesions may also look blue when blood within the lesion contains a large amount of reduced hemoglobin. Shade of blue color may be altered by the thickness of overlying mucosa. Darker blue is seen with most superficial lesion.

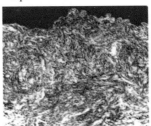

Blue nevus

Blue nevi these are due to benign proliferation of melanocytes. Nevocellular nevi arise from basal layer melanocytes early in life.

B

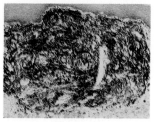

Blue nevus

Blue nevus is common pigmented lesion of oral cavity. These are commonly seen on the mucosal surfaces of hard palate. It is a dome shaped dark blue papule. Cells of blue nevus are elongated, bipolar and spindle shaped. Few pigmented macrophages may be present. These don't change into malignancy and hence surgical resection serves the purpose. Compound nevus presents the combined features of intradermal nevus and junctional nevus. These may be seen at any age. Biopsy is needed simple excision is the treatment of choice.

B-lymphocytes matures without passing through the thymus and matures into plasma cells that produce antibodies.

Body language is the communication of feelings and attitudes/ desires through gesture, postures and facial expression. It is an important relationship between two sexes.

Boil is a lesion where patient presents with a single or multiple painful swelling. It is present in hairy areas and does not occur on palm of hand. Swelling is small and conical having a point. A black dot may be present in the center of swelling.

Boiling is a process of sterilization used when other proper facilities for sterilization is not available. Boiling for 20 minutes may be done. Boiling does not render spores nonviable hence is not very reliable and effective. Needles and syringes are generally sterilized this way.

Bolus is a chewed up mass of food and saliva.

Bonded modified orthodontic brackets are used for fracture with minimal displacement where the fracture can be immobilized with the help of placement of bonded modified orthodontic brackets on to the teeth and applying intermaxillary elastic bands

Bonding-dentin is an establishment of micromechanical bond between cut dentin and the bonding agent.

Bone clamps are another form of external fixation of mandibular fractures. Here instead of pins, the bone clamps are used to secure the fragments of the bone. The clamps are secured on the lower border of the mandible. Pins that project from the clamp, are connected by a system of external rods and universal joints as it is done in external pin fixation.

Bone instruments used in dental surgery includes mallet, bone chisel, bone file and bone forcep.

Bone marrow aspiration is performed when blood picture is not clear about hematological disorder. Marrow biopsy is useful in monitoring the progress of disease. Posterior iliac crest is the preferred site for both marrow aspiration and biopsy. Sternum should be used for aspiration only. Anteromedial surface of tibia is an ideal for infants.

Bone scan is a tracer element study of technetium 99 and then patient is scanned. The tracer localizes to areas of increased metabolic activity such as fracture, infection and cancer.

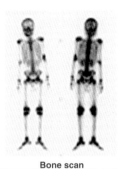

Bone scan

Bonnet's sign is the pain noted on adduction of thigh, seen in sciatica.

Border molding is a technique used in fabrication of denture to adopt the border of the partial or complete denture to the patients soft tissue in order to obtain optimal retention.

Bowel obstruction develops due to hernias. 5-15 % by strangulated hernias and 10 % by neoplasms. Symptoms include abdominal pain, nausea vomiting, and no passing of flatus and distension of abdomen. Abdomen will be tender. In case of hernia tender palpable mass will be felt.

Bowen's disease is localized, intra-epidermal squamous cell carcinoma. It may develop into invasive carcinoma over years. Clinically it is a slow enlarging erythematous patch. Histologically epithelial cells are seen in complete disarray. Many will be of hyper chromatic nuclei. This disease may develop in genital mucosa. Erythroplakia and Bowen's disease both have hairy red patches.

Brachial plexus is a network of nerve fibers formed from the ventral branch of nerves C5-C8 and T1.

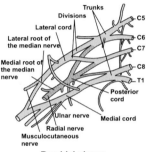

Brachial plexus

Brachial pulse is a throbbing sensation that is felt over the brachial artery located on the inner side of the elbow.

Bracket is small device attached to the teeth that holds the arch wire to the teeth.

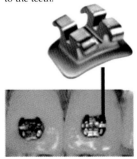

Bracket

Bradykinesia is the slowness of all voluntary movement and speech. It is due to reduced level of dopamine. It is noted in Parkinsonism. Certain drugs may also cause it. There may be tremor and muscle rigidity.

Bradykinin is an endogenous polypeptide released from the inflammatory reaction site. It serves as a powerful vasodilator and excites all types of receptors, sensitizing some high threshold receptors to respond to otherwise innocuous stimuli. It acts only in the presence of prostaglandin.

Bradypnea is a life threatening apnea or respiratory arrest. Respiration is regular but rate is 12 per minute. It may result due to drug overdose.

Brain abscess is an encapsulated pus in brain. It may directly extend from mastoid, skull bones or paranasal sinus. Metastatic brain abscess is secondary to bronchiectasis, empyema or lung abscess. Brain is caused by staphylococcus aureus, staphylococcus viridians and hemolytic streptococci. Abscess manifests with headache, vomiting and convulsions. Hemiplegia may develop. In an event of raised intracranial pressure puncture is not done.

Brain hemorrhage accounts a majority of case of stroke. Hypertension is the main culprit. Blood may be more than 5 cm in diameter.

Brainstem is a lower part of brain which connects the brain with spinal cord. It consists of mid brain, pons and medulla.

Brain tumor headache occur due to rapidly growing brain tumor. Once CSF circulation stops it produces headache. It is worst on

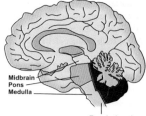

Midbrain
Pons
Medulla

To spinal cord
Brain stem

awakening and is aggravated by sitting, standing and coughing. Supratentorial masses produce frontal or temporal headache while occipital lesions produce occipital headache. Pituitary tumors produce frontotemporal headache. Meningiomas and meningeal sarcomas cause headache at the site. AVMS produce central headache.

Brain wave is a fluctuating electrical activity occurring in brain.

Branchial arches develops during the late somite period (4 weeks IU) the mesoderm lateral plate of the foregut region is segmented to form a series of five distinct bilateral mesenchymal swellings known as the branchial (pharyngeal) arches.

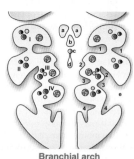

Branchial arch

Branchial cleft cyst develops in lateral aspect of neck in young adults. These are slow growing and symptom free. Cyst is usually lined by stratified squamous epithelium. Surgical removal is a part of treatment.

Brazilian pemphigus is found on tropical regions. It is similar to pemphigus foliaceus.

Breaking cough indicates edema of larynx and surrounding tissue. It may become an emergency.

Breast lipoma is a benign neoplasm. It devops generally as a single lesion. These are soft, movable and fairly well delineated. Treatment is an excision.

Breast pain and nodularity present with complaints of physiological swelling, nodularity and mastalgia. Breast pain is related to menstrual cycle.

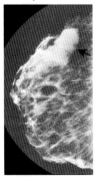

Breast nodularity

Breast traumatic fat necrosis develops in bulky breasts exposed to trauma. It may stimulate carcinoma. Occult fat necrosis is asymptomatic and goes undetected. Such woman have large,dependent breasts. Skin over lesion is red. If tumor develops it is firm and often relatively fixed to the surrounding breasts tissue. Symptoms resemble that of breast abscesses.

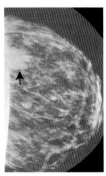

Breast nodularity

Breech loading syringe is an aspirating syringe with a harpoon type of plunger. Thumb ring helps the dentist apply back pressure on the plunger after needle placement in the tissue.

Bridge is a fixed appliance (prosthesis) that replaces missing teeth. A bridge is a series of attached crowns (abutments and pontics). Artificial tooth is known as pontic and supporting teeth are called abutments. The crown on the abutment teeth are called retainers.

Bridge threader is a flexible plastic device used to floss under a fixed bridge to remove plaque from the interproximal surfaces.

Bristle brush is an attachment to the hand piece to remove stain from occlusal surfaces of teeth. Bristle brushes are cleansing and polishing instrument available in wheel and cup shapes. These brushes are used with hand pieces along with a polishing paste.

Brittle bone syndrome can be characterized by thin bones and lack the usual cortex of compact bone. Development of epiphyseal cartilage is unimpaired.

Broadbent's inverted sign includes pulsations in the left posterolateral chest wall during ventricular systole. Put your palm over areas of visible pulsation while hearing for ventricular systole. Rate, rhythm and pulsation will be high. It is due to gross dilatation of left atrium.

Broca's aphasia is striking difficulty with speech though they fully understand what is being said. They can make nonverbal responses. Milder form results in hesistency of speech.

Brodies abscess occurs in patient is between 10-20 years of age. Upper end of tibia and lower end of femur are the common sites. A deep boring pain is the main symptom which may be worst at night. X-ray shows oval lucent area. Treatment is by operation.

Bronchial breathing originates from large airways when lung between these air ways and chest wall is airless due to consolidation, collapse or fibrosis. Sound resembles as listening over trachea. Quality of sound is harsh and of higher frequency. It becomes inaudible just before the end of inspiration.

Bronchiectasis is a congenital or acquired disorder with dilatation and destruction of bronchial wall. Cystic fibrosis and recurrent infection cause it. Symptoms include chronic cough, production of copius amount of purulent sputum, hemoptysis and recurrent pneumonia. Clubbing is frequent and copious foul smelling purulent sputum is characteristic.

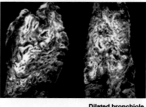

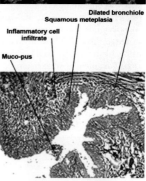

Dilated bronchiole
Squamous meteplasia
Inflammatory cell infiltrate
Muco-pus

Bronchiectasis

Bronchodilator is the dilatation of the bronchi in order to facilitate breathing.

Bronchogenic carcinoma is mostly amongst smokers. Patient presents with anorexia and weight loss. There develops new cough or changes in cough. 25% will show hemoptysis. Some may develop pneumonia or pleural effusion. Sputum cytology is highly specific but not sensitive. CT helps in diagnosis. 5 years survival is only in 5% cases (*see* Figure on page 63).

Bronchopneumonia is a multifocal process which starts in terminal and respiratory bronchioles and

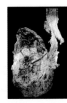

Crushed/compressed tumor cells

Small maligant round cell | Bronchial mucosa | Scanty cytoplasm

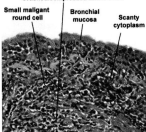

Bronchogenic carcinoma

produces patchy consolidation caused by s. aureus and gram negative organisms.

intra-alveolar infiltrate (peri-bronchiolar)

Unaffected alveoli | Neutrophilic exudate

Bronchial wall

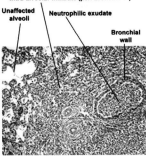

Bronchopneumonia

Bronchopneumonic lesion occurs in scattered nodular fashion around the bronchi. Lesion may be of a few mm to 1 cm. Bronchioles show exudates and lining may show ulceration. Bronchiole is surrounded by a zone of consolidation.

Bronchospasm is a generalized contraction of smooth muscules of bronchi and bronchioles resulting in constriction of bronchi and mucosal edema. Expiratory phase is more involved and may become life threatening.

Brown lesions may be caused by melanin or hemosiderin. Melanin is a substance produced within melanocyte by melanosomes. An increase in brown pigmentation may be brought by increased number of melanocytes. Increased number of melanocytes forms different benign and malignant neoplasms. Heat, ultra voilet rays and X-rays may increase melanin synthesis. Brown color resulting from hemosiderin is associated with crusting and drying of ulcerated lesions.

Brown staining of tooth is a thin, brown delicate pellicle like structure. It may be composed of salivary mucin.

Brown stains due to betel leaf will give rise to stains which can vary in color from dark brown to deep mahogany brown to black. These stains generally contain microorganisms and mineralized content which has the characteristic resemblance to the sub-gingival calculus.

Brown stains due to brown pellicle is smooth and structureless and recurs readily after removal. The pellicle can take on stains of various colors.

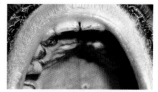

Betal leaf stains

Brown stains due to chlorhexidine mouth rinses are the excellent agents for the plaque control, but repeated use of these agents may give rise to brownish stains on the tooth surfaces generally affecting the proximal surface of the tooth.

Brown stains due to food pigments are resulting from pigments leaching out of the food such as turmeric stains, stains from tea, coffee, and use of artificial colors give rise to various stains.

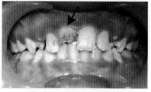

Stains due to trauma

Brown stains due to stannous fluoride appears sometimes as light brown or light yellow, which forms on to the tooth surface after the prolonged or the repeated use of stannous fluoride product which results in the formation of brown tin oxide due to the reaction of the tin ion and fluoride compound.

Bruxism is an involuntary grinding, clinching of teeth specially done during sleep as a result mostly of stress and tension. It causes abnormal wear of teeth. Bruxism is also called a night grinding. It may happen during sleep or during waking hours. Occlusal disturbance may cause it. Emotional tension may be expressed through a number of nervous habits, bruxism is one of them. It may be associated with grinding or grating noise. Bruxism is defined as the grinding of teeth for nonfunctional purposes. Some authors refer to nocturnal grinding as bruxism and grinding during the day as brunomiania. Which could be due to psychological and emotional stresses, occlusal interference or discrepancy between centric relation and centric occlusion can predispose to grinding, pericoronitis and periodontal pain may also trigger bruxism.

Buccal is pertaining to the cheek.

Buccal nerve block is an injection to provide pain control to the soft tissues facial to the mandibular molars.

Buccal object rule is a rule for the orientation of structures seen in two radiographs exposed at different angles used to determine buccal lingual relationship of an object.

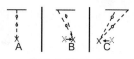

Buccal object rule

Buccal pouch keratosis habit of tobacco chewing may be maintained for decades giving rise to keratosis where there is white thickening and wlinkling of buccal mucosa. There is wrinkling of buccal mucosa. Malignant change can follow after decades.

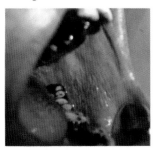

Buccal pouch keratosis

Buccal space refers to the space existing between buccinator and masseter muscle. Infection of this space may lead to swelling of the cheek and may extend to temporal or submandibular space, with which the buccal space communicates.

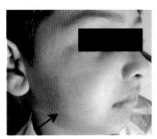

Space infection involving buccal and infraorbital space

Buccal wall refers to cavity wall nearest to cheek.

Buccinator muscle refers to the cheek muscle.

Buccinator is a thin quadrilateral muscle occupying interval between maxilla and mandible. It is supplied by lower buccal branches of facial nerve. It compresses the cheeks against the teeth.

Bullous pemphigoid is a skin lesion and has limited life of five years. Initial defect is in lamina lucida of basement membrane. There is no acanthylosis. Bullae don't extend to periphery. Lesions remains localized and heal spontaneously. Oral lesions are smaller, mild painful and grow slowly. Histologically only one can notice bulla formation in subepithelial region. Systemic corticosteriods are useful. Bullous pemphigoid is basically a disease of an old age. Generalized nonspecific rash develops vesicles and bullae are thick walled and remain intact for some days. Gingival involvement generally occurs much and is painful.

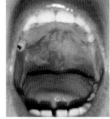

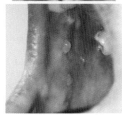

Bullous pemphigoid

Bundle bone is the bone present adjacent to the periodontal ligament that contains large number of Sharpey's fibers.

Bur is smooth tipped hand instrument used to smoothen the occlusal surface of the amalgam restoration.

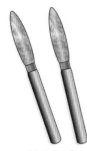

Diamond-Bur

Buried teeth may remain impacted in jaws for many years even without complications. Roots may undergo resorption or hypercementosis ultimately such teeth may be enveloped in dentigerous cyst.

Burn of oral mucosa is a frequent cause of transient nonkeratotic white lesions. Saliva protects mucosa from chemical and thermal burn. Ingestion of caustic liquids results in oropharyngeal burns. Mild thermal burn of anterior tongue is the result of accidental ingestion of hot food. Application of 70% ethyl alcohol to dry mucosa will result in sloughing.

Burning Mouth Syndrome is a painful, burning sensation localized in the tongue or affecting other areas of oral mucosa. The pain of burning tongue is rated similar to that of toothache. Tongue temperature is decreased. Some evidence suggests the existence of oral somatosensory and special sensory deficits.

Burning tongue presents paresthesia of oral mucus membrance a common clinical finding. Pernicious anemia, diabetes, gastric disturbances and psychogenic factors may result in it. Tongue is commonly involved. Pain, burning, etching and stinging of mucus membrane are felt. No satisfactory treatment is available.

Burnishing is smoothing the surface of a dental amalgam after initial carving by rubbing with a metal instrument having a broad surface.

Burns is any injury to skin by an energy source. This source of energy could be heat —which could be by fire or by hot liquids, chemicals, electricity, lasers, friction, and radiation. Burns may involve the different layers of skin and has varied effects on the skin and may be the deeper structures. The amount of damage will be directly proportional to the amount of energy released by the energy source which will depend upon the temperature of the source and the duration of contact. The higher the temperature, greater is the degree and depth of damage.

Burs for low speed hand pieces are made up of steel. These are used to remove caries, trimming dentures and cutting dentine. Burs for air turbine have diamond or tungsten carbide.

Bursa is the fluid sac which reduces friction between two structures.

Burst fracture of vertebra results due to compression force. Fracture is unstable. It may be associated with neurological deficit.

Butterfly cannula is a special needle having flangs to facilitate insertion of it and allow to be

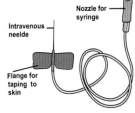

Butterfly intravenous needle (butterfly cannula)

Labels in figure:
- Nozzle for syringe
- Intravenous neelde
- Flange for taping to skin

taped to the skin. It has a flexible tube into which syringe nozzle fits. It arrows additional injections to be given immediately.

By-pass operation is a procedure where coronary vessels which have been blocked through athermatous plaques are literally by passed. Part of vessel is used to connect aorta to a point beyond occlusion in coronary vessel. Vessel can be a vein of leg or an internal mammary artery. It is generally done when at least 3 vessels are blocked.

C fibers are the fibres which carry pain with a speed of 2-3 m/sec.

Cachexia refers to the loss of anorexia due to psychological factors. Anxiety and depression may cause the condition. It may also result in lack of nutrition. Wasting, may develop in course of chronic disease. General weakness is usually associated with cancer.

Caffey's disease generally affects children. High fever, raised ESR and pleural exudate is seen. Child is hyper irritable with soft tissue swelling and pain. There is patchy distribution of lesion characterized by remissions and relapses. Marked cortical thickening of mandible is seen.

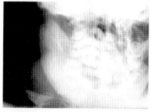

Caffey's disease (infantile cortical hyperostosis) showing gross periosteal thickening of mandible

Calcifying odontogenic cyst is a non aggressive cystic lesion lined by odontogenic epithelium with ghost cell keratinization. Occasionally it may show aggressive behavior. On X-ray it appears as a well defined intrabony lesion that can present as unilocular or multilocular radiolucency. It is well circumscribed. Calcification can occur as radiopaque areas. It is treated by conservative surgical enucleation.

Calcination is a prolonged heating of a substance below its melting point.

Calcined refers to the powdery, friable, dry substance by application of heat.

Calcinosis is the calcification in or under skin. It is of 2 types' calcinosis universalis and circumscripta.

Calcitonin is a peptide hormone secreted by the thyroid gland. It regulates calcium homeostasis.

Calcium homeostasis refers to the process where calcium participates in neuromuscular function, blood coagulation membrane function and multiple enzyme reactions. Human body contains 25 gm/kg of lean body mass. 90% of it is present as calcium phosphate. Daily calcium loss in stool is 100-200 mg contained in intestinal secretion, d3 helps in its absorption.

Calcium hydroxide is a dental material where it can be used as cement for both direct and indirect pulp capping and as a protection barrier beneath composite restoration. It can also be used as antibacterial, root canal medicament, root induction material or an obturating material for primary teeth. The material has an alkaline pH of 11-12 and it functions by stimulating the formation of reparative dentin.

Calcium plays large role in formation of bones and teeth. In blood it ranges from 9 to 11 mg/dl. Low concentrations below 8 mg/dl may produce convulsions. Daily requirement in adults is 500 mg growing child may require a little more. Absorption is hardly 30% of its consumption. Oxalate interferes with calcium absorption forming calcium oxalate. Lactose or milk sugar increases calcium. More than 90% is in bones and teeth. About 1 gm of calcium is found in extra cellular fluids and 4-5 grams in soft tissues. Calcification of deciduous teeth begins by 20th week of fetal life. Permanent teeth begin to calcify when child is between 3 months to 3 years of age. For adults calcium/phosphorus ratio should be 2:1. Daily requirement is 0.5 gram. Milk and dairy products are good sources. Considerable calcium may be lost in preparation of vegetables if thick skins are removed or dark green leaves are discarded. Soyabean is a significant source of calcium. In children lack of calcium affects their growth adversely.

Calculus is an adherent calcified or calcifying mass that forms on the surface of natural teeth and dental prosthesis. Ordinarily calculus consists of mineralized bacterial plaque. It is classified according to its relation to the gingival margin as supragingival and subgingival. It consist of inorganic matter, some water, an organic component made up of desquamated epithelial cells, gram positive filamentous microorganism such as leptotrichia, some gram negative filamentous forms and cocci, leucocytes and an amorphous ground substance. The inorganic component consists mainly of calcium phosphate as hydroxyapatite and other crystalline forms of calcium phosphate such as brushite, whitlockite and octacalcium phosphate. There is also a small

amount of calcium carbonate and magnesium phosphate as well as fluoride.

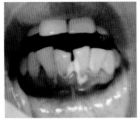
Supragingival calculus

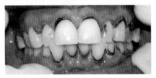
Subgingival calculus

Callus is the structure that unites the two broken ends of the bone. It is composed of fibrous tissue, cartilage and bone. Internal callus is a new bone arising from marrow cavity while external callus is new bone formed around two fragments. As callus formation progresses the cartilage cells begin to mature. Cartilage begins to calcify.

Hematoma | Granulation tissue | Osseous callus
PMNs | Procallus | Remodelling
Callus formation

Calorie equivalent is the number of kilos calories produced per liter of oxygen consumed.

C

Calories is the form of energy present in the body to maintain body temperature for metabolite purposes, to support growth and for physical activity. One kilocalorie is the amount of heat required to raise the temperature of one kilogram of water from 15° to 16°C.

Canalicular adenoma develops in intraoral accessory salivary glands and in upper lip in elderly age group. It is a slowly growing, well circumscribed, firm nodule especially in lip. It is not fixed and is composed of long strands or cords of epithelial cells arranged in double row. Enucleation of lesion is the treatment of choice.

Cancer refers to an abnormal growth of cells that can invade and destroy surrounding normal tissues and sometime spreads to other parts of the body.

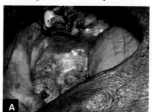

Central necrosis (comedo pattern)

Intraductal component

Invasion in stroma

Malignant cells

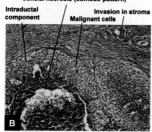

(A) Carcinoma of lower alveolus,
(B) Carcinoma of breast

Candida associated denture stomatitis is a common ailment in wearers of full denture. It is also common in patients wearing orthodontic appliances or Obturators for cleft palate. Patient may be symptom free.

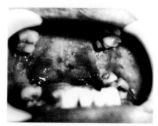

Candida associated stomatitis

Candida hypersensitivity syndrome is a triad of symptoms that includes fatigue, headache/ rashes oral or vaginal infection with candida. Nystatin therapy generally doesn't help.

Canine refers to the third incisor tooth from the midline of the oral cavity. It has the longest crown root with the sharp cusp which performs the tearing action.

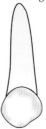

Canine

Canophile is an organism that grows best in the presence of increased concentration of CO_2.

Cap splints are the silver – copper alloy type of splints which fits on to the tooth in a cap or crown form along with locking plates and connecting bars for the immobilization of all types of jaw fractures. The technique is time consuming both clinically as well as in the laboratory.

Capillary hemangiomas are well defined hemangiomas that appear from bright red to purple patches. Common sites are skin, subcutaneous tissue and mucus membrane of oral cavity and lips. Hemosiderin represents the ruptured vessels. These may also be found in liver, bones, stomach and small intestine.

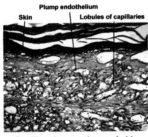

Plump endothelium
Skin   Lobules of capillaries

Capillary hemangioma of skin

Capillary hemorrhage refers to the bleeding occurring from the capillaries. The wound bleeds slowly. The blood is bright red in color and oozes from many points.

Capillary penetration is the movement of a liquid into crevice or tube because of capillary pressure.

Capsule is a fibrous or membranous connective tissue envelop.

Carbohydrate intolerance is the inability of the body to completely process the nutrient carbohydrate into a source of energy for the body, usually because of the deficiency of an enzyme needed for digestion. Lactose intolerance, the inability to digest the sugar found in milk, is widespread.

Carbohydrates are the richest source of energy. About 70-80% of total energy is supplied by carbohydrate. It contains carbon, hydrogen and oxygen. Each gram of it provides 4.1 calories minimum of 100 grams of carbohydrate are needed in diet.

Carbon monoxide is a colorless, odourless and non irritant gas which cannot be perceived by senses. Whenever carbon is burnt some carbon monoxide is formed. It is highly poisoning gas which is absorbed through lungs.

Carbon monoxide poisoning develops by breathing air which is contaminated by coal gas in badly ventilated room. Below 10-20% concentrations will cause lassitude, headache and shortness of breath; 20-30% will have severe throbbing headache, muscular weakness, hurried respiration and defective memory and might faint. 30-40% concentration will produce uncoordinated movement, mental confusion, defective sight and hearing. 40-50% will result in behavior like that of a drunken person and loss of power. Increasing confusion and hallucination will also develop. 50-60% concentration results in comma followed by convulsions. Skin will become pink. 60-70% will result in deep coma. Incontinence of urine and feces will develop. 70-80% concentration will result in quick death.

Carbon steel refers to an alloy of carbon and iron with less than 2% carbon present.

C

Carbuncle is a lesion where there is swelling of short duration. It is present commonly on the neck. It may be bluish red in color. There are multiple openings with pus giving a sieve like appearance. It is diffuse and tender and can be commonly seen in diabetic patient.

Carcinoma *in situ* is a premalignant condition where it is very difficult to differentiate it from dysplasia. There is no individual cell keratinization, no epithelial pearl formation and no hyperkeratosis. Lesions may be flat, red, velvety and granular to look. Lesions of carcinoma in situ are to be treated vigorously with local excision. Wider surrounding area should also be removed but regional nodes are generally not removed. Majority of these lesions occur in floor of mouth.

Carcinoma of buccal mucosa refers to the malignant ulcer affecting buccal mucosa. Chewing of tobacco is commonly involved. Verrucous carcinoma develops in case of chewing tobacco. Leukoplakia is a common predecessor of it. Cheek biting and dental irritation from jagged teeth may rarely cause it. Lesion is painful ulceration. Superficial lesions may grow outwards. Incidence of metastases is high. Maxillary lymph glands are commonly involved.

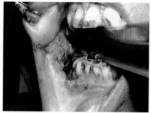

Carcinoma of buccal mucosa

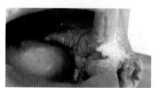

Advanced Carcinoma of Buccal mucosa (intraoral view)

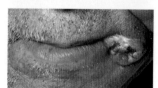

Advanced Carcinoma of Buccal mucosa involving angle of mouth

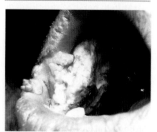

Carcinoma of Buccal mucosa involving angle of mouth

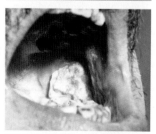

Carcinoma of Buccal mucosa near retromolar pad

Carcinoma of floor of mouth refers to the lesion affecting floor of the mouth. Smoking pipe or cigar is the main etiology. Generally there is indurated ulcer of varying size situated on one side of mid line. It may be painful. Carcinoma may invade deeper structure and may involve sub maxillary or sublingual gland. Involvement of tongue results in slurring of speech. Metastases spread to sub maxillary group of lymph nodes. Even small tumors recur after surgical excision, otherwise prognosis is fair.

Carcinoma of gingiva generally develops after extraction of tooth. Carcinoma initiates as ulceration, purely erosive lesion. Fixed gingiva is more commonly involved. It generally involves maxilla. Mandibular gingiva metastasis occurs more than maxillary gingiva. Metastasis is a common sequel of gingival carcinoma. Prognosis is not very good.

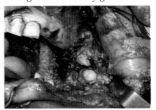

Carcinoma upper gingivobuccal
sulcus

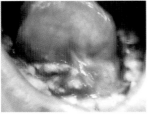

Carcinoma of floor of mouth

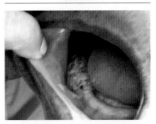

Carcinoma of lower gingival
mucosa in an edentulous patient

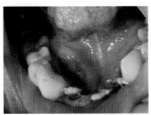

Carcinoma of floor of mouth and
lower gingivobuccal sulcus

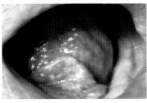

Carcinoma of tongue involving
floor of mouth

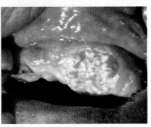

Carcinoma of upper gingival
mucosa

C

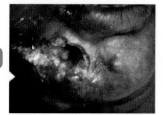

Advanced carcinoma of lower gingivobuccal sulcus with oro-cutaneous fistula

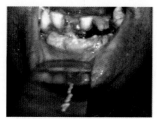

Carcinoma of lower gingivolabial sulcus

Carcinoma of lip refers to the malignant lesion occurring on the lip. Pipe smokers are commonly involved. It involved vermillion border of lip of one side. It starts as area of thickening, indurations and irregular ulceration. Later it may produce an exophytic proliferative growth. Carcinoma is slow to metastasize. Sub mental and sub maxillary nodes of same side are involved. Surgical excision followed by radiotherapy may help.

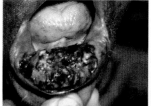

Carcinoma of lower lip

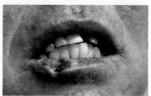

Carcinoma of lip

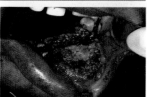

Carcinoma of lower lip

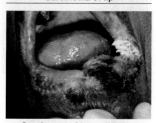

Carcinoma of lower lip also involving angle of the mouth

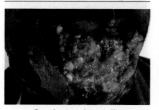

Carcinoma lower lip

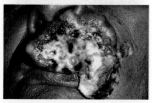

Advanced carcinoma of upper lip

Carcinoma of maxillary sinus is often hopelessly advanced before patient comes to know about it. There is development of swelling and bulging of alveolar ridge, mucobuccal fold and elongation of maxillary molars. Patient complaints of unilateral nasal stiffness along with discharge. Various walls of antrum may be involved. Ulceration into oral cavity may develop. Metastasis generally doesn't occur.

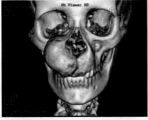

Carcinoma of maxillary antrum

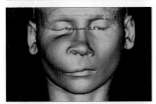

Carcinoma of palate and uvula

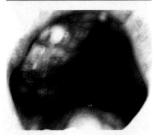

Carcinoma of maxilla with involvement of hard palate

Carcinoma of palate is poorly defined, ulcerated painful lesion on one side of midline. It may invade bone and nasal cavity. Metastasis to regional lymph nodes is common. As treatment both surgery and radiotherapy has been used.

Carcinoma of pancreas occurs most commonly in 50-60 years of age. Tumors of head of pancreas present with weight loss, obstructive jaundice and gastric pain. When mass is palpable surgery loses its use. Liver is enlarged. Gall bladder is palpable. Elevated alkaline phosphatase and bilirubin reflect common duct obstruction or hepatic metastasis. Carcinoma of distal common bile duct present with weight loss, obstructive jaundice and palpable gall bladder.

Carcinoma of tongue is common carcinoma of oral cavity. Leukoplakia may predispose it. There is formation of painless mass or ulcer. Pain develops on infection. There may be development of exophytic mass or to infiltrate deep layers of tongue. It results in indurations and fixation. It develops on lateral border or ventral surface of tongue. Treatment is complicated and prognosis is not good.

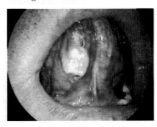

C

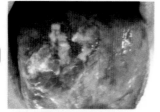

Carcinoma tongue

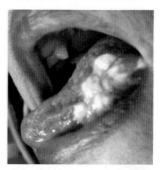

Carcinoma of tongue-exophytic
growth

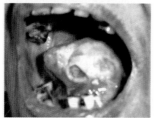

Carcinoma of tongue-ulcerative
growth

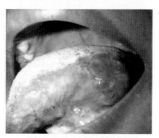

Carcinoma of tongue -
ulceroinfilterative growth

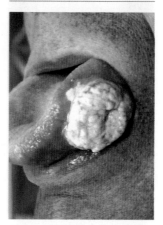

Carcinoma of tongue-exophytic
growth

Carcinoma stomach may be associated with H-pylori. Adenocarcinoma comprises 95% of cases with variable degree of differentiation. Polypoid type is well differentiated (*see* Figure on page 77).

Cardiac arrest is the most serious complication of collapse followed after angina or myocardial infarction. Signs of cardiac arrest include sudden unconsciousness, absence of breathing and pulse and dilated pupils.

Cardiac impulse is an action potential that occurs in the cardiac conduction tissue.

Cardiac muscle is found in heart. Like skeletal muscle cardiac muscle is striated. Cardiac muscle cells are long branching cells and fit tight. These tight fitting

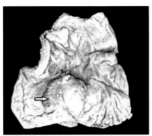

Malignant glands Muscularis propris invaded
Pleomorphism Nuclear atypia

Carcinoma stomach

junctions promote rapid conduction of electrical signals throughout heart. Cardiac muscle is not under voluntary control.

Cardiac edema refers to the right ventricle failure. Edema is systemic in distribution in all tissues and organs. In left ventricle failure the lungs are primarily affected. Edema is in lungs. Cardiac edema is a generalized edema.

Cardinal leprosy includes hypopigmented skin lesions with loss of sensation or absence of sweating. Nerve involvement is manifested by nerve thickening and/or tenderness. Skin smear may be positive for M leprae. When the skin smear is negative presence of other 2 cardinal sign is sufficient to make a diagnosis of leprosy.

Cardiogenic shock occurs when the systolic BP falls to less than 80 mm Hg or 30 mm Hg less than base line. It will result in narrowed pulse pressure. There may be rapid, weak and occasionally irregular pulse. Peripheral vasoconstriction causes cyanosis of extremities giving pale, cool and clammy skin. Person may become restless and anxious. Oliguria and confusion develops.

Cardiomyopathy is a group of disease involving primarily the heart muscle.

Cardiospasm refers to the weak or peristalsis through lower oesophagus and failure of relaxation of cardiac in response to peristaltic wave of swallowing. There develops gradual or sudden onset of dysphagia. To start with food regurgitates and later on when dilatation of esophagus takes place food accumulates. Pain is relieved by drinking cold water. Endoscopy shows chronically inflamed mucosa.

Caries activity test is a quick test that provides information about acid forming microorganisms or their activity in mouth.

Caries severity index was developed by Tank Certrude and Storvick Clara in 1960. This index was developed to study the depth and extent of the caries surfaces and the extent of pulpal involvements. The progress of the dental caries in stages as described by Massler and Schour in 1952, were modified and this caries severity index was devised to measure the extent and depth of decayed surfaces and pulpal involvements based on clinical and radiographic examinations.

Caries susceptibility index developed by Richardson in 1961, for assessing caries susceptibility. This index is based on Bodecker and Mellanby caries indices. There are 2 factors involved in measuring caries susceptibility using the dynamic survey namely: a. Amount of tooth surfaces at risk, b. Amount of caries developing during the period of observation. 'B' divided by 'a' will give a measure of susceptibility.

Caring skills are the nursing skills to maintain patient's health.

Cariogram is, a new method of illustrating an interaction of factors contributing to the development of caries has been introduced by Bratthall et al., (1999) called cariogram. A pie circle diagram is divided into 5 sectors in the following colors. Green - shows and estimation of the chance to avoid caries. Dark blue–'diet' is based on a combination of diet contents and diet frequency. Red-bacteria are based on a combination of amount of plaque and mutants streptococci. Light blue sector – 'susceptibility' is based on a combination of fluoride program, saliva secretion and salivary buffering capacity. Yellow sector–'circumstances' is based on a combination of past caries experience and related disease.

Carotid artery syndrome refers to transient cerebral ischemia with contralateral weakness of arm and leg. Mental confusion and phemisensory disturbance will take place.

Carpus is the proximal portion of hand that contains the eight bones.

Carrier is one who is carrying a disease without being aware of it or is not having clinical symptoms.

Carrying angle is the angle forming at elbow between center line of humerus and forearm. Angle in normal person is 5° in men and 10 to 15° in women. Carrying angle bilaterally should be symmetrical.

Cartilage is a firm, elastic, flexible connective tissue that is attached to articulate bone surfaces forming certain part of skeleton.

Carver is an instrument used to shape restorative material.

Case fatality rate represents the killing power of a disease. It is simply the ratio of death to cases.

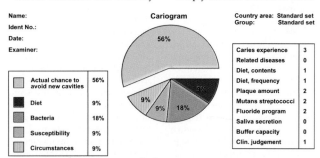

Cariogram

Case study is a method of structuring a qualitative research project by detailed analysis of a well defined unit or case.

Castable ceramic is used to case crowns by the lost wax process. It is used in single anterior and posterior crowns.

Casts in urine are portion of gelled protein like material which are moulds of interior of tubules. Hyaline casts appear as clear cylinders in febrile illness. Red cell casts are RBCs seen in subacute glomerulonephritis. White cell casts are hyaline casts with WBCs seen in chronic pyelonephritis. Epithelial cell casts is seen in tubular necrosis while granular cast is seen in chronic glomerulonephritis. Fatty cast is composed of epithelial cells. Waxy cast is more opaque.

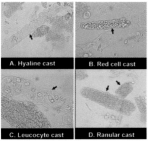

| A. Hyaline cast | B. Red cell cast |
| C. Leucocyte cast | D. Ranular cast |

Casts in urine

Casual comparative research is a non experimental research in which assignment to groups is based on pre existing characteristic or attributes of subjects.

CAT stands for computerized axial tomography.

Catabolism is a metabolic breakdown of complex molecules into simpler molecules. There is the breakdown of food compounds or cytoplasm into simpler compound. Process releases energy.

Catalyst is a chemical that speeds up reactions without being changed. When proteins play a role of catalysts these are known as enzymes.

Catarrh is an inflammation of mucus membrane of nose and throat. It is a non productive cough.

Catatonia is a condition where there is marked inhibition or excitation in motor behavior developing in psychotic disorder. Catatonia stupor and muscle rigidity seen in schizophrenia.

Catheterization is a process where the passage of flexible tube is pushed into bladder through the urethra for the withdrawal of urine.

Cathode is a negative electrode in X-ray tube. It supplies the electrons necessary to generate X-rays.

Cation refers to the positively charged particle.

Caudal means towards tail.

Cauda equine syndrome is a syndrome caused by compression of cauda equine. There will be bladder complaints as well as motor anesthesia with incontinence or urinary retention. Symptoms include low back pain, incontinence of urine and bilateral sciatica. Person may develop fecal retention and saddle anesthesia.

Causalgia is an unpleasant burning type of continuous pain following peripheral nerve injuries. It is more common in hand and arm. Skin of the affected area has spontaneous pain and perspires excessively. Patient will not allow skin to be touched.

Cauterize is to burn, corrode or destroy living tissue by means of caustic soda, heated metal or electric current.

Cavitation is a carious process occuring in a tooth resulting in a cavity or a ditch. It appears as radiolucent lesion on radiograph.

Cavity liners are liquid suspensions of zinc oxide or calcium hydroxide. It can be applied in a thin film to the surface of cavity. Cavity liners neutralize the free acid of zinc phosphate and silicate cements.

Cavity preparation is a mechanical alteration of defective, injured or diseased tooth in order to best receive a restorative material which will reestablish a healthy state for the tooth including esthetic correction where indicated, along with normal form and function.

Cavity primers are used to increase the adaptation of methylmetha-crylate filling materials to cavity walls. It seals the margins.

Cavity varnishes are solutions of one or more resins from natural gums, synthetic resins. It reduces postoperative sensitivity by sealing the open ends of dentin tubules with a glaze like covering but being thin it is insufficient to provide thermal insulation. Varnishes check the microleakage of fluids around the margins of restorations.

Cavosurface margin is the contact between the cavity surface the tooth surface location where the walls and line angles meet the unaltered tooth surface (*see* Figure).

CCD technology is usually made of a chip of pure covalently bonded

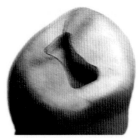

Cavosurface margin

silicon atoms. When the chip is exposed to visible light or X-ray radiation, bonds are broken, and charged electron hole pairs are formed. The electrical charge created is captured, amplified, converted, and displayed as an image.

Cd4 (helper t-cells) promote proliferation, maturation and immunologic function of other cell types.

Cd_{44} are the hematopoietic progenitor cells express the most truncated form of cd44, which bind hyaluronic acid a gag found in ecm. Therefore, a wide variety of adhesive interactions between cell – cell and cell - ecm are critical for hematopoiesis.

Cd_8 (cytotoxic t-cells) are those cells that has an ability to kill cells and that have foreign molecules on their surface.

Cell mediated immunity is a resistance to disease organisms resulting from the actions of cells specially sensitized 't' cells.

Cell-poor zone (Cell-free zone of Weil) is located immediately subjacent to the odontoblast layer, which is 40 mm in width and is relatively free of cells. It is traversed by capillaries and unmyelinated nerve fibres. This zone may be or may not be apparent in young pulps, where dentin forms rapidly or in older pulps, where reparative dentin is being produced.

Cell-rich zone of pulp is located immediately subjacent to the cell-poor zone. It is much prominent in the coronal pulp than in the radicular pulp. This zone is richly populated with fibroblasts, along with macrophages dendritic cells and lymphocytes. It forms as a result of peripheral migration of cells populating the central regions of the pulp, commencing at the time of tooth eruption. Although cell division within the cell-rich zone is a rare occurrence in normal pulps, death of odontoblasts causes a greater increase in the rate of mitosis. It acts as a reservoir for the replacement of irreversibly damaged odontoblasts.

Cellulitis refers to an inflammation of soft tissues. It is a local pain and swelling of acute onset with pyrexia and general debility. Streptococci are particularly potent producing hyalurodinase and causing cellulitis. Cellulitis of face and neck develops mostly due to dental infection. Person is ill with fever and increased WBC count. There is painful swelling of soft tissue. Its boundaries are not very well defined. Skin is of pinkish color and lymph glands are enlarged. Cellulitis is treated by antibiotics. Infection of sublingual space produces swelling of floor of mouth.

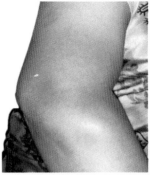
Cellulitis of hand

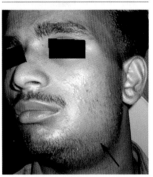
Cellulitis involving floor of the mouth

Cement base is a layer of cement commonly used beneath a permanent dental restoration with purpose to encourage recovery of injured pulp or otherwise protect pulp against thermal injury. Better cement base is zinc oxide eugenol and calcium hydroxide. Glass ionomer cement is polycrylate based and have anticariogenic properties.

Cement sealer is a compound used in filling of a root canal. It is put in plastic form which solidifies after placement. It fills the irregularities of canal.

Cementation is the process where the appliance is glued on to the associated area with the help of cement.

Cementicles are small foci of calcified tissue not necessarily true cementum. It lies free on periodontal ligament. These are developed by calcification of nests of epithelial cells. The pattern of calcification gives appearance of a circular lamellated structure. Cementicles may arise from focal calcification of connective tissue sometimes calcification occurs as small, round or ovoid globules of calcium salt. Cementicles are of no clinical significance.

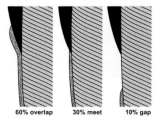

60% overlap   30% meet   10% gap
Cementoenamel junction

is to provide attachment of the tooth to alveolar bone. Union of cementum and dentin is known as dentino-cemental junction. Like dentin, cementum also shows continuous growth. Junction between the enamel and cementum is called Cemento-enamel junction. Cementum has the same hardness that of bone. Composition - 50% of inorganic substance, 50% of organic and water.

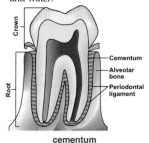

Cementum
Alveolar bone
Periodontal ligament
Crown
Root

cementum

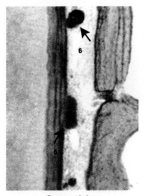

Cementicles

Cementoenamel junction (CEJ) is the line around the visible surface of teeth where the cementum and enamel meet. Actually it is also known as neck or cervix of tooth.

Cementum is the bone like structure which covers the root. The main function of cementum

Cemento ossifying fibroma It is uncommon and is well circumscribed and undergoes slow expansile growth usually in mandibular or molar region. It causes painless swelling between 20-40 years. It is radiolucent with varying degree of calcification in center. Roots of related tooth can be displaced. It may have a definable capsule so can easily be enucleated.

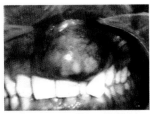
Cemento ossifying fibroma
intraoral view

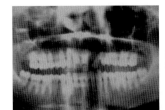
Cemento ossifying fibroma
panoramic view

C

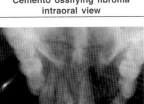
Cemento ossifying fibroma
occlusal view

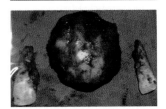
Cementoossifying fibroma
surgically excised

Center of gravity is the center of one's weight, half above and half below. Similarly it is half on left and half on right.

Central buttressing bone formation is the process of compensatory bone formation occurring within the jaw in an attempt to buttress bony trabaculae which is weakened by bone resorption.

Central cementifying fibroma is a neoplasm of bone and may develop at any age. Mandible is more affected. Radiographically one can notice radiolucent area with no radio-opacities. It is composed of delicate interlacing collagen fibres arranged in discrete bundles. Mitotic figures may be present in small number. It has to be excised carefully.

Central giant cell granuloma is a benign intra osseous destructive giant cell lesion. Generally anterior part of jaw bone is affected. It is a reactive lesion. It affects mandible more than maxilla. Some lesions may cross the mid line. It is a small, slow enlarging, bony hard swelling of jaw. Lesion may cause perforation of cortical plate. Teeth in affected region are always vital. Radiographically lesion will slow multilocular radiolucent area in jaw and it gives a soap bubble appearance. When unilocular it will show a drop shaped appearance. Histologically central giant cell granuloma shows multinucleated giant cells. Several areas of hemorrhage and hemosiderin pigmentation are also seen. Around these blood capillaries are also found.

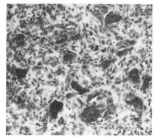

Central giant cell granuloma

Central incisors are used for cutting or biting food, these are the first of the four anterior teeth of either jaw.

Central nervous system includes brain and spinal cord.

Central ossifying fibroma represents a well demarcated expansile jaw lesion. It is well encapsulated. Children and young adults are affected. There is usually a single lesion. There is localized painless non tendered bony hard swelling in jaw. Tumour is slow growing but may disfigure the face. In some cases displacement of teeth may be seen due to expansion and distortion of cortical plates. Histopathologically highly cellular fibroblastic stroma with 'whorled pattern' collagen fibres may be noted. *Central ossifying fibroma* may occur at any age. There is predilection for mandible. Until swelling develops symptom doesn't develop. Displacement of teeth may be one of the early feature. It is slow growing. Lesion contains delicate interlacing collagen fibres. Mitotic figures may be present.

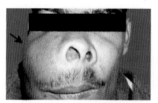

Extraoral view exhibiting a disfigured face

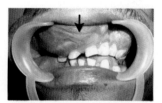

Intraoral view showing movement of maxilla along with the displacement of tooth

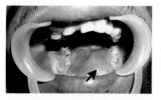

Intraoral view involving mandible

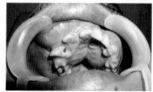

Intraoral involving palate

Central ray is the central portion of the primary beam of radiation.

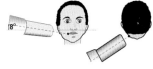

Central ray

Centric occlusion is the relationship of the occlusal surfaces of one arch to those in the opposing arch at physical rest position. Or

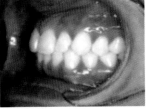

Centric occlusion

Centric occlusion refers to the closing of jaws in a position that produces maximum stable contact between the occluding surfaces of the maxillary and mandibular teeth.

Centric relation is the relationship of the maxillary arch to the mandibular arch when the condyle is in its most retracted position. Or

Centric relation refers to the most cranial position of the mandible along the retruded path of closure

Cephalic vein one of the four superficial veins of upper limb.

Cephalocaudal gradient of growth is an axis of increased growth extending from head towards the feet. In the fetal life, at about the third month, the head takes up almost 50% of total body length. At this stage, cranium is large relative to the face and represents more than half of total head. In contrast, limbs are still rudimentary and the trunk is underdeveloped. By the time of birth the trunk and limbs are grown faster than head and face so that the proportion of entire body devoted to head has decreased about 30%. The overall pattern of growth, there after follows this course with progressive reduction of relative size of the head to about 12% of an adult.

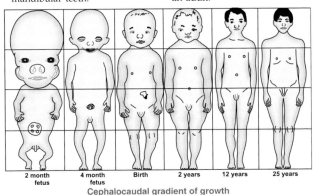

| 2 month fetus | 4 month fetus | Birth | 2 years | 12 years | 25 years |

Cephalocaudal gradient of growth

Cephalometric film is an extraoral X-ray film used to view bony and soft tissue areas of facial profile.

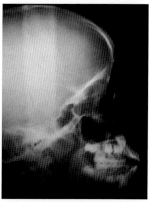

Cephalogram

Cephalometric technique has contributed significantly to the knowledge of human craniofacial skeletal growth. Cephalometry makes it possible to take serial radiographs of a patient's skull in order to study the growth changes taking place.

Cephalosporin is a bactericidal drug which contains a beta-lactam ring. These are broad-spectrum antibiotics. There are many different cephalosporins with varying side chains; these side chains alter the pharmacokinetics, spectrum of activity and beta - lactamase resistance. Cephalosporin's are relatively expensive and, although a good alternative to penicillin's when a broad-spectrum drug is required, but should not be used as first choice unless the organism is known to be sensitive. Cephalosporin's also contains a beta-lactam ring and are bactericidal.

They are broad-spectrum antibiotics. There are many different cephalosporins with varying side chains; these side chains alter the pharmacokinetics, spectrum of activity and beta- lactamase resistance. Cephalosporin's are relatively expensive and, although a good alternative to penicillin's when a broad-spectrum drug is required, should not be used as first choice unless the organism is known to be sensitive.

Ceramic is a compound of metallic and non metallic elements. Dental gypsum, zinc phosphate and porcelains are example of ceramic material. Ceramics are fully oxidized materials and therefore chemically stable. So these don't elicit adverse biological response. Metal they do oxidize. Two types of 'inert' ceramics of interest are carbon and alumina.

Cerebellar ataxia appears in druken patient. Patient walks on a broad base, feet are planted wide apart and placed irregularly. Ataxia is severe in open as well as with closed eyes.

Cerebellar gait the main feature of this gait is wide base, unsteadiness and irregularity of steps. On getting up from chair irregular of swaying of trunk takes place. Standing heel to toe in a straight line is difficult. With lesions of thalamus and midbrain ataxic signs on opposite side develop. It is common in alcoholics, long term dilantin intake and multiple sclerosis. In children tuberculoma may present it.

Cerebellum is a part of the brain that is located in posterior fossa and is separated by tentorium cerebella. It comprises median vermis and two lateral cerebellar hemispheres. It is comprised by a layer of cortex and an internal mass of white matter in which cerebellar nuclei are located. The lesion of flocculonodular lobe causes trunk ataxia, swaying and staggering. Paleocerebellum controls antigravity muscles. Neocerebellum controls fine co-ordinated movements of hands. Extensive lesion of anterior lobe causes hypotonia, postural abnormalities, ataxia and mild weakness of ipsilateral arm and leg. Hypotonia is more apparent with acute lesions.

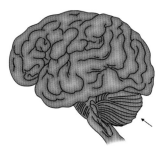

Cerebellum

Cerebral compression is a condition that occurs after head injury. Patient becomes restless and passes into coma. His face becomes flushed and pulse becomes slow. On paralysed side temperature will be more. Pupil on the side of lesion dilates after initial contraction. In last stage both the pupils dilate and become fixed.

Cerebral edema the normal water of grey matter is 80% and of white matter 60% of weight. Brain may also swell due to increase in cerebral volume known as congestive brain swelling.

Cerebral infarction is a disease where contralateral athetosis is accompanied by altered level of consciousness. There may be paralysis of face/limbs of opposite side.

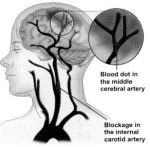

Blood dot in the middle cerebral artery

Blockage in the internal carotid artery

Cerebral infarction

Cerebral ischemia occurs due to deficient supply of glucose to the blood. Usually brain derives the energy from oxidative meta-bolism of glucose. In brain there is no glucose store. Once the CBF (cerebral blood flow) falls below 20 ml/100 gram of brain/minute EEG becomes flat and evoked response disappears signifying the starving neurones. CBF below 10 ml/100 gram of brain tissue per minute leads to infarction and restoration of circulation is of no value as pet shows complete cessation of glucose metabolism. Around the infracted zone, there is potentially viable zone of brain tissue where blood flow is low, function is depressed but recovery is possible. Vasogenic edema starts due to dilation of vessels in infarcted zone. Edema stays maximum by 2-4 days and then subsides.

Cerebral malaria is caused with falciparum infection. Multiple petechial hemorrhages are responsible for CNS symptoms. High fever may be followed by convulsions or unconsciousness. Sensory motor deficits and mental symptoms may occur. Parasite may be recovered from peripheral blood. Mortality is 20-40%. It is a medical emergency. Quinine hydrochloride 600 mg in 5% dextrose is given IV. Oral quinine 350 mg 2 tablets three times a day along with tetracycline is given. Plenty of IV. Glucose is necessary.

Cerebral nuclei are islands of gray matter located in cerebral cortex which are responsible for automatic movements and postures. These are known as basal ganglion.

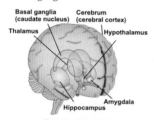

Cerebral nuclei

Cerebral venous thrombosis may develop after pyogenic meningitis, collagen disease, and trauma when superior sagittal is involved it may cause papilloedema and hemorrhagic infarction. Patient may develop papilloedema, extensive bilateral hemorrhagic infarction not confirming to any specific vascular territory. Headache and seizure may develop.

Cerebrospinal fluid (CSF) near about 500 ml of it is produced daily from choroid plexuses of 3rd, 4th and lateral ventricles. It is clear and colorless with slightly opaque hue due to globulin. Specific gravity ranges from 1003-1009.

Cerebrospinal rhinorrhea refers to the escape of cerebrospinal fluid in to the nasal cavity due to communication of ethmoidal bone which occurs due to lefort II and lefort III fractures and the fracture involving nasal complex, which may lead to a dural tear in the region of cribriform plate of ethmoidal bone.

Cerebrovascular accident (CVA) is a focal neurologic disorder caused by destruction of brain substance as a result of intracerebral hemorrhage, thrombosis, embolism or vascular insufficiency. CVA also known as stroke, cerebral apoplexy and brain attack. There are 2 major classes of stroke, hemorrhagic and occlusive. The most prevalent form is the occlusive stroke that commonly results from atherosclerotic disease and cardiac abnormalities. Thrombosis of intracranial and extra cranial arteries and cerebral embolisation from various origins throughout the body are the primary causes of cerebral infarction. Thrombus formation is more likely to occur in other atherosclerotic vessels. Cerebral embolisation is also a causative factor. A major source of emboli is in the heart of individuals with impaired flow or damaged valves–rheumatic heart disease with mitral stenosis and atrial fibrillation is most common case.

Cervical pertaining to the neck of a tooth (*see* Figure on page 89).

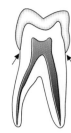

Cervical portion of tooth

Cervical burn out is a radiolucent artifact seen on dental X-ray. It may be confused with dental caries and appears as collar or wedge-shaped radiolucency.

Cervical collar is the splint made of foam or rigid material around the neck.

Cervical erosion is the wearing away of cementum that has been exposed as a result of gingival recession.

Cervical nerve root compression is the compression of cervical nerves supplying upper arm produces chronic arm and neck pain. Prolonged sitting worsen the pain. There will be muscle weakness, paresthesia and decreased reflex response.

Cervical radiculopathy in Latin, radicutus refers to 'by the roots' and when root of nerve is pinched it is called radiculopathy. It causes numbness, and or weakness in arm. Common causes of pinched nerves are calcium deposits from arthritis or herniated disc.

Cervical rib is a congenital disorder. Lowest cervical vertebra is over developed to form a rib. It may be partially or completely developed. It may be symptom free or may cause numbness and tingling.

Cervical spine disc herniation Symptoms include neck pain which may radiate to scalp, shoulder or to extremity certain position may increase the symptoms. One may develop numbness in distal upper extremity. It may result in fasiculations, loss of deep tendon reflex and atrophy of muscles.

Cervicogenic headache describes head pain and occurs as an abnormality in neck. The work genesis means 'to come pain'. So cervicogenic literally means pain coming from neck area. Generally headache is experienced as pain in neck on one side. Certain neck movements may relieve pain.

Cervix is the area that refers to the neck of the tooth; the area where the crown joins the root or the enamel joins the cementum.

Characteristics of lymph node enlargement is of diagnostic valve. In tuberculosis nodes are matted due to periadenitis. Infected nodes are tender and firm. Lymphomas produce symmetrical large, firm and rubbery nodes. These are movable, discrete and non tender. In metastasis one finds fixed, stony hard, localized glands. In children due to throat infection cervical glands are enlarged. Bilateral cervical glands are enlarged in tuberculosis, lymphoma, and leukemias. Nodes in Hodgkin's disease are rubbery, discrete and mobile.

Charcot's joint is more frequently seen in diabetic neuropathy, syringomyelia, spinal cord injury, leprosy and peripheral nerve injury. Prolonged administration of hydrocortisone in bone may cause it charcoal joint. Normal muscle tone and protective reflexes are lost. It is a painless joint with extensive cartilage erosion.

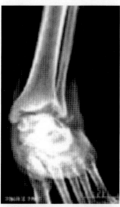

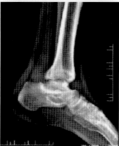

Charcot's joint

Charter's tooth brushing is a method designed to increase cleaning effectiveness and gingival stimulation in the interproximal areas. Bristles are pointed toward the crown of the tooth rather than apically. Tooth brush is positioned horizontally and parallel with the arch in all areas except the lingual area of anterior teeth and the occlusal surfaces. Bristles are placed at gingival margin. These are directed toward the occlusal surface at a 450 angle to the long axis of tooth. Back and forth motion is used for activation. It is good for patients with orthodontic brackets.

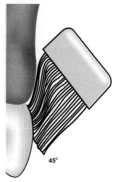

45°

Charter's tooth brushing method

Cheatle forceps is a heavy stainless steel forceps without locking system. It is used to hold sterilized items like bandage, gauze and gloves. It is kept in bottle dipped in savlon solution.

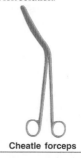

Cheatle forceps

Chediak – Higashi syndrome is an uncommon genetic disease and is fatal in early life. It is transmitted as an autosomal recessive trait. There may be photophobia; nystagmus and albinism. Oral lesions include glossitis, gingivitis and ulceration of oral mucosa. Blood shows giant abnormal granules in peripheral circulating leukocytes. There is no specific treatment. Defect is of granule containing cells as granulocytes and melanocytes. Hypo pigmentation will be seen in skin and hair. Some may develop neuropathy. Child dies before the age of 10 due to recurrent infection. Lymph nodes. spleen, liver and bone marrow are infiltrated with lymphohistiocyte cell. Gingival and periodontal findings are common. Early loss of teeth is noted.

Cheek pouch is the area of the mouth inside the cheek.

Cheilitis granulomatosa develops as a persistent swelling of a lip, facial nerve palsy and fissured tongue. Cause is unknown.

Chelation refers to the decalcification and removal of tooth surface of the lips and angles of mouth.

Chelitis glandularis is a condition where lower lip becomes enlarged, firm and finally everted. Cause is unknown. Labial salivary glands are enlarged. They may become nodular. Orifices of secretary ducts are inflamed and red. These are of three types, simple type, superficial suppurative type and deep suppurative type. Simple type is multiple, pin head size lesion. Central part is depressed. Superficial suppurative type is having painless, induration and crusting ulcerations.

Chemical burn the gingival becomes white and necrotic following injudicious use of caustic agent.

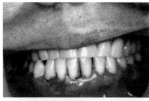

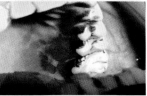

Chemical burn

Chemical cure is a method where the restorative material bonds to the tooth by the means of chemical. It gives good esthetics, more complete cure and curing light is not needed. Disadvantage of it is more porosity, poor color stability and less working time available. Light cure gives better color quality.

Chemical diabetes refers to the asymptomatic diabetes mellitus without any symptoms.

Chemical name refers to the name by which a chemist knows the drug.

Chemical reaction is a process where atoms of molecules or compounds interact to form new chemical combination e.g. Glucose interacts with oxygen to form CO_2, water and energy.

Chemical sterilization is a process where combination of formaldehyde, alcohol, acetone, ketone and steam serves as an effective sterilizing agent. Microbial destruction results from dual action of toxic chemicals and heat.

Chemical test of opium is called marquis test. If the suspect reside is treated with a mixture of 3 c.c. of concentrated sulphuric acid and 3 drops of formalin, it produces purple color changing to violet and finally to blue color.

Chemical theory given by Parmly (1819) rebelled against the vital theory and proposed that an unidentified "chemical" agent was responsible for caries. Support for the chemical theory came from Robertson (1835) and Regnart (1938) who actually carried out experiments with different dilutions of organic acids (such as sulphuric and nitric) and found that they corroded enamel and dentin. He stated that caries began on the enamel surface in locations where the food putrefied and acquired sufficient dissolving power to produce the disease chemically.

Chemiclave is a heat sterilizer that uses heat, chemical vapor and pressure to achieve sterilization.

Chemo–parasitic theory is a blend of the above two theories, because it states that caries is caused by acids produced by microorganisms of the mouth. In a series of experiments Miller demonstrated the following facts, acid was present within the deeper carious lesions, as shown by reaction on litmus paper. Different kinds of foods (bread, sugar, but not meat) mixed with saliva and incubated at 37degree centigrade could decalcify the entire crown of a tooth. Several types of mouth bacteria (at least 30 species where isolated) could produce enough acid to cause dental caries. Lactic acid was an identifiable product in carbohydrate –saliva incubation mixtures. Different microorganisms (filamentous, long and short bacilli and micrococcus) invade carious dentin. Miller concluded that no single species of microorganism caused caries but the process was mediated by an oral microorganism capable of producing acid and digesting protein.

Chemoreceptors are the receptors that respond to chemicals and are responsible for taste and smell.

Chemotaxis is a process in which substance attracts cells or organism in its vicinity.

Chemotherapeutic agent is a term used for a chemical substance that provides a therapeutic benefit

Chemotherapeutic index is the ratio of minimal effective dose to the minimal tolerated dose.

Chemotherapeutic is an agent of a chemical nature which exerts an antimicrobial effect.

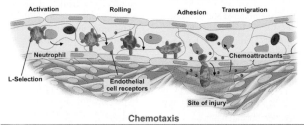

Chemotaxis

Cherubism is an uncommon disease involving teeth. It appears at the age of three. It generally develops bilaterally. Mostly mandible is involved. Deciduous teeth shed suddenly at the age of three. Permanent dentition is defective with the absence of numerous teeth. Oral mucosa remains normal. Some teeth look like floating in cyst like space.

Chest pain the most common cause in winter is fibrostitis. Chest pain may be caused by pleurisy and pneumonia. Most prominent is the pain of angina and myocardial infarction. Myocardial pain may be referred to arm. Pain of pericarditis is felt in center. In some cases anxiety and stress may also cause chest pain.

Chicken pox causative virus is similar to herpes virus. Incubation period is 14 days. Prodromal symptoms include headache, nasopharyngitis followed by maculo papular or vesicular eruptions. Eruptions start on trunk and spreads to involve face and extremities. Small blisters develop on oral mucosa. Tongue, gingiva and palate may be involved. These rupture soon and ulcer develops. Complications are not common and mortality rate is low.

Chief complaint is complaint recorded by a medical professional in patients own words.

Child psychology is the science that deals with the mental power (or) an interaction between the conscious and subconscious element in a child.

Childhood is the period an from 15 months until 12-13 years. During early childhood there is active ossification, but the child grows older, the rate of growth slows down.

Chills are extreme, involuntary muscle contractions. There may be violent shivering and teeth shattering. There may be fever, pneumonia produces a single chill and malaria produces a recurring chill with high fever. Chill can be produced by transfusion reactions and exposure to cold. Certain drugs may also cause it.

Chime is partially digested food mixture leaving the stomach.

Chin-neck contour is the mentocervical angle formed by the intersection of the e-line and a tangent to the submental area. (110-120°). The Submental neck angle is formed between the submental tangent and a neck tangent at points above and below the thyroid prominence.

Chiropractice was known to Hippocrates, 2500 years ago. It is concerned with treatment of mechanical disorder of joint especially spinal joints.

Chisel scalers are the set of double ended instruments with the curved shank at one end and straight shank at the other end, although the blades are slightly curved and has a straight cutting edge bevelled at 45 degrees.

Chitin is a polysaccharide found in fungal cell wall but not in any other micro organism.

Chloasma is the hypopigmentation of skin specially cheeks. Ladies taking estrogen tablets as family planning measure may also develop it. Lesions are distributed symmetrically over bridge of nose, upper lip, cheeks and forehead. Disease is asymptomatic. Local use of hydrogen peroxide may be useful. Lesions may disappear after delivery.

Chloramphenicol is a broad spectrum antibiotic with a range

C

similar to tetracycline. Side effects include agranulocytosis. It is used in the treatment of typhoid fever.

Chlorhexidine is a bis-biguanide 0.012%with a broad antimicrobial spectrum. It acts by binding to the hydroxyl apatite of enamel, the pellicle, the bacteria, extracellular polysaccharides and the mucous membrane owing to its cationic nature. After binding, the agent is slowly released in an active form over a 12-24 hour period. This property of chlorhexidine is an attribute to its substantiality. It can be delivered as a rinse, a syringe for subgingival application and incorporated in chewing gum. Disadvantages include brownish–black discoloration of the teeth, restorations and tongue, temporary aberration of taste sensation (dysgeusia), burning lips and mucous membrane discoloration.

Chlorhexidine stain is extrinsic stains caused by prolong use of a mouth wash containing chlorhexidine.

Chloride compounds are oxidizing agents and end products are inactive chlorides. Strong hypochlorite solutions have a penetrating and irritating odor due to release of chlorine gas. It may corrode metals.

Chloride shift is a diffusion of chloride ions into red blood cells as bicarbonate ions diffuse out. It maintains electrical neutrality of red blood cells.

Chlorine dioxide is a stronger oxidizing agent than other chlorine disinfectants. Sporicidal action is independent of pH over 6-10.

Chlorine is closely related with that of potassium and sodium maintaining water balance.

Average daily consumption is 6-9 gm. It is excreted through kidney. Normal blood plasma concentration is 550-650 mg/dl. It activates salivary amylase. Large quantities may lead to convulsions. In reference to dentistry, chlorine is a potent germicide widely used as disinfectant of water. Sodium hypochlorite in 0.5% solution is an effective anti septic and will dissolve necrotic tissue. It is useful for irrigation of root canals. One percent solution of sodium hypochlorite diluted with 3 times hot water is useful irrigating in dry sockets.

Chloroquine is a drug used for the prevention of malaria. It may be used as antirheumatic drug. It is the main drug in case of acute malaria. Side effects include nausea, headache, diarrheal and abdominal cramps.

Chloroxylenol is a 0.2% chloroxylenol with menthol and diluted 1 in 50 is a pleasant mouthwash as reported by Dilling and Halam. It is active against streptococci and less against staphylococci.

Chlorpromazine is a drug that induces emotional sedation. Patient becomes completely isolated from outside environment. These develop apathy, lethargy and reduced motor activity. Large doses produces fall in body temperature. It has a moderate anticholinergic and antihistaminic effect. It is rapidly absorbed form G.I.T.

Choking agents include ammonia, chlorine, hydrogen chloride and chemicals which irritate throat, airway and lungs. Onset may be immediate or delayed. There will be irritation to eyes, coughing chest tightness, shortness of breath and dizziness. Cyanosis and ventilation failure may develop.

Cholecystectomy is a surgical removal of gall bladder.

Cholecystitis is the inflammation of gall bladder.

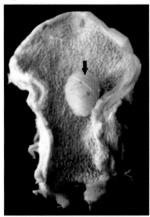

Rokitansky-Aschoff   Thickened
Chronic   sinus   perimuscular layer
inflammation   Cholesterolosis

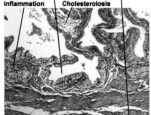

Chronic cholecystitis with cholelithiasis

Cholecystokinin is a peptide hormone secreted by intestinal mucosa. It regulates several gastrointestinal activities including motility.

Cholera is caused by coma shaped actively motile flagellated gram negative bacillus vibrio cholera. The bacilli proliferate in small intestine without invasion producing a potent protein. Incubation

period varies from a few hours to 6 days. Disease has 2 phases. Evacuation phase is of acute, painless profuse diarrhea with vomiting. Stool is rice watery odourless. In collapse phase there develops cold clammy skin, hypotension and tachycardia. Patient becomes dull and apathetic, prompt rehydration is the only remedy. Chemoprophylaxis with 500 mg helps.

Cholesterol is present as free sterol in most tissues except for adrenal cortex, plasma and athermatous plaques. Most of the tissues are capable of synthesizing cholesterol; most of plasma cholesterol originates from liver and distal small intestine. Increase in ldl and decrease in HDL cholesterol are related to atherosclerosis in dependently.

Cholestremia refers to the increased amount of cholesterol in blood, more than 225 mg %.

Choline was first used in 1939 when it was shown to relieve a condition known as fatty liver. Prevention of fats and cholesterol in the body is the function of choline. It maintains integrity of myelin sheath. Daily requirement is 10 mg.

Cholinergic nervous system includes nerve fibres which release acetylcholine as a neurotransmitter.

Cholinesterase is an enzyme which splits acetylcholine into acetate and choline.

Chondral fracture is a fracture of an articular surface in a synovial joint.

Chondrocyte – Cartilage cell.

Chondrolysis is a degeneration of cartilage cell.

Chondroma is a painless slowly progressive swelling of jaw and is composed of mature cartilage. It seldom develops in membranes. It may develop at any age. Radiographically one notices an irregular radiolucent or mottled area. Root resorption may be seen surgical excision is advanced because it is resistant to X-rays.

Chondromyxoid fibroma was first described by Jaffe in 1946. Majority of cases develop in long bones. It exhibits swelling and pain is severe. Foci of calcium are sometimes found. Conservative surgical excision is done.

Chondrosarcoma is a malignant neoplasm of bone. There is formation of abnormal cartilage tissue is formed but no osteoid bone is produced. Peak age is 30-40 years. Males are more affected. In mandible it develops in posterior region. It produces a painless swelling of jaw. Later on it becomes painful and tender. It is very fast enlarging causing severe expansion. Radiologically it shows moth eaten radiolucent area in bone with ill defined borders. Blotchy areas of radiopacities are also found. Even wide surgical excision gives poor prognosis.

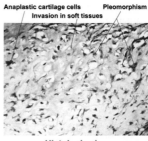

Histologic view
of Chondrosarcoma

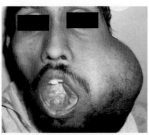

Chondrosarcoma of jaw involving
mandible

Chorea is a brief, rapid, involuntary, non repetitive irregular arrhythmic that can affect any part of body but are more pronounced in digits, unpredictable burst of rapid jerky movements. But these movements remain purposeful. It can affect both sides of body. It may disappear during sleep otherwise excitement may increase. It may be hereditary with Wilson's disease. Anticonvulsants, cocaine and amphetamine may also result in this condition.

Choroid plexus is a specialized group of capillaries in ventricles of the brain that secrete cerebrospinal fluid.

Chroma is a term used in munsell color system to describe the intensity or extent of saturation of a certain color.

Chrome is colour intensity

Chromosome analysis is a procedure that is undertaken at 16-18 weeks of pregnancy. The amount of desquamated fetal cells are obtained and cell culture is necessary before a chromosomal diagnosis is made.

Chronic alveolar abscess is a local mild inflammation of infection. It occurs around the roots of tooth. It may result due to pulpitis. Sinus may be present and pass through alveolar bone to open into mucosa.

Chronic atrophic rhinitis is of two varieties simple atrophic rhinitis and ozaena associated with fetor. In ozaena fetor comes from presence of dry cysts formed from viscid secretions. Surface epithelium is thinner than normal. The overlying crusts are made up of dense inspissated neutrophilic exudates, necrotic debris and bacteria.

Chronic bacterial sialadenitis is a non specific inflammatory disease of salivary gland generally occuring in children after the obstruction of duct. Usually parotid gland of one side is affected. There is sudden onset of unilateral swelling at the angle of mandible. Fever or leukocytosis is not marked. There is mild pain and disease responds to antibiotics. There may develop recurrent, tender swelling. Salivary flow is decreased. Treatment includes massage and antibiotics.

Chronic cholecystitis is mostly associated with gallstones. There will be ill defined epigastric discomfort and a dull ache in right hypochondrium. Fat intolerance may occur. Plain X-ray may show gallstones. Sometimes cholecystectomy may be done.

Chronic desquamative gingivitis was first recognized in 1894 but the term was coined by Prinz in 1932 and described this term as a desquamative and ulcerative lesion of free and attached gingiva. The lesion is generally limited to gingiva though the involvement of other areas are also reported. Gingiva is red, swollen and glossy with multiple vesicles. Distribution is patchy, buccal mucosa may also be involved. Patient is not able to eat hot, cold or spicy food. It is more commonly found in women between the age group of fourth to fifth decade of life.

Chronic diffuse sclerosing osteomyelitis is a chronic infection that may develop at any age. PE may develop vague pain and bad taste. Radiographs show diffuse sclerosis of bone. Lesion may be bilateral. Look is of 'cotton wool' appearance. Lesion shows dense, irregular trabeculae. Focal areas of osteoclastic activity are seen and polymorphs are in plenty. Lesion is too big to be removed surgically.

Chronic discoid lupus erythematosis can be described as irregularly thickened red plaques with well defined margins develop as an important localizing stimulus. After sometime atrophy or scarring may develop in these areas, these can also be seen as hyperkeratosis and warts.

Chronic disease refers to that kind of disease which lasts for longer duration including diabetes, hypertension, cancer, asthma etc.

Chronic focal sclerosing osteomyelitis generally develops in adults. First molar of mandible is involved. Radiograph will show well circumscribed radiopaque mass of sclerotic bone. It consists of dense mass of bony trabeculae with interstitial marrow tissue.

C

Chronic gingivitis is slow in onset but is of long duration. It is a painless condition unless complicated by acute exacerbations.

Chronic glomerulonephritis is a renal condition where these patients develop loss of appetite, weakness, hypertension and vomiting. In terminal stage proteinuria may diminish but specific gravity of urine is fixed at 10 which is otherwise of plasma. Kidneys are symmetrically contracted with diffusely granular cortical surfaces.

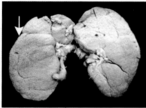

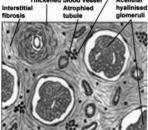

Chronic inflammatory cells
Thickened blood vessel / Acellular
Interstitial   Atrophied   hyalinised
fibrosis   tubule   glomeruli

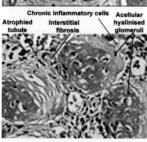

Chronic inflammatory cells   Acellular
Atrophied   Interstitial   hyalinised
tubule   fibrosis   glomeruli

Chronic glomerulonephritis

Chronic hyperplastic pulpitis generally occurs in young children. Affected pulp appears as pinkish. Deciduous molars are affected more. Hyperplastic tissue is a granulation tissue made up of delicate connective tissue fibres with small capillaries. Condition is not reversible and extraction of tooth to be done.

Chronic laryngitis refers to the repeated acute attacks which may develop due to singing, teaching, speaking, nasal obstruction and mouth breathing.

Chronic leukemia refers to the increased number of WBC count in children. Disease may be present for months and may be diagnosed incidentally. Patient may remain totally asymptomatic. Lymph node enlargement is common in lymphatic leukemia but is uncommon in myeloid leukemia. Enlargement of salivary glands and tonsil may take place. Skin may show petechiae or ecchymoses. Finally nodular lesions composed of leukemic cells may occur.

Chronic lymphocytic leukemia is never seen in children. There is a permanent lymphocytosis. Half of CLL patients show decreased immunoglobin production. High risk patients require chemotherapy.

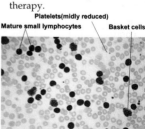

Platelets(midly reduced)
Mature small lymphocytes   Basket cells

Chronic lymphocytic leukemia

Chronic lymphoedema swelling starts from most dependent part. Swelling pits on pressure to start and later on edema pits less and less due to fibroedema. Overlying skin becomes thick and rough.

Chronic maxillary sinusitis may not be symptomatic and may be discovered radiographically. There may be pain and stuffiness on the affected side. Breath may be fetid. Sinus mucosa is thickened and polyps may develop. Antibiotics help.

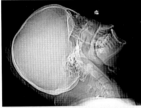

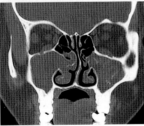

Maxillary sinusitis

Chronic mercurial poisoning is a condition that occurs due to presence of excessive amount of mercury in the body. Symptoms include loss of appetite and colicky pain in the abdomen and occasional vomit Gingiva become tender, swollen and ulcerated. Tongue and cheeks are also ulcerated. There may be necrosis of jaw. Teeth become loose,

anemia develops and skin eruptions are common. Speech becomes stammering, muscles of arm and leg may have tremor.

Chronic myelocytic leukemia is a condition where cells retains the capacity for differentiation and are able to perform essential function. There is marked shift towards granulocytic differentiation at the expense of erythroid differentiation. Anemia is present. Mass of myeloid tissue is greatly increased. Myeloid cells have a striking propensity for malignant blastic transformation. It has three phases. (i) Chronic phase lasting for 3 years. (ii) Accelerated phase which lasts for 1½ years. (iii) Final phase of 3-6 months which usually ends in death.

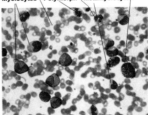

Chronic myeloid leukemia

Chronic obstructive pulmonary disease is the chronic lung disease that results in narrowing of air ways, emphysema and bronchitis.

Chronic osteomyelitis with proliferative periostitis Garre in 1893 described the lesion as thickening of periosteum. Maxilla and mandible are often affected in children. Patient complains of pain in tooth and jaw. Radiograph will show caries tooth against bony mass. X-ray shows focal growth of bone. Mass is smooth and well calcified. Periosteal reaction of carious tooth is the remedy.

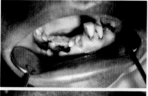

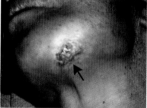

Intraoral and extraoral view of chronic osteomyelitis

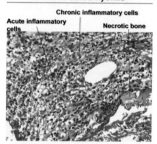

Histologic view of osteomyelitis

Chronic pain is associated with long standing disease and may persist for a longer period of time.

Chronic pancreatitis is a condition that results due to excessive alcohol consumption. There is deposition of protein plugs within pancreatic ducts. Chronic pancreatitis is not reversible. Only it can be arrested. There will be a chronic pain radiating to back. It is deep seated and antacids don't give any relief. Protein plugs calcify to give pancreatic calcification. Pain is to be controlled and surgical resection may be needed.

Chronic periodontitis/adult periodontitis/chronic adult periodontitis is a slowly progressing disease and is defined as an infectious disease resulting in inflammation within the supporting tissues of the teeth, progressive attachment loss and bone loss. Clinically supragingival and subgingival plaque accumulation can be seen which is frequently associated with calculus formation, gingivitis, pocket formation, loss of periodontal attachment and alveolar bone. Loss of stippling along with spontaneous bleeding and suppuration can be appreciated

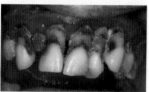

Periodontitis

Chronic pulpalgia refers to the pain of pulpal origin. The pain is diffuse and patient may not be able to locate the site of pain. The pulp involved is not affected by cold. Pain persists till irritant is there. These are the lesions which cause pain until irritant is dislodged. Radiograph often reveals interproximal or root caries or recurrent caries under a restoration. The apices of involved roots also show external resorption. Thermal tests are of little value in a positive sense. Pulp extirpation and endodontic therapy if the tooth is to be saved, otherwise extraction is the line of treatment.

Chronic pulpitis is a pain of pulpal origin where pain is not an important feature of chronic pulpitis. Reaction to thermal change is dramatically reduced. Pulp may become totally necrotic without pain. There is infiltration of pulp tissue by varying number of mononuclear cells specially lymphocytes and plasma cells.

Chronic pyelonephritis is a chronic tubulointestinal disease resulting from repeated attacks of inflammation and scarring with pelvicalyceal damage. Most of patients develop hypertension. Kidneys are small and irregularly scarred. Involvement is symmetrical in both kidneys. Hallmark of disease is coarse, discrete large scars with flat surface. Pelvic and calyceal walls are thickened and distorted mucosa becomes granular or atrophic.

Chronic sclerosing sialadenitis is a chronic inflammation of salivary gland tissue. It results in degeneration and subsequent replacement of acini by fibrous tissue. Trauma, infection and autoimmune all may cause it. Major or minor gland all may be affected. Affected gland is enlarged and remains freely movable. More the fibrosis develops more the firm it becomes. Once the acini are lost the gland parenchyma undergoes progressive sclerosis. Then sialodectomy has to be done.

Chronic suppurative osteomyelitis is a chronic form of acute stage.

Symptoms will be mild with slight leukocytosis. Tooth may not be loose and patient may be able to chew food. Symptoms may develop periodically. Fistula may be formed.

Chronological age refers to the age in years.

Chuck is a small screwdriver type of instrument to replace burs in hand piece.

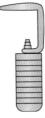
Bur chuck

Chvostek's sign is an abnormal spasm of facial muscles which can be elicited by lightly tapping the patient's facial nerve. It can develop in lower calcium level.

Chyle is a fatty material taken up by the central lacteals in the villi of duodenum after a fatty meal.

Cicatricial pemphigoid is an autoimmune disease and is also known as benign mucus membrane pemphigoid. Mucus membranes including oral and conjuctival surfaces develop lesions. There develops transient vesicles and bullae formation which on rupture gives ulcers. Ulcers of cicatricial pemphigoid tend to heal more with scarring. Oral lesions can be widespread. Long term management requires local and systemic corticosteroid.

Cicatrization refers to the formation of scar tissue.

C

Cingulum refers to a raised area on the lingual surface of anterior teeth.

Circular fibers are those which through the marginal and interdental gingiva encircle the tooth in a ring like fashion

Circumcision is a surgical removal of foreskin or prepuce.

Circumferential wiring is technique for intermaxillary fixation where oblique fractures of the mandible can be managed by passing a soft stainless steel wire circumferentially.

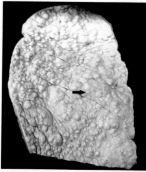

Ductular hyperplasia   Chronic inflammation
Regenerating   Nodularity
nodule   (variable-size)

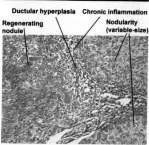

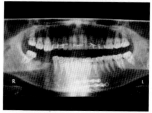

Circumferential wiring

Chronic inflammation   Nodularity
Fatty change   Fibrous septa (small-sized)

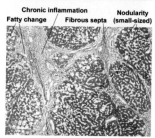

Cirrhosis liver

Cirrhosis of liver is an irreversible pathological state of liver with widespread hepatic cell necrosis. Diffuse scarring, shrinkage and nodular regeneration is seen. Alcohol, hepatitis B, C, biliary cirrhosis all may lead to it. Regenerating nodules are smaller than 3 mm is called micronodular cirrhosis and when larger than 3 mm it is known as macronodular. Liver may be large or shrunken, firm to hard in consistency. Hepatocellular dysfunction includes jaundice, palmer erythema. Raised aminotransferases, low serum albumin, raised serum bilirubin helps in diagnosis. Prothrombin time may be prolonged.

Citatrix refers to a scar, fibrous tissue left after healing of a wound.

Class I caries refers to the lesions that occur in pits and fissures of all teeth, but this class is essentially intended for bicuspid and molars.

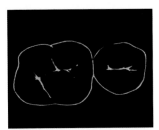

Class I (carious lesion) involving occlusal surfaces

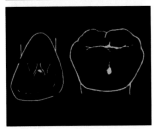

Class I (carious lesion) involving buccal and lingual pit

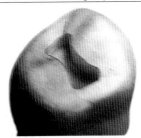

Class I cavity preparation

Class I molar relationship is the mesiobuccal cusp of the maxillary first permanent molar occludes with the buccal groove of the mandibular first molars. This is considered as the normal relationship of these teeth.

Class II lesion refers to the lesion that can involve either mesial and distal surfaces or only proximal surface of a tooth and is referred to as a Mesiocclusal (MO), Distocclusal (DO) or Mesiocclusodistal (MOD).

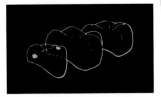

Class II carious lesion

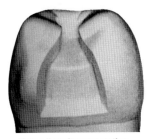

Class II cavity preparation

Class II molar relationship is the mesiobuccal cusp of the maxillary first permanent molar occludes mesial to the buccal groove of the mandibular first molar.

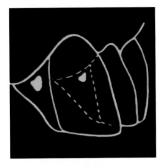

Class III carious lesion

C

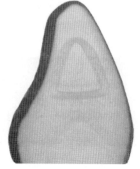

Class III Cavity preparation

Class III lesion refers to the cavity which may occur on mesial and distal surface of any incisor/cuspid.

Class III molar relationship is the mesiobuccal cusp of the maxillary first permanent molar occludes distal to the buccal groove of the mandibular first molar.

Class IV refers to the lesion that are found on the proximal surfaces of anterior teeth that involves the incisal edge – is a lesion on the proximal surface of an anterior tooth, in which the incisal edge is also involved.

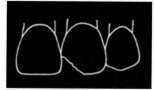

Class IV carious lesion

Class V caries found at the gingival third of the facial and lingual surfaces of anterior and posterior teeth – can occur on either the facial or the lingual surfaces; however the predominant occurrence of these lesions is adjacent to the lip and cheeks rather than tongue.

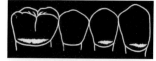

Class V carious lesion

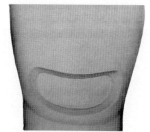

Class V cavity preparation

Class VI refers to the lesion that involves occlusal cusps of posterior teeth and incisal edge of anterior teeth. Defects are found on incisal edges and cuspal tips. Also found on premolars and molar cuspal tips.

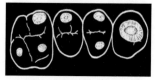

Class VI carious lesion

Classical conditioning is a behavioral theory put forward by a Russian physiologist. Ivan Pavlov in 19th century. During his studies of reflexes that apparently unassociated stimulus could produce reflexive behavior. Pavlov's classic experiment involves a presentation of food to a hungry animal, along with some other stimulus like ringing of a bell. The sight with sound of food elicits the salivation by reflex mechanism. If a bell is rung every time the auditory stimulus is associated with food presentation stimulus. In short time, the ringing of a bell by itself will elicit salivation. Classical conditioning then operates by the simple process of association of one stimulus with another. It is unusual for child to see a people with white coat if the unconditioned stimulus of painful treatment comes to be associated with conditioned stimulus of white coat, a child may cry withdraw immediately of first sight of white coat. Later on child learns to associate these stimuli on seeing white coat is enough to produce a pain.

Classical migraine is described as periodic headache, usually unilateral in onset but which later on becomes generalized. It is associated with nausea, photophobia or diarrhea. Prodromic phase includes visual disturbance. Usually it attacks half the visual field. At times it induces typical toothache. It may last from a few hours to several weeks. It may occur at any age.

Classification variable is a variable created not by manipulation but through division of subjects into groups based on an existing attribute such as sex or age.

Claude's hyperkinesis signs involves the increased reflex activity of paretic muscles elicited by painful stimuli.

Clavicle sign is a swelling, puffiness or edema at the medial third of right clavicle seen in congenital syphilis.

Clear cell carcinoma is found in major salivary glands especially parotid. Clear cell carcinoma is composed of cluster of cells surrounded by thin septa of fibrous connective tissue. These are treated by surgical excision.

Cleft tongue or complete bifid tongue is rarest. Partial cleft is the result of incomplete merging and failure of groove obliteration by mesenchymal proliferation.

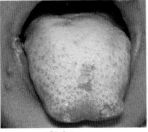
Cleft tongue

Cleidocranial dysostosis is an autosomal dominant disorder caused by mutation of chromosomes. Person presents with large head, small face and drooping shoulders. Chest is narrowed. There is delayed or absent ossification of calvaria. Pelvis is small or under developed. There may be agenesis of middle or lateral portion of clavicle.

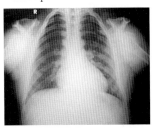
Cleido-cranial dysostosis showing hypoplastic absent clavicles

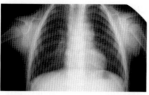

Cleido-cranial dysostosis with nearly absent clavicles

Clenching is the term used when the person holds the teeth together firmly with significant force

Cleoid refers to a dental hand carving instrument with a blade shaped like a pointed spade.

Clinical crown refers to that portion of the tooth visible in the mouth, extending from the occlusal or incisal edge to the crest of the free gingiva. Any unerupted area is not a part of clinical crown.

Clinical pocket depth/ probing depth is a distance to which probe penetrates in to the pocket. The measurement of this depth is dependent on variable factors such as size, force, direction of probe penetration and resistance given by the tissues.

Clinician refers to a practicing physician.

Clip true copy refers to the clones of cells descended from one original cell. Clones of organisms can be produced by removing the nucleus from a cell of one individual and transplanting it into egg cell of another individual.

Closed anchor suture is used to close a flap in edentulous area present mesial or distal to the tooth and consist of tying a direct suture that closes the proximal flap, carrying one of the threads, around the tooth to anchor the tissue against the tooth.

Closed chain exercise refers to an exercise in which distal segment of extremity is fixed to the ground.

Closed coil spring refers to orthodontic springs that are stretched between teeth and exert a pulling force on selected teeth.

Closed format item questionnaire refers to items which require a specific type of response such as yes or no.

Closed wound is the one in which there is no outside opening to skin/mucous membrane.

Cluster headache is also known as migranous neuralgia. It is a recurrent unilateral headache. Pain starts 2-3 hours after falling asleep during the phase of REM sleep. Headache is intense, non throbbing, unilateral and around the orbit. Stress, strain and alcohol may precipitate it. Prednisolone 60-80 mg daily helps.

Cluttering is produces abnormal speech characterized by excessive speed, repetition, and interjections. Cause is unknown.

CO_2 laser is a gas active medium laser that must be delivered through a hollow-tube like wave–guide in continuous or gated pulse mode. It has a wavelength–10,600 nm. It is will absorbed by water, there is rapid soft tissue remover and has a shallow depth of tissue penetration, which is important when treating mucosal lesions especially useful for cutting dense fibrous tissue-focused onto the surgical site in a non-contact fashion. Loss of tactile sensation is disadvantageous, but the tissue ablation can be precise with careful technique.

Coadaptation refers to proper adaption of ends of fractured bone or the edges of a wound without overlap.

Coaggregation is the ability of two genetically distinct bacteria to recognize and adhere to one another is called co-aggregation and the term was first coined in 1970. Co-aggregation is based on specific interaction of a proteinaceous adhesion produced by one bacteria and a respective carbohydrate or protein receptor found on the surface of another bacterium.

Coagulation refers to it is changing of a soluble into an insoluble protein process of changing into a clot.

Coarctation of aorta (COA) is a congenital heart disease where infants may have severe heart failure. Adults may have only hypertension. There will be absent or weak temoral pulse. Systolic pressure is higher in upper extremity then lower and diastolic pressure remains the same. Harsh systolic murmur may be heard in back. ECG shows left ventricular hypertrophy.

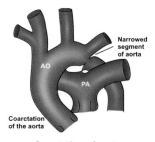

Coarctation of aorta

Coated hairy tongue is a yellow, whitish or pigmented covering on all or a portion of the tongue's dorsal surface. Normally keratinized surface layers of filliform papillae are continuously desquamated due to friction of food and anterior upper teeth. These are replaced by new epithelial cells from below. When tongue movements becomes restricted during illness the papilla enlarges and become heavily coated. Longer papilla entangles food particles of different colors. Tobacco smoke colors it black. Mid dorsum is first to be affected. Dehydration and terminally ill patients also develop thick coatings. Nicotinamide deficiency may produce black hairy tongue in experimental animals. Systemic antibiotics may also produce hairy tongue. Through scrapping and cleaning of tongue is advised.

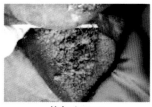

Hairy tongue

Cobalt-chromium-nickel wire constitutes 40% cobalt, 20% chromium, 15% nickel, 15.8% iron, 7% molybdenum, 2% manganese, 0.15% carbon and 0.04% beryelium. These are available in foru tempes, soft, ductile, semi resilient and resilient. Soft temper wires are popular with clinicians because they are easily deformed and shape into appliance. Heat treated wires have increased values yield strength and resilience.

Cobalt is a part of vitamin B_{12} molecule and is incorporated in many enzymes. Human body contains 100 to 150 mg of it. Generally there is no deficiency of cobalt in human being Daily requirement is of 2 microgram. Its deficiency leads to anemia, abnormalities of hair and skin pigmentation. Its deficiency may cause hepatolenticular degeneration. Acute cobalt poisoning leads to diarrhea, tinnitus and loss of hearing. Chronic administration may cause polycythemia.

Cocaine is an alkaloid derived from leaves of erythroxylon coca and its varieties. It is a colorless, odourless, crystalline substance and has bitter taste causing numbness of tongue and mucus membrane of mouth. It is slightly soluble in water but dissolves readily in alcohol. It reduces hunger. Small doses develop euphoria. There is exhilaration, excitement and restlessness.

Cocaine poisoning first stimulates then depresses the central nervous system, paralyses the nerve centers of the brain and spinal cord. Small doses develop euphoria. There is exhilaration excitement, restlessness, talkativeness and reflexes. Increased temperature may suddenly rise with rigor. Later on dryness of mouth and throat, feeling of numbness and tingling in hand and feet, quick irregular pulse develops. Lastly person may start gasping, convulsion and coma may follow. 10 to 15 grains orally is sufficient to kill a person. A grain injected hypodermically may kill an adult. Death may occur within a few minutes to a few hours.

Coccidioidomycosis causative organism is Coccidiodes Immitis. It is of 2 types, primary non disseminated and progressive disseminated. Patient develops cough, pleural pain, headache, and loss of appetite. Disease may be self limiting in nature.

Coccus spherical bacterium.

Cocoa is obtained from the seeds of plant theobroma cocoa. Fat content of seeds is removed and then dried. Theobromine is stimulating principle. It is nutritive as well as stimulating. It has a palatable taste. Chocolate is a preparation of it which is made from ripe seeds of cocoa beans. It lessens the feelings of hunger but does not prolong life in starvation.

Codeine is a poor analgesic. It is an effective antitussive and is useful in controlling diarrhea due to its spasmogenic effect on gut. Overdose of it produces, vomiting, dizziness and confusion.

Codman's sign occurs due to pain resulting from rupture of supraspinaturs tendon. Have a patient relax the arm on the affected side while you abduct it. If patient reports no pain until you remove your support and the deltoid muscle contracts sign is positive.

Coefficient of thermal expansion all metals when cooled they shrink or contract when heated they expand. Coefficient of thermal expansion is the change in volume in relation to change in temperature.

Cofactor is a non protein factor attached to an enzyme molecule that enables the enzyme to function well.

Cognition refers to giving attention.

Cognitive theory in the year 1952, Jean Piaget; A Swiss psychologist formulated a theory on how children with adolescent think and acquire knowledge. He derived his theories from direct observation of children by questioning the about their thinking. Like other theories it also passes through relatively distinct stages and its development is based on one dominant individual. This process of adaptation is made up of 3 functional variants. Assimilation concerns with observing, recognizing taking up an object and relating it with earlier experiences (or) categories. Accommodation accounts for changing concepts and strategies as a result of new assimilated information piaget calls the strategies and mental categories as schemes. Equilibration: refer to changing basic assumptions following adjustments in assimilated knowledge so that the facts fit better.

Coherency is a property unique to lasers. The light waves produced by a laser are a specific form of electromagnetic energy. A laser produces light waves that are physically identical. They are all in phase with one another; that is, they have identical amplitude and identical frequency.

Coherent scatter is one of the interactions of X-radiation with matter in which the path of X-ray photon is altered by matter without a change in energy.

Cold abscess is a slow forming abscess. It can develop anywhere in the body. Patient is usually a young person with swelling of insidious onset. It is hemispherical, smooth, soft and non-tender. Edges are soft and may not be well defined. Fluctuation may be present. Patient may have an evidence of tuberculosis.

Cold injury develops due to localized tissue damage due to cold. Frost bitten area becomes hard and white. At high altitude in snow it may develop so. Blood restriction to the area may cause gangrene. Amputation has to be done.

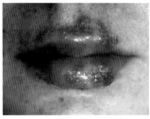
Cold sores

Cold intolerance happens due to damage of body's temperature regulating mechanism. Hormonal deficiency may result it. It may happen in old age too.

Cold sterilization is a process of disinfecting instruments by using a liquid chemical germicide. It requires exposure up to 10 hours. Aseptic rinsing with sterile water and drying should follow.

Cold sweat When person is emotionally upset sympathetic nervous system is stimulated and it results in sweating. Occurs sweating is regulated by sympathetic nervous system. This sweating is not associated with exercise or with high temperature then it is called a cold sweat.

Cold therapy is the application of cold in the tissues after injury it is an old technique. Now ice therapy is done to reduce pain, spasm and spasticity. It reduces swelling, promote repair and provides excitatory stimulus.

Colitis is any inflammatory condition of colon or rectum.

Collagen is a protein which is basically composed of different type of amino acids such as glycine, proline, hydroxylysine and hydroxyproline. The cells mainly responsible for the synthesis of collagen are fibroblasts, chondroblasts, osteoblasts and odontoblasts.

Collagenases is a bacterial enzyme that causes the breakdown of collagen.

Collapsing pulse refer to water hammer pulse.

Collimation refers to the beam having specific spatial boundaries. These boundaries ensure that there is a constant beam size and shape that is emitted from the laser unit.

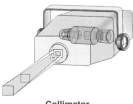
Collimator

Colloid is a material in which a constituent in a finely divided state is invisible to the eye but is capable of scattering light if suspended.

Colon is a part of large intestine that is 2.5 inches wide and 4.5 feet long M shaped loop in abdomen. It is irregular in outline. It consists ascending, transverse, descending and sigmoid colon. Ascending colon starts at cecum and extends upto liver. Point is known as hepatic flexure. Then it passes to spleen and bend is known as splenic flexure. From here it comes to pelvis and becomes 's' shaped sigmoid colon.

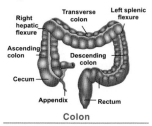
Colon

Colorado stains was the name given by Dr Frederick S. Mckay for the condition dental fluorosis and described it in the literature as mottled enamel. Ingestion of excessive fluoride leads to enamel hypo mineralization due to toxic damage to the ameloblastic cells. This may lead to development of pitting or crack in the tooth. The stains may range from isolated white flakes to smudged dark brown stains.

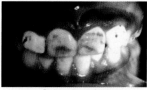
Colarado stains

Color content is relative intensity at each wave length.

Color doppler of heart is a diagnostic test that shows patterns and direction of flow. It is better for evaluation of heart disease. It can frequently detect clinically insignificant valvular regurgitation.

Color fatigue refers to decrease in response to one color due to constant stimulus.

Color rendering index is a measure of the degree to which illuminant can impart the color of an object as compared to the reference source.

Colostomy is the opening of the colon.

Colubrine snake bite is clinically marifested within 15 minutes. Patient complains of burning pain which passes off with local redness, erythema and local paresis. There will be nausea, progressive weakness, staggering gait and feeling of intoxication with loss of power. There may be general paralysis of all voluntary muscles and person will not be able to swallow. Death occurs due to paralysis of respiratory center in medulla.

Coma is the stage of unconsciousness resembling deep sleep and involves stoppage of action of brain. Consumption of excess of barbiturates, alcohol, and opium or brain injury may result in it. In the actual stage of coma reflexes are absent. Sphincters are relaxed and there is intoxication of urine and feces. Body temperature becomes subnormal and breathing becomes slow and irregular.

Comminuted fracture involves compound fracture with extensive communition.

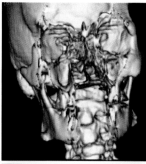

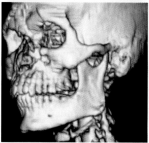

Comminuted fracture

Commissural lip pits are epithelium lined blind tracts located at corners of mouth. Tracts may be shallow or of several millimeters deep. These are common developmental anomalies. No treatment is advised.

Commissures refer to the corner of mouth.

Common bile duct is a duct from liver going to duodenum. It is made up of right and left hepatic duct.

Common cold is a viral disease and lasts for 5-7 days. Large virus of 5 micro millimeter causes upper respiratory tract infection. Smaller than this causes pneumonitis and bronchiolitis. Person develops sore throat and nasal obstruction. Diagnosis is on the basis of symptoms so is the treatment.

Communicable disease are those diseases which are capable of being transmitted from one person to another.

Communicable is a term which signifies a capacity for the maintenance of infection by various means of spread such as by direct contact or by air borne route

Communication is a two way process of exchanging and shaping feelings, ideas and information. It is more than mere exchange of information. It is an interdisciplinary science. Communication gaps produce problem.

Community dentistry encompasses the dental health of the public and use of dental services by public. It involves identifying and addressing the oral health needs of a particular population.

Community oral health is the oral health education and promotion aimed at meeting the specific oral health needs of a people, group, community, state or nation.

Community organization is a process aimed at developing the skills and abilities for the betterment of group.

Community water fluoridation is defined as the controlled adjustment of the concentration of fluoride in a community water supply so as to achieve maximum caries prevention and a clinically insignificant level of fluorosis.

Compact bone is a dense bone, contains structural units called haversian systems.

Complement (c) pathway is an interacting network of about 30 membrane associated cell receptors and soluble serum of about 30 membrane associated cell receptors and soluble serum glycoprotein's.

Complete radiolucent radiopaque areas. Radiolucent and radiopaque areas may show sun burst appearance. Peak age of incidence is around 25. Jaw lesions have fewer tendencies to metastasize hence better prognosis.

Complex caries refers to lesion involving three or more than three surfaces.

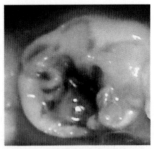

Complex caries

Composite faced crowns these crowns are also used as long-term provisional restorations. The laboratory grade composite is cured by an intense light and sometimes with additional heat and pressure.

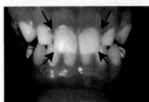

Composite faced crown

Composite is a tooth colored restorative material. The word "composite" refers to the mixture of filler particles in a liquid resin. Commonly, the resin used is BIS-GMA (bis-gammamethyl-metacrylate). Filler particles are added to alter the color and wear characteristics. Common filler particles are silica, aluminium, zinc, tin, copper and iron.

Composite resin cement are liners having antibacterial effect with reparative dentin. Calcium hydroxide mixed with resins is initially less irritating but are able to stimulate the formation of reparative dentin. It acts as a contract dressing in the event of exposure of pulp. There is an evidence that these material breakdown in time and create a gap between the restoration and the cavity wall.

Composite syringe is a device which helps to dispense composite into tooth preparation.

Compound caries refers to lesion involving two surfaces of a tooth.

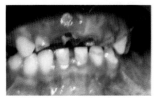

Compound caries

Compound fracture involves overlying skin and adjacent tissues including bone.

Comprehensive fluoride therapy refers to the use of both systemic and topical fluoride therapies to maintain a caries free oral environment.

Compression plates are plates designed on the same principle, for anatomical reasons, it is only used on convex surface of the mandible towards its lower border. These are applied on the bone surface using screws which engages itself in the inner cortical plate hence it should be placed below the inferior dental canal.

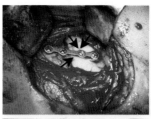

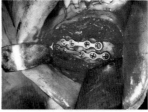

Compression plates

Compton scatter refers to one of the interactions of radiation.

Compulsive eating is an uncontrolled episode of overeating without other signs of eating disorder. Most compulsively overeat in response to stress or feelings of depression.

Compulsive habits are deep rooted habits that have acquired a fixation in the child to the extent that the child retreats to the habit whenever his security is threatened by events which occur around him. The child tends to suffer increased anxiety when attempts are made to correct the habit.

Concave refers to the curving inward away from the viewer.

Concept is a phenomenon expressed in words sometimes used as a more concrete term than construct.

Conceptualization is the process of developing a mental configuration of a concept.

Concordant refers to a condition where a disease occurs in both twins.

Concrescence is union of two adjacent teeth by cementum alone without union of the underlying dentin. Unlike fusion and gemination, concrescence can be developmental or post developmental inflammation. More frequently in posterior maxilla. Usually it occurs between maxillary second and third molars.

Concurrent disinfection is a measure taken to keep the patient's environment clean on a daily basis.

Condensation polymerization is a polymerization process in which a by product such as water or alcohol is formed as chain grows.

Condenser refers to a dental hand instrument used to pack plastic type restorative material into a cavity preparation.

Condensing osteitis is well defined radio opacity below the apex of a non-vital tooth suffering from long standing pulpitis.

Condiments refer to the agents those besides giving flavours and stimulating the flow of digestive juices. Condiments relieve flatulent distension occurring from the fermentation in the intestines. Black pepper, cloves, chillies and coriander are all used in the preparation of different foods to give color, flavor and taste. Condiments are known as food adjuncts. These should be used in strict moderation. If taken in excess, they tend to irritate and inflame the mucosa of stomach. Vinegar is a well known antiseptic and preservative. It is used for pickling fish, fruits and vegetables. It also softens hard muscle fibres of meat and cellulose of green vegetables.

Condylar hyperplasia is an unilateral overgrowth of mandibular condyle. Face becomes asymmetrical up. On opening, face deviates towards unaffected side. Pain is variable. One may develops crossbite.

Condyle is a rounded projection on a bone.

Condyloma Acuminatum is an infectious disease caused by virus (HPV). It is transmissible and auto inoculable viral disease. It presents as soft pink nodules which proliferate and coalesce. These lesions appears as small in size, multiple and white or pink nodular. Surgical excision may be required.

Cone cut is a clear, unexposed area on a dental radiograph that occurs indicating that device is misaligned and X-ray beam is not centered over the film.

Confabulation is fabrication to cover gaps in memory. It is most commonly seen in alcoholism.

Confidentiality is the ethical requirement to restrict disclosure of client information outside therapy session. Confidentiality can also be explained as the right of the patient to have information about his illness remain private.

Confusion is an altered state that can result from fluid and electrolyte imbalance or due to lack of oxygen. It may result due to many diseases and may even be irreversible. It is the inability to think quickly and coherently. It is aggravated by stress.

Confusional insanity is characterized by unstable attention and poor perception of present reality, disorientation and inability to act coherently. It results from mental or physical exhaustion and fever.

Congenital epulis is a lesion present at birth as a protuberant mass of maxilla or mandibular gingiva. Size varies from a few mm to a few cms. Histologically it is similar to granular cell myoblastoma. Capillaries are numerous. Surgical excision is the treatment of choice. Recurrence is known.

Congenital erythropoietic porphyria results in the deposition of types I and III porphyrin pigments in bone and teeth. Although this is a rare in born error of metabolism, the dental effects are more pronounced.

Congenital lip pits are pits present congenitally.

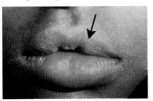

Lip pits

Congenital syphilis is contracted in utero from a mother who had treponemal infection. Syphilis produces classic patterns of hypoplastic dysmorphic permanent teeth. Saber shins, frontal bossing and saddle nose are common structural anomalies. Congenital syphilis clinically will present with (1) interstitial keratitis, (2) deafness, (3) tooth anomalies (Hutchinson's triad).

Congenitally missing teeth is meant those teeth whose tooth germ did not develop sufficiently to allow the differentiation of the dental tissues. The teeth most frequently found congenitally missing mandibles second bicuspids, maxillary lateral incisor, and in maxilla are second bicuspids. Complete absence of all teeth is called Anodontia and Oligodontia is partial presence of teeth.

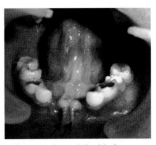

Hypodontia and double frenum

Connation refers to joined teeth.

Conscious sedation is a minimally depressed level of consciousness. Patient maintains airway and respond to verbal command.

Consensus refers to generally accepted view.

Consent is a patient agreement with a physician doing surgery or certain tests. Consent is valid when patient has been told about implications, side effects of

procedure in clear terms. When patient is not fit consent can be given by near relatives.

Consent of sexual intercourse refers to a women of and above the age of 16 years who is capable of giving consent, to an act of sexual intercourse. But the consent must be conscious free, voluntary and given in full command of senses.

Constrictive pericarditis is a healed pericarditis which may cause marked thickening of visceral and parietal layers of the pericardium making it thick and rigid. Cage closely developing the heart hampers the filling of cardiac chambers. Tuberculous pericarditis is the most important caused. Areas of caseation necrosis may be recognized. Pericardial fluid is thick, opaque and consists of fibrin, caseous material and blood. Heart is reduced in size. Stroke volume is low and progressive heart failure results.

Contact angle is an angle formed between the surface of a liquid drop and the solid surface on which it rests.

Contact area refers to that portion of the proximal surface of a tooth that touches the adjacent tooth.

Contact dermatitis can be described as itching or burning sensation at the site of contact. Mucosa becomes remarkably inflamed and edematous. Small vesicles may form. On rupture areas erosion and ulceration develops. Certain dental material has been implicated causing contact dermatitis. Acrylic when used as a denture material may produce allergy. Treatment includes withdrawal of offending material.

Contact hypersensitivity is characterized clinically by eczema at the site of contact with the allergen seen maximally at 48 hours. The most common Ag are haptens such as nickel, chromate, chemicals found in rubber and poison oak. It is the major cause of occupational disease. Small haptens which induce hypersensitivity need not by themselves be antigenic. However, these low molecules weight compounds penetrates epidermis and become conjugated either covalently or non covalently to body proteins.

Contact precautions is a the measure taken to block transmission of pathogens by direct or indirect contact.

Contagious disease refers to an infective disease that can be transmitted to another person.

Contaminated refers to not sterile material.

Content analysis is a process by which the text of archival records is reduced to quantifiable information.

Continence training is the process of restoring control of urination.

Continuous fever occurs when fever does not fluctuate more than 1 to 1.5 degree Farenheit during 24 hours but never touches normal.

Continuous sutures is a method of suturing. One thread runs from one end to final end and is tied at last.

Continuous variable is a variable that theortically can be measured to finer degrees.

Continuous wave is the laser beam emitted at one power-level continuously as long as the device is activated by pressing the foot switch.

Contracture refers to shortening or distortion. It is a permanent damage due to shrinkage of muscles.

Contralateral refers to opposite extremity.

Contrast film refers to the characteristic of film that influences radiographic contrast.

Contrast medium is the substance that adds density to a body organ such as barium/iodine.

Contrast refers to comparison of two means specifically multiple comparison tests conducted as part of complex analysis of variance tests.

Contrast short scale refers to radiograph with two densities of gray a black and white. It results from the use of lower kilovoltage range.

Contributory negligence describe a patients contribution to the disease. He has not take drugs as advised. In this way patient contributes to the negligence.

Control tooth refers to healthy tooth used as a standard to compare questionable teeth.

Contusion refers to a bruise. It is a superficial injury usually painful produced by impact without laceration.

Conventional finger rest is a type of rest which is established on tooth surfaces immediately adjacent to the working area

Convex refers to curving outward toward the viewer.

Cooley peg is a device used to seat a crown or bridge restoration into tooth preparation.

Coping is a thin metal covering or cap placed over a prepared tooth.

Coping material is a thin sheet of plastic sometimes used for fabricating a temporary bridge with a custom acrylic material.

Copper cement was widely used as temporarily filling material in children's teeth. It has strong germicidal property. In human it produces inflammatory cell infiltration, hemorrhage and necrosis with destruction of odontoblasts in pulp. This effect is due to soluble copper ions which are dissolved in acid.

Copper is needed for normal erythropoiesis as well as for absorption of iron. Other metalloenzymes require copper included tyrosinase and lysyl oxidase.

Copper sulphate poisoning is known as 'neela thota' poisoning. Symptoms develop within 15-30 minutes. There is a metallic taste in the mouth. There is sense of burning with abdominal pain. Vomiting and diarrhea develops. Vomited matter is green or blue colored. Convulsions and coma precede death. 30 gram is fatal dose and person may die within 3-5 days.

Core is a preparation built upon a tooth on which a crown will be fitted. It is usually made of amalgam, metal or glass ionomer.

Core temperature is the warmth at the center of body.

Corneal abrasion symptoms include significant eye pain, foreign body sensation, photophobia and tearing. Person will develop edema of eyelid and redness of conjunctiva.

Corneal ulcer will produce pain in eye, lacrimation, photophobia and blurring of vision. Marked blephrospasm is present. There is rough and yellowish white area on cornea. Surrounding cornea may be hazy. Ciliary congestion is present. Small amount of pus may be visible in lower part of anterior chamber.

Corneal xerosis is due to deficiency of vitamin A. Liquefaction of cornea is a medical emergency. Cornea may become soft. Process is rapid and is an important cause of blindness.

Coronal divides the body into anterior and posterior.

Coronal dentin dysplasia is inherited as autosomal dominant type. Primary teeth are translucent with amber color. Primary teeth present normal color and normal crown. Permanent teeth may or may not have pulp stones.

Coronary arteries refers to those arteries which carry blood to the muscles of heart. Left and right coronary arteries arise from aorta. In coronary thrombus obstruction and narrowing takes place. This reduces the blood supply to the part which is a major cause of heart disease.

Coronary embolism refers to the blocking of a coronary blood vessel by a clot.

Coronary sinus refers to the area that receives deoxygenated blood from the coronary veins and empties into right atrium.

Corrective orthodontics refers to reduce the severity of an existing malocclusion or to eliminate it.

Corrosives are those substances which cause destruction of the parts with which they come in contact due to protoplasmic coagulation and extraction of water. Corrosives include acids and alkalies. There will be burning pain in mouth and throat.

Bowels are constipated. There may be tenesmus. Voice become hoarse and husky.

Cortical plate refers to the compact bone covering the alveolar process.

Cortical refers to the outer layer of bone which appears radio opaque.

Corticosteroids inhalers are used as the choice of treatment in bronchial asthma. Oral prednisolone and inhalational steroids like beclomethasone, betamethasome are used in the prophylactic treatment of moderate cases. Exact mechanism is not known but there is stabilization of most cells, inhibitions of release of inflammatory mediators. These reduce edema of submucosal tissues.

Cortisol deficiency can lead to relatively rapid onset of clinical symptoms, including loss of consciousness and possible death. Adrenocortical deficiency is called Addison's disease.

Cortisol refers to the steroid secreted by adrenal cortex. It is one of the stress hormones.

Cosmetic dentistry is the branch of dentistry that deals with the aesthetic improvement of the color and shape of teeth performed by a general dentist.

Cost benefit ratio is the difference between the expense of having a program or not to have a programe.

Costen's syndrome is a condition in which severe shooting pain radiates down to cover jaw. Pain may be in temple area on chewing. It is due to malocclusion.

Cotton pellets are one of the most common products used in dentistry. These are small balls of plain cotton used to clean cavity preparations, apply intraoral medications and control minor bleeding.

Cough formula is a prepration that is commercially available. It includes preparations of centrally acting cough suppressants, expectorants and mucolytics. These may also be combined with antihistamines, antiadrenergics and bronchodilators like salbutamol.

Cough is a reflex action to clear the airways of mucus or foreign body. It may be a symptom of underlying disease. In bronchitis cough contains large amount of phlegm. Bronchospasm as in asthma produces dry cough. Pneumonia will produce cough with pain. Bronchiectasis causes large amount of foul smelling cough in morning.

Cough lozenges are disc shaped tablets taken to treat the irritation of pharyngeal mucosa. It develops in much diseases like influenza, common cold and pneumonitis. Irritation of mucosa results in cough.

Coupling agent is a chemical attached to the filter surface for the purpose of creating a bond with the resin matrix upon polymerization. It improves strength and wearing resistance.

Cowden's Syndrome refers to hamartomas involvement of many organs with a potential of neoplastic transformation. It is inherited as autosomal dominant character. Multiple cysts over lips and gingiva are seen. Tongue is also fissured. Hemangiomas and neuromas are also seen.

Cracked tooth syndrome referes to development of a crack in a restored or an unrestored tooth due to excessive occlusal forces as one of the main cause. There is sharp pain on biting. Pain is similar to that of trigeminal neuralgia. Radiographs are unable to show cracked tooth.

Cranial is towards head.

Cranial arteritis occasionally causes ischemic pain in masticatory muscles after the age of 55. There is weakness, low grade fever and loss of weight. Temporal artery becomes red, firm, swollen and tortuous. Healing is by fibrosis specially of media with thickening of intima.

Craniometry is the metric study of cranial dimension in dry skulls.

Craniopharyngioma these arise from hypophyseal duct. Being suprasellar they present with visual loss and hydrocephalus. Size may vary from small rounded nodule to large multi-locular cyst. Suprasellar calcification is seen. Cystic tumors require evacuation.

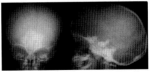

Extensive supra-sellar calcification in a child due to craniopharyngioma

Craniosynostosis is a premature fusion or closure of one or more sutures of skull. It may be primary or secondary. Skull may show silver beaten appearance (*see* Figure on page 120).

C

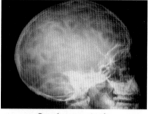

Craniosynostosis

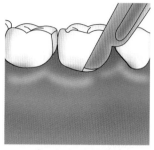

Crevicular incision

Crazing is a formation of fine cracks on the surface of material due to stresses built up by dimensional changes with in the structure. Denture base is crazed by alternate drying and soaking.

Crede maneuver is the act of bending forward and applying hand pressure over the bladder to stimulate urination.

Creep is a time dependent deformation of an object subjected to a constant stress, i.e. marginal fracture of dental amalgams.

Cresol is three times potent as phenol and is equally toxic. Lysol is a 50% cresol in linseed oil and is widely used for disinfecting floors. It is fairly an efficient bactericide. It is a popular root canal antiseptic. It is lesser irritant then phenol. It is a popular phenol derived root canal medicine.

Crest refers to a prominence or ridge.

Crevice corrosion is an accelerated corrosion caused by differences in concentration of O_2 and pH levels within a crevice compared with sites outside the crevice. It is mostly found at margin of metallic restorations.

Crevicular incision is made from the base of the pocket, to the crest of the bone. This incision forms a v- shaped wedge ending near the crest of the bone.

Critical instruments used to penetrate soft tissues and bones known as critical and are to be sterilized after every use. Such instruments include forceps, scalpels, bone chisel and surgical burs.

Critical pH is the pH at which a solution is just saturated with respect to a particular mineral, such as tooth enamel. If the pH of the solution is above the critical pH, then the solution is supersaturated with respect to the mineral, and more mineral will tend to precipitate out. Conversely, if the pH of the solution is less than the critical pH, the solution is unsaturated, and the mineral will tend to dissolve until the solution becomes saturated. The concept of critical pH is applicable only to solutions that are in contact with a particular mineral, such as enamel.

Crohn's disease is a disorder characterized by non specific, sub mucosal alteration of the gastro intestinal tract, accompanied by stenosis, necrotic breakdown and scarring of mucosa. Oral manifestations includes aphthous ulceration, cobblestone appearance of oral mucosa, confined to buccal mucosas ie diffuse erythematous granular enlargement. Gingival lesions are seen with edematous, fissured and ulceration.

Cross arch finger rest is a type of rest which can be established on the other side of the same arch.

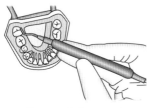

Cross arch finger rest

Cross contamination refers to passing of disease indirectly from one patient to another through the use of improper sterilization procedures.

Cross linked polymer refers to a polymer with a three dimensional network structure.

Cross sectional study refers to measurements made of different samples and studied at different periods of time.

Crossbite refers to malocclusion in which the facial aspects of the maxillary teeth are located labial to mandibular teeth (ref figure of anterior cross bite).

Crowing respiration is slow deep inspiration accompanied by high pitched crowing sound.

Crown a collar senare italics are short beaked and are used to trim metal matrix bands.

Crown is an artificial restoration and replaces at least ¾th of natural crown of tooth. These are made up of various materials. Temporary crowns are used to maintain appearance and avoid pain. Metal

crown of aluminium or stainless steel are used on back teeth. Temporary crowns are cemented with an adhesive which can easily be removed and cleaned for fitting of permanent crown.

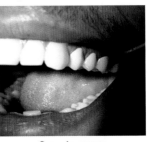

Ceramic crowns

Crown-cast refers to a cast restoration that covers the entire anatomic crown of the teeth.

Crude death rates are defined as the number of deaths per 100 estimated midyear populations in one year, in a given place.

Crude fibre is that part of a plant which is not broken down by boiling repeatedly in weak acid and weak alkali. It is a part of cellulose and part of lignin which makes wood harder. Dietary fibre is which passes through the small intestine completely undigested. Bran and whole wheat flour are a good source of it.

Cryosurgery refers to surgery performed with the use of low temperature.

Crystal habit refers to the external geometrical shape of a crystal.

Crystals in urine are seen in normal as well as in abnormal urine. Calcium oxlate crystals are small, colorless resembling envelops seen in chronic renal disease. Uric acid and urate crystals are four

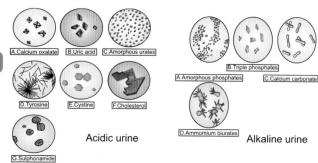

A.Calcium oxalate B.Uric acid C.Amorphous urates

D.Tyrosine E.Cystine F.Cholesterol

G.Sulphonamide

Acidic urine

A.Amorphous phosphates B.Triple phosphates C.Calcium carbonate

D.Ammomium biurates

Alkaline urine

Crystals in urine

sided yellow or brownish seen in gout. Phosphate crystals are colorless 3 to 6 sided prisms having little clinical significance.

Cullen's Sign includes irregular, bluish hemorrhagic patch on the skin around the umbilicus and occasionally around abdominal scars. It may be due to trauma or hemorrhage.

Cumulative index is an index that measures all the evidence of a condition, past and present, e.g. DMF index for dental caries.

Cumulative trauma disorder is the term used to identify the group of musculoskeletal disorders involving injuries to tendon, bones and muscles.

Cure is to harden.

Cure stage is a stage at which an impression material hardens and may give off heat.

Cure-dual is a process where hardening of restorative material is brought about by both self curing and light curing.

Curettage refers to scraping of epithelial lining of the periodontal pocket to separate diseased soft tissue.

Curettes are the fine instruments used for subgingival scaling, root planning and removal of soft tissue lining of the periodontal pocket. The instrument has a cutting edge on both the sides with a rounded toe. The instrument is finer than the sickle scaler and therefore easy to use in deep pockets.

Curing refers to the act of polymerization of a chemical compound.

Curve of Wilson refers to the cross arch curvature of posterior occlusal plane.

Cushing's syndrome results from glucocorticoids. When this excess is secondary to ACTH producing primary tumor it is called Cushing's disease. In practice one of the commonest cause is exogenous administration of corticosteroids. Clinical features include obesity, amenorrhea, muscular weakness and fatigue and symptoms of depression. Polyuria, headache and hyperpigmentation may develop. Face becomes round, like full moon. Osteoporosis may be severe to cause vertebral collapse. Pathological fractures are common. Patient may be hypertensive and hypoglycemic. Gingiva, palate and buccal mucosa may be blotchy due to melanin granules.

Cusp of carabelli's most common example is that the cusp of carabelli located on the palatal surface of mesiolingual cusp of a maxillary molar. It is most obvious on first molar.

Cusp refers to the elevated projection on the crown of a tooth that makes up a divisional portion of occlusal surface.

Cuspid refers to the third tooth from the center of the mouth towards the back, also known as canines (figure refer canine).

Cuticle is a thin edge of skin at the base of nail.

Cutting end of burrs are made of different shapes. Round shape is used for reaching to cavities at low speed. Pear shape is used for outlining the cavity (*see* Figure).

Cyanosis is a bluish coloring of skin owing to insufficient oxygen in blood.

Cyclamate is another sucrose substitute about 30 times sweeter than sucrose with a pleasant taste.

Cyclic Neutropenia is an unusual form of agranulocytosis with periodic or cyclic diminution in polymorphs. Etiology of disease is not known. Infants and young children suffer more. Symptoms are milder than agranulocytosis. Patient exhibits severe gingivitis, stomatitis and ulceration. Isolated painful ulcers occur that may last for 10-14 days. These heal with scarring. There is mild to severe loss of superficial alveolar bone. For 4 to 5 days patient may show normal blood count. At the peak of disease, neutrophils completely disappear. There is no specific treatment for the disease.

Cyclopropane is the only alternate gas to nitrous oxide. It is stored under pressure. It is inflammable and explosive in both air and oxygen. It tends to cause increased salivation.

Cyclosporine was first isolated in switzerland in 1970 as a metabolite of the fungus specious talypocladium but have little nature as an antifungal antibiotic. It is also used in the treatment of autoimmune disorder like Behcht diseases, rheumatoid arthritis, SLE, bullous pemphigoid and pemphigus, crowns disease and insulin – dependent disables.

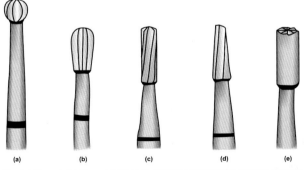

(a)   (b)   (c)   (d)   (e)

Bur (a) Round; (b) Pear; (c) Fissure; (d) Tapered fissure; (e) End-cutting

Cylindroma is a malignant tumor of salivary gland. It is not capsulated and infiltrates surrounding tissue. Tumor is composed of deeply stained, small uniform epithelial cells. These cells are arranged in oval islands. Complete surgical excision is the remedy.

Cylopia is a single or partially divided eye in single orbit; absence of nose or presence of proboscis, severe microcephaly with no division between anterior lobes of brain.

Cynacobalamine (Vitamin B$_{12}$) is a red crystalline substance containing the metal cobalt. It is necessary for the synthesis of DNA. It is not present in food of vegetable origin. It is only available in food of animal origin. It is synthesized by bacteria in human colon but is not being able to absorb. This is relatively heat stable and little is lost in cooking. Daily requirement is 0.5 to 2 microgram. Generally its deficiency is not seen except in malabsorption syndrome, post gastrectomy or Crohn's disease. It develops neurological symptoms in 10% of cases of pernicious anaemia. Sub acute degeneration of spinal cord may occur. Deficiency of it may lead to sore tongue with or without depapillation

Cyst is a closed sac or pouch lined with epithelium containing semisolid or fluid. Fluid may or may not be infectious.

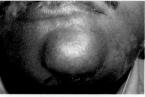

Soft tissue cyst

Cystic duct is a duct from gall-bladder. It joins the hepatic duct to form the common bile duct.

Cystic fibrosis is an autosomal recessive inherited disease. There develops deficiency of pancreatic enzyme and increased susceptibility to respiratory infections. Sodium content increases in sweat.

Cysticercosis is most common parasitic infection. It is a condition that affects central nervous system. Man is the usual definitive host of Taenia solium. Infection occurs by consuming raw or improperly cooked pork. Cysts evoke intense inflammatory reaction which resides after the death of scoleces. Signs and symptoms include seizures, raised intracranial pressure and chronic meningitis. If lodged in brain parenchyma symptoms may include aphasia, ataxia, sensory loss to motor palsy. Average interval between infection and manifestation is 5 years. MRI show circular cystic lesions or calcified nodules. Albendazole 15 mg/kg/daily for 30 days are effective calcified cysticerci don't respond to the therapy (*see* Figure on page 125).

Cytogenetics is an area of biology concerned with chromosomes and their implication in genetics.

Cytokeratins are those filaments which are typically expressed in the epithelium. Ten cytokeratins are specific to 'hard' tissues (e.g. nail and hair). Approximately 20 cytokeratins are found more generally in epithelial lining internal body cavities.

Cytokines molecules are released by host cells into the local environment, providing

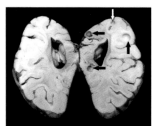
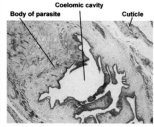

Coelomic cavity
Body of parasite   **Cuticle**

Cysticercosis brain

molecular signals to other cells thereby affecting their function.

Cytoskeleton is a system of proteins that supports the topography of the cell membrane and organizes the arrangement of the cytoplasmic components into defined areas. The cytoskeleton is composed of three types of filaments: actin (microfilaments), microtubules, and intermediate filaments. Its major functions are: determining cell shape, organelle anchoring and polarity determination, motility (and migration), anchoring of the cell to external structures, metabolic functions, separating duplicated chromatids and homologous chromosomes into separate cells.

Czechoslovakian caries index the czechoslovakian caries index was introduced by Poncova, Novak and Matena in 1956. This index is mainly used to compare caries experience in one group with that of the other groups with a similar population density but living in different environments. In this index, the "variables" seems to be controlled. In all examination studies and tests in which this index is used, the average number of teeth, tooth surfaces and tooth areas and the condition of previously extracted or crowned teeth were considered.

D

Dead space is the part of lung where air is moved in and out but no exchange of gas occurs. **Dean fluorosis index** is an index for assessment of dental fluorosis introduced by Trendley H. Dean in 1934 - known as 'dean's classification system for dental fluorosis or 'dean's fluorosis index'. Dental fluorosis is shown on a seven point scale; 'normal', 'questionable', 'very mild', 'mild', 'moderate', moderately severe', and 'severe'. This first description of fluorosis index could be considered an ordinal scale, although no numbers were used. Dean revised version of his fluorosis index in 1942 where he used a six point scale, i.e., "normal", "mild", "very mild", "moderate" and "severe" where he combined the "moderately severe" and "severe" in 1989.

Death certificate is a legal document confirming a person's death.

Debridement refers to the treatment of a bacterial infection by removing irritants (bacteria, calculus) from the periodontal pocket so as to allow healing of adjacent tissues.

Decalcification refers to the loss of calcium from your teeth, thereby weakening the teeth and making them more susceptible to decay.

Decayed-missing-field-surface index (DMFS) refers to when the DMFT index is employed to assess each individual surface of each tooth, it is termed as "decayed-missing-filled-surface index" (DMFS index). The only difference here is that the surfaces are examined. Each posterior tooth has five surfaces examined and recorded; facial, lingual, mesial, distal and occlusal. Anterior tooth has four surfaces for evaluation; facial, lingual, mesial and distal.

Decayed-missing-filled index (DMF index) the decayed-missing-filled index was introduced by Henry Klein, Carrole E. Palmer and Knutson J.W. In 1938 DMF index was the most universally employed index for measuring dental caries. This index is based on the facts that the dental hard tissues are not self-healing, established caries leaves a scar of some sort. The tooth either remains decayed, or if treated it is extracted or it is filled. The DMFT index is therefore an irreversible index, meaning that it measures total lifetime caries experience.

Deciduous teeth are the baby teeth; teeth that exfoliate or shed.

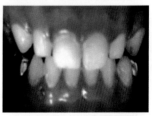

Deciduous dentition

Deep cementopathia is a condition where there is inhibition of continuous cementum formation. It was hypothesized that cementopathia was a disease of eruption and a foreign body response was initiated by the cementum, as a result the host attempted to exfoliate the tooth which consequently results in bone resorption and pocket formation.

Deep dermal burns refer deep partial thickness burns.

Deep partial thickness burns are the one which involves the epidermis and papillary dermis and reticular layer of dermis to varying depths. A few sweat glands and hair follicles are left behind in the reticular dermis from which there is marginal spread of epithelium which gradually covers the wound. This process usually takes more than 6 weeks and the healing takes place by extensive repair which lead to hypertrophic scarring.

Deep sedation refers to a controlled state of depressed consciousness accompanied by partial loss of reflexes. Person is unable to respond verbal command.

Def' index was described by Gruebbel A.O. In 1944, it was used as an equivalent index to dmf index, for measuring dental caries in primary dentition. As defined by Gruebbel, d = decayed

teeth, e = indicated for extraction, f = filled teeth. The basic principles and rules for def index are the same as that for dmf index.

Deflouridation refers to the removal of excess fluoride from water.

Deformation refers to an alteration in shape, form or structure of a previously normally formed part e.g. Clubfoot.

Deglutition refers to swallowing.

Dehiscence can be expressed as the denuded areas along with the loss of marginal bone. Such defects are more common on facial surfaces and on anterior teeth (*see* Figure on page 128).

Delayed eruption of teeth in some cases of fibromatosis gingiva will not allow eruption due to the presence of connective tissue. Systemic diseases doing so include rickets, cretinism and cleido – cranial dysplasia.

Delayed reaction refers to an allergy causing skin eruptions in response to certain drugs. It is caused by sensitized lymphocytes and not by antibodies.

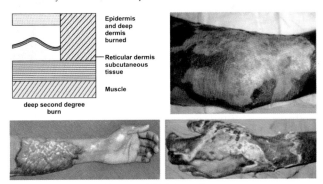

deep second degree burn

Deep partial thickness burn

D

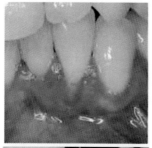

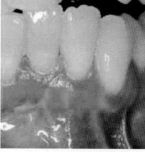

Dehiscence

Delayed union refers to the time taken for a mandibular fracture to unite is delayed beyond the expected time for that particular fracture, it may be assumed that the healing process is disturbed.

Delinquent is one who shows deviation from normal behavior. He has the tendency to committ an offence e.g. Theft, sexual offence, murder and burglary. It is a problem of many communities.

Delirium is a disturbance of consciousness or an acute confusional state in which orientation is impaired, the critical faculty is blunted or lost and thought content is relevant or incoherent. Patient becomes restless, uneasy and sleepless. Delusions and sometimes hallucinations are present. It may develop in high fever, due to overwork, mental stress and drug intoxication and metabolic disorders.

Delirium tremens refers to a disorientation of time and place and a peculiar kind of delirium of horrors resulting from hallucination of sight and hearing. Patient imagines insects crawling under the skin. There may be coarse muscular tremors and may develop loss of memory and insomnia. He may commit suicide, homicide or violent assault.

Delta hepatitis is a defective virus that can replicate only in those who are already infected with HBV. Its transmission and epidemiology is similar to HB virus.

Delusion is an exaggerated belief in one's importance, wealth or talent.

Dementia is a clinical syndrome having failing memory and loss of other intellectual functions. There develops behavioral and personality changes also. Loss includes memory, verbal facility, and ability to deal with mathematical symbols. Patient develops lack of initiative, irritability loss of interest and inattentiveness. There is loss of coordination between speech, thought and action. Delusions and hallucinations may occur. Locomotion may fail.

Demianoff's sign is a lumbar pain caused by stretching the sacrolumbalis muscle. Place the patient supine on table and raise the extended leg. Lumbar pain which prevents lifting the leg high enough to from a 10° angle is a positive sign.

Demineralization is the dissolution or removal of mineral content of enamel or cementum by acid.

Demineralization refers to the loss of mineral from tooth enamel just below the surface in a carious lesion usually appearing as a white area on the tooth surface.

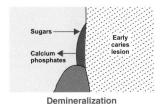

Sugars

Calcium phosphates

Early caries lesion

Demineralization

Dendrite is the process that conducts impulses toward the cell body of a nerve.

Dendritic cells are accessory cells of the immune system. Similar cells are found in the epidermis and mucous membranes (Langerhan's cells). They increase in number during inflammation and may also play a role in repair processes of the pulp. Dendritic cells are primarily found in lymphoid tissues but they are also widely distributed in connective tissues, including the pulp. These cells are termed antigen presenting cells and are characterized by Dentritic cytoplasmic processes and the presence of cell surface class ii antigens. They are known to play a central role in the induction of T cell dependent immunity. They engulf protein antigens and then present an assembly of peptide fragments of the antigens and class ii molecules.

Dens evaginatus (accessory cusps/ supernumerary cusps) can be defined as a tubercle or protuberance from the involved surface of the affected tooth. This is also referred by other terms like occlusal tubercle, Leong's premolar, tuberculated premolar, occlusal enamel pearl. This protuberance has an outer layer of enamel, a core of dentin and may also contain pulp extension into it. Most commonly it is seen on occlusal surface of premolars and also may occur in the form of a drop, nipple or cylindrical cone. Occur predominately in people of mongoloid origin. This condition is clinically important because fracture or wear of the tubercle frequently leads to the major complications like pulp necrosis, periapical infection, often before the root completion.

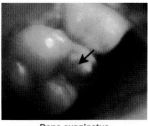

Dens evaginatus

Dens invaginatus/dens in dente/ dilated odontome is a deep surface invagination of the crown/root that is lined by enamel. Dens invaginatus can be divided into coronal and radicular type. Coronal type has been further divided into three types (Oehler 1957), type I – invagination confined to the crown, type II – extends to the root portion and ends in a blind sac that may or may not communicate with the adjacent dental pulp, type III – extends through the root and perforates in the apical or lateral root surface without any communication with the pulp. Radicular type is rare. Strip of enamel lined invagination extends into the root surface. In most cases dens invaginatus is detected by chance on radiograph. Clinically an unusual crown morphology in the form of dilated peg shaped, barrel shaped crown or deep foramen coecum may be important hint. As maxillary lateral incisors are commonly involved, these teeth should be investigated thoroughly clinically and radiographically, at least in case of deep pit in foramen coecum region. If one tooth is involved contralateral tooth also should be investigated. In case of coronal type, pulpal involvement can occur shortly after the eruption of tooth, early diagnosis is mandatory.

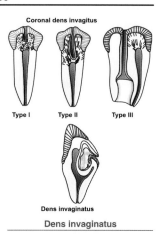

Coronal dens invagitus

Type I   Type II   Type III

Dens invaginatus

Dens invaginatus

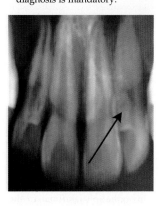

Density of material refers to the amount of mass of a material in a given volume. Common unit of density is grams/cubic centimetres. High density of material makes them heavy.

Dentaire Internationale (FDI) numbering system refers to a numbering system that uses a two digit tooth recording system. The first digit indicates the quadrant and the second indicates the tooth within the quadrant. The numbering is from the midline toward the posterior. The permanent teeth are numbered as follows: maxillary right quadrant is #1, maxillary left quadrant is #2, mandibular left quadrant is #3, and mandibular right quadrant is #4.

Dental amalgam refers to an alloy of a silver tin alloy containing other metals; usually copper and zinc at will be mixed with mercury forming an amalgam.

Dental caries can be defined as a microbial disease of the calcified tissues of the teeth, characterized by demineralization of the inorganic portion and destruction of the organic substances of the tooth resulting in cavitations. Dental caries can occur on any aspect of the tooth but the surfaces which are more prone to the accumulation of plaque and bacteria, are the one which are more susceptible to caries. Closely knitted plaque has a very complex structure and harbors variety of microorganisms. Formation of cavity requires acid producing bacteria, substrate, plaque, and host susceptibility factor.

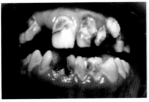

Dental decay

Dental caries severity index for primary teeth was introduced by Aubrey Chosack in 1985. This reproducible caries severity index for primary teeth is based on clinical examinations only, which could be used in surveys of dental caries and give information in addition to 'def' figures, especially when investigating preventive measures.

Dental chair refers to the chair which is used by patient to obtain treatment.

Dental composite is a mixture of silicate glass particles with an acrylic monomer that is polymerized during the application.

Dental compound is a wax like material used to stabilize the rubber dam clamp.

Dental diagnosis is the act of identifying diseases or problems for which dentist provides the treatment.

Dental discoloration is the term given to the discolored tooth. A tooth presenting with smooth and shiny surface, depicts a healthy tooth. Tooth color varies from individual to individual i.e. It can range from pearl white to pale yellow. Any deviations from these colors and smooth surface anatomy can be termed as dental stains or dental discoloration.

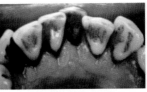

Staining of the teeth

Dental duplicating materials are used to prepare duplicate casts for prosthetic appliances and orthodontic models. These are used to make an impression of original dental cast. Agar hydrocolloid duplicating materials are used most frequently. Their composition has higher water content.

Dental endoscope is recently introduced system which is used subgingivally in the diagnosis and treatment of periodontal disease. The instrument consists of a 0.99 mm diameter reusable fibreoptic endoscope, over which is fitted a sterile sheath. This fiberoptic endoscope fits on to the periodontal probes designed to accept the system. This device allows clear visualization, deep in to the gingival pockets and furcation areas.

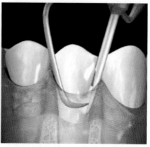

Dental endoscope

Dental fluorosis is a hypoplasia or hypomaturation of tooth enamel or dentin produced by chronic ingestion of excessive amount of fluoride during the period when the teeth are developing. The enamel exhibiting dental fluorosis is called "mottled enamel". G.V. Black and Fredrick S. McKay were the first to coin the term "mottled enamel" in 1916 in Colorado, USA.

Dental groove originates in the incisive papilla region and extends backwards to touch the gingival groove in the canine region and then laterally to end in the molar region.

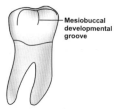

Mesiobuccal developmental groove

Developmental groove

Dental health index (DHI) was developed by Carpay J.J., Neiman F., Konig K.G., Felling A.J.A. and Laminers J.G.M in 1983. The DHI uses selected teeth for developing the index. Any number of teeth may be examined and the denominator is adjusted accordingly. The DHI was developed to minimize the difference between sound and affected (or extracted) teeth. The sound teeth were given a score of "+1" and the affected (or extracted) teeth were given a score of "-1".

Dental home is a place, a source of comprehensive dental care.

Dental hygiene action refers to the interventions performed by dental hygienists that are meant to meet the needs of day today.

Dental hygiene clinician refers to the role of dental hygienist, to identify their problems and to help patients to get rid of these.

Dental hygiene research refers to an application of the scientific methods to develop new knowledge and to keep a proper record of it.

Dental hygienist refers to a licensed preventive oral health professional who provides educational, clinical and therapeutic patient service. Dental hygienist are trained for 2 years. Under guidance of a dental surgeon they can do cleaning, polishing teeth, application of fluorides and fissure sealants.

Dental implants are titanium implants placed directly into alveolar bone and used to anchor fixed restorations or removable prosthesis.

Dental index (Pamela Zarkowski) is an abbreviated measurement of the amount or condition of disease in a population; a numerical scale with defined upper and lower limits designed by the same criteria and method.

Dental mirrors as know as mouth mirrors are the diagnostic hand instruments that are used for indirect vision, illumination and retraction. These are available in sizes of 2 to 6.

Dental nurse is a professional who is trained in preparing, mixing filling and using impression material. She also helps in suction, illumination and retraction. She keeps the operating field clean and dry.

Dental percussion test conducted by gently tapping a tooth with tip of dental mirror handle. There may be tenderness to percussion or dull percussion note on the buccal or palatal aspect of tooth that shows inflammation of periodontal ligament and periodontitis. Greater tenderness to percussion in an apical direction on percussing the occlusal aspect of tooth is suggestive of pulpal and periapical infection.

Dental pliers are forceps used to place of retrieve small objects in oral cavity like cotton balls or rolls. These are available in both locking and unlocking styles.

Dental practice act is a law that regulates the practice of dentistry, dental hygiene and individuals.

Dental public health is an art of preventing and controlling dental diseases and promoting oral health and prevention of dental disease including control through organized community efforts where the whole community is treated as patient. It promotes dental health through organized community efforts.

Dental pulp organ can be defined as a firm, cohesive and resilient unit and this is because pulp is composed principally of gelatin like substance called ground substance, which is reinforced throughout by irregularly arranged and interlaced collagen fibbersand fibre bundles. Embedded in its stroma are cells, blood vessels and nerve fibers that make up loose connective tissue.

Dental record refers to a complete record of health and dental status which will help in treatment and comparing the effect of it.

Dental resin refers to a dental material applied to the tooth which is used in cases of severe dentinal hypersensitivity; usually not used unless all other treatment attempts have failed.

Dental sclerosis exact process of deposition of calcium is not understood. Increased mineralization of tooth decreased conductivity of odontoblastic process.

Dental shade guides are used in determining the color of natural teeth so that substitutes restorations will have similar color and esthetics.

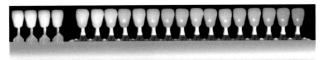

Dental shade guide

Dental tape is a polishing paste used for polishing proximal surfaces that are inaccessible to other polishing instruments; care should be taken to avoid injuring the cementum and the gingiva. The area should be cleansed with warm water to remove the remnants of paste.

Dental technician is highly skilled craftsmen who construct crown, bridges, inlays, splints and orthodontic appliances. They are not allowed to undertake any form of dental treatment.

Dental therapist is an auxiliary dental worker who has completed 2 years course. He can do cleaning and polishing of teeth, application of fluorides and fissure sealants, simple fillings and extraction of deciduous teeth. He can also administer local infiltration analgesia for extractions, fillings and scaling.

Dental unit refers to a control center for the dental hand pieces, oral evacuator, air water syringe, saliva ejector, ultrasonic scaler and light probe.

Dental varnish is a fluid used for hypersensitivity treatment which sometimes contains sodium fluoride applied to the tooth surface, covering the outer surface of dentin and thus blocking transmission of stimuli to the pulp.

Dentate alveolus fracture is the term which implies fracture of alveolus with associated damage of teeth.

Dentifrice is the substances used with a tooth brush or other applicator to remove bacterial plaque, materia alba and debris from gingiva and teeth for cosmetic and sanitary purposes, and for applying specific agents to the tooth surfaces for preventive and/or therapeutic purposes.

Dentigerous cyst is the most common odontogenic cyst. It has a lumen lined with epithelium. Most commonly affected tooth is mandibular premolar and maxillary third molar. Multiple dentigerous cysts may be accompanied with basal cell nevus syndrome or cleidocranial dysostosis. Cyst varies from 2 cm in diameter to large expansion of jaws. Cysts usually yield a straw colored thin liquid. Cyst is painless and causes delayed eruption of tooth. Painless cyst is

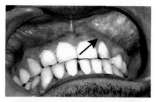

Dentigerous cyst with missing canine

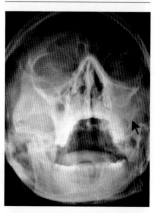

Para nasal sinus view showing dentigerous cyst

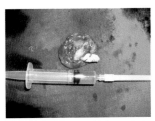

Dentigerous cyst with impacted canine and aspirator

D

forming a new dentin called as secondary dentin. Composition - 70% inorganic substance, 30% organic and water.

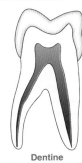

Dentine

indicative of some infection. It generally does not expand so much so that it may press sensory nerve. Pain is localized but may be referred to any part of face. Smaller lesions can be surgically removed.

Dentin bonding is the type of retention that occurs between dental material and the dentin of a tooth. It can include micro mechanical retention and chemical adhesion.

Dentin dysplasia is a rare disturbance of dentin formation. There is normal enamel with atypical dentin formation with abnormal pulpal morphology. Radicular type appears clinically normal except slight amber translucency. Eruption pattern is normal. Tooth is mobile while type II of coronal type is amorphous with atubular dentin. There is no treatment.

Dentin forms the main portion of the tooth which is covered by enamel in the crown region and cementum in the root region. Dentin is hard, dense, calcified tissue similar to the enamel however it is softer than enamel and but hardest than the cementum. Dentin is yellow and elastic in nature and capable of

Dentin secondary refers to a dentin formed after the eruption of tooth.

Dentinal tubule refers to microscopic canals that run from the outside of the dentin to the nerve inside the tooth.

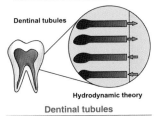

Dentinal tubules

Dentinogenesis imperfecta is a developmental defect, inherited as an autosomal dominant trait. In this condition the permanent and primary dentitions are involved, enamel appears to be normal, roots are also affected. Post eruption, and there is a rapid calcification of the pulp chambers and root canals which will lead to the darkening in the color of the clinical crown. Characteristic findings consist of a peculiar opalescent purplish-brown or gray color of the teeth. Rapid attrition of the crowns, and reduction in carious lesions. Enamel, cementum, and periodontal membrane show no microscopic abnormalities, but there are many changes noted in the dentine. The dentinoenamel junction is straight rather than scalloped which probably accounts for the weak attachment of the enamel to the dentine and the tendency for the enamel to chip, leaving exposed dentine. Irregular tubular arrangement can be seen. Smaller number of tubuli, decreasing toward the pulp. Occasional larger diameter of tubuli and cellular inclusions. Numerous branching of the tubuli. Poor calcification of the teeth. The circumpulpal dentine picture resembles irregular secondary dentine formation. The teeth are much smaller than normal, about one-half the dimensions or one-eighth the volume. Enamel appears as a very thin layer, and is quickly worn away in the mouth. Pulp chambers and canals show in the radiographs of deciduous teeth during formation, but are almost completely obliterated in erupted teeth of the permanent set. The teeth are not sensitive to grinding, indicating that the dentine does not contain vital fibrils. Enamel hypoplasia is a disorder affecting the structure of the teeth. It is often seen as one component associated with many syndromes or enamel hypoplasia may be mild enough resulting in a pitting of the enamel surface or a horizontal line across the enamel of the crown.

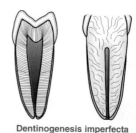

Dentinogenesis imperfecta

Dentinoma is rare tumor. It develops in central mandible in molar area. Radiographic findings are not specific. It is large, solitary, opaque mass. Masses of calcified material are seen. It consists of irregular dentin as there is lack of enamel formation. Surgical excision with thorough curettage helps.

Dentition refers to the natural teeth as a unit.

Dentition consist of the natural teeth in the jaw bones that consist of primary and permanent dentition. The dentition is of three type's i.e. Primary dentition, mixed dentition and primary dentition.

Dentoalveolar anterior cross bite are the one in which one or more maxillary anterior teeth are in lingual relation to the mandibular anteriors termed dento-alveolar anterior cross bite. This is often manifested as single tooth cross bite and usually occurs due to over retained deciduous teeth that deflect the erupting permanent teeth into a palatal position. They can be effectively treated using tongue blades, catalans appliance and double cantilever spring with posterior bite plate.

Dentoalveolar fractures are those that involve avulsion, subluxation, displacement or fracture of teeth in conjunction with fracture of the alveolus. They may occur alone or in association with mandible.

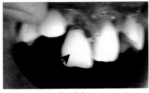

Avulsion

Dentrifice is a paste used to clean the tooth, i.e. tooth paste.

Dentulous areas refer to area with teeth.

Denture adhesive is an adjunct to stabilize and retain denture by increasing peripheral seal. It is commonly available in powder and paste form.

Denture base is a material used to contact the oral tissues and support artificial teeth.

Denture hyperplasia is a chronic inflammatory tissue reaction to ill fitting dentures with overextended or sharp denture border. It develops in 5-10% of elderly denture wearers. It is painful when traumatized and ulcerated. It is seen as single or several folds of pink tissue in the sulcus related to periphery of a denture. Lower jaw is more frequently affected. After adjustment of dentures, the inflammation and edema may subside and produce clinical improvement.

Denture induced fibrous hyperplasia refer denture hyperplasia.

Denture irritation hyperplasia refer denture hyperplasia.

Denture porcelain is defined as a white translucent ceramic fired to a glazed state. It has an excellent biocompatibility, natural appearance and high resistance to wear and distortion. Disadvantages include brittleness; require mechanical attachment and produces clicking sound on contact. Higher density increases weight of teeth.

Denture sore mouth is a diffuse inflammation of maxillary denture bearing area. Pain and burning are usually reported during periods of exacerbation although raw area will persist for years till denture is born. Raised antibody titres against Candida Albicans are found in salvia and serum. Three clinical varieties are found, a localized simple inflammation or pin point hyperaemia, a more diffuse erythema granular type.

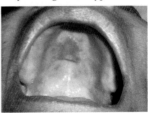

Denture sore mouth

Denture stomatitis is an inflammation of oral mucosa associated with wearing dentures. It is generally found under maxillary mucosa. Mucosa becomes red and velvety appearance. There may be burning sensations (*see* Figure on page 138).

Deontological ethics is an ethical theory that focuses on morality rather the consequences of action.

D

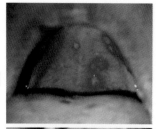

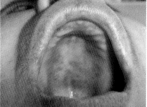

Denture stomatitis involving palate

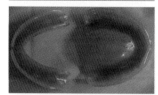

Ill fitting denture surfaces

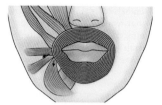

Depressor angular oris

Depressor labii inferioris is a facial muscle. It is quadrilateral and arises from oblique line of mandible. It draws the lower limb downwards and laterally during mastication.

Dermoid cyst is a painless slow growing swelling at the site of lines of embryonic fusion. It is generally seen above the outer canthus of eye, behind the ear, root of nose and midline of body. Majority of these develop during adulthood. It produces a bulge in mouth causing difficulty in eating. It is smooth, soft and non tender when infection develops, sinus may be formed. Overlying skin remains free but is attached to deeper tissue. Once removed surgically these don't recur.

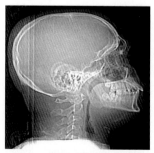

Dermoid cyst

Deposition refers to a process of laying down of new bone.

Depression is an abnormal psychological state. There develops a low mood, interest and vitality. It differs from normal sadness in the severity of symptoms.

Depressor angularis oris is a facial muscle that arises from oblique line of mandible below and lateral to depressor labii inferioris. It draws the angle of mouth downwards and laterally in opening the mouth and in sadness.

Descriptive study is a research that involves describing, analyzing and interpreting data to evaluate a current population event or situation.

Desensitization refers to the blocking of painful stimuli which causes dentinal hypersensitivity.

Desiccate is to make dry; to remove all moisture.

Desmin are the filaments that are found predominantly in muscle cells. It forms an interconnecting network perpendicular to the long axis of the cell. Desmin fibres anchor and orientate the z bands in myofibrils, thus generating the striated pattern.

Desmoplastic fibroma is benign neoplasm arising from mesenchymal tissues of jaw bone. It develops in younger age group. Mandible is affected more. These are generally asymptomatic neoplasm. Neither teeth nor lesion is tender. Treatment includes local excision and curettage.

Development (Moyers) includes all naturally occurring unidirectional changes in the life of individual from its existence as a single cell to its elaboration as multi-functional unit terminating in death.

Development (Todd) refers to progress towards maturity.

Developmental anomaly is an abnormality in which a tooth has deviated from its normal form due to aberration in odonto-genesis. The dental anomalies have been reported more often in Eskimos, Mongols and Orientals. Such variations can be traced to ancestral times and have been reported to have a genetic basis.

Developmental depression is a concavity in a surface that formed while the tooth was developing.

Devitalization pulpotomy is a two stage procedure and involves the placement of devitalizing paste over the pulp exposure in the first sitting to fix the entire coronal and radicular pulp tissue. The basic technique, first introduced by Witzel in 1898, used a true paraformaldehyde paste.

Dewels method is a three-step extraction procedure. In first step the deciduous canines are extracted to create space for the alignment of the incisors. This step is carried out at 8-9 years of age. A year later the deciduous first molars are extracted so that the eruption of first premolar is accelerated. This is followed where in the first premolars are enucleated at the time of extraction of the first deciduous molars. This is frequently necessary in the mandibular arch where the canines often erupt before the first premolars.

df index is another method of getting around the exfoliation problem the 'df' index in which the missing teeth are ignored. This is the method of choice of the world health organization in their basic survey technique. The 'df' index can be applied to the whole tooth as the decayed-filled-tooth ('dft' index) or to the individual surfaces as the decayed-filled-surface ('dfs' index)

Dhatura seeds are used to stupefy travellers in railway stations, places of pilgrimage in order to commit theft, robbery and rape. These are mixed with colored food, cereals, vegetables curry etc. An average size fruit contain 400-500 seeds. Seeds are similar to of brinjals. Its poisoning results in giddiness, vomiting and staggering gait. Face is flushed, pupils are dilated. Patient makes pill rolling movements. Stomach is to be washed with weak solution of potassium permanganate or 2-4% tannic acid. Emetics are to be given.

Diabetes insipidus is a disease resulting from an inadequate secretion of antidiuretic hormone marked by great thrust and passage of a large volume of urine.

Diabetes mellitus represents a syndrome of disordered glucose metabolism and inappropriate hyperglycemia that results from an absolute deficiency in insulin secretion, a reduction in the biologic effectiveness of insulin or both. Predisposing factors includes: genetic disorder of primary destruction of islets of Langerhan's in the pancreas caused by inflammation, cancer or surgery, an endocrine condition, such as Hyperpituitarism and hyperthyroidism, administration of steroids, resulting in iatrogenic diabetes. Classification of diabetes mellitus includes insulin dependent diabetes mellitus (IDDM) – type 1, non insulin dependent diabetes mellitus (NIDDM) - type II

Diabetes mellitus type I the primary form of diabetes is genetic. This is a more severe form. In type I, circulating insulin is essentially absent, plasma glucagon levels are elevated and pancreatic β-cells do not respond to insulinogenic stimuli. Human lymphocyte antigen (HLA) which is located on 6th human chromosome adjacent to immune response genes are closely associated with development of type I diabetes.

Diabetes mellitus type II describes a heterogeneous group composed of milder forms of diabetes that occurs most frequently in adults and only occasionally in children. Most type II diabetics do not require exogenous insulin therapy to sustain life.

Diabetic gangrene occurs in a diabetic patient of above the age of 50 years who presents, pain, ulceration and discharge. Lesion starts with boil or trauma, usually great toe is involved. In moist gangrene affected part is swollen with offensive discharge. It spreads extensively with sloughing of tissues. There is no line of demarcation.

Diabetic kidneys refers to the specific lesions of diabetes include diabetic glomerusclerosis and exudative lesions. Others lead to pyelonephritis. Microalbuminuria is indicative of kidneys involvement. Kidneys are enlarged. External surface may show scars due to hypertension.

Diabetic nephropathy incidence of nephropathy is between 10-20%. All such patients having diabetic nephropathy, there is proteinuria with progressive renal failure. There develops enlargement of kidney. Patients of diabetic type I develops more of nephropathy. There should be protein restriction with curtailment of sodium and potassium. Hypertension is to be controlled along with diabetes (*see* **Figure** on **page 141**).

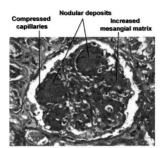

Histological section of Diabetic nephropathy

Diabetic peripheral neuropathy microangiopathy with obliteration of vasanervorum or poor myonisitol uptake and increased nerve accumulation of sorbital and fructose are pathological mechanisms of diabetic neuropathy. It manifests with symmetric, pain and loss of tendon jerks.

Diabetic retinopathy changes are either simple or proliferative. In background lesions there is micro–aneurysm formation, venous dilatation and dot hemorrhages. In proliferative form new vessel are lost. Senile cataracts develop 10-15 years earlier in diabetics. Snow flake cataracts are characteristic in young diabetics. In proliferative type photocoagulation is the only answer.

Diagnodent is a new method of caries detection introduced by KaVo, Germany in 1999, which is based on the principle of fluorescence. It enables to recognize pathological changes that are difficult or even impossible to detect, such as initial lesions, demineralization, changes affecting the tooth enamel. The incidence of fissure, approximal and residual caries can be identified. It is also useful in determining the amount of carious involvement/decalcification in different areas of the same tooth.

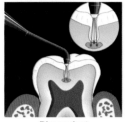

Diagnodent

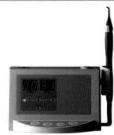

Diagnodent

Diagnosis is identification of health related problem determination of the nature of disease.

Diagnostic and statistical manual of mental disorder (DSM III-R) (1987) defined habit as a mental disorder which is non goal directed, repetitive and intentional behavior often performed rhythmically, that are of sufficient severity to cause physical injury to or to interfere markedly with the normal activities of the child, adolescent or adult.

Diagnostic cast are replicas of the tissues of the maxillary and mandibular arches made from impressions. (*see* **Figure on page 142**)

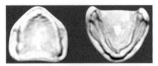
Diagnostic cast

Diagnostic refers to the procedures performed by the dentist to identify what's going on in the mouth.

Dialysis is a process of separating crystalloids from colloids by the difference in their rates of diffusion through a semi permeable membrane.

Diaphragm is a membrane and partition that separates one thing from another. It is a flat muscular sheet that separates chest from abdomen.

Diaphragmatic breathing is the breathing that promotes the use of diaphragm.

Diarrhea is the passage of watery stool.

Diastema is a space or reparation between two teeth especially between the upper central incisor.

Diastema refers to an abnormal space between two adjacent teeth.

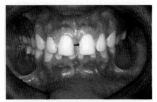
Midline diastema

Diastolic dysfunction is an inability of the heart to fill with blood during diastole at a normal filling pressure.

Diazepam is a barbiturate and was introduced fifty years back and was used for minor insomnia and anxiety. Dose dependent mild cardiovascular depression may occur. Chances of dependence increase if drug is used for longer period. Diazepimes are used in the management of mild anxiety and tension. Librium and valium are commonly used. It is rapidly absorbed and acts for 3-4 hour. Drowsiness, lethargy and ataxia are common. Minor dependence of physical dependence may develop.

Differential diagnosis is the process of listing out the various diseases having common signs and symptoms of which only one could be attributed to patients suffering.

Differentiation is the change from generalized cells or tissue to more specialized kinds during the development.

Diffuse atrophy of alveolar bone is a periodontal disease reported by Gottlieb in 1923 characterized by loss of collagen fibers in the periodontal ligament and was replaced by loose connective tissue and severe bone resorption leading to widened periodontal space.

Diffuse gingivitis is said to occur when the marginal gingiva, interdental gingiva and attached gingiva all are affected.

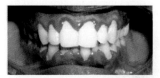
Diffuse gingivitis

Diffuse lesion is said to have occur when the border of lesions are not well defined and it is not possible to define exact parameters of lesions.

Diffusion refers to spreading, spreading of dissolved particles.

Dilaceration is an abnormal angulation or bend in the root or less frequently the crown of a tooth. It is caused by trauma to the root development. Any tooth may be affected. Dilaceration do not interfere with eruption. Dilacerated tooth erupt into complete occlusion, but follow altered path. Minor dilacerations of normal teeth requires no treatment. If eruption is delayed or abnormal, surgical exposure and orthodontic movement is required. Caution must be exerted during endodontic treatment of dilacerated teeth to avoid perforation of the root.

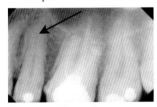

Dilaceration

Dilantin sodium is an anticonvulsant drug used in epileptic seizures. But it causes fibrous hyperplasia of gingiva.

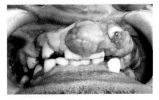

Dilantin induced hyperplasia

Gingival hyperplasia begins as early as 2 weeks after drugs. There is increase in size of gingiva which is painless. Gums may become warty. It has tendency to bleed. Discontinuing drug is best treatment.

Diode lasers have a solid active medium. It is a solid-state semi conductor laser that uses some combination of al, gallium and arsenide to change electric energy into light energy. It has a wave length range from 800-980 nm. Laser energy is delivered fiberoptically in continuous-wave and gated – pulse mode used in contact with the tissue. It is poorly absorbed by tooth structure so that soft tissue surgery can be performed safely in close proximity to enamel, dentine and cementum. It is an excellent soft tissue surgical laser indicated for cutting and coagulating gingiva and mucosa and for soft tissue curettage, or sulcular debride-ment.

Diphodont refers to having two successive sets of teeth.

Diphtheria is an acute infection caused by *cornyebacterium diphtheria*. Direct or droplet infection may cause it. Incubation period is only for a few days. It is a disease of childhood. After a short incubation period of 4 days. Child becomes restless, headache, fever, sore throat and mild redness and oedema of pharynx may takes place. Patchy deptheric membrane often begins on tonsils and around. Fever may be very high. On examination one finds uniform greyish or yellowish white membrane covering tonsil. It may extend to pharynx and soft palate. Membrane is adherent to underlying mucosa. Cervical glands are enlarged. In severe case membrane may show hemorrhagic areas and there may be bleeding. Neurological complications include palatal paralysis, ocular paralysis and peripheral neuritis within 6-8 weeks but all three are reversible. Throat swab will confirm the diagnosis.

Diplococcic refers to Cocci arranged in pairs.

Direct contamination refers to direct contact with impurities or germs.

Direct current refers to current in which electron flows in one direction.

Direct digital radiography is a method of obtaining a digital image currently, digital radiographic images may be obtained by video recording and digitization of a conventional film radiograph or by direct digital radiography. The first digital dental radiograph introduced in dentistry is called radio-visiography (RVG). According to Wenzel (1998), the sensitivities are relatively high for detection of occlusal lesions into dentin with a false-positive fraction to 5% to 10%. The imaging system uses a charge-coupled device (CCD) or storage phosphorus screen.

Direct ground microscopy is a microscopic procedure where specimen is illuminated obliquely by a special condenser organism appears bright as light rays hit them.

Direct suture loop is a type of interdental ligation where the needle is passed from buccal interdental papillae, which then comes out from the lingual aspect of interdental papilla, the two are gently pulled together and conventional knot is given. The knot is generally placed on the labial/buccal aspect for the ease of accessibility.

Direct wiring is a technique where the middle portion of the 6 inch wire is twisted around a suitable tooth and free ends of wire is twisted together to produce a plaited wire. Similarly it's done throughout the upper and lower arch, then after the reduction of the fracture the plaited ends of the upper and lower wires are twisted together.

Disability refers to a physical or mental impairment that substantially limits one or more of an individual's major life activities.

Disaccharide is a carbohydrate composed of two monosaccharide's lined together.

Disclosing agent is an Erythrosine based solution. Dr Sumter Arnin (1963) introduced disclosing agents into preventive dentistry in the form of 'wafers', which are tablets of erythrosine food dye, termed F.D.C. Red. No. 3 (a 6% solution in water). Other brands are 'ceplac' disclosing tablet, rose pink food dye, red cote solution, c-red solution. Disadvantages include indiscriminate staining of lips, cheeks and tongue. Iodine based solution contains. Talbot's iodine comprises of iodine 1.6g, ki 1.6g, water 13.4 mld glycerin to make 30ml. Plaque is stained brown or black.

Disclosing solution will discolor plaque accumulation as stained areas on teeth. It is available in tablet form also.

Discoid is a spoon shaped dental hand instrument with a cutting edge around the total periphery.

Discoid lupus erythematosis is a mixed red and white lesions. A radiating pattern of very delicate white lines is seen. Alternate red, white and red zones provide a characteristic appearance. Histological changes consist of hyperorthokeratosis with keratotic plugs. Most of the intra-oral lesions in DLE occur on the cheeks with the gingival tissues and border of lip. Hot and spicy food will produce burning sensation. It responds to cortisone well.

Discoloration of teeth occurs due to varios reasons yellow is due to heavy plaque build up. Green color is due to poor oral hygiene and is difficult to remove. Black is due to iron compounds from oral fluid. Tobacco stain is rare but develops with chromogenic bacteria.

Disease eradication literally means to 'tear out by roots'. Today smallpox is the only disease which has been eradicated. India is trying to eradicate polio, measles and dracunculous infection.

Disease index The'd (decay) portion of the dmf index best exemplifies a disease index. The indices measuring gingival / sulcular bleeding are essentially symptom indices. This type of index measures the 'number' or 'proportion' of people in a population with or without a specific condition at a specific point in time or interval of time.

Disinfectant is an agent used to kill pathogenic micro organisms without sterilizing the material.

Disinfectant refers to a chemical agent which is applied onto inanimate surfaces to destroy germs.

Disinfection is a lethal process killing disease producing micro organisms but not bacterial spores.

Disinfection is the chemical destruction of most forms of micro-organisms. Disinfectant does not kill all micro-organisms regardless of amount of time they are exposed to chemical.

Disinfection refers to a cleaning process which destroys the majority of micro-organism, but not highly resistant forms such as bacterial and mycotic spores.

Displaced flaps are the ones, when the flap is placed apically, coronally or laterally to their original position.

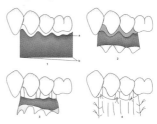

Apically displaced flap

Displacement is the movement of whole bone away from one another creating space within which enlargement of each of the separate bone takes place.

Disposable materials refer to materials intended for one time use and then to be discarded.

(e.g.: gloves, paper gowns, cotton rolls, etc.)

Distal refers to the surface of the tooth farthest from the midline of the dental arch.

Dissecting aneurysm is a condition where blood from lumen of vessel enters the substance of wall and extends along the wall of the vessel resulting in blood filled channel. No true aneurysmal dilatation is present. Onset is sudden and may be fatal.

Distal step terminal plane is characterized by the distal surface of the lower second deciduous molar being more distal to that of the upper. Thus the erupting permanent molars may be in angle's class II occlusion.

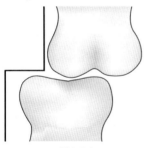

Distal step

Distal wedge procedure is used for deep periodontal pockets distal to last molar.

Distomolar refer supernumerary teeth.

Distortion geometric is a characteristic that refers to a variation of true size and shape of the object being radio graphed. Radiograph distortion is influenced by object film alignment and X-ray beam angulation.

Distraction is intentional diversion of attention.

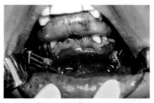

Intraoral distractor

Distraction osteogenesis is the process of generating new bone by streching.

Diuretic is a substance which increases urine secretion.

Divergent refers to spread.

Diverticulitis coli colonic diverticula are acquired and are false containing mucosa and submucosa herniated through muscular coats. Lack of fiber in diet, high intraluminal pressure results in diverticula formation. Sigmoid colon is generally affected when inflamed. These produce pain, discomfort and tenderness in left iliac fossa. Diarrhea is a common feature. Bleeding per rectum may be severe. Severe cases may result in intestinal obstruction. Barium enema shows outpouching of colonic mucosa.

dmf index is for use in children before ages of exfoliation - for children over 7 years and up to 11 or 12 years, the decayed, missing and filled primary molar and canines, have been used to determine decayed - missing - filled teeth (dmft), or decayed-missing–filled surfaces (dmfs), when surfaces are counted.

DNA probe is an advanced diagnostic aid that helps to

identify the organism associated with periodontal disease. It identifies species and specific sequence of nucleic acids that make up DNA, thereby permitting identification.

Doctor-Nurse relationship makes a team although doctor role is to diagnose and cure the patient while nursing role lies in the process of care helping, comforting and guiding.

Doctor-Patient relationship Patient comes unbidden to a doctor and enters voluntarily into a contract to agree to follow doctor's advice. Doctor exercises an authorative role because being superior in professional knowledge. If doctor communicates well on an emotional plane, on a cultural plane and at intellectual plane he is a successful doctor and patient will develop confidence in him.

Doll's eye reflex infant holds the fixation of faces, on the movements or changing intensity of light within their visual fields.

Doppler stethoscope is a device that help in directing sounds by the velocity of blood moving through a blood vessel.

Dorendorl's sign is a fullness of supraclavicular groove. This sign may occur in aneurysm of aortic arch.

Double teeth refers to two conjoined teeth. However this term should not be applied to teeth joined only through their root cementum. They are referred by other terms like "bifid teeth"

Douche is a procedure for cleaning the vaginal wall and cavity.

Down syndrome/ Mongolism / Trisomy 21 is a congenital disease caused by chromosomal abnormalities, it is characterised by mental deficiency and growth retardation. Oral manifestation present are periodontal disease with periodontal pockets, diastema, crowding, high freenal attachment.

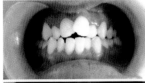
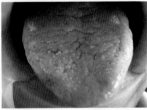
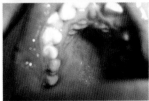

Down syndrome

DPT vaccine helps to immunize simultaneously against 3 diseases diphtheria, pertussis and tetanus which is an administrative gain. In addition pertussis component in DPT vaccine enhances the potency of diphtheria toxoid. There are 2 types of vaccine plain and adsorbed.

Dracunculiasis is caused by largest viviparous nematode, the dracunculus medinesis popularly known as guinea worm. Larvae liberated by female worms are ingested by an intermediate host cyclops. People consuming the contaminated water with cyclops develop dracunculiasis. The lesions are usually seen in various parts of body, feet, nape of neck and back. During removal of worm it is broken. The affected part becomes swollen, painful and inflamed. Death of adult female worms results in serious and grave complications. Arthritis, abscess formation and fibrosis of joints develop.

Drifting is a process when tooth is lost, surrounding tooth will move out of position.

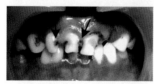

Drifting of teeth

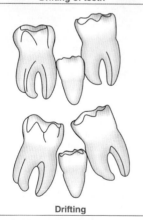

Drifting

Drop attack begin in childhood and are associated with diffuse brain lesions. Patient may suddenly fall on ground. Attacks may occur many times a day. These are common in old age due to weakness, ataxia and gait disorder. Event is unexpected but consciousness is retained

Drowning is a form of death in which atmospheric air is prevented from entering into lungs by submission of body in water/liquid. Drowning person feels auditory and visual hallucinations. Asphyxia supervenes within 2 minutes after complete submersion and heart stops in 2-5 minutes afterwards. A fine white leathery froth is seen at mouth and nostrils. Skin may be goose skin and grass, gravels sticks may be found firmly grasped in hands due to cadaveric spasm. On post-mortem lungs are distended and pit on pressure of fingers. Water cannot get into left side of heart if body is thrown into water after death.

Drug allergy is a hypersensitive adverse reaction. Oral reactions include stomatitis medicamentosa. In early reactions vesicles or bullae may be found. Occasionally purpuric spots appear. Involvement of gingiva, palate, lips and tongue are common. On discontinuation of drug, allergic reaction subsides.

Drug eruptions are an eruption of skin or mucus membrane after oral or systemic administration of drugs. Drug eruptions vary in severity from a mild rash to toxic epidermal necrolysis. Onset may be sudden or delayed. Lesions may be local or generalized. Well define edematous wheels are seen in aspirin reaction. From a few small oral vesicles or urticaria lesion to painful oral ulcerations are seen in case of sulfonamides and barbiturates. Fixed drugs are well circumscribed dusky red or purple lesions on mucus membrane mostly seen in tetracycline, sulfonamide. Lichen planus like eruptions are seen in antimalarials and chlorpromazine.

Drug induced hyperplasia is caused due to prolong use of phenytoin. Calcium channel blockers can also cause the similar condition.

Drug tolerance is a diminished effect of a drug at its usual dosage range.

Drugs after delivery certain drugs can be excreted in milk affecting the infant. We should avoid the use of aspirin, benzodiazepines ciprofloxacin, cytotoxic drugs, corticosteroids, diuretics, lithium etc.

Dry cough is produced as a result of stimulation of irritant receptors in the pharyngeal wall. These receptors are distributed throughout the tracheobronchial tree. Character of cough is hacking and it can be disturbing. In some common conditions such as pertussis and tracheobronchitis it may be associated with whoop sound.

Dry gangrene generally affects lower limbs and is due to slow occlusive vascular disease such as atherosclerosis and thromboangitis obliterans. Spread is very slow. Affected area becomes cold and clammy. Part becomes black, dry and shrivelled. A well demarcated line of separation is noted (*see* Figure).

Dry heat sterilization oxidizes the microbes. It penetrates less well

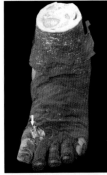

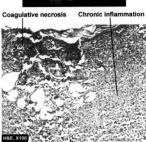

Coagulative necrosis   Chronic inflammation

Dry gangrene foot

and is less effective than moist heat. It takes 45 minutes to reach 160°C.

Dry socket mostly occurs as a postoperative complication of the extracted tooth. It can develop after human extraction wound. It generally takes place in lower bicuspid and molar socket. Dry socket is extremely painful and is treated by packing of zinc oxide eugenol dressing. Healing of such wound is very slow.

D-speed film is an intraoral film. Letter 'd' identifies the film speed.

Dual arch tray is an impression tray that takes an impression of the desired upper and lower teeth at one point of time. It is best for a posterior quadrant.

Dual-cure bond agent is an adhesive material which can be changed to its final hardened state by light curing or by a chemical cure.

Dual energy X-ray absorptiometry (DEXA) is a body composition analysis used to provide regional estimates of fat mass with minimal radiation. Dexa measures the differential attenuation of two main X-ray photon energies as they pass through the body. Total tissue mass is separated into fat, bone, mineral and lean according to measured X-ray attenuation.

Ductility is the characteristic of a material to undergo significant plastic or permanent deformation under stress before fracturing.

Ductless glands are specialized glands that secrete hormones directly into blood.

Due care is a legal term for just, proper and sufficient care. No negligence.

Due cause is to show justifiable reason an action.

Dug's sign is a sign of dislocated shoulder. Ask the patient to place affected hand on opposite shoulder and elbow toward the chest. Inability to do so is a sign of shoulder dislocation.

Dunlop beta hypothesis states that best way to break a habit is by its conscious, purposeful repetition. He suggests that the child should be asked to suck his thumb observing himself as he indulges in the habit. This procedure is very effective if the child is asked to do the same at a time when he is involved in an enjoyable activity.

Duodenal ulcer pain is absent in morning. Pain develops 2-3 hours after meals and is eased by food. Pain generally develops in night during 12-2 a.m. Pain is aggravated by coarse foods, alcohol, and nervous tension. Antacids give relief. Recurrent nausea and vomiting suggests possibility of duodenal ulcer. There develops deep tenderness over lesion. Superficial tenderness may be present.

Duties of patients – he should furnish all the relevant information to doctors about the facts, circumstances and duration of illness. Patient should obey instructions to carry out direction of doctor as regards diet, medicine and mode of life. He should pay the fee to the doctor and should not exploit the doctor in any way.

Dye lasers use complex organic dyes, such as rhodamine 6g, in liquid solution or suspension as lasing media. They are tuneable over a broad range of wavelengths.

Dysarthria anarthria is a complete loss of speech due to a disorder of neuromuscular lesion. It is rare but dysarthria which is an impaired articulation is common. Speech is slurred and indistinct. Lesion at highest level may cause it.

Dyskeratosis congenital (Zinssner – Engmann Cole Syndrome) is a rare X-linked disorder characterized leading to atrophic, leukoplakic oral mucosa. Tongue and cheek are adversely affected. Oral lesions start before the age of 10 as vesicles and white necrotic patches with candida, ulcerations and erythroplakic changes. *Dyskeratosis congentia* nail changes are the first manifestation of disease. Skin may become atrophic, face starts appearing red. There may be mental retardation, small sella turcica, eye lid infections and dental abnormalities. Tongue and buccal mucosa are involved. There is no possible treatment.

Dysmenorrhoea is the pain and cramps in back and lower abdomen associated with menstruation.

Dysphoria is an unpleasant emotional state. It is a mixture of sadness with low grade anxiety and negativity. It is a normal spectrum of human experience.

Dysplasia is an abnormal formation of cells of a particular tissue. Dysplasia is characterized by a proliferation of cells with altered nucleus size and shape. Dysplasia can vary in grade. Not all dysplasia are associated with malignancy.

Dystonia is abnormally increased muscular tone causing fixed abnormal postures. There is sustained contraction of both agonist and antagonist muscle. Focal dystonia is spasmodic torticolis and writers cramp. Spasms are slower and involve trunk more than limbs. It can be seen in Wilson's disease and Huntingtons disease.

Dystrophic Epidermolysis Bullosa includes extensive bulla formation due to trauma and desquamation. Hands, feet, oesophagus and oral cavity are involved. Oral mucosa becomes thick, gray and inelastic. Lesions are smooth. Buccal and lingual sulci become obliterated. Scarring develops. Lips may become immobile. Person may be dwarf. There may be associated conjunctival scarring, laryngeal stenosis and hoarseness of voice.

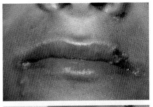

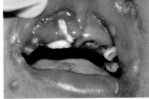

Epidermolysis bullosa

Dystrophic refers to disorder developed due to defective or faulty nutrition.

Dysuria is a painful urination, usually it is associated with inflammation. Pain is referred to the lip of the penis.

Early adolescence is a stage of development that includes casting off childhood role and emergence into adolescence. It also includes developmental changes and the onset of puberty, initiated and indicated by the growth spurt.

Early shift occurs during the early mixed dentition period. The eruptive force of the first permanent molar is sufficient to push the deciduous first and second molars forwards in the arch to close the primate space and there by establish a Class I molar relationship. Since it occurs early in the mixed dentition period it is called early shift.

Ebola virus infection is a member of the Filoviridae, causing hemorrhagic fever. It is transmitted from person to person. Virus spreads through blood. Mucosal bleeding is common. Patients die in intractable shock. Patients in high fever become delirious. No antiviral therapy is effective.

Eburnation refers to the term where radiographically bone end appears sclerosed or rounded off. Eburanation can be observed in cases of non union of fractures.

Ecchymoses is a condition occurring due to erythrocyte extravasation into submucosa, the lesion will appear of brown color i.e. when haemoglobin is degraded to hemosiderin. Patients on anti-coagulant therapy may produce it. Traumatic ecchymosis is common on lips of face.

Eccrine sweat glands are more and widely distributed of sweat glands. These are located throughout body specially palms and soles. Sweat plays an important role in temperature regulation. These sweat glands function throughout life.

Echinococcosis hydatid disease is caused by Echinococcus graunlosus. Dogs and cattle are the definite hosts where man is an accidental host. The cyst contains hydatid fluid which is colorless with a specific gravity of 1005 to 1010. The fluid is antigenic, toxic and can cause severe allergic reactions. Most common sites are liver, lung, spleen and brain. Development of hydatid is slow.

Echocardiography (ECG) is a diagnostic test which provides measurement of left ventrical, function and thickness. Size of all four chambers can be determined. Morphology of heart valves can be examined. Hypertrophic cardiomyopathy, pericardial effusion, mitral value prolapse can be diagnosed.

Ecologic plaque hypothesis (Marsh PD 1994) proposes that the organisms associated with disease may also be present at sound sites, but at levels too low to be clinically relevant. Disease is a result of a shift in the balance of the resident microflora drives by a change in local environmental conditions. The bacterial composition of plaque remains relatively stable despite regular exposure to minor environmental perturbations. This microbial homeostasis is due to a dynamic balance of both synergistic and antagonistic microbial interactions. However, homeostasis can break down, leading to shifts in the balance of the micro flora, thereby predisposing sites to disease.

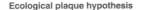

Excess sugar — Neutral pH — S. sanguis, S. gordonii — Health

Stress | Environmental change | Ecological shift | Disease

Acid production — Low pH — Mutans-streps lactobacilli — Caries

Ecological plaque hypothesis

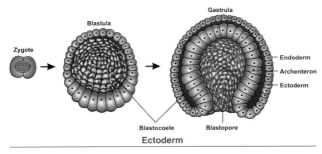

Zygote → Blastula → Gastrula

- Endoderm
- Archenteron
- Ectoderm

Blastocoele   Blastopore

Ectoderm

Ectoderm is the outermost layer of three germ layer of an embryo.

Ectopic lingual thyroid nodule is a small mass of thyroid tissue located at tongue. Clinically it appears as a smooth nodular mass at the base of tongue. It may be asymptomatic causing feeling of fullness in throat or difficulty in swallowing. Sometimes it may require surgical removal.

Eczema is a superficial skin inflammation characterized by vesicles, redness, oozing, crusting, scaling and itching. Scratching or rubbing may lead to lichenification.

Edema refers to swelling resulting from fluid accumulation in gingival tissues.

Edentulous refers to area bearing no teeth.

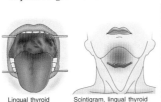

Lingual thyroid   Scintigram, lingual thyroid

Ectopic lingual thyroid

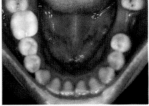

Edentulous space

Effector cells are the unique cells specialized to secrete large amount of Ig proteins into surrounding. Secreted Ig retains the ability to bind the specific ligand and are then referred to as antibodies which constitute 7-26g/L in adult and 25% of total serum protein. In human, approximately 109 B-cells are generated each day. Plasma cells are oval or egg shaped with abundant cytoplasm and an eccentrically placed round nucleus. Clumps of dark staining chromatin are distributed around inner aspect of membrane giving the nucleus a characteristic *'Pin wheel/ Clock face'* appearance. Protein secretary organelles include golgi apparatus. Ig is not present on surface of plasma cell but produced in copious amount in cytoplasm and secreted into extra cellular space. Plasma cells are terminally differentiated and have a short life span of days to weeks.

Efferent refers to the nerves that carry motor messages away from the brain or to take away from a central point.

Efficacy means biological effects of treatment delivered in carefully controlled conditions usually determined by randomized controlled trial.

Ego is a part of psychosexual theory. In Latin it means 'I'. Ego develops out of Id in 2nd and to 6th month of life when infant learns to differentiate between itself and outside world. Ego is a mediation between Id and superego. Unlike Id, Ego is governed by the reality, concerned with memory and judgement. It develops after birth, expands with age and it delays, modifies and controls Id impulses on realistic level.

Ehler's–Danlos Syndrome is a group of hereditary disorder of connective tissue. There is hyper elasticity of skin, hyper-extensibility of joint, fragility of skin and blood vessels. Oral mucosa gets bruised easily and is excessively fragile. Gingival tissues appear fragile and bleed after tooth brushing. Tooth mobility is not increased. There will be hyper mobility of temporomandibular joint causing repeated dislocation of jaw. Hypoplastic changes in enamel have been noted. There is no known treatment.

Ejaculation is a subjective response to emission.

Elastic modulus is the measure of rigidity or stiffness of a material.

Elastic refers to the capability of sustaining deformities without permanent change in size or shape.

Elastomers are the impression material. The advantage of this material is their elasticity which makes it suitable for all types of impressions. It is stronger than alginate and less subjected to change in dimension on standing.

Electra complex is said to have occurred when the young girls develop an attraction towards their father and they resent mother bring close to the father. Freud has reported that little girls have a comparable Electra complex to resolve this.

Electric heating pads are available of various sizes. Heating is by conduction so effect is superficial.

Electric pulp test is a diagnostic tool which uses electric current to stimulate nerve fibres in the pulp to test vitality.

Electric shock refers to the shock that result from passing current through the entire body. It usually does not produce cutaneous burns but has more severe affects on central nervous system cardiovascular system and other systems of the body. The patient usually suffers from trembling, sweating, pallor. Intracranial pressure may be raised and patient may become unconscious because of cerebral edema. There may be temporary deafness, auditory hallucinations, paralysis, and stiffness of limbs, sudden blindness from retinal detachment or cataract occurs at a later stage. Delayed neurological affects are rare. Apnoea or cardiac arrest is the most severe presentation which requires immediate manual cardio pulmonary resuscitation (CPR).

Electric tooth brush is a powered tooth brush which either uses electricity or battery to simulate the brushing action of a patient.

Electrical flash burns are the electrical burns that results from fire or resulting from electrical sparks or flash. Degree of damage depends upon the time duration of exposure to the flash or the proximity of the patient to the actual flash.

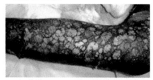
Electrical flash burns

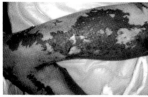
Electrical flash burns

Electro surgery is a surgical method which uses a tiny arch of electric current to make the incision in the gingiva.

Electro thermal burns are the type of electrical burns that results from accidental contact with elements of electrical instruments. These are specially seen amongst children.

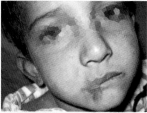

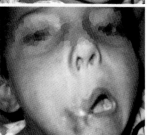
Electro thermal burns

Electrocoagulation is a procedure performed to obtain hemorrhage control by using electrocoagulation current with the help of fine tungsten wire used for electrosection.

E

Electroencephalogram is a recording of the electrical activity in the cerebral cortex that is sometimes used as an index of arousal or anxiety. Electrodes are placed over scalp. Arousal and agitation is associated with rapid, irregular, low amplitude impulses. While relaxation is associated with slow, steady, high amplitude impulses.

Electroencephalography involves the detection, amplification, filtering, storage and analysis of small changes in electrical potential produced by brain, the underlying cortex. Recording are made with electrodes in specific scalp locations. Accuracy of EEG diagnosis is over rated.

Electrogustometry refers to a procedure where taste bud fields can be stimulated by low voltage anodal and cathodal currents applied by means of battery. Instrument is known as electro-gustometer.

Electrolyte refers to a substance that ionizes in solution rendering the solution of conducting a current.

Electromyogram is a recording of electrical activity of a muscle that sometimes is used as an index of tension and anxiety. Mostly electrodes are placed over skin.

Electromyography is a study of voluntary and spontaneous electrical activity of muscle. The potentials generated by stimulation of motor unit are recorded by concentric needles. In neuropathy, when axons are lost then surviving axons sprout and take over nearby denervated muscle fibres resulting in larger and longer EMG record while in myopathy some fibres cannot be activated and recorded muscle potential is smaller. Electromyography is one of the major criteria in diagnosing Myofacial pain. Electromyography finds out the changes in muscle activity and knowing the process of muscle pain and monitoring the effect of treatment.

Electron microscopy is a microscopic procedure where Light waves are replaced by a beam of electrons which allows resolution of extremely small organism such as several of 0.001 micro millimeter size.

Electronic apex locator is a tool to determine the location of the apex of the tooth.

Electronic pulp tester refers to a diagnostic device used to determine tooth vitality.

Electroplating is the process of depositing metal from solution on to the surface of an impression using an electric current.

Electrosection is the term used for incisions, excisions and tissue planning with the help of single wired active electrodes that can be bent or adapted to perform any kind of cutting procedures.

Electrosurgery is a surgical technique performed on soft tissue using controlled high frequency electrical currents.

Elephantiasis is an infectious disease that starts below the malleolus and then spreads to involve foot but thigh is rarely involved. Swelling pits on pressure to start with but later on overlying skin may become rough and thickened.

Elevators are the surgical hand instruments that are used to elevate a retained root or impacted tooth out of socket. Many types are available. Warwick James elevators are straight left and right curved. Cryer elevators are used for retained roots and impacted teeth. These have a triangular sharp end made in a set of two left and right. Coupland chisel dilates the socket and facilitate extraction.

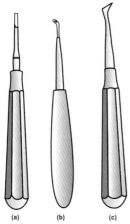

Elevators (a) Coupland; (b) Warwick James; (c) Cryer

E-line (Esthetic plane) (Rickett's E-line) Normally the upper lip is about 4 mm behind E-line while the lower lip lies about 2 mm behind it.

Elongated styloid process associated with pain and is known as eagle's Syndrome. There is a unilateral pain extending from ear to neck. Persons develop a feeling of foreign body in throat.

Embedded teeth refer to those teeth that don't erupt on its own, owing to a lack of eruptive force.

Emboli is the moving clot.

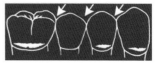

Embrasure

Embrasure refers to the space between two teeth created by the sloping away of the mesial and distal surfaces.

Eminence refers to a prominence

Embrittlement refers to objects susceptible to breakage under slight pressure.

Embryo is the earliest stages of development, the first 8 weeks.

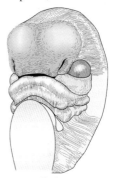

Embryo

Embryology is a study of the development of an individual from conception to birth.

Emesis basin is a basin basically kidney shaped for receiving expectorated or vomited material.

Emission of radiation includes that once an electron moves to a higher-energy orbit, it eventually wants to return to the ground state. When it does, it releases its energy as a photon — a particle of light. This phenomenon is

E

termed spontaneous emission of radiation.

Emotion is a complex reaction by the whole organism, often to an abrupt shift in social circumstances, involving widespread bodily change in visceral function such as heart beat, breathing and glandular secretion and characterized mentally by strong feelings, excitement, agitation and turmoil. Emotion is a state of mental excitement characterized by physiological, behavioral changes and alterations of feelings.

Empirical therapy is prescribed without the benefit of laboratory test getting done.

Empty habits are those habits that are not associated with any deep-rooted psychological problems.

Emulsion is the suspension of very small droplet of one immiscible liquid in another.

Enamel hypocalcification is a developmental anomaly that results in a disturbance of maturation of enamel matrix. It appears as a localized white chalky spot on the middle third of smooth crowns. Underlying enamel may be soft and susceptible to caries. Remedy improves aesthetic appearance.

Enamel hypoplasia is the incomplete formation of enamel resulting in alteration of tooth form or color. It results due to damage to ameloblasts during enamel matrix formation. Due to tetany hypoplasia is pitting. Due to infection there may be any type of hypoplasia from a mild brownish discoloration to a severe pitting irregularity. There when single tooth is involved it is known as Turner's tooth.

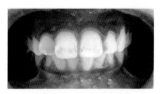
Enamel hypoplasia

Enamel pearl is small, spherically shaped enamel located on a root surface. It develops due to abnormal displacement of ameloblasts during tooth formation. It is usually found on maxillary molars. It does not require any treatment.

Enamel refers to the outermost surface of the anatomical crown. It is thickest at the top of the crown and becomes thinner and ends in a knife edge at the cervical line. The color of the enamel varies with its thickness and mineralization. The color varies from yellowish white to grayish white. Enamel appears whiter if it is thicker. The more mineralized enamel shows more translucency. The translucency gives yellowish

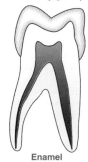
Enamel

color to the tooth. Enamel is densely mineralized, hardest and highly polished in the human body. This dense mineralization gives the enamel ability to resist wear and tear of the crown. Composition- Inorganic content 96-97% by weight (Calcium, Magnesium, Po_4, $NaCo_3$) Organic content Soluble proteins, insoluble proteins, peptides, citric acid and water.

Encephalitis is inflammation involving cerebral hemispheres, brain stem and cerebellum is known as encephalitis. Viral encephalitis is more common. Viral encephalitis may be primary, para or post infections. Onset is abrupt with lethargy, drowsiness, confusion and behavioral abnormality. It may progress to stupor or coma. Cerebral hemispheres when involved cause aphasia and sensory loss.

Enchondroma it is a benign bone tumor of residual islands of cartilage specially of bones of hand. It is painless, develops between 10 and 30 years of age. Radiographycally it presents areas of radiolucency that expands and deform bone.

Margins are well defined. Cortex remain intact. Stippled or punctate calcification may be found.

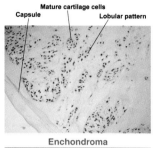

Enchondroma

Endemic disease refers to a disease that is always present in a particular region.

Endemic is a disease present in a community or among a group of people, the continuing prevalence of a disease as distinguished from an epidemic.

Endocrine system consists of a series of ductless glands found in body. These glands which then produce hormones to regulate the rate of metabolism, growth and sexual development. Hormones are secreted directly into blood.

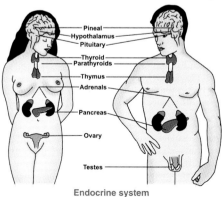

Endocrine system

E

Glands include thyroid, parathyroid, ovaries, testes, pituitary, pancreas and adrenal medulla.

Endocrine therapy is the treatment with hormones and drugs to interfere with hormone production. There may be surgical removal of endocrine glands.

Endodontia refers to within a tooth.

Endodontic file is a hand instrument used to smooth, shape and enlarge root canal.

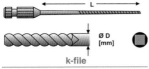

k-file

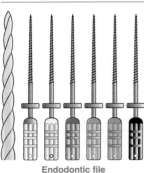

Endodontic file

Endodontics is a branch of dentistry that consists of all forms of root canal therapy including root filling, pulpotomy, pulp capping and apicoectomy. Aim of treatment is to remove the inflamed pulp and replace it with permanent obturation.

Endogenous intrinsic Stains refers to those stains that get incorporated within the tooth structures that have occurred to take place during the development of the tooth and are more suggestive of developmental anomalies of tooth. As the name suggests these tooth cannot be removed by regular prophylactic procedures.

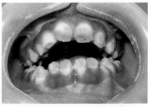

Endogenous intrinsic stain due to amelogenesis imperfecta

Endorphins are chemicals present in CNS that influences pain perception and acts as a natural pain killer.

Endoscopic method for caries detection is potentially sensitive diagnostic tool, which involve the use of endoscopic methods. This method gives a magnified image of the carious lesion to be viewed. Initial studies on the potential benefits of endoscopic examination, either with white light (VMV) or with filtered fluorescence excited by a blue curing light (VFF), it may detect a greater number of carious lesions than do conventional methods. One advantage of endoscopy is a 5 to 10 fold magnification of the sites. Disadvantages include meticulous drying and isolation of teeth taking about 5 to 10 mins for an examination, as compared with 3 to 5 min. for conventional methods.

Endosseous Implant is an implant placed directly with in the maxilla or mandible.

Endosteum can be described as tissue lining the internal bone cavities. Unlike periosteum, the Endosteum is composed of single layer of osteoblasts and sometimes a small portion of connective tissue.

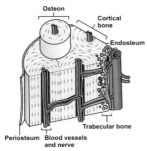

Endosteum

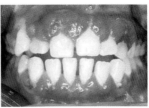

Enlargement due to puberty

Endotoxins are cell wall lipopolysaccharide of gram negative cocci and bacilli and are not actively released from cell. These cause fever, shock and other symptoms.

Energy refers to capacity for doing work.

Enlargement due to puberty refers to gingival enlargement may be seen in males and females during puberty, in area of plaque accumulation. Enlargement is usually confined to marginal gingival with bulbous interproximal papilla seen more frequently on facial aspect than the lingual aspect. Features of inflammatory enlargement are seen and it undergoes spontaneous reduction after puberty if plaque and calculus is removed (*see* Figure).

Enlargement due to vitamin C deficiency Vitamin C deficiency does not cause gingivitis but increases the severity of inflammation in minimal amount of plaque. Clinical features appears as gingival enlargement is marginal appears bluish red in color, tender, grossly swollen and boggy. It is soft and friable in consistency with a smooth and shiny surface. Hemorrhage occurs spontaneously or on slight provocation in long standing cases. Gingiva develops a purple hue and surface necrosis with preudomembrane formation is common feature.

Eosinophil is a blood cell. These comprise 1-3% of all blood leukocytes. These are weak phagocytes. The function of these is to detoxify the proteins before they can damage the body. These help in dissolution of old clots. Eosinophils collect at the site of antigen antibody reaction. In trichinosis large number of eosinophils develops (*see* Figure on page 162).

Eosinophilic enteritis is a condition where blood shows eosinophilia with eosinophilic infiltration of gut wall. Some may show steatorohea with malabsorption, hypoalbuminemia or intestinal obstruction and some show ascites with eosinophilia. Corticosteroids help. Barium study may show mucosal edema, nodular masses, sawtoothed mucosal pattern. Parasite infestation should be excluded.

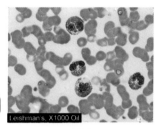

Leishman's, X1000 Oil

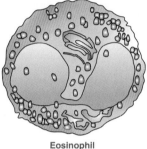

Eosinophil

Eosinophilic granuloma was introduced by Lichenstein and Jaffe in 1940. There may not be any symptoms. Patient may develop local pain and swelling. Radiographically lesion appear as irregular radiolucent area involving superficial alveolar bone. Cortex is destroyed, pathological fracture may develop. When lesion matures, fibrosis occurs. Prognosis is good.

Eosophageal varices are tortuous and dilated veins at the junction of lower end of esophagus and cardia of stomach. These occur in cirrhosis of liver. Rupture and hemorrhage is the cause of death.

Ephebodontics is the science of dentistry which deals with the children who are in the process of growing up from childhood to manhood or womanhood. Medically adolescence can be considered as the period beginning with the appearance of the secondary sex characters and terminating with the cessation of somatic growth.

Epidemiologic indices (Irving Glickman) are attempts to quantitate clinical conditions on a graduated scale, thereby facilitating comparison among populations examined by the same criteria and methods.

Epidemiology (Nikki Foruk) has been defined as a study of health, disease states, effects of ecological or extrinsic factors and intrinsic factors on these states.

Epidemiology can be defined as the frequency and severity of health problems in relation to age, sex, geography, race, economic status, nutrition and diet. This information is obtained from different kind of research epidemiological studies such as mortality rates, morbidity, effects of treatment and prevention.

Epidermal burns refer first degree burn.

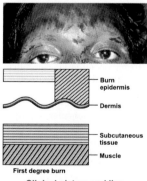

Burn epidermis
Dermis
Subcutaneous tissue
Muscle
First degree burn

Clinical picture and line diagramme for epidermal burns

Epidermoid cyst is a painless slowing growing swelling of skin of insidious onset. It usually occurs over scalp, face, neck and scrotum. Palm and soles are not affected. It is hemispherical in shape. A black dot called punctum may be present on the top of swelling. It is mobile over deeper tissues but fixed to skin. It is not transilluminant. Overlying skin may not have hair.

Epidermolysis Bullosa is a genetic skin disease which causes oral ulceration. Ulcers develop recurrently. Skin lesions are bullae which rupture to give ulcers. Oral ulcers vary in frequency and severity. Complications include ankyloglossia. These cannot be cured or effectively controlled. Only supportive line of treatment is given.

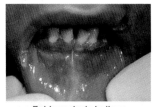

Epidermolysis bullosa

Epiglottis is the cartilaginous appendage overlying the opening of larynx.

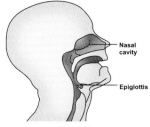

Epiglottis

Epilepsy is a sudden, transient disturbance of cerebral function due to abnormal, chronic, recurrent and paroxysmal neurological discharge in brain. Each episode of such neurological dysfunction is called a seizure.

Epinephrine is the substance that causes blood vessels to constrict.

Epinurium refers to tough fibrous sheath covering the whole nerve.

Epithelial adaptation is the close approximation of the gingival epithelium to the tooth surface without the complete obliteration of the pocket.

Epithelial rests of Malassez are the remnants of Epithelial Hertwig's root sheath ie after the formation of radicular portion as the tooth elongates, the root sheath breaks up and begins to partially disappear and the remaining portion is termed as epithelial rests of Malassez.

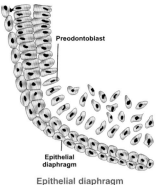

Epithelial diaphragm

Equine gait includes regular steps, gait is due to paralysis of pretibial and paroneal muscles. There develops a slapping noise as foot strikes the floor.

Er, Cr:YSGG and Er:YAG lasers
Er,Cr:YSGG (2790 nm) has an active medium of a solid crystal of yttrium – scandium-gallium-garnet that is doped with erbium and chromium. Er:YAG (2940 nm) has an active medium of a solid crystal of yttrium-Al-Garnet that is doped with erbium. Both are delivered fiber optically in the free running pulsed mode. The fibers are air-cooled and have a larger diameter than the other lasers mentioned, making the delivery system somewhat less flexible. They have the highest absorption in water of any dental wave length and have a high affinity for hydroxyapatite .These lasers are ideal for caries removal and tooth preparation when used with a water spray.

Erb's palsy is a paralysis of arm due to the damage to cervical nerve roots 5th and 6th brachial plexus.

Erben's reflex is a slowing of pulse when head and trunk are forcibly bent forward. It shows vagal excitability.

Erg refers to unit of energy equivalent to 10×10^{-7} joules or 2.4×10^{-8} calories.

Ergonomics is the study of person's environment, his abilities and limitations.

Erogeneous zones are different external areas of body which are exceptionally sensitive to sexual stimulation including breasts, buttocks, thighs, ear lobules etc.

Erosion (soft tissue) is the term often used for breach of the epithelium in which there is little damage to the underlying lamina propria. Such lesions, if penetrating the epithelium only partially, usually have a red or red and yellow appearance. If they penetrate the full thickness of the epithelium, however, they are typically covered by a fibrinous exudate and may then have a yellowish appearance.

Erosion (Hard tissue) is a loss of tooth substance by a chemical process. There is no bacterial erosion. Smooth lesions with no chalkiness appear on labial and buccal surface of teeth. Proximal surfaces may also be eroded. It may affect the labial surfaces of anterior teeth; erosion may also involve the dentin. It may occur due to decalcification of tooth.

Erosive lichen planus is an erosive bullous lesion of lichen planus occur in severe form. It has been associated with drug therapy and reaction to dental restorations. The association between erosive lichen planus and squamous cell carcinoma remains controversial. To start it will start as vesicles or bullae. There is formation of vesicles, bullae, irregular shallow ulcers of oral mucosa. Biopsy is needed for correct diagnosis. Treatment of choice is of tropical ointment.

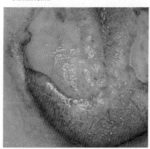
Erosive lichen planus

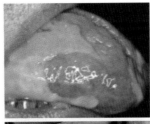

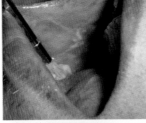

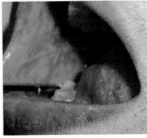

Erosive lichen planus

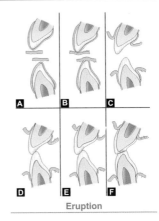

Eruption

Eruption cyst is a cyst that is found in the soft site around the crown of an erupting tooth.

Eruption refers to migration of tooth into functional position (*see* Figure).

Eruption sequestrum is a tiny irregular sequel of bone overlying the crown of an erupting permanent molar just following eruption of tips of the cusps. On X-ray it appears as tiny irregular opacity which lies over central occlusal fossa.

Erythema induratum is a type of panniculitis. Lesions appear as erythematous, slightly tender nodules. Skin over nodule ulcerates. Caseation necrosis is to identify lesion. Granuloma is observed in the septae. Gradually fibrosis sets in.

Erythema migrans tongue in it there is recurrence appearance and disappearance of red areas on tongue. Its cause is unknown. An irregular, smooth, red area appears with a sharply defined edge. It remains for a few days and then heal. Soreness may be psycogenic. There is thinning of epithelium.

Erythema multiformae is an acute dermatitis of unknown etiology. It is a non viral condition. It can affect skin and submucosa separately or in combination. It occurs chiefly in young adults. Individual symptoms vary in size. In skin central vesicle is surrounded by concentric erythematous skin colored rings. Ulcers are painful and most commonly located on lips, tongue and buccal mucosa. A concentric ring like appearance of lesions looks like bull's eyes. The hyperaemic macular, papules or vesicles may become eroded or ulcerated and bleed freely.

Erythematous candidiasis is a poorly understood condition associated with corticosteroids, topic or systemic broad spectrum or HIV disease. It is generally seen on the dorsum of tongue, palate or buccal mucosa. There may be associated or angular candidiasis.

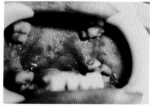

Erythematous candidiasis

Erythroblastosis fetalis is a clinical condition where Rh incompatibility occurs due to destruction of fetal blood that results in congenital hemolytic anemia. Some infants may be stillborn. Jaundice, edema and compensatory erythropoiesis may develop. Blood pigment may be seen in the enamel and dentin of developing teeth. One can see green, blue or brown line. Strain is intrinsic. No treatment for teeth stain is necessary. Erythroblastosis fetalis is actually a congenital anemia due to Rh incompatibility. It results due to the destruction of fetal RBC. Oral manifestations includes: discoloration of milk tooth, Enamel hypoplasia, Defect in tooth crowns also known as Rh hump.

Erythromelalgia is a paroxysmal bilateral vasodialatory disorder of unknown etiology. Symptoms include erythema, warmth and bilateral burning pain lasting minutes to hours on feet and palms. Relief may be given by cooling and elevating the limbs.

Erythromycin is a potent antibiotic which is active against gram positive organisms. Gram negative bacteria except hemophilus influenza all are resistant. Clindamycin is better tolerated. Better it is used in upper respiratory tract infections.

Erythroplakia is a lesion of oral mucosa presenting as bright red, velvety plaque which cannot be classified as any other disease. It is less common than white lesion leukoplakia. Several clinical variant have been described. It develops in an elderly age group. Biopsy is needed. After removing the irritant toludine blue staining should be done. A lesion that stains is likely to be precancerous in nature.

Eschapyramidal signs and symptoms includes movement and posture disturbances resulting from disorders of basal ganglia and cerebellum. It includes ataxia, athetosis, dysarthria, dystonia and muscle rigidity and spasticity.

Eschar refers to a slough produced by burning or corrosive application.

Escharotics are the corrosive which can produce sloughing.

Esophagitis is a condition that is extremely common in symptomatic HIV patient. Symptoms include odynophagia, dysphagia, chest pain, heart burn, fever and abdominal pain. Anorexia, fever and white lesions on tongue will develop.

Essential fatty acids are selective in promotion of growth as well as the maintenance of dermal integrity i.e. Linoleic, Linolenic and Arachidonic acid. These are present in vegetable oils in large quantities than in animal fats. Phrenoderma is attributed to essential fatty acid. The disease characterized by horny popular eruption on the posterior and lateral aspect of limbs, back and buttocks.

Esthetic refers to appearance.

Etch refers to treating enamel with 37% of phosphoric acid to provide retention for resin sealants.

Etchant refers to acid solution to etch tooth structure.

Etched porcelain veneers are aesthetic porcelain facings that are placed on anterior teeth.

Etching process involves the use of 30 to 50% phosphoric acid which is applied to pits and fissures to seal. Acid removes inorganic materials and creates tiny crevices or micropores into which sealant material can flow. Mechanical bonding is the force which holds the sealant to the enamel.

Ethical dilemma is a situation that includes, two or more important opposing ethical principles.

Ethics refer to rules of morals, principles and rules governing standards.

Ethnographic research refers to the type of research whose purpose is to develop an in depth picture of the culture of a group.

Ethyl alcohol is an antiseptic that is used on skin and kills vegetative forms of bacteria. It is in effective against spores. It is effective in concentration of 50 to 70% by weight. In higher concentrations it is less effective.

Ethylene oxide is a room temperature gas used to sterilized instruments and equipment.

European system (Conservative) systems, that is used for diagnosing pit and fissure caries, which consists of certain conservative criteria's, was described by Backer-Dirks O., Houwink B., and Kwant, C.W., in 1961. Description of the system: In upper molars, the mesio-occlusal and disto-occlusal-palative fissures are assessed seperatively. In lower molars, the occlusal fissures and the buccal pits are assessed separately. Teeth are dried, sharp new explorer are used for assessment Caries is diagnosed in four categories: C. I - Minute black line at base of fissure, C. II - In addition, a white zone along margins of fissure [dark in transmitted light), C. III - The smallest perceptible break in the continuity of the enamel, C. IV - Large cavity more than 3 mm wide

Eustachian tube is the tube extending from inside the ear to the throat to equalize air pressure.

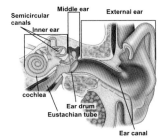

Eustachian tube

Eutectic is an alloy or solution whose components are proportioned to the melting point which is the lowest possible for those components.

EVA system is the most efficient system used for the correction of overhanging and overcontoured proximal alloy and resin restoration.

Evidenced based dentistry is an oral health care that requires judicious integration of systemic assessment of clinically relevant scientific evidence about patient's oral and medical condition.

Ewing's sarcoma is a highly malignant neoplasm with destructive lesion of bone. Tumor may arise from undifferentiated cells of reticuloendothelial system. It develops in very young age. Pain develops of an intermittent nature. Swelling of bone is noted. Facial neuralgia, lip paresthesia. Low grade fever is seen. Radiographs shows formation of layers of new bone giving an onion peel appearance. Osteophyte formation may be seen. Some cases may show sunray appearance. Neoplasm is radiosensitive clinically. It develops between 5 to 25 years. Mandible is affected more than maxilla. Patient develops fever, leukocytosis, ESR is raised. Jaw bone is expanded. Mobility of tooth is a common feature. Neoplasm develop surface ulcer. There is radiolucent area with ill defined margins. Periosteum shows lamellar layering. Radiotherapy and chemotherapy is the line of treatment (*see* Figure).

Excavators are sharp double ended hand instruments. These are used to remove carious dentine. Spoon like cutting edges are having oval outline.

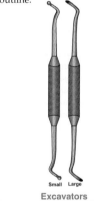

Small   Large

Excavators

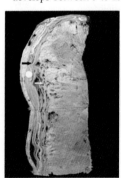

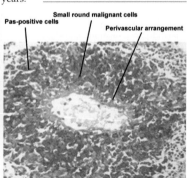

Pas-positive cells   Small round malignant cells   Perivascular arrangement

Ewing's sarcoma

Excimer lasers (the name is derived from the terms excited and dimers) use reactive gases, such as chlorine and fluorine, mixed with inert gases such as argon, krypton or xenon. When electrically stimulated, a pseudo molecule (dimer) is produced. When lased, the dimer produces light in the ultra violet range.

Excisional biopsy refers to the removal of entire lesion plus some adjacent normal tissue.

Excisional new attachment procedure (ENAP) is a technique developed by U.S Naval Dental Corps and is a definitive subgingival curettage procedure performed with a knife.

Excoriation is a chemical skin injury

Excursive movement refers to any movement away from ICP.

Exercise electrocardiography is done to confirm diagnosis of angina and to determine severity of limitation of activity due to angina. It is useful to evaluate response of therapy. It may also be used to screen asymptomatic population for silent coronary disease.

Exercise tests is the measure of the performance of a controlled physical task with increasing workload physical task with increasing work load to examine a person's maximal physical capacity.

Exfoliate refers to shed.

Exfoliative cytology is a type of biopsy procedure that is widely used for the diagnosis of carcinoma of uterine cervix. These days for oral cancer, cytology are done because it is quick, simple, painless and blood less procedure. It helps to confirm false negative biopsies or where biopsy is not desirable.

Exhaustion psychosis is a condition that results from exhaustion of nervous system in older people. Insomnia, dyspepsia, anorexia, loss of physical activity, irritability, altered power of hearing occurs. Patient loses self interest. Self control and memory deteriorates. Later on mental confusion and depression occurs.

Exhumation is a lawful digging out of a buried body from the grave. It is necessary to identify the dead body or to determine the cause of death in a doubtful case. Only a magistrate can issue order for this.

Exocrine glands are the glands that secrete their products into ducts that empty onto a surface or into a cavity.

Exodontia is the area of dental practice which deals with removal or extraction of teeth.

Exodontics is the science and practice of removing teeth.

Exogenous intrinsic stains refers to those stains are present within the tooth substance but come from an outside source and not from within the tooth itself, such stains present themselves as exogenous intrinsic stain.

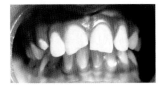

Exogenous intrinsic stains due to use of obturating material

Exogenous malodour refers to halitosis at other times of the day is often the consequence of eating various foods such as garlic, onion or spices (in curries), durian, cabbage, brussels sprouts, cauliflower, radish or habits such as smoking or drinking alcohol. Avoidance of these foods and habits is the best means of prevention.

Exostoses are the outgrowths of bone of varied size and shape. They can appear as small nodule, large nodule, sharp ridges, spike like projections or any combination of above.

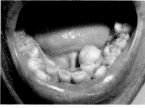

Exostoses

Exothermic refers to heat releasing.

Exotoxins are both gram positive and gram negative bacteria that secrete exotoxins. Exotoxins are polypeptides. These are highly toxic. These are good antigens and induce synthesis of antitoxin useful in disease like tetanus.

Expansion appliance refers to the type of fixed or removable appliance that is used for the expansion of the constricted arch.

Experimental epidemiology refers to the study of epidemics among colonies of experimental animals such as rat/mice.

Experimental research in which at least one independent variable is subject to controlled manipulation.

Experimental study means research officer controls the condition.

Explanatory stroke is a vertical motion performed by probes and explorer to detect calculus, pocket depth, caries and the general contour of tooth surfaces.

Explanatory theory refers to the one which examines the why and how questions that undergrid a problem.

Explorer refers to a hand instruments used to locate caries as well as hard deposits. These are available in various size and shapes for the variety of uses.

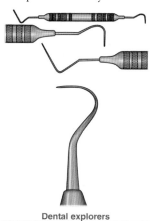

Dental explorers

Exposure button is a component of dental X-ray machine control panel, activates the dental X-ray machine to produce X-rays.

Exposure light is a component of dental X-ray machine control panel providing a visible signal when X-rays are produced.

Exposure refers to a measure of ionization produced by radiation in air.

Exposure time refers to the time interval during which X-rays are produced.

Expressed consent refers to the permission given in written or verbal form.

Extended shank curettes are the modification of standard Gracey curettes. The terminal shank is 3 mm longer which allows the deeper penetration into deep periodontal pockets. The blades are also comparatively smoother and thinner to allow easy subgingival insertion.

External pin fixation is a method of achieving immobilization where extensive communition of the whole or the large part of mandible is required. The stainless steel or the titanium pins are inserted into each major bone fragment which diverge from each other but are connected by a cross bar which are attached to each pin by the mean of universal joints. They are mainly indicated for infected fracture line, for extensively communited fractures and for the treatment for bimaxillary fractures

External refers to the outer surface.

Exteroceptors are the pain receptors which are stimulated by the immediate external environment; with most of the impulses being sensed at conscious level, e.g. Free nerve ending – tactile and superficial pain. Krause's corpuscles are cold receptor, Meisssner's corpuscles are tactile skin receptors. Merkel's corpuscles are tactile receptor in the oral mucosa and sub mucosa of the tongue. Ruffini's corpuscles are pressure and warmth receptors

Extrachromosomal are the structures that are not part of chromosomes. DNA units in the cytoplasm that control cytoplasmic inheritance.

Extraction elevators are lever like instrument used for luxation of a tooth from its socket.

Extraoral refers to outside the mouth.

Extraoral film refers to type of dental X-ray film that is placed outside the mouth during X-ray exposure. These are used to examine large areas of skull or jaws.

Extripation refers to complete removal or eradication of pulp from the pulp chamber or root.

Extrusion is term given to migration of teeth in an incisal or occlusal direction

Exudates is the accumulation of material in a body cavity or on a body surface.

Eye strain headache refers to uncontrolled visual refractive error is present. Pain is relieved by proper spectacles.

Fabricated wounds refer of wounds that are produced by a person on his body or by another person with his consent. These are called fictious, forged or inverted wounds. Intention of these is to charge enemy with assault or attempted murder. Woman may inflict on her reproductive organs to bring a charge of rape.

Face mask is the disposable or non disposable item designed to protect the face from microorganisms. Although these masks are permeable to microorganisms, mask should ideally have at least 95% infiltration efficiency for particles 3 to 5 micro millimeter and should be changed for each patient. When dealing with TB patient mask with greater filtration capacity should be worn.

Facial hemiatrophy is a progressive atrophy of some or all tissues on one side of face. Exact cause is not known but it may be due to atrophic function of cervical sympathetic nervous system, trauma and hereditary. There may be hollowing of cheek and eyes may be depressed. Loss of facial hair is common. Hemiatrophy of lips and tongue is also reported.

Facial hemihypertrophy is a condition where exact etiology is not known but may be due to hormonal imbalance, incomplete turning and chromosomal abnormality. Familial occurrence has been reported in a few cases. Dentition of hypertrophic side is abnormal in regard to crown and root size and rate of development. On the developed side permanent teeth erupt before their counterpart. Tongue may be enlarged.

Facial nerve is the seventh cranial nerve having a medial motor root and a lateral sensory root. Sensory root carries taste fibres from anterior two third of tongue, floor of mouth and the palate. Motor root supplies muscles of face, scalp and auricle (*see* Figure on page 173).

Facial neuritis (Bell's palsy) results from the inflammation of facial nerve. Location is usually but not necessarily within facial canal. Taste aberration may also be seen. Angioneurotic edema may also put pressure on the nerve in facial canal to cause pain.

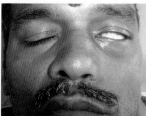
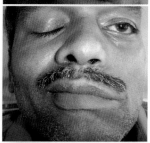
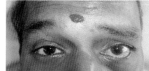

Facial neuritis

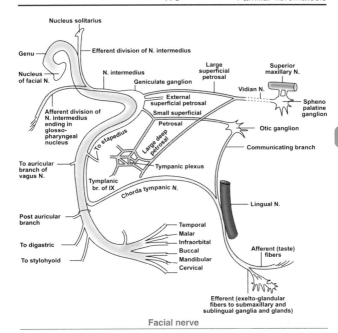

Facial nerve

Facial pain may occur due to maxillary sinusitis, neoplasia of maxilla, caries, dental abscess, atypical facial neuralgia, trigeminal neuralgia etc. Pain provoked by cold and hot is of dental origin.

Facial refers to the surface next to the face; the outer surface of a tooth resting against the cheeks or lips.

Factor analysis is a multi variate correlational technique used to reduce a large number of variables into a smaller number of factors clustering related variables.

Fainting is actually a loss of consciousness caused by reduced blood supply to the brain. It is known as syncope too. In most of the dental patient cause is psychological or due to fear of bleeding and pain.

Familial fibromatosis is kind of enlargement generally characterized by slowly progressive, non hemorrhagic enlargement of the maxillary and mandibular gingiva or may be localized to either jaw. Enlargement may be bilateral, thus the name, symmetrical gingival fibromatosis has been suggested by Wiktop, 1971, But since, the enlargement is not always symmetrical, the name was given as focal gingival fibromatosis. Gingiva are grossly enlarged and pink color, firm, lathery in consistency and a minutely rebelled surface. Secondary inflammatory changes may be present.

Fan sign is a component of Babniski's reflex. This sign refers to the spreading apart of patient's toes after his foot is firmly stroked.

Fastidious bacterium is a bacteria that is difficult to isolate or grow in the laboratory owing to its complex nutritional requirement.

Fat soluble vitamins are not excreted when consumed in excess; rather these are stored in liver and adipose tissue. These can be toxic when consumed in large doses over a long time specially vitamin A and vitamin D. Deficiency of fat soluble vitamins occurs in malabsorption syndromes, pancreatic and biliary diseases. Fat soluble vitamins include Vitamin A, D, E and K.

Fatal dose of snake venom – 12 mg of dried Cobra venom and 15 mg of Daboi venom is fatal. Average dry weight of lyophilized venom in one bite was 0.2 gm from a cobra, 0.15 gm from a russel viper, 0.022 gm from krait and 0.0046 gm from echis carinata.

Fats contain carbon, hydrogen and oxygen padding around the organs and keep them in place. It protects nerve. Fat insulates body avoiding rapid change of body temperature. It carries vitamin A, D, E and K. Fats are concentrated source of calories each gram giving 9 calories.

Fatty acids are of two types. Saturated fatty acids are palmitic acid, stearic acid and chidic acid. While unsaturated fatty acids are oleic acid, linoleic acid, linolenic acid and arachidonic acid. Saturated fatty acids are harmful to heart.

Fatty liver is a mild injury due to changes in metabolic activity of hepatocytes. It is seen more on occasional drinking. Liver is enlarged, pale or yellowish in color. Microscopically central and mid zones are involved more. Variable fatty change of hepatocytes gives vacuolated appearance.

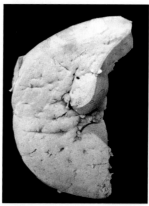

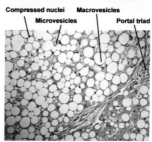

Fatty liver

Favorable fractures are the one where the vertical fracture or the horizontal fracture lines are unopposed by the action of the muscle around them. However, these types of fractures are easier to reduce and stabilize.

F-distribution is a distribution of squared t statistics, the basis of analysis of variance.

Febrile refers to pertaining to fever.

Febrile seizures refers to the type of seizure , those occurring after the age of one month these are associated with a febrile illness not caused by CNS infection. These occur without previous unprovoked or neonatal seizures. These may be generalized or partial.

Feeble mindedness refers to those kind of people who are better than imbecile but are still incapable of protecting themselves, hence require care and supervision. They don't show any physical defect. They are frequently impulsive as regards sexual acts, murders and assaults.

Female ejaculation is not a correct term used for secretion of lubricating fluid by glands adjacent to vagina during sexual stimulation. As sexual stimulation and excitement build up the flow of lubricating fluid increases. In certain cases sudden contraction of vaginal wall causes fluid to spurt which is commonly mistaken as female discharge.

Fenestration can be described as the isolated areas in which the root is denuded of bone and the root surface is only covered by periosteum and overlying gingiva along with the intact marginal bone.

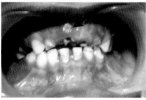

Fenestration

Fergusson gag It is an adjustable prop. used to force open the mouth and keep the jaws apart.

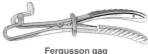

Fergusson gag

Fermentation is a process that occurs without oxygen. It is an anerobic biochemical pathway in which substances are broken down and energy + reduced compounds are produced. It also refers procedures like making curd out of milk. Another example could be making idli, rice is to be fermented. Here microorganisms multiply with great rapidity. Enzymes acts in the starch present producing carbon dioxide.

Festinating gait is a type of gait that is peculiar to Parkinsonism. Arms are flexed in front of the body. Legs are stiff and bent at hips and knees. Steps are short and shuffling. The upper part of body advances ahead of lower

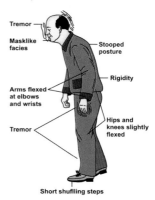

Festinating gait seen in parkinsonism

part. Patient can run better than walking. Patient bents forwards and advances with rapid, short and shuffling gait. Arms don't swing. When pulled he may walk backwards.

Fetishism is a psychosexual disorder in which sexual gratification is repeatedly or exclusively achieved through fondling, kissing or licking inanimate objects such as women's bra, hair, undergarments etc. Handling these objects is often accompanied by sexual fantasies and masturbation.

Fever hypoplasia refers to a linear alteration of enamel that may be manifest as the result of a febrile episode during the chronological point in tooth development such that the distribution of enamel changes will vary between teeth at different stages of crown formation. Some studies have indicated that the exanthematous diseases, including measles, chickenpox and scarlet fever are etiological factors. In general, it might be stated that any systemic disease is potentially capable of producing enamel hypoplasia, since the ameloblasts are one of the most sensitive groups of cells in the body in terms of metabolic function. The type of hypoplasia occurring from these disease states is usually of the pitting variety. Clinical studies indicate that most cases of enamel hypoplasia involve those teeth that form within the first year after birth.

Fiber reinforced denture base material is a material used for fabricating dentures. It has high stiffness, very good impact strength and good fatigue life. it gives good surface finish. Disadvantage is of poor color and poor surface.

Fibre optic transillumination (FOTI) is an advanced diagnostic aid that has been designed for the detection of approximal caries by Freidman and Marcus in 1970. The principle of transillumination is that there is a different index of light transmission for decayed and sound tooth structure. Illumination is delivered by means of fibre optics from the light source to the tooth structure. The resultant changes in light distribution as the light traverses the tooth are then recorded as an image for analysis. Since tooth decay has a lower index of light transmission than the sound tooth structure, an area of decay shows up as a darkened shadow that follows the decay along the path of dentinal tubules.

Fibre refers to the thread like structure. The walls of every cell are composed of fibre. It is more abundant on outer sides of seeds, fruits, peas and beans. Daily requirement of fibre is 6 gram.

Fibrin is the main fibrous protein in a blood clot.

Fibro sarcoma is a malignant soft tissue neoplasm of an old age. It tends to invade locally producing a fleshy, bulky lesion. Great variation occurs. There is proliferation of fibroblasts and formation of collagen and reticulin fibers. Cells are spindle shaped with elongated nuclei. Mitotic figures are common. Radical surgical excision is done.

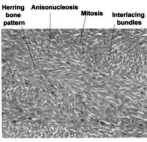

Fibro sarcoma

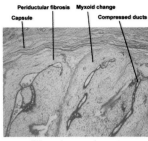

Fibroadenoma breast

Fibrocytes are the mature form of fibroblasts. Their Quantity increases with maturity of the pulp and their primary function is the maintenance of collagen fibres (*see* Figure).

Fibroadenoma breast is a common benign neoplasm of younger age. It is a round or ovoid rubbery, discrete, movable non tender mass, 1-5 cm in diameter. It does not occur after menopause. Excision helps.

Fibroma is the most common benign soft tissue neoplasm. It is an elevated lesion of normal color. It is well circumscribed, smooth and pedunculated about 1-2 cm in diameter. It may be firm and nodular and might be soft in nature, when infected superficial ulceration may be seen. Soft fibroma are spongy otherwise may be hard fibroma. Conservative surgical excision may help (*see* Figure on page 177).

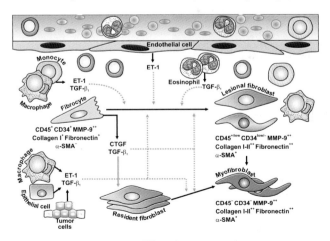

Fibrocytes

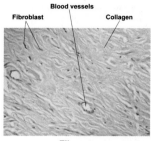

Fibroma

Fibromatosis gingivae is a diffuse fibrous overgrowth of gingival tissues. It is dense, diffuse, smooth or nodular overgrowth of gingiva. Tissues are not inflamed. As there is no inflammation, haemorrhage takes place. Crowns of teeth look hidden. It may require surgical correction due to cosmetic purpose.

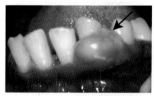

Fibromatosis gingivae

Fibromyalgia affects about 2% adults and is a condition causing increased sensitivity to pain in many parts of body. These are especially sensitive to touch and pressure. Other symptoms include fatigue, sleep disturbance, stiffness, depression and anxiety.

Fibrosarcoma develop from fibroblast cells. It commonly arises from cheek, tongue, gingive and floor of mouth. Among the jaw lesions mandible is most commonly involved. To start it is asymptomatic. Soon it enlarges into a large, painful fleshy mass. Lesion is firm and indurated. These are not capsulated tumors. Radiograph shows sharply defined radiolucent area. Radical surgery+chemotherapy is the treatment of choice.

Fibrosseous integration can be described as relationship between endosseous implants and bone in which soft tissue such as fibers or the cells are interposed between the two surfaces.

Fibrotic pocket wall is said to be occurred where there is relative predominance of newly formed connective tissue cells, fibers and the pocket wall is more firm and pink.

Fibrous dysplasia is lesion of bone developed as a result of abnormal proliferation of fibrous tissue. As lesion matures it destroys trabeculae. Radiographs in early stage will show radiolucent lesion. Intermediate lesion will be smoky, mottled or hazy pattern. Intense aggregations will be distributed throughout lesion. In mature stage, picture will be of salt and pepper type, ground glass or orange peel appearance. It may result in irregularity of bone without pain. There may also be malocclusion (*see* Figure on page 179).

Fibrous epulis is a pain free swelling on the gum. There is a firm, pedunculated or sessile mass. It is of the same color as the adjacent gingiva. Biopsy confirms the diagnosis.

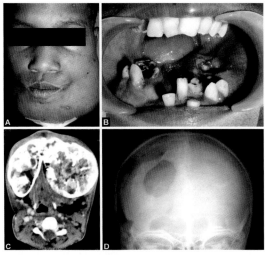

Fibrous dysplasia: (A) Extraoral view of fibrous dysplasia, (B) Intraoral view of fibrous dysplasia showing displacement of teeth causing malocclusion, (C) CT scan section of fibrous dysplasia, (D) Radiograph showing polyostotic lesions of fibrous dysplasia of skull

Fibrous gingival hyperplasia refers to gingival enlargement where often single papilla or several papillae will be enlarged. Sometimes inflammatory changes are superimposed on the fibrous hyperplasia. Chronic low grade irritation of gingival tissue can result in localized hyperplasia of fibrous tissue. Treatment includes removal of local irritation.

Fibrous hyperplasia is the commonest tissue reaction to chronically ill fitting denture. There is development of elongated rolls of tissue in the mucobuccal fold. It is slow in development. Inflammatory fibrous hyperplasia is to be surgically excised.

Fibrous nodule refer Fibroma.

Field block is a method of obtaining anesthesia by injecting the anesthetic agent solution close to large terminal nerve branches. More circumscribed, most often involving one tooth and the tissues surrounding it.

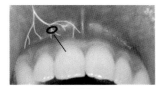

Field block

Fifth branchial arch refers to the fifth arch which is a transitory structure that disappears, almost as soon as it forms and bequeaths no permanents structural elements (see Figure on page 180).

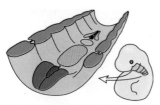

Fifth pharyngeal arch and pouch

F

Fifth pharyngeal pouch appears as a diverticulum of the fourth pouch. The endoderm of the fifth pouch forms the ultimobranchial body. The calcitonin secreting cells of this structure, however, are derived from neural crest tissue and are eventually incorporated into the thyroid gland. The laryngeal ventricles could present the remnants of fifth pharyngeal pouch.

Figure eight suture is also a type of interdental ligation where the suture given is in the shape of eight hence the name and is indicated the two flaps are not in close apposition to each other.

Filament circuit is the circuit that regulates the flow of electric current to the filament of X-ray tube.

Filariasis is caused by two species Wuchereria bancrofti and Brugia Malayi. Microfilariac mature in lymph nodes and rarely produce visible damage. Lymphadenopathy is characteristic but not diagnostic. Scrotal swelling is due to Wuchereria bancrofti. Allergic manifestations are due to toxic metabolites released by worm. Incubation period is one year. Acute stage shows fever with inflammation of lymphatic vessels and swelling of affecting part of body. Fever subsides but swelling persists. In chronic stage typical elephantiasis develops. Swollen part becomes thick and rugose/papillomatous.

Files are periodontal instruments which have series of blades on the base and their main purpose is to fracture or crush the tenacious calculus. As files can

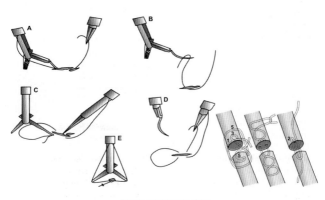

Figure eight suturing

gouge easily and roughen the root surface if used improperly, therefore these are not the ideal instruments for fine scaling.

Filling refers to a restoration placed on a tooth to restore its function and appearance.

Film badge is a device to measure and monitor radiation exposure worn by persons frequently exposed to radiation.

Film hanger is a stainless steel device equipped with clips used to hold films during manual processing.

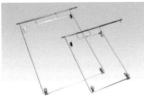

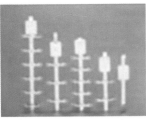

Film hanger

Film mount refers to a card board, plastic or vinyl holder used to support and arranges dental radiographs in anatomic order.

Film over exposed is an exposure error resulting in dark film due to excessive exposure to X-ray time, kilovoltage or milliamperage or a combination of these.

Film speed is the sensitivity of film to radiation exposure.

Final diagnosis is a diagnosis based on clinical laboratory data or biopsy analysis.

Fine needle aspiration cytology (FNAC) is a convenient and expeditious means of differentiating cyst from solid tumors and getting cytological specimen. It is performed with a 21 gauge needle fitted to a 10 ml syringe.

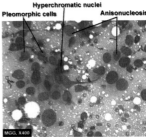

Pleomorphic cells — Hyperchromatic nuclei — Anisonucleosis
MGG, X400

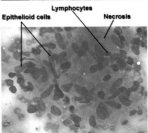

Epithelioid cells — Lymphocytes — Necrosis

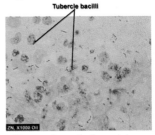

Tubercle bacilli
ZN, X1000 Oil

Fine needle aspiration cytology (FNAC)

Fine particle composite resins contain fine sized filler particles of 0.5 to 3 micro mm. It is more polishable than micro filled composites.

Finger nail artifact is a film handling error, a black finger print when the film has been touched by fingers contaminated with developer.

Finger prints and ridges The surface of the palms, fingers, soles, and toes are marked by series of ridges and grooves. They appear either as straight lines or as a pattern or loops and whorls, as on the tips of the digits. These epidermal ridges develop during the third and fourth fetal months as the epidermis conforms to the contours of the underlying dermal papillae of the papillary region. The ridges increase the surface area of the epidermis and thus function to increase the grip of the hand or foot by increasing friction. Because the ducts of sweat pores, the sweat and ridges from fingerprints (or footprints) when a smooth object is touched. The ridge pattern is genetically determined and is unique for each individual. Normally, the ridge pattern does not change during life, except to enlarge, and thus can serve as the basis for identification. Comparing the structural features of the papillary and reticular region of the dermis.

Finger rest stabilizes the hand and the instrument by providing a firm fulcrum as movements are made to activate the instrument, this helps in preventing injury and laceration to the gingiva oc-curring due to poorly controlled movements. The fourth/ring finger is most commonly used as rest. The finger rest are of two types: the intraoral rest and the extra oralrest.

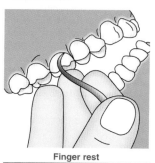

Finger rest

Finger sweep is an insertion of index finger into mouth along the inside of the cheek deep into throat to the base of the tongue.

Finger-on-finger rest is established on the index finger or thumb of the non operating hand

Finishing disks are small abrasive disks of sand paper used to contour and polish various restorations.

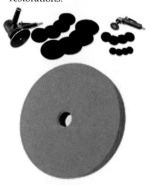

Finishing disk

First branchial arch is the first mandibular pair of branchial arches the precursor of the jaws, both maxillary and mandibular and appropriately bound the lateral aspects of the stomodeum which at this stage is merely a depression in the early facial region. The maxilla is derived from a small maxillary prominence extending cranio-ventrally from the much larger mandibular prominence derived from the first arch. The cartilage skeleton of the first arch known as Meckel's cartilage, arises at the 41st to 45th day providing a template for subsequent development of the mandible but most of its cartilage substance disappears in the formed mandible. The mental ossicler is the only potion of the mandible derived from marked cartilage by endochondral ossification. Persisting portions of Meckel's cartilage from the basis of major portions of two ear ossicles, the head and neck of the maleus, the body and short crus of the incus and two ligaments, the anterior ligament of the malleus and Sphenomandibular ligament. The musculature of the mandibular arch is subdivided and migrates to form: The muscles of mastication, mylohyoid muscle, anterior belly of the digastric, Tensor tympani, Tensor Veli Palatini muscles all of which are innervated by the nerve of the first arch, i.e. the mandibular division of the Vth cranial or trigeminal nerve.

First degree burns are limited only to the most superficial layers of epidermis and heal sponta-neously within 7 days because of abundance of epithelial cells which regenerate very fast. So this healing is by regeneration only and does not leave any scars.

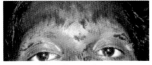
First degree burn

First pharyngeal pouch is obliterated by the developing tongue. The dorsal diverticulum deepens laterally as the tubotympanic recess to form the auditory tube, widening at its end into the tympanum or middle ear cavity separated from the first branchial groove by the tympanic membrane. The tympanum occupied by the dorsal ends of the cartilages of the first and second branchial arches develop into the ear ossicles. The tympanum maintains contact with the pharynx via the auditory tube throughout life. The proximal portion of the expanding and elongating auditory tube becomes lined with respiratory mucous membrane and fibrous tissue and cartilage form in its walls. Chondrification occurs in the 4th month of influence. From four centre in the adjacent mesoderm growth of the cartilaginous portion of the tube

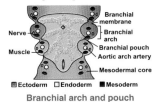

Branchial membrane

Nerve — Branchial arch

Branchial pouch

Muscle — Aortic arch artery

Mesodermal core

▨ Ectoderm   ▢ Endoderm   ▬ Mesoderm

Branchial arch and pouch

is greatest between 16 and 28 weeks intrauterine. These after increase in tubal length is primarily in the osseous portion of the tube. The changing location of the opening of the auditory tube reflects the growth of the nasopharynx. The tubal orifice is inferior to the hard palate in the fetus, is at level it at birth, and well above the hard palate in the adult.

First transitional period is characterized by the emergence of the first permanent molars and the exchange of the deciduous incisors with the permanent incisors.

Fissure is defined as deep clefts between adjoining cusps. They provide area for retention of caries producing agents. These defects occur on occlusal surfaces of the molars and premolars, with tortuous configuration that are difficult to assess from the surfaces. These areas are impossible to keep clean and highly susceptible to advancement of the carious lesion (Orbans, 1990).

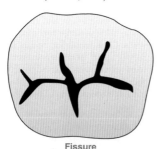

Fissure

Fissure sealant is a material that is placed in the pits and fissures of teeth in order to prevent or arrest the development of dental caries.

Fissure sealing is a procedure done to seal the occlusal fissures. Occlusal fissures are natural stagnation areas where caries occurs. In the past fissure filling was done using amalgam. In it one has to cut a cavity in sound enamel. But new glass isonomer cement allows fissure sealing to be done without any cavity preparation.

Fistula is an abnormal opening between an internal structure and the surface of body.

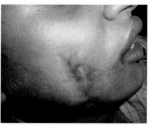

Parotid fistula

Fixation of film is a procedure done to fix a film, i.e. when fixer solution removes the unexposed under developed silver halide crystals from the film emulsion.

Fixed drug eruption is the lesion which appears at same site each time a drug is taken. Reaction subsides when the drug is discontinued. Reaction causes vasculitis and subsequent damage to the vessel wall giving rise to erythema and edema of superficial layers of skin and mucosa.

Fixed functional appliances are those appliances that are fitted on the teeth by the operator and cannot be removed by the patients.

Fixed habit breakers are the fixed appliance that helps in breaking the deleterious habit of the child. Heavy gauge stainless steel wires are designed to form a frame that is soldered to bands on the molars.

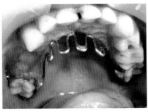

Fixed habit breaking appliance

Fixer spots refer to a chemical contamination error white spots appear on film as a result of fixer solution contacting the film before processing.

Flap surgery is a procedure used for deep periodontal pockets to remove the diseased lining of the periodontal pocket and the marginal gingiva.

Flash refers to the excess material that extrudes beyond the intended margins of a restoration.

Flat foot in the young child the foot appears to be flat because of the pressure of a large amount of subcutaneous fat on the sole. Otherwise medial margin of foot from heal to the first metatarsal head is arched above the ground because of medial longitudinal arch. Medial longitudinal arch consists of calcaneum, the talus navicular bone and three cuneiform bones and the first three metatarsal. Flat foot person is not able to run fast for long.

Flatus is a gas which is formed in the intestine and released from rectum.

Florescence refers to emit visible light in the blue or green spectrum.

Florid osseous dysplasia is a disease of disordered cementum and bone development. Radiopaque masses may involve multiple quadrants. Cause is not known. No treatment is indicated.

Floss is thinner than dental tap and passes more easily in between teeth. The wax coating on dental floss helps make passing floss through the contact area easily. Polytetrafluoro ethylene floss is made of Gore-Tex type of material and it slips easily and resists fraying.

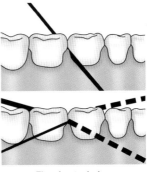

Flossing technique

Flow is a plastic deformation that occurs while the material is setting and in the process of developing its final strength.

Fluorescence is the emission of light by an object at different wave lengths. Dental porcelains are also fluorescent under ultraviolet light.

Fluorescence microscopy is used in immunology. It employs the principles of emission of a different wavelength of light each wavelength strikes a fluorescent object.

Fluoride electrode coupled with standard pH meter is the most recent and universally acceptable fluoride estimation method. Fluoride electrodes of different make such as Orion (Model 94-09). Radiometer (Model F 1052 F fluoride electrode) are available. This method allows fluoride in aqueous solutions to be measured quickly simply, economically and accurately.

Fluoride mouth rinse is done weekly rather than monthly, some recommended on daily basis for limited period. It reduces caries by 20 to 30% and are inexpensive.

Fluoride probe is a computerised periodontal probe consisting of a probe, handpiece, a digital readout, a foot switch and a computer. It is used to measure the pocket depth and has a high degree of accuracy.

Fluoride refers to topical application of a gel or liquid that prevents decay.

Fluoride tablets are effective means of fluoridation that act both systematically and topically at different times of tooth eruption. Guidelines for their use have been laid down by Joyston-Bactal with the recommended dosage being: 6 months to 2 yrs-0.25 mg, 3 Yrs to 4 yrs - 0.50 mg, Above 4 yrs - 1.0 mg.

Fluoride toothpaste is a method of topical fluoridation. Most of the tooth pastes now a days contains fluoride to prevent caries. Only a pea sized amount of tooth paste is used but it has to be kept in mouth. It should not be rinsed out immediately after brushing.

Fluoride varnish is a preventive procedure in which highly concentrated varnish is painted over teeth. Semiannual application is sufficient.

Fluorides topical are the ones where fluorides applied in direct contact of teeth through mouth rinses and tropical fluoride application.

Fluorine is an essential element, about 95% of fluoride in the body is found in bones and teeth. It is essential for formation of dental enamel. Drinking water contains 0.5 mg/L but in endemic areas of fluorosis water contains 3 to 12 mg of fluoride. Sea fish, cheese and tea are rich in fluorides. 0.5 to 0.8/L in water is considered safe limit in our country. Deficiency of it leads to dental caries.

Fluoroscopy is a form of radiography in which image is displayed in real time.

Fluorosis leads to a permanent damage to the enamel, which consists of white or brown spots that appear on the children's teeth. When fluoride reaches the cells, which make enamel, ameloblasts, become poisoned. As they degenerate they lay down irregular enamel. Instead of the regular hydroxyapatite, they will produce mottled, porous and thin enamel. As the poisoning worsens the enamel may even be absent. At the same time the enamel is being mottled other hard and ligament tissues are being affected as well. Fluorosis also refers to discoloration of the enamel due to excessive fluoride absorption (greater than one 1 part per million) into the bloodstream, also called enamel mottling.

Fluorosis risk index (FRI) was introduced by David G. Fendrys, in 1990. The FRI, is designed to permit a more accurate identification of associations between age-specific exposures, fluoride sources and the development of enamel fluorosis. The FRI divides the enamel surfaces of the permanent dentition into two developmentally related groups surface zones, designated either as having begun - (I) formation during the first year of life ("Classification I") or (ii) formation during the third through sixth years of life ("Classification II).

Flush terminal plane is the mesiodistal relation between the distal surface of the upper and a lower second deciduous molar is called the terminal plane. A normal feature of deciduous dentition is to find a flush terminal plane where the distal surface of the upper and lower second deciduous molars are same in the same vertical plane.

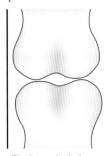

Flush terminal plane

Flushing is sudden redness of skin.

Flux is a substance that promotes the flow of solder over the metal parts by cleaning the surfaces and removing oxides during welding.

Focal dermal hypoplasia syndrome is an autosomal dominant disease. There is focal absence of dermis with herniation of subcutaneous fat into defects, skin atrophy and streaky pigmentation. Mental retardation is present. Papilloma of lip is a striking feature. Teeth are defective in size. Microdontia is common, cleft/lip/cleft palate may be seen.

Focal epithelial hyperplasia is a condition where lesion occurs primarily in lips and check. It is 0.1 to 0.4 cms. Flat, raised, whitish plaques are seen. Histologically local acanthosis is seen. Dyskeratosis is not present. Lesions may regress suddenly.

Fogged film is a processing error. It appears gray and lacks detail and contrast. Improper safelight in dark room may result it.

Folic acid was discovered in 1941. Word comes from folium means leaf. Folates are essential for synthesis of DNA. Richest source are liver, eggs and leafy vegetable. Commonest cause of nutritional anemia is folate deficiency especially in pregnancy hence 500 micro gram of folic acid is given to pregnant leady. Deficiency of it causes irritability, forgetfulness and mental sluggishness. 90% alcolics are said to suffer from it.

Fontanelles are the cartilages that bridge the gap between the bones. They are made up of dura mater, primitive periosteum and the aponeurosis from inside outwards. Fontanelles present at birth are Anterior fontanelle: between the two parietal bones and the frontal bone, Posterior fontanelle: between the two parietal bones and the occipital bone, Sphenoid fontanelle: between the fontal, parietal, temporal and the sphenoid bone, Mastoid fontanelle: between the parietal, occipital, temporal bone.

Food and caries Carbohydrate + bacteria → Acids (dental plaque) + susceptible tooth → Decay.

Foot and Mouth disease is a viral infection. Transmission is through contact person develops fever, nausea, vomiting and ulcerative lesions of oral mucosa. Lesions of oral mucosa may develop anywhere. Lesions begin as small vesicles which rapidly rupture and heal within 14 days.

Foramen refers to an opening in bone.

Force delivery refers to the force produced by an orthodontic wire against a tooth.

Force refers to change of state of rest or motion of a substance.

Fordyces Granules Normal oral mucosa contains many tubulo-acinar sebaceous glands in vermilion border of lip and buccal mucosa. Histologically these are similar with sebaceous glands except hair follicle as they contain lipase secretion. Function of Fordyces Granules is not known. They appear small, white submucosal plaques.

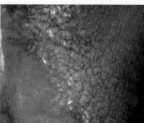

Fordyces granules of buccal mucosa

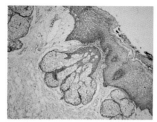

Histological view of Fordyces granules

Forensic dentistry is that branch of dentistry that relates and applies dental facts to legal problems, dental identification, malpractice, litigation and dental licensure.

Formaldehyde is a highly toxic irritant gas which precipitates and destroys protein. It is effective against vegetable bacteria, fungi and viruses. It is used to disinfect rooms. In addition it can be used to disinfect blankets, beds, books and other articles which cannot be boiled.

Forward decay refers to a type of lesion where the caries starts in the enamel and then it involve the dentin i.e. wherever the caries in enamel is larger than in dentin.

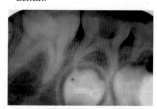

Forward decay

Fossa refers to a shallow depression on the lingual (tongue) surfaces of some front teeth (*see* Figure on page 189).

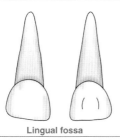

Lingual fossa

Foster miller probe is a diagnostic probe that determines pocket depth along with detection of CEJ from where level of clinical attachment level is automatically detected.

Four handed dentistry is the delivery of the dental treatment by the dentist and assistant working together at chair side.

Fourth branchial arch the cartilage of this arch probably forms the thyroid cartilage. The arch muscles develop into the cricothyroid and constrictors of the pharynx, the palatoglossus muscle of the muscles of the soft palate and the palatoglossus muscle of tongue. The nerve of the fourth arch is superior laryngeal branch of the vagus (Xth cranial nerve), which innervates these muscles. The fourth arch artery of the left side forms the arch of the aorta, that of the right side contribute to the right subclavian and branchocephalic arteries. The para aortic bodies of chromaffin cells that secrete noradrenaline arise from the ectomesenchyme of the fourth and sixth branchial arches.

Fourth degree burns refers to a type of burn where the damage extends beyond the skin till muscle, fascia or bone. However,

this is not a universally accepted term and is not used.

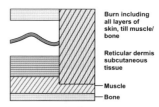

Burn including all layers of skin, till muscle/bone

Reticular dermis subcutaneous tissue

– Muscle
– Bone

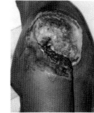

Line diagram of clinical section of fourth degree burn

Fourth pharyngeal pouch the fate of the endoderm of the ventral diverticulum is uncertain; the lining membrane may contribute to thyhmus or thyroid tissue.

Fracture of teeth is a cause of sudden severe trauma such as fall, blow or road accident. There are several classifications of fractured teeth. If crown is fractured but pulp is maintained the teeth remains alive. There may not be severe pain. Tooth may be sore and slightly loose. Fractured crown exposing pulp is more serious. Pulpotomy or pulpectomy may be required.

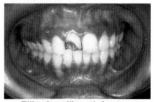

Ellis class III tooth fracture

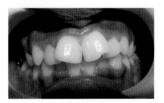
Ellis class I fracture

F

Fracture refers to the breach in continuity.

Fracture stress strength is a limit of applied force which a material can withstand without fracture. It is the strength of material. The stress at fracture is normally used to characterize the strength of a material.

Fracture toughness is a measure when crack is present.

Frankel's sign in tabes dorsalis the excessive range of passive motion at the hip joint. It takes place due to decreased tone of foot and ankle.

Free (uncapsulated) receptors are the predominant form of nociceptors, especially in the cutaneous tissues, oral mucosa and periodontal tissues.

Free flowing solder is the one that flows the solder over the metal parts readily and penetrates small openings and joints by capillary action.

Free graft refers to a tissue for grafting is completely removed from its donor site.

Free radical is any atom (e.g. oxygen, nitrogen) with at least one unpaired electron in the outer most shell, and is capable of independent existence. Free radicals are highly reactive due to the presence of unpaired electrons

Free running pulsed mode is unique in that large peak energies of laser light are emitted for an extremely short time span, usually in micro seconds, followed by a relatively long time in which the laser is off. For example, a free running pulsed laser with pulse duration of 100 µs with pulses delivered at 10 pulses per second would mean that the energy at the surgical site is only present for 1/1000 of a second and absent for the remaining 99.999% of that second.

Frenectomy refers to complete removal of a frenum.

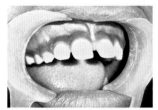
Frenectomy

Frenum refers to a fold of mucus membrane attaching the cheeks and lips to upper and lower arches.

High frenum attachment

Frequency distribution refers to tally of number of times each individual score is represented in a data set. It can be presented visually as a histogram of a stem and leaf plot.

Fresh whole blood transfusion – The advantage of it is simultaneous presence of red blood cells, plasma and fresh platelets. It is used in cardiac surgery and massive hemorrhage when more than 10 units of blood is required in 24 hours.

Friable refers to easily breakable.

Friction blister occurs due to excessive friction. Epidermis separates from dermis and plasma oozes in for example blister of ill fitting shoes.

Frictional keratosis is an isolated area of thickened whitish oral mucosa which can be identified to local irritant. Histological studies show various degrees of hyperkeratosis, parakeratosis and acanthosis. Within 2 weeks of treatment lesion will start reducing in size. Frictional keratosis occurs due to some local irritant an isolated area of thickened whitish oral mucosa develops. Histologically these show varied hyperkeratosis and acanthosis. Broken and rough edges may cause it. Majority of lesions will be reduced, if irritant is removed. Biopsy will help.

Frigidity is the inability to initiate or maintain the sexual pattern.

Front teeth see anterior teeth.

Frontal lobe tumor It develops slowness of comprehension, memory disorder, childish behavior and impaired judgement. Tumor or medial surface of frontal lobe may cause urinary urgency. Ataxic gait and profound mental changes appear. With the left frontal lesion intelligence is reduced. Motor aphasia develops.

Frost bite symptoms of frost bite develop when skin temperature drops from 20 to 14° F. It may be due to impaired circulation, injury or shock. Blisters form within 24-36 hours and become hard and black in two weeks. Tissues up to bones may be involved. There may be discoloration from blue to violet.

Frozen blood – RBCs can be frozen and stored for up to 3 years but the technique is costlier. It is to maintain a supply of rare blood type. In it plasma components are being removed.

Full mouth indices are those indices that measure the patient's entire periodontium or dentition. Eg: Russel's Periodontal Index (PI).

Full mouth X-rays refers to those X-rays showing all the teeth. It includes 14 periapicals and 4 bitewings, also known as a complete series.

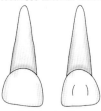

Anterior tooth

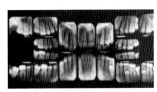

Full mouth X-ray

Full thickness flap/Mucoperiosteal flap refers to the flap where all the soft tissue including the periosteum is reflected to expose the soft tissue.

Fumigation theory is given by Guy de Cahuliac (1300-1368), was the greatest surgeon of Middle Ages believed that worms caused dental decay. He advocated fumigation with seeds of leek, onion and hyoscyamus as a cure for dental caries. The fumigation was also used in earlier times by Chinese and Egyptians.

Function of spinal cord – Each nerve is attached to spinal cord by two roots. Dorsal roots consists of sensory pathways and anterior root the motor pathways. Spinal cord provides a pathway for sensory information travelling from periphery to brain. It also provides a pathway for motor information coming from brain and going to periphery. In addition spinal cord acts as a major reflex center.

Functional anterior cross bite is seen in pseudo class II malocclusion where the mandible is compelled to close in a position forward of its true centric relation. It occurs as a result of occlusal prematurities that cause the deflection of the mandible into a forward position during closure. These can be treated by eliminating the occlusal prematurities.

Functional matrix theory refer Moss Hypothesis.

Functional measure index (FMI) was proposed by Sheiham A., Maizels J., and Maizels, A. in 1987, as one of the two alternative indices, which were modifications of the DMFT index. In FMI, the "Filled and the "Sound' teeth are weighted equally, while, the 'Decayed and 'Missing' teeth are given zero weight. The FMI is calculated by adding the Filled and sound teeth and then dividing by total number of teeth present.

Functional tongue thrust is said to be present when the tongue thrust mechanism is an adaptive behavior developed to achieve an oral seal, it can be grouped as functional.

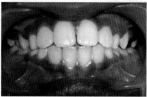

Functional tongue thrust

Functions of proteins, these provide material for growth, wear and tear of tissue. These provide energy and stimulate metabolism. These are source of enzyme needed for digestion. Antibodies which are defence against infections are protein in nature. These maintain acid-base balance.

Fundal height and gestation is just above symphysis pubis at 12 weeks gestation, at umbilicus at 22 weeks and at xiphisternum at 36 weeks.

Fungal infection of lung is generally opportunistic infection. They develop in patients with suppression of immune status. It develops in chronic congestion and edema where fungi gets comfortable environment. Histoplasmosis, Aspergillosis, Cryptococcosis are common diseases.

Furcation involvement is the term given when there is invasion or bony destruction of bifurcation or trifurcation of multirooted tooth due to periodontal disease. The bone loss around the each tooth may be horizontal and angular; furcation involvement is a stage progressive periodontal disease

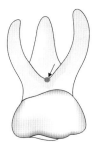

Furcation area

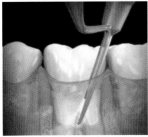

Furcation

Furcation refers to an area where the root divides.

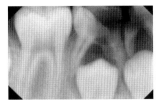

Gross caries involving furcation of primary teeth

Furrow refers to a groove.

Fusion refers to union of two separate tooth germs during their formation. They may be joined only by enamel and/or dentin. Pulps may also be fused. Extent of union depends on the stage of development of teeth at the time of fusion. Fused teeth appear broader. They also frequently exhibit incisal notch or groove which may continue on to the root surface. Whereas fusion takes place at an angle causing crooked appearance. Pulpal anatomy: fused teeth tend to have double pulpal space and

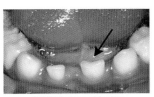

Clinical view of fusion

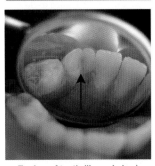

Fusion of teeth (lingual view)

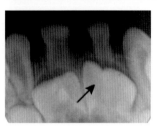

Radiographic view of fusion

However, in both gemination and fusion the pulp spaces may or may not be separated. Location in the jaw: Double teeth in the mandible would almost exclusively represent fusion crowding: fused teeth occupy less space than separate teeth would, causing spacing in the arch. In case of fusion there will be reduction in tooth number.

F

G (Glabella) is the most prominent anterior point in the midsagittal plane of the forehead.

Gabapentin is a drug that is used in the treatment of partial seizures. It is a GABA analogue. Its mechanism of action occurs at calcium channel. It is generally well tolerated. It is well absorbed after oral administration and is eliminated by renal excretion. Average half life is 5-7 hours.

Gag reflex is seen at 18 1/2 week of I.U. life. In the buccal cavity and pharynx, the ectoderm/endoderm zone is towards the posterior third of the tongue. Touching here elicits a gag reflex, a protective reflex.

Gait is the period between successive points at which the heel of the same foot strikes the ground. 60-65% time of one cycle foot remains in touch to the ground. Gait has four components, antigravity support of body, stepping, maintenance of equilibrium and means of propulsion.

Galactorrhea refers to the bilateral, spontaneous, multiple ducts, and milky type of discharge in child bearing age. It is caused by increased production of prolactin and is most commonly seen after pregnancy. Normal levels of prolactin range from 1 – 22 mg per ml.

Galactosemia is an inability to metabolise galactose. It leads to high blood and tissue galactose level and galactosuria. Each one of three types develops due to deficiency of specific enzyme. Classical galactosemia is due to galactose – 1 phosphate uridyl

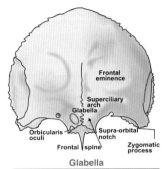

Glabella

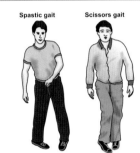

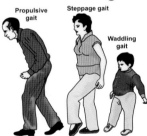

Different types of Gait

transferase deficiency. Manifestations include cataract, cirrhosis and mental retardation.

Gallium amalgam is a product formed by the reaction of an alloy powder, silver-tin-copper with a gallium based liquid alloy i.e. gallium – indium – tin.

Galvanic current refers to a current of electricity produced by chemical action between two metals suspended in liquid.

Gardner's syndrome is carcinomatous transformation of adenomatous intestinal polyps. There may be osteomas of jaw and accompanying cysts are indictors of Gardner's syndrome and bowel should be examined.

Gas gangrene is caused by C Perfrigens, C Histolyticum. Onset is sudden with pain and swelling in affected area, tachycardia and hypovolemic shock. There develops foul smelling blood tinged discharge from wound. Red fluid filled vesicles develop around wound. Palpable crepitus shows gas formation at the site. Hemolytic jaundice and renal failure are common. Radiograph may show gas.

Gas lasers (Helium and Helium-Neon, HeNe, are the most common gas lasers) have a primary output of visible red light. CO_2 lasers emit energy in the far infrared, and are used for cutting hard materials.

Gastrointestinal bleeding is the most common cause including gastric ulcer, gastric erosion duodenal ulcer and esophagitis. Red or coffee ground hematemesis with or without malena indicates upper G.I. bleeding. Bright red rectal bleeding may be due to lower G.I. bleeding. Signs include hematemesis, gross occult blood in stool. Hypotension occurs in late cases. Tachycardia develops earlier.

Gate control theory of pain is still the most accepted mechanistic theory of pain. It was devised by *Melzack* and *Wall*. According to this theory noxious stimulation of the Substantia Gelatinosa (SG) functions as a gate control system that modulates the afferent pathways before they influence the transmission cells. The afferent patterns in the dorsal column system therefore function

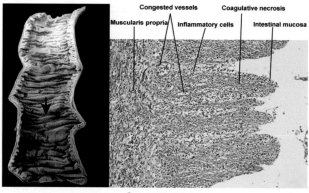

Congested vessels   Coagulative necrosis
Muscularis propria   Inflammatory cells   Intestinal mucosa

Gas gangrene

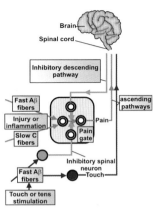

Gate control theory

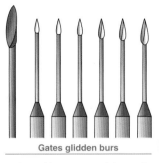

Gates glidden burs

in part as a control trigger which activates selective brain process that influence the modulating properties of the gate control system.

Gated pulse mode are periodic alterations of the laser energy being on and off, similar to a blinking light. This mode is achieved by the opening and closing of a mechanical shutter in front of the beam path of a continuous wave emission. Duration of on and off time normally is as small as a few milliseconds.

Gates-Glidden burs are elliptically shaped burs with very long shanks. These are used to retrieve broken instruments and preparation of post endodontic procedures.

Gaucher's disease is the most common lysosomal storage disorder (incidence 1 in 25,000 live births). Inheritance is autosomal recessive, with a high incidence seen in Ashkenazi Jews, who have a carrier frequency of 1 in 60. There is a deficiency of glucosidase, resulting in accumulation of its substrate glucocerebroside. The enzyme is encoded on chromosome. There are three types of Gaucher's disease. Type I - adult type, non-neuronopathic. Type II - severe infantile, rare, neurological signs seen at 3 months, die by 2 years of age. Type III - subacute, neuropathic, variable presentation from childhood to 70 years of age.

Gel is a colloidal system in which the solid and liquid are continuous phases. Gel is usually flexible.

Gelatine is a sponge. It can be left adherent to the bleeding surface. It will be completely absorbed in 1-2 weeks. It can be used in treatment of bleeding tooth sockets.

Gemination refers to a double teeth originated from one tooth bud. This is the result of incomplete splitting. In case of gemination, fused crowns exhibit mirror image. Pulpal anatomy geminated teeth usually have an undivided pulp. Germinations are more common in maxilla. Gemination results in extra tooth hence require more space thereby likely to cause crowding. Fusion of normal tooth bud with a supernumerary would result in crowding. Hence neither crowding nor diastema seems decisive. Gemination does not reduce the tooth number.

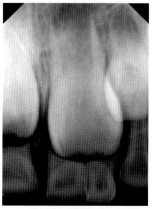

Gemination

Gene therapy is a treatment of inherited diseases by introducing wild type copies of defective genes causing the disorder into the cells of affected individuals.

General anesthetics are the drugs having the capability to depress excitable tissue at all levels of CNS. There are different stages of anesthesia, analgesia and respiratory paralysis. Course of general anesthesia includes three stages, induction of anesthesia which is the period in which concentration of anesthetic agent in blood tissue increases. During maintenance of anesthesia operation is performed. Anesthesia is controlled to maintain constant depth of it. Third stage is emergence from anesthesia, cessation of anesthetic agent ending with complete recovery of reflexes.

General anesthesia is a procedure done by giving an inhalation drug before a surgical procedure to relieve the sensation of pain.

Generalize periodontitis is said to have occurred when more than thirty percent of the areas assessed in mouth demonstrate the bone loss and loss of attachment.

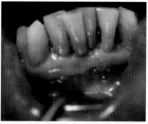

Severe gingival recession with generalized periodontitis

Generalized aggressive periodontitis usually occurs in the individuals of below the age group of thirty. Clinically there is generalized interproximal attachment loss affecting three permanent teeth other than first molars and incisors. The destruction occurs is episodic in nature with the period of advanced destruction followed by the variable stages of remission.

Generalized diffuse gingivitis involves the entire gingiva

Generalized gingivitis is said to occur where inflammation involves the entire mouth (*see* Figure on page 199).

Generalized infection is an infection which has spread throughout the body.

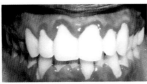
Generalized gingivitis

Generalized marginal gingivitis involves the gingival margins in relation to all the teeth.

Generalized seizures are the seizures involving the whole body. Grand mal epilepsy also known as tonic clonic seizure and is the most common form of seizures disorder. This is produced by idiopathic neurologic disorders or may develop in a neurologically sound brain; secondary to a systemic, metabolic or toxic disturbance. Causes include drug withdrawal, menstruation, fatigue, falling asleep or awakening. Neurologically induced generalized tonic clonic seizure usually last about 2-3 minutes and seldom more than 5 minutes, the entire seizure – lasts 5-15 minutes.

Genetic theory is one of the earliest concepts of growth and development put forward by Brodie.

Genetics is the science that studies inheritance and expression of inherited traits. Genetics is the history of individual and biological and temperamental effects given in birth and development.

Geniculate neuralgia is characterized by pain in ear and anterior tongue. Location of pain is similar to sensory distribution of the nerve i.e. external auditory canal, posterior auricular region and the soft palate. If motor root is also involved then facial palsy may develop. Pain is not too severe.

Short course of high dose steroid therapy is beneficial.

Genital tubercles are the tiny bumps of bone in the anterior region of mandible that serve as attachment sites for genioglossus and geniohyoid muscles. These appear as radio opaque.

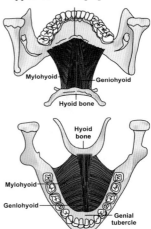
Genital tubercles

Geographic tongue is also known as migratory glossitis. It refers to irregularly shaped, reddish areas of depapillation. There will be thinning of dorsal tongue epithelium. There is spontaneous development and regeneration of affected area. There may be associated fissured tongue. Etiology of geographic tongue is not clear. An immunologic reaction is suggested. No inheritance pattern is noted. The disease is asymptomatic but some may complaint of burning pain and stinging. Clinically irregularly shaped red patches with white patterns look like a map. Red patches are smaller to start surrounded by a white rim. Red patches go on enlarging and regressing and pattern goes on changing every week.

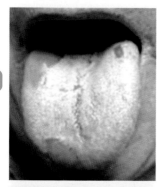

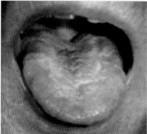

Geographic tongue

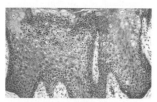

Histological view of geographic tongue

Geometric teeth refer to non anatomic posterior teeth.

Geotrichosis is a fungal disease caused by Geostrichum species. Oral lesions are similar to candidiasis or thrush. It is white, velvety covering of the oral mucosa. It may be isolated or diffuse organisms are small rectangular shaped spores 4 to 8 microns.

Gerber space regainer is a space regaining appliance where a seamless orthodontic band or a crown is selected for the tooth to be distalized. This space regainer consists of 'U' shaped tubing and a 'U' shaped rod that enters the tubing. The rod is soldered or welded on the mesial aspect of the first molar to be moved distally. The 'U' shaped wire or rod is fitted into the tube, in such a way that the base of 'U' rod contacts the tooth mesial to the edentulous area. Open coil springs of adequate length are placed around the free ends of the 'U' shaped rod and inserted into the tubing assembly. The forces generated by the compressed open coil springs bring about a distal movement of the first molar.

German measles is an acute specific fever characterized by sub occipital and posterior cervical glandular enlargement. Macular rash starts on first day. Fever is moderate with malaise. Rash consists of small, pink, discrete macule. Occasionally patient may complain of joint pain. There is typical enlargement of lymph gland and mild coryza.

Germicides refer to anything that destroys bacteria.

Gerontology is the scientific study of factors affecting the normal aging process and the effects of aging.

G

Gerstmann's syndrome is a combination of right left disorientation finger agnosia and constructional apraxia. Acalculia and dyslexia are common.

Ghomphoses joint movements are minimal. Example includes teeth and jaw.

Ghost teeth are an unusual developmental problem in which one or several teeth in the same quadrant shows marked reduction in radiodensity. Very thin enamel and dentin are present. Such teeth if erupt are malformed and non functional.

Giant cell epulis is found of gingival margin between teeth anterior to permanent teeth. Numerous multinucleate cells lie via vascular stroma of plump spindle shaped cells. It should be excised with its gingival base and underlined bone curetted.

Giant cell fibroma develops from fibrous connective tissue, mandibular or maxillary gingiva is mostly affected. Lesion is pedunculated. It has papillary or warty surface. Some may be painless, smooth nodular growth. Histologically multiple multi-nucleated giant cells are seen. Nuclei are large of giant cells. Numerous small capillaries are noted. Surgical excision is the line of treatment.

Giant cell granuloma is hyper-plastic than neoplastic. It is seen in young person. There develops painless swelling. It forms a proliferating vascular connective tissue packed with giant cells. Fibroblastic proliferation and prominent osteoid and bone formation are common. Curettage is sufficient although recurrence follows incomplete removal.

Giardiasis is protozoal infection of small intestine caused by flagellate Giardia Lamblia. Cysts are transmitted as a faecal contamination of water or food by person to person contact. It may result in acute diarrhea and malabsorption. Incubation period is 1-3 weeks. There may be marked weight loss. Single dose Tinidazole is effective in 90% cases.

Gifford sign is a resistance to everting the upper eyelid.

Gingiva is a masticatory type of oral mucosal membrane that forces the covering of the teeth. It is divided into three zones for descriptive purpose.

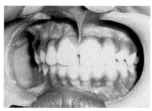

Healthy gingiva

Gingival abscess is a localized purulent infection involving marginal gingiva or interdental papilla. It is a localized, painful rapidly expanding lesion that is usually of sudden onset. It is generally limited to marginal gingiva or interdental papilla. In early stages, it appears as a red swelling with a smooth, shiny surface. Within 24 hr to 48 hr the lesion usually become fluctuant and pointed and forms a surface orifice from which purulent exudates may be expressed.

Gingival crevicular fluid (GCF) is the fluid which is present in gingival sulcus. Sulcular fluid

G

seeps into it from the gingival connective tissue through the thin sulcular wall. The gingival fluid is believed to Cleanse material from the sulcus, contain plasma proteins that may improve adhesion of the epithelium to the tooth. It has antimicrobial properties, exert antibody activity in defense of the gingiva.

Gingival cyst develops either in free or attached gingiva. It may develop at any age. It is a soft tissue lesion and does not show on radiographs; when bigger in size, it may bulge the cortical plate of bone. Otherwise it presents a small well circumscribed painless swelling of gingiva. It resembles a superficial mucocele. Surgical excision is the remedy.

Gingival fibers are the connective tissue of marginal gingiva which are densely collagenous in nature and mainly composed of type I collagen. Their main function is to hold the marginal gingiva firmly, to provide rigidity so that the tooth can withstand masticatory forces and to unite marginal gingiva with the cementum of the root and adjacent attached gingiva.

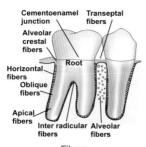

Fibres

Gingival graft is a surgical procedure that removes gingival tissue from one area of the mouth to place it in another area of the mouth which is deficient in gingiva.

Gingival groove is the groove separating the gum pad from the palate.

Gingival hyperplasia is an increase in size of gingiva and soft tissue that overfills the interproximal spaces. Hyperplasia may be inflammatory, noninflammatory or mixed. In inflammatory hyperplasia the enlarged gingiva are soft, edematous and sensitive to touch. While noninflammatory is hard firm, dense and paler.

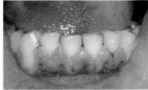

Gingival hyperplasia due to cyclosporin

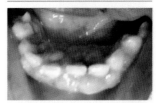

Gingival hyperplasia due to nifedipine

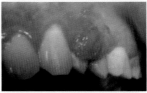

Gingival hyperplasia due to pregnancy

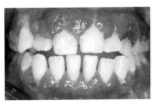

Gingival hyperplasia due to oral
contraceptives

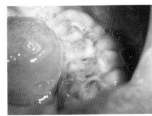

Gingival hyperplasia

Gingival margin trimmer (GMT)
is a dental hand instrument
designed to bevel the cervical
cavosurface walls of the cavity
preparation.

Gingival overgrowth can occur
due to variety of reasons that
induces drugs such as
cyclosporin nifidipine and
calcium channel blocker. Tooth
brush trauma may cause localized
thickened gingiva with a more
linear appearance. Chronic
inflammation can cause firm,
rolled and fibrotic gingiva. Poor
oral hygiene can lead to chronic
inflammation and thickened
gingiva.

Gingival pocket usually occurs
due to enlargement of gingival
tissue without any underlying
destruction of periodontal
tissues.

Gingival recession refers to the
apical movement of gingiva. Histologically there is thinning of

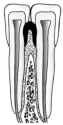

Gingival pocket

gingival tissue. Etiology of gingival recession includes: Improper
brushing bone loss, peuodontion
trauma to occlusion and again.

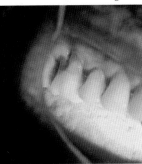

Gingival recession

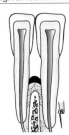

Gingival recession

Gingival sulcus is the shallow
crevice or space around the tooth
bounded by the surface of the
tooth on one side, and the

epithelium lining, the free margin of the gingival on the other. The clinical determination of the depth of the gingival sulcus is an important diagnostic parameter. It is V-shaped and under normal physiological condition, it barely allows the penetration of the periodontal probe. The so-called probing depth of a clinically normal gingival sulcus in humans is 2 to 3 mm. The sulcus depth around the primary teeth is comparatively greater those that found around the permanent teeth. The mean values range from 1.4 mm to 2.1 mm.

Gingivectomy refers to the excision of the gingiva.

Gingivitis refers to inflammation of gingiva and may occur as acute or in subacute form. Plaque or plaque derived endotoxins act as irritants. Food impaction and general oral neglect may result it Gingiva becomes deeper pink to red as the hyperaemia and inflammatory infiltrate develop. Inflammatory swelling produces a bulbous appearance. In chronic gingivitis pus may be expressed on pressure. Irritants are to be removed.

Gingivodental fibres are those present on the facial, lingual and interproximal surfaces. They are embedded in the cementum just beneath the epithelium at the base of the gingival sulcus.

Gingivodental fibres

Gingivoplasty refers to reshaping of the gingiva, to create physiologic gingival contours. The procedure is performed with the help of periodontal knife, scalpel, rotary diamond stones or electrodes.

Gland of Blandin and Nuhn is the anterior lingual gland lying close to inferior surface and lip of tongue. Five to seven of its ducts open on small protuberances of mucus membrane under the tongue.

Glandular cheilitis is not very common and lower lip becomes enlarged, everted and firm. Use of tobacco and constant exposure of sun may result it. Emotional disturbance may also result in glandular chelitis. There are three types: *Simple* - these are multiple, pin headed and painless lesions. *Superficial suppurative type* - there will be painless swelling, crusting, induration and superficial ulceration of lip. *Deep suppurative type* – there is deep seated infection with abscess and fistula. Mucosal surface shows numerous dilated salivary duct orifices surrounded by a red macular area. Person notes a mucus secretion at the orifice of duct. In severe form, lip is considerably and permanently enlarged and develops pain and tenderness. Volkmann's chelitis is a severe form and epidermoid carcinoma may be associated. Vermilionectomy is the line of treatment.

Glandular fever is caused by Epstein Barr Virus. Chiefly young people are affected. Deep kissing may transmit it. Person develops fever, sore throat, headache and lymphadenopathy.   Cervical glands enlarge to start with. Pharyngitis and tonsillitis are common. Some cases may be symptomless. Oral lesion includes gingivitis and stomatitis. There may be occasional oral ulcers and palatal petechiae. Some may develop hemorrhagic tendency. Blood may show atypical lymphocytes. Abnormal forms may be oval, horseshoe shaped. Nuclei may be indented and irregular. Thrombocytopenia may be present. There is no specific treatment of this disease.

Glasgow coma scale (GCS) was first described by Teasdale and Jennett in 1974. This scale relates the clinical observation under the three categories: motor response, verbal performance and eye opening allowing any changes over a period of time to be appreciated.

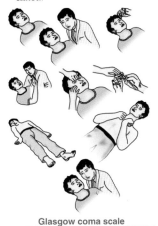

Glasgow coma scale

Glass blowers' white patch is a variant of traumatic keratosis affecting cheek and lip. Histologi-

cally it resembles cheek and lip bite.

Glass ionomer cements (GICs) are the one that consists of a basic glass and an acidic water-soluble powder that sets by an acid–base reaction between the two components. These cements bond chemically to tooth and posses' anticariogenic properties, Non-irritant to the tissue, low thermal diffusivity and biocompatible.

Glenoid fossa is a concave depressed area of the temporal bone of which mandibular condyle rest.

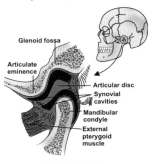

Glenoid fossa

Glial fibrillary acidic protein (GFAP) is a type of filament found in Glial cells surrounding neurons.

Gliomas are very common measuring 50% intracranial neoplasms of brain. Symptoms of increased intracranial pressure may get developed. Intellectual decline, personality changes, emotional liability, seizures and headache may also over. Focal lesions depend on the site of lesion (*see* Figure on page 206).

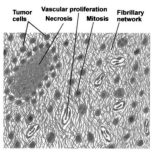

Tumor cells | Vascular proliferation | Necrosis | Mitosis | Fibrillary network

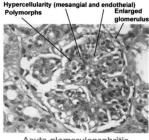

Hypercellularity (mesangial and endotheial) | Polymorphs | Enlarged glomerulus

Acute glomerulonephritis

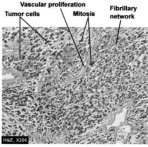

Tumor cells | Vascular proliferation | Mitosis | Fibrillary network

H&E, X200

Gliomas (Astrocytoma) brain

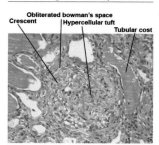

Crescent | Obliterated bowman's space | Hypercellular tuft | Tubular cost

Rapidly progressing Glomerulone-phritis

Globulin zinc insulin is most active upto 8 hour following subcutaneous injection and action fades out by 18 hours.

Globulomaxillary cyst is a well defined pear shaped radio-lucency found between the roots of maxillary lateral incisor and cuspid. These are found within the bone at the junction of globular portion of medial nasal process and maxillary process. It is found accidentally being symptom free. Radiographically it appears as inverted pear shaped.

Glomerulonephritis results in hematuria, dysmorphic red cells, casts and mild proteinuria. Edema is found in periorbital and serotal lesions Hypertension may develop.

Gloss is the optical property that produces a lustrous appearance. Luster is the proportion of specular reflection to diffuse reflection. When the incident beam is scattered by the object there is decrease in gloss. Gloss is an important appearance property of dental restorative material.

Glossopharyngeal nerve is a ninth cranial nerve having motor and sensory part. Sensory fibres supply posterior 2/3rd of tongue and pharynx. Motor fibres supply the stylopharyngeus muscle (*see* Figure on page 207).

Glossopharyngeal neuralgia is neuralgia of 9th cranial nerve. Its pain is paroxysmal but less severe than trigeminal nerve pain. Location of trigger zone and pain

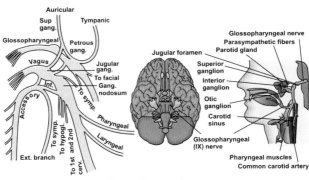

Glossopharyngeal nerve

G

sensation follows distribution of the nerve. It includes posterior tongue, pharynx and infra auricular area. Pain is triggered by chewing and swallowing because all this stimulate pharyngeal mucosa. Glossopharyngeal neuralgia may be associated with trigeminal neuralgia. Sometimes it may be associated with vagal symptoms. Intra or extra cranial tumors may compress cranial nerve. Treatment is similar to trigeminal neuralgia.

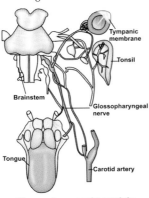

Glossopharyngeal neuralgia

Glossy polymer is an amorphous polymer that behaves as a brittle solid.

Gloves are a disposable item that gives protection to health care worker through cuts and abrasions. Gloves should be changed for each patient. Surgical gloves are not to be washed before or after being used.

Glucometer is a small instrument that measures the amount of glucose in capillary blood.

Glutraldehyde It is a high level disinfectant. 20 minutes immersion in 2% alkaline glutraldehyde solution for disinfection and 6-10 hours immersion for sterilization of instruments is recommended. It has a pungent odour, irritating to eyes.

Glycerol is a three carbon carbohydrate which combines with fatty acids to form triglycerides.

Glycogen is also known as animal starch. It is highly branched poly saccharide similar to plant starch. Glucose is stored in human body as glycogen. When blood sugar lowers down the glycogen is converted in the liver to glucose. Glucose released in blood restores normal blood sugar levels.

Goitre is an enlargement of thyroid occurring due to deficiency of iodine leading to goitre which is marked by swelling of the neck with the enlargement of thyroid gland. Babies born to these mothers may be physically or mentally deformed. Endemic goitre is a public health problem. Common salt fortified with small quantities of sodium and potassium iodate has been widely used in reducing the prevalence of goitre. A simple goitre secretes low levels of thyroid hormones. Other types of goitre hyper secrete thyroid hormones and are known as toxic goitre.

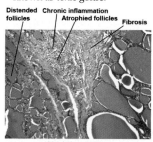

Distended follicles Chronic inflammation Atrophied follicles Fibrosis

Nodular goitre

Gold filling makes an excellent filling material. It is most malleable filling material therefore it can be directly inserted and adopted to cavity wall. It brings hardness to cavity. It is insoluble in oral fluids and will not tarnish to corrode. It maintains high polish.

Gold foil takes longer to build up than other gold filling materials due to softness and lack of mass. It can be used throughout the cavity and is suitable as a surface material. But it takes considerable time to build up restoration.

Gold inlays are used on amalgam fillings. These are used where teeth have lost cusps or otherwise are too weak. Advantage of gold is that is does not tarnish and has great strength.

Gold is used as the restorative material. The pulp reaction to gold crown is a result of type of cement used to retain the restoration. The condensation of cohesive gold is a factor in pulp response. Mild to severe response is seen in 10-20 days. If a base in required pulpal inflammation is reduced. There are no irreversible changes and use of cohesive gold may be found biologically sound. Gold foil shows the least marginal leakage.

Golden proportion is the guidelines which dentists use in determining the most esthetic appearance of a particular tooth (teeth need to maintain a certain height to width ratio to look their best.)

Gold-palladium alloys were introduced in 1970 and were developed to avoid color change due to silver. The only disadvantage of the gold palladium group is thermal expansion incompatibility with some of higher expansion porcelains. Otherwise rigidity is increased and corrosion resistance is excellent.

Gonial angle (A-Go-Me) is the angle formed by the tangents to the body of the mandible and posterior border of the ramus. This not only expresses the form of the mandible but also gives information on mandibular growth direction. If this angle is acute the growth is horizontal. This is a favorable condition for anterior positioning of the mandible with an activator. In skeletally derived malocclusion, a casual type of treatment is possible only by channeling basal growth pattern to provide the morphologic and functional changes needed to establish a normal structural and functional pattern.

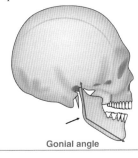

Gonial angle

Gonorrhea is a venereal disease generally affecting genito urinary parts. Oral – genital sex affects oral cavity. Lips may develop acute painful ulceration. Gingiva may become erythematous with or without necrosis. Gonococcal pharyngitis and tonsillitis are well recognized lesions.

Good cholesterol named HDL is capable of transporting cholesterol back to liver where it is disposed. So it is called good cholesterol and elevated levels are helpful to heart.

Gout may be primary or secondary. Primary is inherited metabolic disorder. There is hyperuricemia resulting from over production or under excretion of uric acid. Depostis of urate crystals can occur in subcutaneous tissues, joints and kidneys. Secondary gout results due to drugs i.e. thiazides, frusamide or diseases like lymphoma. Colchicines are most effective agent when given within 24 hours of acute attack.

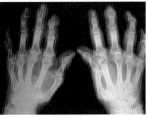

Multiple, punched-out lytic lesions of phalanges in gout

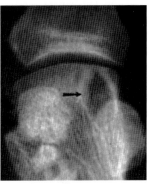

Gout

Gracey curettes is a periodontal instruments that consists a set of four mini – bladed curettes; the sub 0 and number 1–2 are used for anteriors and premolars, number 11–12 are used for posterior mesial surface and number 13–14 are used for posterior distal surface. The length of blade is nearly half of the conventional Gracey curette and is slightly curved upwards which helps in adapting the instrument more closely to the tooth surface (*see* Figure on page 210).

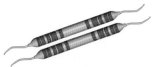

HuFriedy Mini five extended shank

Grandmal seizures are a type of epileptic seizures involving whole body. There is no aura but sudden loss of consciousness with falling to the ground is there. Cry may be heard due to forced expiration. Finally the muscles are relaxed but patient remains unconscious for some time. Tongue biting and urinary incontinence is not rare. Headache and drowsiness may remain for a few days.

Granulocytes are the precursor and mature form of leukocytes characterized by neutrophilic, eosinophilic or basophilic granulocytes in their cytoplasm.

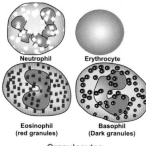

Neutrophil   Erythrocyte

Eosinophil   Basophil
(red granules)   (Dark granules)

Granulocytes

Granuloma gravidorum is a gingival lesions associated with pregnancy. 30 to 40% women show mild gingival enlargement. Post delivery enlargement subsides on its own.

Granuloma Inguinale is caused by Donovania Granualomatosis. It is considered to be a venereal disease. External genitalia are affected more. Papule/nodule ulcerates soon. Lips, buccal mucosa or palate are affected. Painful ulcerated lesions sometimes bleed. Mucus membrane is inflamed and edematous. Fibrous scar formation may be extensive.

Granuloma is described a type of nodule which contains granulation tissue. On gingiva it occurs as a swollen mass.

Granulomatous chelitis is also known as Miescher's syndrome of unknown etiology. Young females are more affected. Histologically, there is focal non caseating granuloma formation. There will be epitheloid cells with Langhans type of giant cells. Lower lip is diffusely swelled up. There may be fever, headache and visual disturbances. Some may develop scales, fissures and pustules. Swelling is non pitting. Swelling may be hard as rubber. Regional lymph nodes may be enlarged. It may be associated with Melkerson Rosenthal syndrome consisting of fissured tongue and facial paralysis. Differential diagnosis includes angioedema and sarcoidosis. Angioedema appears suddenly. History of recurrence is there. Sarcoidosis will be excluded by absence of any other manifestation and by a negative Kveim test. It is managed by repeated injection of corticosteroid every few weeks and cheiloplasty.

Granulomatous hypersensitivity is the most important form of delayed hypersensitivity, causing many of the pathological effects in diseases, which involve, T-cell mediated immunity. It results from the presence within macrophages of a persistent agent usually a microorganism, which the cell is unable to destroy. It may also be due to presence of immune complexes, which results in 'Epitheliod Cell granuloma' formation.

Grasp is a precise control of movements during the instrumentation or performing any other dental procedure.

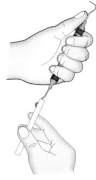

Pen grasp

Grasp reflex means when the body's palms are stimulated the hand closes. This is also a corresponding plantar reflex. But movements disappeare by 24 months of age.

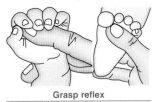

Grasp reflex

Gray lesions are not only due to biologic pigment but also due to

the deposition of foreign material in connective tissue. It may be localized or diffuse. Color may be due to amalgam particles encountered in oral mucosa. Diffuse gray pigmentation is seen in silver, lead, and bismuth.

Green stain appearance varies from light or yellowish green to very dark green. These stains are generally embedded in the bacterial plaque. Generally facial one third of the maxillary anterior teeth are involved. These stains appears to be soft and is difficult to remove. Stain of long standing may cover a decalcified area of enamel. No micro-organism has been identified to stain green.

Green stick fracture when only one cortex is discontinued.

Greincspan's syndrome is a triad of lichen planus, diabetes mellitus and hypertension. It may predispose to squamous cell carcinoma.

Grit size is a numerical grading of particle size. Larger numbers denote fine particles while small numbers denote coarse particles.

Groove refers to a long, narrow depression.

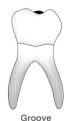

Groove

Ground nut is known as poor man's dry fruit. It contains about 25% proteins and 40% fat. It does not contain vitamin C but contain

G

high quantity of thiamine and nicotinic acid. In humid area it may develop aflatoxin which is harmful to body.

Ground substance (sol-gel colloidal system) is an amorphous matrix in which the connective tissue cells and fibres of the pulp are embedded. It is generally regarded as a gel rather than a solution and therefore is considered to differ from tissue fluids, because of its content of polyelectric polysaccharides, the extracellular matrix is responsible for the water holding properties of connective tissues. It occupies the space between formed elements.

Growth according to Krogman refers to increase in size change in proportion and progressive complexity.

Growth according to Meridith refers to entire series of sequential anatomic and physiological changes taking place from the beginning prenatal life to senility.

Growth according to Moss refers to change in any morphological parameter which is measurable.

Growth according to Moyers refers to quantitative aspect of biological development per unit of time.

Growth according to Todd refers to an increase in size.

Growth curve is a graphic representation of the change in size of a bacterial population over a period of time, including a phase of log phase, a stationary phase and a death phase.

Growth field can be explained as follows i.e. the bone doesn't grow by generalized uniform deposi-

tion of new bone on all outside surface with corresponding resorption from all inside surface because of the topographically complex nature of each bone's shape. The bone must have a differential mode of enlargement. Some of its parts and areas grow much faster and greater extent.

Growth site refers to fields that have some special significance or noteworthy role in growth process are often called.

Growth spurts refers to the periods when sudden acceleration of growth occurs. This sudden increase in growth is termed as growth spurts. The growth spurts in the prenatal period and the infantile period involves the division of the cells. On the other hand, the physiological alteration in the hormonal secretion is believed to be the cause of pubertal growth spurts. The timing of growth spurts differs in boys and girls.

Gubernacular canal refers to the holes seen in a dry skull from lingual to primary teeth in jaws that represent openings of Gubernacular cord.

Gubernacular cord refers to the connective tissue overlying a successional tooth that connects with the lamina propria of the oral mucosa by means of a strand of fibrous connective tissue that contains remnants of dental lamina.

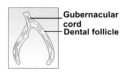
Gubernacular cord
Dental follicle

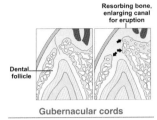

Gubernacular cords

Gubernacular foramina are the small openings in mandible and maxilla an evidence of eruption pathways of permanent teeth. Gubernacular foramina are sites for Gubernacular cords

Guillain Barre Syndrome is caused by progressive demyelinating neuropathy. It is an autoimmune following a non specific disease. Impaired swallowing or parasthesia of mouth and face is the early sign. There may be ascending anesthesia and paralysis of legs and trunk. In severe case respiration is compromised.

Gulland's Sign is a quick, flexion of hips and knee in response to pinching of the contralateral quadriceps's muscle. It indicates meningeal irritation.

Gunning type splints is a type of intermaxillary fixation introduced by Gunning in 1866 where the vulcanite overlay of the natural teeth which he used as a splint for fractured dentate mandible. Properly constructed gunning splint should hold jaws in a slightly over closed relationship as the fracture of mandible are effectively used in this position. The splints are constructed in acrylic resin and the fitting surface is lined by black gutta percha.

Gustatory sense refers to sense of taste therefore called gustatory sense and taste buds are special organs of taste. Taste receptors are located on tongue and are known as chemoreceptor's. Basic taste sensations are sweet, salty, sour and bitter.

Gutta percha is clay like material used in the filling of root canals. The material is used due to its stability and easy manipulation. Material is inert so action is not chemical one. Because it is put after being heated, injury may be thermal. It provides a poor seal of the cavity margins hence saliva may leak and irritate the pulp.

Habit can be defined as the tendency towards an act that has become a repeated performance, relatively fixed, consistent and easy to perform by an individual or habit According to *Butters-worth (1961)* it is a frequent, constant practice or an acquired tendency which has been fixed by frequent repetition. Habit according to *Finn* is an act, which is socially unacceptable. Habit according to *Hogem boom (1953)* was also defined as the methodical way in which mind and body act as a result of the frequent repetition of certain definite set of nervous impulses. Habit according to *William James (1972)* is an acquired habit from a psychological point of view, is nothing but a new pathway of discharge formed in the brain by which certain incoming currents tend to escape. Habit according to *Boucher (1982)* was also defined as a tendency towards an act that has become a repeated performance relatively fixed, easy to perform and almost automatic.

Habitual cheek/lip biting refers to a more of a superficial lesion produced due to constant trauma by rubbing, sucking or chewing

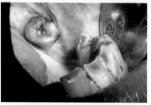

Habitual cheek biting

movements which abrade the area of lip cheek. It does not produce ulceration. These are poorly macerated and reddened areas. It is a subconscious nervous habit.

Habitual mouth breathing refers to a condition where oral breathing persists as habit even after the removal of the nasal obstruction or any other underlying etiology. Interceptive procedures should involve identification and removal of the cause. Persistence of habitual oral breathing is an indication to use a vestibular screen to intercept the habit.

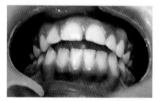

Habitual mouth breather

Habitual tongue thrust refers to a condition where the tongue thrust swallow is present as a habit even after the cessation of the malocclusion.

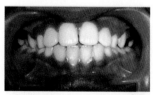

Habitual tongue thrust

Hair papilla refers to a small, cap shaped cluster of cells located at the base of follicle where hair growth begins (*see* Figure on page 215).

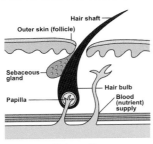

Hair papilla

Hair source – Hair from head is usually long and soft and taper gradually. Hair from female head is thinner. Hair from beard and moustache are usually thicker than those from any part of body. Hair from chest, axilla and pubic region are short and thicker. Pubic hair and from axilla show split ends. Hair from eyebrows, eye lashes and nostrils are stiff, thick and bristly. Hair from body surface is fine, short and flexible. They don't show pigment cells in cortex. Medullary canal is small. The fine downy hair of new born infant has no medullary canal or pigment cells.

Hairy leukoplakia is highly indicative of HIV infection.

Hairy tongue is an unusual condition characterized by hypertrophy of filliform papillae of tongue. Normally keratinized surface layers of filliform papillae are continuously desquamated due to friction of food and anterior upper teeth. These are replaced by new epithelial cells from below. When tongue movements becomes restricted during illness the papilla enlarges and become heavily coated. The color of papilla varies from yellowish white-brown black depending upon the type of stains, the tongue is exposed to. Longer papilla entangles food particles of different colors.

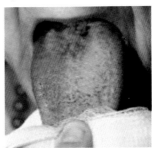

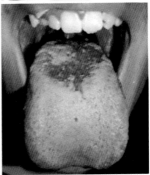

Hairy tongue

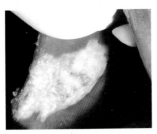

Hairy leukoplakia of buccal mucosa

Tobacco smoke colors it black. Mid dorsum is first to be affected. Dehydration and terminally ill patients also develop thick coatings. Nicotinamide deficiency may produce black hairy tongue in experimental animals. Excessive exposure of radiation to head and neck area and systemic antibiotics may also produce hairy tongue. Because the condition is benign, the treatment is also empirical, in such cases, thorough scrapping and cleaning of tongue is advised to promote desquamation and removal of debris.

Halitosis in general means bad breath, and is also known as oral malodor. The term halitosis originated from the Latin word halitus, breath, and the Greek – osis, meaning abnormal condition Oral malodor is a common complaint that may periodically affect people of all age groups.

Halothane is a non-irritating, potent anesthetic agent which can produce profound anesthesia without hypoxia. Its induction and recovery is quick. It is a poor analgesic but is used in dentistry with 70% N_2O/30% O_2 concentration. Skeletal muscle is relaxed and uterine contractions are depressed. In dental practice it relaxes the masseter muscle and inhibits salivation. Laryngospasm is inhibited Classical signs of anesthesia are lacking.

Hamartomas are tumor like malformations. These are usually congenital. Once achieved adult dimensions these don't increase in size.

Hand Schuller Christian disease occurs in early life. Oral manifestations are often nonspecific. It includes sore mouth, gingivitis and suppuration. There develops an unpleasant taste. Lesions in skull are sharply outlined. Leucopenia and thrombocytopenia is often found. Prognosis is good.

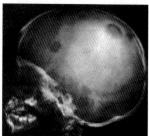
Hand shuller christian disease

Hand, Foot and Mouth disease is an endemic disease of very young children. There is formation of maculo papular, exanthematous and vesicular lesions of skin. Low grade fever, lymphadenopathy, diarrhea and vomiting develop. oral manifestation includes small, multiple vesicular and ulcerative oral lesions. Hard palate, lips and gingiva are involved. Intracytoplasmic viral inclusions can be shown in vesicular scrapings. No specific treatment is needed.

Handpiece low speed hand pieces upto 4000 revolutions a minute are driven by a miniature compressed air. Contrangle hand piece is used because it provides access to every tooth. Air turbine hand pieces are driven at a speed of 40,0000 revolutions a minute. These are contrangled and are used with a built in water spray to counter act the heat generated by high speed cutting. There is abscence of vibration. Disadvantage is of high pitched whistling noise.

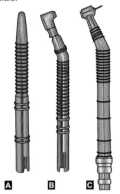

Handpieces, (A) Straight; (B) Contra-angle; (C) Air turbine

Hanging is a form of asphyxial death produced by suspending body with a ligature around the neck. The constricting force is the weight of the body. It takes a few seconds when knot is over cricoid cartilage and 1-2 minutes when it is over larynx. Neck is found stretched and elongated. Head is always inclined to opposite side of the knot. Face is pale but may be swollen. Tongue is caught between teeth, protruded and bitten. Bloody froth may be seen at mouth or nostrils. Hands are often clenched. Escape of urine or faces is often found.

Hard lasers (High level energy) refer to thermal lasers emitted at wavelength in the visible infra red and UV range. Example: Er:YAG laser ; Nd: YAG laser.

Hard palate is the anterior portion of roof of mouth.

Hardness refers to a material's resistance to penetration when indented by a hard material. The hardness of dental material is reported in Knoop hardness number. Larger the indentation, smaller will be the hardness number. Enamel and porcelain are two of the hardest material and have highest numbers Hardness of certain material is enamel 350, dentine 60, Acrylic resin 20, dental amalgam 100, porcelain 450, Alloys 420.

Harmful habits refers to those habits that have a deleterious effect on the teeth and their supporting structures, such as thumb sucking, mouth breathing, tongue thrusting etc.

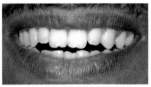

Enamel notching due to bobby pin habits

Harmonal sialadenosis is associated with menarche, menses and pregnancy. Hypogenitatlism, gynecomastia and menopause may also cause it. Diabetes results in retromandibular enlargement of parotid.

Haversian canal is a canal in bone tissue containing nerve and blood vessels surrounded by concentric layers of calcified bone tissue (*see* Figure on page 218).

Headache is produced by stimulation of pain sensitive structures within the cranium or the extra cranial tissues. Cranial bones are insensitive. Within the skull sensitive areas are meninges, walls of venus sinuses and large arteries. Most of the cerebral substance itself is insensitive to stimuli which are painful.

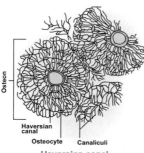

Haversian canal

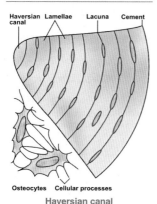

Haversian canal

Headache of intracranial origin is due to inflammation, compression and distortion of or traction upon the pain sensitive meninges and blood vessels within skull.

Healing of fracture refers to formation of blood clot due to damaged blood vessels in medulla, cortex and periosteum. Within 24 hours the hematoma is converted into vascular, fibroblastic granulation tissue. After about 7 days cartilage and osteoid tissues are laid down by osteoblasts. It forms callus. Provisional callus is converted into normal bone. After a period of time bone is moulded by osteoclasts and osteoblasts.

Health history is a structured format and must be recorded as it is.

Health promotion is the science of art of helping the lifestyle of individuals and society to attain optimal health.

Health refers to state of complete physical, mental, social and spiritual well being not merely the absence of disease.

Hearing acquity is the ability to hear and identify the sound.

Heart attack is expressed by sudden onset of a severe crushing pain across the chest pain and may radiate to shoulder, left arm and jaw. It is caused by coronary heart disease.

Heart block is a blockage of impulse conduction from atria to ventricles so that the heart beats at a slower rate than normal.

Heat capacity is the amount of energy it takes to raise the temperature of that object by one degree. Some metals require more energy than others.

Heat cramps develop in those who are doing heavy muscular work in high temperature and humidity. There are painful and spasmodic contractions of calf muscles. Sodium chloride level in blood goes down.

Heat cure silicone is the dental material. Advantages include adequate bond strength to acrylic resiliency and more resistant to aqueous environment. Disadvantages include low tear strength and poor resistance abrasion.

Heat cured acrylic denture base is the denture base material used for fabricating denture. It has a good appearance with high glass transition temperature, easy fabrication, low capital cost and good surface finish. But it has low impact strength and fatigue life is too short.

Heat exhaustion is a mild form due to failure of thermo regulation. It is a mild form of heat stroke. It is due to inadequate replacement of water and salt lost in perspiration due to thermal stress. Body temperature does not go very high. Symptoms include dizziness, weakness and fatigue. *Heat exhaustion* is said to have occurred when attack is gradual and patient feels giddiness, nausea and anorexia. Headache is of throbbing character, but patient remains conscious. Heat exhaustion is caused by dehydration and salt deficiency, sweating may cause a fluid loss of 3 to 4 litres per hour.

Heat of fusion is the amount of energy required to melt a material.

Heat of vaporization is the amount of energy required to boil a material.

Heat sterilizing refers to the use of an autoclave or dry-heat sterilizer to kill all potential disease-causing agents that remain following patient treatment. Any instruments that is not heat stable and cannot tolerate high temperatures should be thoroughly cleaned and soaked in disinfectant chemicals.

Heat stroke is said to have occurred when there is feeling of heat, headache confusion, disorientation, emotional bursts, giddiness and vomiting. Excessive thirst may be felt. Temperature of body may arise up to 106° F. Face will be flushed and pupils dilated. When in shock, hypotension, tachycardia and hurried respiration will set in. Urine becomes scanty. Heat cramps occur due to loss of sodium chloride.

Heat syncope is a mild effect of hot environment. Person standing in sun becomes pale, his B.P. falls and he collapses suddenly. There is no rise in body temperature.

Heath education is a communication activity aimed at enabling individuals to achieve positive health.

Heck's disease is focal epithelial hyperplasia described by Archard Heck and Stanely in 1965. It presents as multiple nodular lesion with a sessile base on lower lip, buccal mucosa and tongue. Nodular lesions are of 1-5 mm in diameter, soft in consistency of buccal mucosa. There is spontaneous regression after 4-6 months. It does not require any treatment.

Hemangioendothelioma is a malignant angiomatous neoplasm of mesenchymal tissue. It is more common in younger age group. Oral lesions are not very common. It is a fast enlarging. There is presence of localized, nodular, painful swelling. Surface ulceration is present. Teeth become mobile and bleed on pressure. Jaw shows destruction. Lesion is expansible with cortical expansion. It is angiomatous in origin. Lips, palate and gingiva may be involved. Endothelial cells are seen. Lesion is firm, round and nodular. When vascular it looks reddish. These grow fast. Surgical excision and radiotherapy is the treatment.

Hemangioma develops due to proliferation of blood vessels. There is variety of hemangiomas. It appears as a flat or raised lesion of mucosa. Lips, tongue and buccal mucosa are commonly involved. Central hemangioma of maxilla or mandible occasionally occurs. It may be by birth. In oral cavity these frequently occur. These are raised, red/blue/purple lesions. Lesions are raised, but are easily blanched on pressure. These are soft and pulsatile. Capillary hemangioma are characterized by small, numerous, endothelial lined pyogenic granuloma. Cavernous hemangioma reveals large, irregularly shaped, dilated endothelial lined sinuses. Such blood pooled sinuses are communicating with each other. These lack muscular coat. Local excision is the treatment. In case of large lesion sclerosing agents may be given earlier to reduce the size.

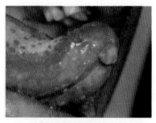

Lingual hemangioma

Hemangioma of tongue is a painless and slowly growing swelling of tongue. It is diffuse and bluish in color. It is compressible extending into floor of mouth and cheek.

Hematoma refers to a collection of pooling blood.

Hematopoiesis is the process by which blood cells grow, divide and differentiate in bone marrow. There are three general classes of blood cells derived from a pool of *pluripotent hematopoietic stem cells (HSC)*, which reside in the marrow and have the unique ability to give rise to all of the different mature blood cells types: RBC, Platelets and WBC.

Hematopoietic stem cells (HSC) are defined by their abilities to self renew throughout life and give rise to committed progenitors that can differentiate along all of the possible hematopoietic lineages. HSC are self-renewing cells; when they proliferate, some of their daughter cells remain as HSC, so they are not depleted. HSC daughter cells can commit to any of several alternative differentiation pathways that lead to production of one or more of types of blood cells. Progression along these pathways is coupled to cell division. The more mature forms greatly outnumber the less differentiated precursors. Most types of hematopoietic cells lose their replicative capacity altogether, by the time they are fully mature and are said to be terminally differentiated. Progressively HSC initially commit to one of three main alterative different pathways or lineages. The most primitive cell in each lineage called 'Lineage committed progenitors'.

Hematospermia is the presence of blood in the ejaculate resulting from inflammation of prostate or seminal vesicle. Blood in initial portion of ejaculate suggests involvement of prostate while terminal hematospermia implies seminal vesicle origin.

Hemiplegic gait is a spastic gait in which only one leg is involved. Spasticity does not allow leg to flex freely at hip, knee and ankle. Leg rotates outwards and makes a semicircle. Each leg is advanced slowly. Scissors gait is noted. It is the manifestation of cerebral diplegia, ischemic brain damage and compressive myelopathy.

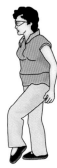

Hemiplegic gait

Hemisection/Bicuspidization is the splitting of two rooted tooth into two separate portions.

Hemiseptum can be described as one – wall bony defect.

Hemochromatosis is a iron storage disease and is of two types. One is idiopathic and secondary form. Normal body contains 2 to 4 gram of iron when it reaches 15-40 gram clinical signs and symptoms of hemochromatosis appear. There is slow progressive enlargement of liver with fibrosis and ending up in cirrhosis. Hemosiderin deposit in skin gives slate gray color. Cardiac arrhythmia and heart failure may develop. Serum ferritin may go > 300 mg/L.

Hemolysin is a destruction of red blood cells in such a manner that hemoglobin is released.

Hemolysis refers to destruction of RBC Jaundice caused by hemolysis often have known sickle cell disease, G6PD deficiency or other hemoglobino-pathies. Hemolysis can be induced by infection, acidosis or drug abuse. Symptoms include fatigue, weakness, light headed-ness, dyspnea on exertion, upper abdomen pain and nocturnal hemoglobinuria. Person will develop pallor, jaundice and splenomegaly.

Hemolytic anemia is said to have occurred when the circulating red blood cell lacking a nucleus is unable to synthesize protein for growth and repair. It may be inherited or acquired. Destruction may be episodic or continuous. Reticulosis is a clue to disorder. Hemolysis increases the indirect bilirubin. Serum LDH levels are strikly elevated. Hereditary causes include thalassemia, hereditary spherocytosis, sickle cell anemia, acquired auto-immune hemolysis and Erythro-blastosis fetalis. Certain chemical agents can also damage to RBC's. Clinical features include pallor, weakness and fatigability; Jaundice, dyspnea may also occur. Oral Manifestations include pallor of oral mucosa, discoloration of teeth in the event of erythroblastosis. Blood hemo-globin level goes down to 10 mg/dL and average survival of RBC

H

comes down to 12 days instead of 120 days. Reticulocyte count is raised. Treatment includes blood transfusion in severe cases, splenectomy in cases of spherocytosis.

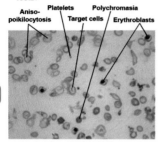

Hemolytic anemia

Hemolytic uremic syndrome – For 1 to 10 days develops anuria. Patient may develop diarrhea, abdominal pain, purpura and fever. BP may be high with edema and hematuria.

Hemopericardium refers to the presence of blood and blood stained fluid in the pericardial sac. Causes include transmural myocardial infarct, ruptured aneurysm of aorta and penetrating injuries. When bleeding is rapid death may take place. Treated pericardium may produce thickening of pericardium and adhesions.

Hemophilia is a sex linked recessive disease characterized by a prolonged coagulation time and hemorrhagic tendencies. It is due to deficiency of plasma proteins needed for conversion of fibrinogen to fibrin. It is a sex linked recessive trait. It is of two types: Hemophilia A, classic hemophilia, Hemophilia B, Christmas type. Hemophilia type A is caused by deficiency of clotting factor called factor VIII. Type B or Christmas disease is less common. This defect is due to defect in Factor IV. In type C there is less severe bleeding and is due to deficiency of factor IX. Disease is hereditary. Hemorrhage into subcutaneous tissues, joints and some internal organs are common. Hemorrhage from many sites in oral cavity is seen. Gingival hemorrhage is massive. Serious bleeding may occur from umbilical cord. Easy bruising and prolonged bleeding occurs with spontaneous bleeding in subcutaneous tissue. Fatal Epistaxis may develop rarely. Gastric bleeding from ulcer may develop. Spontaneous intracranial hemorrhage may develop. Gingival tissue may bleed after extraction, recurrent sub periosteal hematoma of jaw may develop, High caries index, with severe periodontal disease. Dental extraction remains problematic and should be done with lot of caution.

Hemoptysis refers to coughing of blood. It may be in the form of frank hemorrhage. Commonest cause is tuberculosis and pneumonia. Frank blood indicates rupture of blood vessels. It has to be differentiated from hematemesis.

Hemorrhoids refers to varicosities of the hemorrhoidal venous plexuses. Commonest place to occur is anal sphincter. These may be caused by increased intrabdominal pressure as in pregnancy, rectal tumours and constipation.

Hemostasis is arrest of bleeding.

Hemostat is a multipurpose instrument. It is to clamp blood vessels that may be severed during surgery. Narrow beaks are serrated and handles have locks. It can be used to grasp unwanted tissue which are to be removed during surgical procedure. Different shapes and sizes are available.

Hepadnaviruses are small, spherical DNA viruses causing hepatitis, chronic, liver infections and liver cancer. Their mode of transmission along with blood is via saliva too.

Heparin is found in large amount in mast cells of liver and lung. It is a strongest organic acid in body. It is released with histamine in anaphylactic shock. It prevents the conversion of prothrombin to thrombin. It may also decrease the conversion of fibrinogen to fibrin.

Hepatic encephalopathy is a life threatening disorder. It causes mild personality changes and slight tremor. Person becomes lethargic with aberrant behavior. Lastly patient becomes stuporous and hyperventilation sets in. There may develop bradycardia, decreased respiration and seizures.

Hepatitis A virus is non enveloped 27 nm RNA virus enterovirus group. It is excreted in feces and transmission is by fecooral route. The antibody to HVA is detected during first week of infection and IgM type. Incubation period varies from 2-6 weeks. Nausea, vomiting, loss of appetite precedes 1-2 weeks. Dark urine and stool may be noticed. Liver is enlarged and becomes soft. During recovery appetite improves. Management includes restrictions of fat and increased glucose intake. B complex supplements help.

Hepatitis B is a 42 nm DNA virus with 3 antigenically distinct components. HBsAg can be detected in blood during prodrome and remains during the entire icteric phase. The spread is by infected blood, blood products, and breast milk. Incubation period lasts six weeks to six months.

Hepatitis C 90% cases are of post transfusion hepatitis. Hepatitis C virus is a single stranded RNA virus. It has properties similar to falvi virus. No vaccine is available. Treatment of HCV is with low dose alpha interferon with 30-50% success over 3-12 months. After treatment relapse is very common.

Hepatitis G is closely related to HCV and is transmitted through blood. Blood donors suffer most upto 1-3%. Not much is known about it because it does not cause any specific disease.

Hepatocellular carcinoma arises from parenchymal cells. It is associated with cirrhosis in general and hepatitis B and C in particular. Liver becomes tender with palpable mass. Friction rub over tumor may be heared. There will be anemia with leucocytosis.

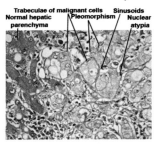

Hepatocellular carcinoma

Hereditary benign intraepithelial dyskeratosis appear as white, spongy macerated lesions of buccal mucosa. These are present on floor of mouth, tongue, gingiva and palate. There may be white plaques overlaying the cornea producing blindness. Buccal mucosa exhibit thickening of epithelium with pronounced hydropic degeneration. *Hereditary Benign Intraepithelial Dyskeratosis* is also known as Witkop – von sallman syndrome. It is an autosomal dominant trait. Patient shows oral mucosal thickening plaques occur on bulbar conjunctiva. Histologically peculiar intraepithelial dyskeratosis, in addition to acanthosis is seen. Cell with in cell phenomenon occurs.

Hereditary fructose intolerance (HFI) is caused by remarkably reduced levels of hepatic fructose-1-phosphate aldolase, which splits fructose-1-phosphate into two 3-carbon fragments for further metabolism. Persons affected with this rare metabolic disorder have learned to avoid any food that contains fructose or sucrose, because the ingestion of these foods can cause nausea, vomiting, malaise, tremor, excessive sweating, and coma due to fructosemia. Most of the symptoms are due to a secondary hypoglycemia. These persons live quite comfortable on other foods (glucose, galactose, and lactose-containing foods like milk, bread, dairy products, rice, and noodles). Although there have been only a limited number of cases reported in the literature, the dental caries prevalence in these subjects has been extremely low.

Hereditary hemorrhagic telangietasia are characterized by multiple round or oval purple papules. The size is below 0.5 cms in diameter. Number may even be one hundred. Purple papules are seen on lips, tongue and buccal mucosa.

Hereditary mucoepithelial dysplasia is an autosomal dominant disorder. Whole of the oral mucosa is involved and oral lesion is a fiery red. Gingival and hard palate are commonly involved. Fissured tongue is seen.

Herpe's Zoster is an acute infectious viral disease. It is very painful and of incapacitating nature. Virus causing it is similar to chicken pox. General malaise, pain and tenderness along with the involved sensory nerve are the symptoms. Often trunk is affected. Patient has a linear popular or vesicular eruption of the skin or mucosa supplied by affected nerves. It is unilateral and dermatomic in distribution. It may affect face due to infection of Trigeminal nerve. Extremely painful buccal mucosal lesions occur. Antiviral drugs are to be continued.

Herpengina is a viral disease of summer caused by coxsackie group of virus. Symptoms are mild and of short duration. It includes sore throat, headache, vomiting and abdominal pain. Small ulcer shows greyish base and inflamed periphery. There may develop fever, pain and enlargement of lymph glands. Lymphocytosis is constant. Disease spreads from one person to another. No treatment is needed as the lesion is self limiting.

Herpes labialis may be caused by common cold and febrile injection. Prodromal paresthesia, burning sensation and then erythema develops. Vesicles form after an hour or two. Vesicles enlarge, coalesce and weep exudates. After 2 days these rupture and coalesce. Aciclovir cream helps.

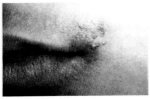

Herpes labialis

Herpes simplex is a viral infection occuring in, patients on immune suppressed drugs are most likely to develop chronic oral ulcers. On these response of T lymphocytes changes. There is formation of small, round, symmetric lesions associated with recurrent herpes infection. Lesions last from weeks to months. Larger lesions have raised white borders of small vesicles.

Herpetic conjunctivitis is a serious disease because it may cause blindness.

Herpetic whitlow is a lesion generally present on finger can be transmitted through saliva. Incubation period is 2 to 12 days. It causes tingling, fever, chills and general malaise. Infected area becomes red and swollen with severe pain.

Herpetiform aphthae are multiple, painful, recurrent mouth ulcers. Ulcers are multiple; shape is irregular with ill defined edges. Floor is grey. Size is small up to 1 to 3 mm.

Heterodont refers to different types of teeth within the same dentition i.e. Incisors, canines, molars.

Heterograft is graft obtained from another species. Usually porcine skin is used .Though used very rarely because it is very expensive.

Hexachlorophene is an anti bacterial, bacteriostatic effect. It is used as presurgical scrub. It has been incorporated in tooth paste.

Hiatus hernia is a sliding type stomach with esophago gastric junction slides upwards through the hiatus into chest. In paraesophageal type esophago-gastric junction is fixed below the diaphragm and a part of stomach herniates through the hiatus besides the esophagus. There will be retro sternal chest pain especially on stooping or lying down soon after meals. Nocturnal regurgitation may cause chocking attacks.

Hierarchy of needs is a theory given by Maslow in the year 1954 believed in self-actualization theory, i.e., the need to understand the totality of a person. The general requirements were arranged in a hierarchy. If one basic requirement is satisfied then next one emerges in the order. The desire for the most basic biologic needs to the more psychological ones becomes secondary after basic needs have been satisfied. Motivation is constantly required and is a never endings, fluctuating complex present in almost all organisms. Pain avoidance, tension reduction and pleasure acts as source of motivating behavior.

High copper alloy is a dental alloy with a relatively high copper content by 10% weight. It is a corrosion free.

High gold alloys are composed principally of gold and platinum group metals with minor addition of tin, indium and iron. Gold content is 78 to 87% by weight. Tin, indium and iron are added to promote a good porcelain bond. The alloy is light yellow in color. Corrosion resistance of gold alloy is excellent.

High risk patients are the patients where the frequency of infectious disease is higher. High risk patients groups include patients requiring frequent blood transfusions, patients of renal dialysis units and immune deficient individuals. Intravenous drug users are also at risk.

High points are used in reference to sealants and restorative areas with sealant and restorative material that interferes with occlusion.

High voltage burns are the electrical burns that are caused by contact with high voltage electric lines ranging from 10,000 to 32,000 volts. The tissues are so extensively and rapidly damaged that they usually involve amputation of a limb either partly or completely. In these cases the damage actually extends into the normal tissues quite proximal to the apparently affected areas. This is to be kept in mind while doing amputation that the level of amputation can be higher than what is planned because of proximally damaged muscles below the normal skin.

High-stepping gait is adopted to avoid tripping from the toes catching the ground. It develops when there is weakness of extensor muscles of feet as in perineal nerve palsy.

Hill's sign occurs if femoral systolic pulse pressure 60 to 100 mm. higher in right leg than right arm. It is indicative of aortic insufficiency.

Hirsuitism is a condition where there is growth depending on the testosterone. Cells of hair follicle secrete in enzyme which acts on testosterone and makes it active.

Histamine is a vasoactive amine that acts as a vasodilator and increases the permeability of the small blood vessels and functions as a central nervous system neurotransmitter.

Histiocytosis develops due to proliferation of histiocytic cells occurring in bone marrow, spleen and liver. Lesions around jaw are common. Localized destructive lesion occurs. Tooth buds may be destroyed.

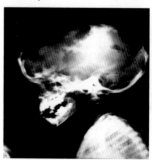
Histiocytosis

Histoplasmosis is a fungal infection caused by *Histoplasma capsulatum*. It is a demographic fungus. Inhaling infected dust may cause the infection. Person develops low grade fever, productive cough, lymphadeno-pathy and enlargement of liver and spleen. Oral lesion develops after pulmonary involvement. Oral manifestations appear as nodular, ulcerative or vegetative lesions on buccal mucosa, tongue palate or lips. Ulcerated areas are covered by gray membrane. Organisms may be easily isolated. Nodule may ulcerate and grow slowly. Cervical lymph glands may be enlarged and firm. Culture of infected tissue may give appropriate diagnosis. Treatment includes Ketoconazole for 6-12 months.

Historical research is a type of research in which past events are documented because they can provide a perspective that can guide decision making in present.

HIV related gingivitis appears as typical redness in gingiva extending into the alveolar mucosa also known as linear gingival erythema.

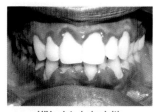

HIV related gingivitis

HIV related myelopathy usually occurs in AIDS subject. It is less common than encephalopathy. It may develop due to methyl group deficiency and is of 3 types. One is vascular myelopathy in which features are similar to acute combined degeneration. Secondly degeneration restricted to

gracile tracts has also been known. Finally HIV specific multi nucleate giant cell infiltration is seen in brain in HIV encephalopathy and may extend to spinal cord.

HIV related oral melanosis occurs due to involvement of Addison's disease. Progressive hyper pigmentation of skin, nails and mucus membrane may take place. Etiology remains undetermined. Buccal mucosa, gingiva tongue and palate may be affected.

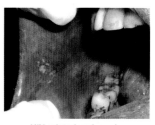

HIV related melanosis

Ho: YAG lasers has solid active medium, a crystal of YAG doped with Holmium. Fiberoptically delivered in contact with the tissue in free-running pulsed mode. Wavelength is 2120 nm. Ho laser has little affinity for pigmented tissue; its hemostatic ability is decreased because of its lower absorbency into hemoglobin and other similar pigments. Absorbency by tooth structures is low. Frequently used for arthroscopy surgery on the TMJ.

Hoarseness is defined as roughness of voice resulting from variations of periodicity and intensity. To have normal voice. Vocal cords should be able to approximate properly. It should also have a proper size, stiffness and be able to vibrate regularly.

Hodgkin's lymphoma is a malignant histiocytic origin arising from lymph nodes. It is a disease of young adults. It may present with asymptomatic lymphadenopathy. Glands are painless, discrete and rubbery. Mediastinal lymph glands or retroperitoneal lymph glands provide clues. Clinical features includes, malaise, pyrexia, night sweats, weight loss and pruritus. Lower cervical glands are mostly enlarged with axillary nodes. Nodes are discrete, non tender, mobile and firm. Feel is like of rubber. Dysphagia and syphonea may develop.

Hodgkin's lymphoma is not a common disease. Males between the ages of 15-35 years are affected. Generalized lymphade-nopathy is the hallmark of the disease. Enlarged lymph nodes are firm, and rubbery in consistency. Fever, weight loss, pain abdomen are the features. There may be persistent cough due to pressure on trachea. Liver and spleen is enlarged. Oral lesion

includes submucosal swelling with ulceration. Pain is present. Lesion may be fixed to underlying bone. Chemotherapy with radiotherapy helps.

Hoe and chisel are the instruments used to remove tenacious subgingival calculus and altered cementum.

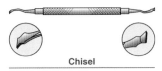

Chisel

Hoe scalers are the hand instruments used for scaling of ledges or removal of rings of calculus. The blade is bent at 90° angle thus forming a cutting edge at the junction of flattened terminal surface with the inner aspect of the phase. The blade is slightly bowed so that it can maintain contact at two points on a convex surface.

Holding solution is a disinfecting solution used to cover conta-minated instruments before they are processed for sterilization.

Homan's sign is said to have occured where pain is felt in calf when the foot is pulled upwards. This indicates venous thrombosis.

Homodont refers to the presence of only one type of tooth in the dentition.

Homograft is obtained from any other human being except the patient himself. Usually the patient's own relatives are chosen as donors, i.e. the best donors being siblings followed by the parents. However, fresh cadaveric skin can also be used if prior permission has been taken.

Eosinophils   Macrophages
Lymphocytes   Reed-sternberg cell   Plasma cells

Hodgkin's lymohoma, mixed cellularity

In such donors, HIV and HBsAg is tested prior to donation as the contraindications for homograft use in hepatitis, AIDS and disseminated fungal infections. Usually fresh skin is used but skin stored for less than 2 weeks can also be used. Older skin can be used in early phases of wound debridement and preparation for auto grafting. A good 'Take 'of homograft is a good test for wound readiness to accept auto graft.

Hopewood house children is the study done to assess the dental status of childhood between 3 and 14 years of age residing at Hopewood House, Bowral, New South Wales, longitudinally for 10 years. All lived on a strictly institutional diet that, with the exception of an occasional serving of egg yolk was entirely vegetable in nature and largely raw. Except for weekends between-meal snacks were limited to milk, fruit, and raw vegetables. The dental caries prevalence in young children in Hopewood House was almost negligible in the primary dentition, and approximately one tenth that seen in the permanent teeth of the average Australian child. A total of 25 out of 82 children remained caries free over a 5-years study period.

Horizontal bone loss is a bone loss that occurs in a plane parallel to the cementoenamel junction of adjacent teeth.

Horizontal brush scrubis the technique of tooth brushing commonly used. But unlimited scrubbing motion exerts pressure on the facial tooth prominence. It result in gingival recession, gingival and tooth abrasion.

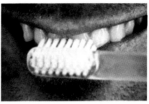

Horizontal brusing

Horizontal fibres extends at right angles to the long axis of the tooth from cementum to alveolar crest.

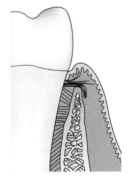

Horizontal fibres

Horizontal mattress suture is often used for the interproximal areas of diastema or for wide interdental spaces to properly adapt the interproximal papilla against the bone. The horizontal mattress suture can either be incorporated with continuous, independent sling suture (*see* Figure on page 230).

Horner's syndrome comprises contraction of pupil of eye, ptosis or drooping of eye lid, anhidrosis and vasodilatation over face. Features depend on the degree of

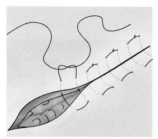

Horizontal mattress suture

damage of sympathetic path to head and site of the damage.

Horse shoe kidney is produced by fusion of two ureteric buds. It may remain functionally normal except hydronephrosis or stone may develop.

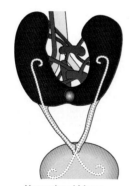

Horseshoe kidney

Host factors are the factors with in an individual host that can influence disease.

Host resistance is the ability of an individual to resist a pathogen or the ability of the person to fight off disease.

Hot air sterilization is done by hot air produced in an electrically heated oven called hot air sterilizer. Contents are kept at 160° C for two hours. It is utilized for sterilizing large batches of instruments overnight. Root canal instruments which are to be kept dry can be sterilized.

Human development Index is defined as a composite index combining indicators representing three dimensions, longevity, knowledge and income.

Human fibrin foam is an anticoagulant used in case of bleeding tooth socket. It can be packed into the socket and sutured if needed. Socket is then kept undisturbed.

Humerus is the second largest bone of body. It is a long bone of arm.

Humidity is always present in atmosphere. It depends on air's temperature. If the air is cooled excessive moisture precipitates which is known as dew point for that temperature.

Humor's theory statics that the ancient Greeks considered that a person's physical and mental constitution was determined by the relative proportions of the four elemental fluids of the body-blood, phlegm, black bile, and yellow bile which corresponds to the four humors–sanguine, phlegmatic, melancholic and choleric. All diseases, including caries could be explained by an imbalance of those humors.

Humoral immunity is the one in which antibodies play the predominant role.

Huntington's disease is characterized by choreoattetatic moments, personality changes and progressive dementia. Symptoms appear between 35 to 40 years of age. Choreic movements are diagnostic and involve distal as well as axial musculature. Person drops the objects. Walking is associated with more brisk arm and leg movements.

Hurler syndrome is a disturbance of mucopolysacchrides metabolism. Its excretion in urine increases. Symptoms develop within 2 years of life. Head is enlarged with prominent forehead, broad nose and puffy eyelids. There is shortening and broadening of a mandible, thick lips, large tongue. Open mouth and nasal congestion. Short neck and spinal injuries are common. Teeth are small, widely spaced and with altered morphology. Gingival hyperplasia is developed. There is no treatment for the disease.

Hutchinson's Wart generally occurs in an adult who presents with a warty swelling of tongue. Onset is insidious and is mostly situated in midline. It is soft and painless.

Hyaline degeneration is a translucent homogeneous material staining pink with eosin. This calcification is common in leiomyoma.

Hybrid composite resins are the type of composites containing colloidal silica of 0.01-0.12 micro millimetre in addition to fine sized particles.

Hydatid cyst of liver for two species of cystodes echinococcus granulaosus and echinococcus mulitlocularis human being act as intermediate host. Hydatied cyst of E.granulosus is usually solitary involving right lobe of liver, while E. multilocularis is having germinal membrane which permits formation of new cysts on its outer surface. Renal involvement produces lumbar pain and hematuria. Calcification occurs in 40% cases. Eosinophilia is usual. Complement fixation and indirect hemagglutination tests are positive.

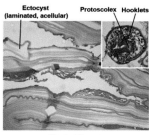

Ectocyst (laminated, acellular)   Protoscolex   Hooklets

Hydatid cyst

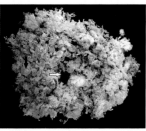

Hydatidiform mole

Trophoblastic hyperplasia   Hydropic change
Chorionic villi   Stromal core

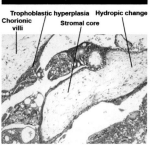

Hydro densitometry is a method of measuring body composition.

Body mass divided by body volume reflects the body's fat content. Body density can be estimated by dividing its mass in air by a volume obtaining its mass in air by a volume obtained by weighing a subject both in air and under the water.

Hydro phosphate cement is an innovation of compounding of zinc phosphate cement the mixing of dehydrated dihydrogen phosphate of zinc calcium and other materials. These cements have no marked advantage over the conventional zinc phosphate material.

Hydrogen peroxide is an unstable compound. It breaks down to yield to give water and oxygen. Its antibacterial effect is brief and is useful in mouthwashes against ulcerative gingivitis. Ten volume of hydrogen peroxide with equal amount of water is useful in debridement of root canals during root canal therapy.

Hydronephrosis refers to the dilatation of renal pelvis resulting into atrophy of parenchyma. It may be congenital or acquired. It can be unilateral when condition involves the renal pelvis and a ureter, while those involving bladder outlet and urethra hydronephrosis can be bilateral. Bilateral hydronephrosis leads to renal failure and uraemia. Kidney may be massively enlarged. One or both ureters may be enlarged depending on level of obstruction.

Hydrophilic liner is a soft liner that is readily wet by water.

Hydrophobic is a water repellent showing a high contact angle.

Hydrostatic pressure is a pressure caused by the weight of a column of water.

Hygiene is the science that deals with the preservation of health.

Hygroscopic is pertaining to the absorbing of water.

Hyper immunoglobulin is the preparation containing specific antibodies used to prevent disease after exposure to a pathogen.

Hyper kinesis refers to excessive motility.

Hyperactive pulpalgia is characterized by short, sharp shock. It is never spontaneous. Pain is of short duration so long irritant is there-may be cold or hot, sweet or sour. Icecream excites the nerve in teeth and pain is referred to eyes. Hyperactive pulpalgia is common following the placement of new restoration. Patients also complain this after curettage. It may be associated with caries of tooth. Fractured teeth are more hyper reactive. In maxillary sinusitis maxillary teeth are involved.

Hypercalcemia refers to the increased levels of calcium in blood. In mild cases it may be asymptomatic. Person may develop constipation and anorexia. In moderate high person develops polyuria, nocturia and polydipsia. In severe high cases person develops emotional liability, confusion, delirium and psychosis. In late stage acute renal failure may develop.

Hypercementosis refers to deposition of excessive amount of secondary cementum on root surfaces. It covers the entire root area. It may be caused by accelerated elongation of a tooth inflammation, tooth repair and osteitis deformans. It shows no signs and symptoms. Cemental spikes may be seen. There is no increase or decrease of sensitivity. Radiographically bulging and thickening of rods is noted. No treatment is indicated.

Hyperdontia is the presence of extra teeth beyond the normal complement. Also refer supernumerary teeth

Hyperemia is an increased blood flow in the pulp. The increased pressure against the sensory nerve endings in the pulp produce the sensation associated with hyperemia. It will explain why the pain appears to be of different intensity and character with application of cold or heat, the cold producing hypersensitivity response and the heat producing true transient hyperemia.

Hyperkalemia is recognized by increased levels of potassium. It may be the result of extensive tissue breakdown, severe dehydration, or excessive amount of potassium. Symptoms include numbness, mental confusion, cold skin and disturbed cardiac rate.

Hypermangesemia refers to the increased serum levels of magnesium in acute and renal failure. Deep tendon reflexes are lost and necrosis, hypotension, respiratory paralysis occurs with serum level 10 mEq/L. Treatment includes 100-200 mg of calcium.

Hyperocclusion is when occlusal surface of a tooth or restoration is raised above the occlusal plane of the teeth in arch.

Hyperparathyroidism refers to excess of circulating parathyroid hormone. Bone and kidney are the target organs. Serum calcium level is elevated. Clinical features include emotional instability, painful bones and joints, crampy abdomen, bowing of long bones, pigeon chest, collapse vertebra, muscle weakness, fatigue, polyuria and polydipsia. Radiological Features include Ground glass appearance, moth eaten appearance with varying intensity, punctate and nodular calcification may develop in kidney and joints, pepper pot skull due to osteopenia, Teeth may become mobile and migrate, Loss of lamina dura which may be complete or partial.

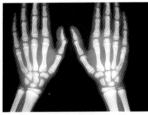

Hyperparathyroidism with subperiosteal erosion

Hyperpituitarism result due to hyperfunction of the anterior lobe of pituitary gland producing growth hormone. Before closing of epiphysis, gigantism occurs and after closure, acromegaly. In this condition, bone overgrowth and thickening of soft tissue causes a coarsening of facial features. Head and feet become large with clubbing of toes and fingers. There will be enlargement of sella turcica, paranasal sinuses and thickening of outer table of skull. Angle between ramus and body of mandible is widened. There is enlargement of inferior dental canal. Radiograph will show increased tooth size specially of root due to secondary cemental hyperplasia. Oral manifestations include prominent mandibular condylar growth, Overgrowth of mandible leading to prognathism, Lips become thick like Negro's, Teeth become more spaced, Body and root may be longer than normal.

Hyperplasia is defined as an increase in number of cells in a tissue or organ. Pathological hyperplasia is common in oral cavity. Increase in number of epithelial cells and increased thickness of epithelium due to chronic irritation or abrasion.

Hypersecretion of cortisol leads to increased fat deposition in certain areas, such as face and back, elevated blood pressure, and alters blood cell distribution. Clinically cortisol hypersecretion is referred to as Cushing's syndrome, a condition usually corrected through surgical removal of part of adrenal gland.

Hypersensitivity is a condition in which there is an exaggerated or inappropriate immune reaction that causes tissue destruction or inflammation.

Hypersensitivity of drug is an unwanted drug reaction related to abnormal individual susceptibility. It is related to genetic factors. Drugs can act as antigens causing immunologically induced inflammatory response. Topical administration may cause a greater number of reactions than oral and parental. However, parental administration will result in wide spread reaction and patients with multiple allergies will have more reaction to drugs.

Hypersensitivity of teeth is caused by the initiating factors of a hypersensitive pulp and is usually cold food or drink or cold air or stimulation of exposed dentin on the root surface by cold, sweet or sour substances. Fruits and salts may also result in hypersensitivity. The sensation disappears as soon as electrolyte is diluted away or metal is removed. Actually pain can be evoked from dentin by applying solutions to it which exert high osmotic pressure. A sharp, sudden painful reaction is seen when a tooth is exposed to hot, cold, chemical, mechanical or osmotic (sweet or salt) stimuli.

Hypersensitivity Type II reaction is caused by IgG and IgM antibodies and is capable of causing type III hypersensitivity reaction as well. The main distinction is that type II reactions involve antibodies directed to Ag on the surface of specific cells or tissues whereas type III are due to antibodies against widely distributed antigen or soluble Ag in serum. While damage caused by Type II localizes reaction to a particular tissue or cell type, damage caused by type III react affects those organs where Ag-Ab complexes are deposited. These hypersensitive reactions are related to normal immune responses seen against micro-organism and parasites. In the reaction against pathogens, exaggerated immune reaction may be as damaging to the host as the effects of the pathogen itself. These reactions are seen in autoimmune disease, trans-plantation reactions.

Hypersensitivity Type IV is a delayed type of reaction. In the original classification by Coomb and Gell in 1968, Delayed hypersensitivity or type IV was used as a general category to describe all those hypersensitivity reactions, which took place more than 12 hrs to develop. DTH cannot be transferred from one to another by serum. It is associated with T- cell protective immunity.

Hypertensive arteriosclerosis shows thickening of arteries in case of hypertension. Medium and large sized arteries show hypertrophy of media due to increased number of smooth muscle cell and elastic fibres. In later stage hyalinisation of vessel wall may occur.

Hypertensive brain hemorrhage are putamen and around internal capsule, thalamus, pons and cerebellum. It generally does not occur in white matter. Putaminal hemorrhage is characterized by contralateral hemiplegia. In bigger hematoma there may be development of bilateral motor palsy, irregular respiration and dilated fixed pupil. Thalamic hemorrhage develops hemi sensory defect, unequal pupils. Pontine hemorrhage produces deep coma, pinpoint reactive pupil, quadriplegia and hyper- thermia. Cerebellar hemorrhage presents with ataxia, headache and hydrocephalus.

Hyperthyroidism is known as thyrotoxicosis, due to overpro- duction of thyroxine. It may be caused by Graves' disease. Hyperthyroidism Symptoms are due to increased metabolic activity of tissues or body. BMR is increased. Thyroid is enlarged, Enlargement may be asym- metrical and nodular, Thyroid may be tender, Liver and spleen may be enlarged, Nervousness, muscle weakness and fine tremors, cardiac palpitation, irregular heart beat and excessive perspiration develops. Tachycar- dia, and increased pulse pressure, Ankle edema and systolic hypertension, Amenorrhea, infertility, decreased libido and impotence are noted. There may be lymphadenopathy and osteoporosis. There may be alveolar resorption, Trabaculae may be of greater density, faster eruption and premature loss of primary teeth, early eruption of permanent teeth, early jaw development, generalized decre- ase in bone density is seen with loss of edentulous alveolar bone.

Hypertonic is a solution containing a higher level of salt i.e. NaCl than is found in living RBC which is 0.9% NaCl.

Hypertrophic Lichen planus may occur on oral mucosa as a well circumscribed elevated white lesion like leukoplakia. Biopsy is required to confirm diagnosis.

Hypertrophy is overgrowth of tissue.

Hyperventilation is a condition caused by rapid respirations leading to acapnia i.e. carbon dioxide depletion and subsequent respiratory alkalosis. Person develops light headedness, trembling, tingling and numb- ness. It may be caused by excessive nervousness or hysteria.

Hypervitaminosis D refers to excess of vitamin D in body. Toxicity has been found to result when daily doses of between 10,000 and 50,000 i.u. are taken over a prolonged period of time. This vitamin is resistant to heat and cooling process. Being fat soluble it is stored in body. Excessive intake of vitamin D results in anorexia, nausea, vomiting, excessive thirst and drowsiness. Cramps and tingling of finger and toes are also noted.

Hypervitaminosis is an excess of specific vitamins accumulated in the body to the level of toxicity. Commonest is vitamin A and vitamin D.

Hypnotics are drugs which are used to induce sleep and drowsiness. They depress the central nervous system acting on central cerebral cortex.

Hypocalcaemia refers to where serum calcium falls below 8 mg %. It may be due to decreased bone resorption of calcium, decreased intestinal calcium resorption calcium binding and sequestration. Clinical features include numbness, cramps, anxiety and tetany followed by convulsions, laryngeal stridor, dystonia and psychosis. 10 ml of 10% calcium gluconate IV followed by 10-40 ml of 10% calcium gluconate in 5% dextrose gives relief. Oral vitamin D and calcium are needed.

Hypocalcification is the lack or deficiency of initial calcification of organic enamel matrices.

Hypocalcified type of amelogenesis imperfecta is characterized by enamel of normal thickness which is poorly calcified. These are of two types; one is inherited as an autosomal dominant trait and other as autosomal recessive trait. At eruption teeth presents as yellow to orange enamel which is soft and rapidly lost. It leaves exposed dentin. Radiographically enamel has moth eaten appearance and is less radio-paque than dentin. Cervical enamel is better calcified.

Hypoglossal nerve is a twelfth cranial motor nerve. It supplies muscles of tongue controlling its shape and movement (*see* Figure on page 237).

Hypoglycaemic encephalopathy refers to when blood sugar level falls below 25-30 mg causes confusion, convulsion, hemi paresis and coma. Overdose of insulin may result in the condition. Initial symptoms are headache, palpitation, anxiety, trembling and profuse sweating. When blood sugar falls below 10 mg/dL patient develops deep coma, dilated pupils, hypotonia and shallow respiration. Prompt correction of hypoglycaemia before the onset of medullary phase reverses the symptoms.

Hypoglycemia is when blood sugar falls below 40 mg %. It occurs when liver glucose output falls below the glucose uptake by peripheral tissues and when brains requirement is not met, patient shows neurological symptoms like psychiatric disorder, fits, epilepsy and cerebrovascular disease. Patient may feel tired and weak; palpitation, sweating and hunger may develop. Later headache, confusion, visual disturbance, ataxia and personality changes appear. Lastly convulsions and coma may develop. Blood sugar may be very low in polycythemia and leukaemia.

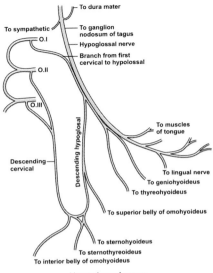

To dura mater

To sympathetic

To ganglion nodosum of tagus

O.I

Hypoglossal nerve

Branch from first cervical to hypolossal

O.II

O.III

Descending hypoglossal

To muscles of tongue

Descending cervical

To lingual nerve

To geniohyoideus

To thyreohyoideus

To superior belly of omohyoideus

To sternohyoideus

To sternothyreoideus

To interior belly of omohyoideus

Hypoglossal nerve

Hypokalaemia refers to low level of potassium in the body. Patient becomes listless with slow and slurred speech with intense drowsiness. Tone of muscles is reduced. The reflexes become absent. Patient may develop incontinence of urine. Abdomen is distended and bowel sounds become absent. Pulse may become irregular.

Hypomagnesemia refers to low level of magnesia. In this condition patient may complaints of anorexia, weakness and apathy. One may feel tremor, ataxia and vertigo along with depression/irritability and psychotic behavior. Hence twice the estimated deficit is to be given.

Hypomaturation can be explained as lack of secondary mineralization or maturation.

Hypomaturation amelogenesis imperfecta refer to a developmental disturbance of teeth where enamel is normal in form but is opaque and white to brownish yellow. Teeth are mottled. Teeth are soft and develop attrition.

Hypoparathyroidism refers to when there is insufficient secretion of parathyroid hormone. It may result from autoimmune destruction, surgical damage to parathyroid, parathyroid damage from radioactive iodine I-131. Clinical features include stiffness in hands, feet and lips, parasthesia around mouth, tingling in fingers and toes, anxiety and depression and intelligence is lowered. Oral Manifestations are delayed eruption of teeth and hypoplasia of enamel.

Hypopituitarism may be congenital or due to destructive disease. Space occupying lesions like craniopharyngioma, adenomas may result it. There is symmetrical underdevelopment but in some cases there may be disproportionate length of long bones. Hypoglycemia may develop due to growth hormone and cortisol deficiency. Onset of puberty is delayed. Patient becomes lethargic, fat mass is increased. Skull and facial bones are small. Tooth eruption is hampered, dental arch is smaller than normal, so overcrowding of teeth results, Eruption of teeth is delayed, and so is the shedding of deciduous teeth.

Hypoplasia due to congenital syphilis is contracted in utero from a mother who had treponemal infection. Syphilis produces classic patterns of hypoplastic dysmorphic permanent teeth. Saber shins, frontal bossing and saddle nose are common structural anomalies. Congenital syphilis clinically will present with (1) Interstitial Keratosis (2) Deafness (3) Tooth anomalies (Hutchinson's triad). The hypoplasia involves the maxillary and mandibular permanent incisors and the first molars. The anterior teeth affected are called "Hutchinson's teeth" while the molars are referred to as "Mulberry Molar" (Moon's molars, Fournier's molars). The upper central incisor is "screw – driver" shaped, the mesial and distal surfaces of the crown tapering and converging towards the incisal edge of the tooth rather than towards the cervical margin. As a result, diastema is occasionally observed between the central incisors. The cause of the tapering and notching of the maxillary incisor has been explained on the basis of the absence of the central tubercle or calcification center. The crowns of the first molar in congenital syphilis are irregular and the enamel of the occlusal third of the tooth appears to be arranged in an agglomerate mass of globules rather than in well-formed cusps.

Hypoplasia of parotid gland is seen with Melkerson – Rosenthal syndrome. It consists of orofacial granuloma, facial paralysis and fissured tongue.

Hypoplastic amelogenesis imperfecta main defect is in formation of matrix. Enamel is irregular pitted but hard and translucent. Defects become stained but caries don't develop easily.

Hyposensitization is the therapy involving the injection of increasing doses of allergen. Following treatment there is an increase in serum levels of allergen specific IgG and suppressor T cell activity while specific IgE levels tend to fall. However, since allergic humans are clinically diagnosed after sensitization and this may explain the relative lack of success of desensitization in many subjects.

Hypothesis is a proposed explanation of an observed phenomenon or it is a conjectural statement of the relationship between variables.

Hypothyroidism is a condition where secretion of thyroid is diminished. It may be due to atrophy of thyroid gland or failure of thyrotropic function of pituitary gland. It may lead to three types: Cretinism- hormone failure occurs in infancy, Juvenile myxedema- it occurs in childhood, Myxedema- it occurs after puberty. Clinical features: cretinism and myxedema may be present at birth, constipation and hoarse cry may result, delayed fusion of epiphysis, hair becomes dry and sparse cretinism leads to mental defects, generalized edema and other changes. Base of skull is shortened. Face fails to develop in longitudinal direction. Mandible is underdeveloped. Tongue is enlarged by edema fluid. Development of teeth is delayed.

Hypoxia is low oxygen level.

Hysteric tremor tends to involve a limb or the whole body and is worsened by the examiner's attempt to control it.

H

Ice immersion is a procedure in which the part to be treated is immersed in an ice solution such as hand, feet and elbows. Solution is made up of 50% water and 50% ice. It has to be single less than 10 minutes immersion or shorter immersion making a cumulative time of 10 minutes.

Ice packs – Crushed or flanked ice placed inside a specially made terry towel bag. It may be done by folding towel into an appropriate shape. The wet ice pack is placed on the top of the part to be treated. It should not put pressure to obstruct the circulation. Reduced circulation may lead to ice burn.

Id was described by Sigmond Frued in 1905 in psychosexual theory. In Latin it means 'it' Greek- primal urges, it is the basic structure of personality which serves as reservoir of instincts (or) their mental representative. Present at birth, impulse ridden and drives immediate pressure gratification.

Ideal occlusion is a complete harmonious relationship of the teeth and masticatory system.

Identification dot is a small raised dot that appears in one corner of intraoral film. It is used for film orientation.

Idiocy is the result of congenital defective mental faculty. The person may have negative existence and may be devoid of any will power, memory, emotion and initiative power. He is not able to protest himself. IQ is between 0 to 10.

Idiopathic dysguesia like atypical facial pain and idiopathic xerostomia is considered a manifestation of depression. Taste dysfunction is reported as a complaint by burning mouth syndrome.

Idiopathic thrombocytopenic purpura is an uncommon disease of remissions and exacerbations when platelet count is low, excessive bleeding may occur after dental extraction. Bleeding time is prolonged.

Idophor is a disinfectant used in different strength as a surgical scrub and as a surface disinfectant. These are intermediate level hospital disinfectants with tuberculocidal action. These are effective with in 5-10 minutes. These may discolor surface or metals.

Idoxuridine is used as anti herpetic agent in treatment of mouth and eye infections due to herpe's simplex ions.

IL-1 (Interleukin-1) is a pro-inflammatory, multifunctional cytokine, which among its many biological activities enables ingress of inflammatory cells into sites of infection, promotes bone resorption, stimulates eicosanoid (specifically PGE_2) release by monocytes and fibroblasts, stimulates release of Matrix metalloproteinases, that degrade proteins of the extracellular matrix, and participates in many aspects of the immune response.

IL-6 -1 (Interleukin-6) is a cytokine that stimulates plasma cell proliferation and therefore antibody production and is produced by lymphocytes, monocytes and fibroblasts. Levels of IL-6 have been shown to be elevated in inflamed tissues, higher in periodontitis than in gingivitis tissues and higher in Gingival crevicular fluid (GCF) from refractory periodontitis. IL-6 has been shown to stimulate osteoclast formation. Thus, this cytokine may in large part account for both the predominance of plasma cells in periodontitis lesions as well as bone resorption.

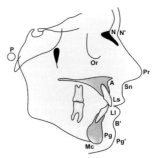

Inferior labial sulcus

IL-8 (Interleukin-8) is a chemo attractant that is mainly produced by monocytes in response to lipopolysaccharide, IL-1 or Tumor necrosis factor alpha (TNF-α). It is present at high levels in periodontitis lesions, mainly associated with the junctional epithelium and macrophages. In addition to serving as a chemo-attractant for neutrophils, it appears to selectively stimulate matrix metalloproteinase activity from these cells, thus in part accounting for collagen destruction within periodontitis lesions.

Illegitimate child is the one which is born out of wedlock or not within a competent line after the cessation of relationship of husband and wife or when procreation by the husband is not possible due to congenital defect or getting vasectomy done.

ILS (Inferior labial sulcus) is the point of greatest concavity in the midline of the lower lip between labrale inferiour and soft – tissue pogonion.

Imbecility – These are more or less idiots but can speak in articulated language. They are intellectually poor and often dangerous to society. Their IQ is between 20-40.

Imipramine is a drug used in treatment of mental depression and effect is produced in 4-10 days. It can be given once daily. It results in papillary dilatation, paralysis of accommodation, dryness of mouth, postural hypotension and urinary retention.

Immunity is a resistance exhibited by the host towards injury caused by micro-organisms and their products. Certain white cells release antibodies and antitoxins into blood plasma. Many causative factors such as micro-organisms, bacteria and animal toxins can produce antibodies and antitoxins. All such factors are known as antigens.

Immunization is a procedure when delibrate artificial exposure to disease to produce acquired immunity.

Immunodeficiency is a type of immunopathological condition that involves deficiency in number, function or inter relationship of involved WBCs and their products. It may be congenital or acquired. When person's immune system is not functioning opportunistic infections invade the host.

Immunogen is any substance capable of inducing an immune response called an immunogen and is said to be immunogenic.

Immunology is the study of the ways in which the body defends itself from infectious agents and other foreign substances in its environment. It encompasses many layers of defense including physical barriers like skin, protective chemical substances in the blood and tissue fluids and the physiologic reaction of tissues to injury or infection.

Impacted tooth can be discribed where teeth cannot erupt due to physical obstruction.

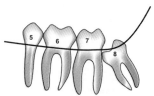

Impacted lower third molar

Impaction-bony refers to the tooth that is blocked by both bone and tissue.

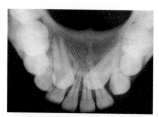

Bilaterally impacted canines

Implant is a titanium post that is implanted into bone. A crown, bridge, or denture is then placed over the implant to restore function and esthetics. Overdentures and bridges rely on presence of teeth for retention. If there are no tooth roots for an overdenture artificial tooth roots are to be implanted into alveolar bone. Implants are made up of titanium and consist of threaded cylinders which are screwed in bones.

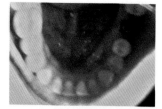

Implant placed in the Alveolar bone

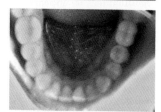

Postoperative picture of implant along with the placement of Crown

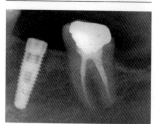

Radiographic view of an implant

Implantation is the procedure where the placement with in body tissue of a foreign substance.

Implied contract is established between patient and doctor. An expressed contract is informed consent given in writing or verbally. Gardian's consent is given when patient is minor or is not mentally competent to do so. Written consent is an expressed consent.

Impotence is the inability to have sexual intercourse. While sterility is the inability of male have the child. A person can be sterile without being impotence.

Impression is the negative replica of an oral cavity.

Impression material is used to make an accurate replica of oral tissues area involved varies from a single tooth to the whole dentition. Impression gives a negative reproduction of tissue and by filling it, positive case is made. Die is used to prepare inlays or bridge.

Impression compound is a solid material which is softened by heat to a plastic consistency suitable for recording impression. Upon cooling it hardens rapidly in oral cavity. Slab form is softened in hot water and sticks which are softened over a flame. It gives a full denture by means of a perfect peripheral seal. Disadvantage is that it cannot be withdrawn from undercut areas without distortion.

Impression paste is a material used to make impression of dentures. It is supplied in 2 tubes. One containing white zinc oxide mixture and the other containing red eugenol mixture. Equal length of mixtures are mixed together with a spatula to give an uniform pink mix. Disadvantage of it is not very useful for partial impressions.

Impression tray is a tray that is made up of either stainless steel or plastic formed in the general shape of the mouth, used for taking impressions. These are of two types. Partial trays are used for impressions of partial dentures and edentulous trays are used for full dentures. These are semicircular in cross section.

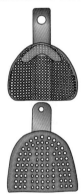

Impression tray

Impulse is an action potential transmitted along a nerve or muscle fibre.

In vitro means outside living body or in a test tube.

In vivo means in the living body, plant or animal.

Inborn immunity refers to the immunity to disease that is inherited.

Incidence is defined as the number of new cases occurring in defined population during a specified period of time. It is calculated as **Incipient interproximal lesion** extends less than halfway through the thickness of enamel. The term incipient means beginning to exist. An incipient lesion is seen in enamel only.

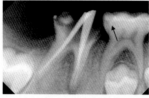

Incipient proximal caries

Incipient malocclusion may be defined as a condition, which shows a tendency to develop into a deviation from the normal dentofacial or occlusal relationship.

Incisal edge is the cutting edge, ridge, or surface of anterior teeth.

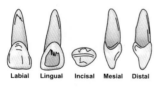

Labial   Lingual   Incisal   Mesial   Distal

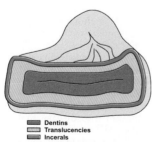

Dentins
Translucencies
Incerals

Incisal edge

Incisive foramen is an opening or hole in bone located at midline of the anterior portion of hard palate, posterior to maxillary central incisor. It appears radiolucent.

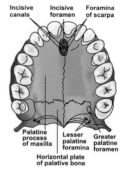

Incisive foramen

Incisive nerve is the nerve that originates at the mental foramen and innervates those teeth anterior alveolar nerve.

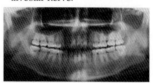

Incisive canal

Incisor liability is the size difference between the four permanent maxillary incisors teeth and four primary incisor teeth. According to Baume it is 7.6 mm in maxilla and 6.0 mm in mandible.

Incisors refer to the central and lateral incisors; the first and second teeth from the midline of the mouth. In permanent and primary dentition, they are 8 in number four upper, i.e. 2 central

The trigeminal nerve and its branches

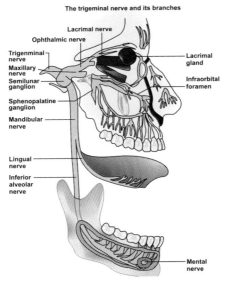

Incisive nerve

2 lateral and four lower, i.e. 2 central, 2 laterals.

Inclination angle gives an assessment of the indication of the maxillary base. It is the angle formed by the Pn line and palatal bone. A large angle expresses upward and forward inclination, whereas small angles indicates down and back tipping of the anterior end of the palatal plane and maxillary base. This angle does not correlate with growth pattern.

Inclination of the nasal base is angle formed between true vertical (e.g. SnV) and the long axis of the nostril varies from about 90° in men to as much as 105° in women.

Incontinentia pigmenti develops vesicobullous lesions on trunk and extremities. The pigmentation begins to fade with in a year. There may be associated local and generalized baldness and optic atrophy. There is delayed tooth eruption. No treatment is required.

Independent 't' test is a parametric test of differences between two independent samples.

Independent variable is the presumed cause of a measured effect. In experimental research at least one independent variable is manipulated.

Index (Esther M. Wilkins) is an expression of clinical observation in numerical values which is used to describe the status of the individual or group with respect to a condition being measured

Index (Russel A.L) has been

defined as a numerical value describing the relative status of a population on a graduated scale with definite upper and lower limits, which is designed to permit and facilitate comparison with other populations classified by the same criteria and methods.

Indirect transmission of disease occurs through dirty hands, soiled laundry, contaminated instruments touching during dental procedure.

Indomethacin is an anti nflammatory agent with analgestic and anti pyretic effect and is absorbed well when given orally. Bone marrow depression has been reported. Side effects includes GIT upsets, headache and dizziness with oral ulcerations. It is not given in dental disorder.

Inert refer to the no inherent power of action, motion or resistance.

Infancy (Soother or Nursing Bottle) Caries: is a rapidly progressing type of dental caries that affects the primary teeth of children, usually during the first 2 years of life and as early as the first year. In infant there is a unique distribution of dental decay. The 4 maxillary anterior incisors are affected first; these teeth are anatomically so positioned in the mouth as to be most frequently bathed by a feeding and if unchecked the decay may extend to the maxillary and mandibular molars. Initially, the lower anterior teeth may not be involved because of the protective environment of the mandibular salivary secretions and the cleansing action of the tongue muscles. Infancy caries is most often seen in children with an unusual dietary history such as the addition of syrup, honey or sucrose to the formula of the use. It has been reported that prolonged and unrestricted night time breastfeeding can result in increased caries rates.

Infancy refers to the 1st year after birth and the first 4 weeks of which are designated as the new born or neonatal period.

Infantile beri beri is a condition that results in infants between second and sixth month deficiency of to day of vit B_6 (Thiamine). Illness develops acutely and is rapidly fatal. Child becomes restless, often cries, passes less of urine and becomes puffy. He may develop convulsions and coma. Child may become cyanosed suddenly with tachycardia and dies within 24-48 hours.

Infantile swallowing is a non congenital conditional reflex. During the normal infantile swallowing the tongue lies in between the gumpads and the mandible is stabilized by an obvious contraction of the facial

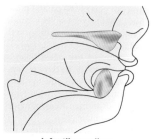

Infantile swallow

muscle. The buccinator muscle is strong in infantile swallow as it is during nursing. The normal infantile swallow is such in the neonate and gradually disappears with the eruption of molars in the primary dentition.

Infectious mononucleosis also called kissing disease include, fever, sore throat, malaise and glandular enlargement. Fauces may show exudates. Spleen is enlarged. Hepatitis may be seen. Liver may be enlarged. In severe cases myocarditis, neuritis and encephalitis may develop.

Infective conjunctivitis presents with red eye with discomfort and a foreign body sensation in the eye. There is sticking together of lid margins during sleep. Chemosis of conjunctiva is present. Mucopurulent discharge is seen at the inner canthus, lower fornix or at the root of eye lashes.

Infective oral ulcer occurs mostly due to tuberculosis usually dorsum of tongue. Shape is angular or stellate. Floor is pale in color with thick mucus like material in base of ulcer. Edge is irregular with undermined border. No extra specific treatment is required.

Inferior alveolar nerve is nerve that descends medial to the lateral pterygoid muscle then passes downward to the medial surface of the ramus and pterygomandibular space where it enters in mandibular foramen (*see* **Figure**).

Inferior alveolar neuritis involves the mandibular dental nerve within the mandibular canal. It may result due to trauma,

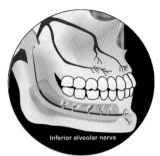

Inferior alveolar nerve

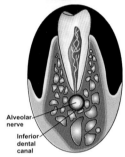

Inferior alveolar nerve

surgery or dental sepsis. Pain may be felt in all structures innervated by these nerve fibres. No autonomic or muscle symptoms are present.

Inferior Vena Cava is one of the two large veins carrying blood into right atrium (*see* **Figure on page 248**).

Inflammation is the reaction of the body to the irritation. It is a defence reaction and not actually a disease. White cells are body's main defence mechanism hence there is always a increase of blood flow to the infected part. WBCs fight against invading bacteria. Cardinal signs of inflammation are swelling, redness, heat, pain and loss of

Right hepatic vein
Inferior phrenic vein
Middle hepatic vein
Left hepatic vein
Inferior vena cava (IVC)
Right suprarenal vein
Inferior phrenic vein
Left suprarenal vein
To azygos vein
To azygos vein
L1 vein
L1 vein
Right renal vein
Left renal vein
L3 vein
L2 vein
Left testicular (or ovarian) vein
L3 vein
Right testicular (ovarian) vein
L4 vein
Right and left common iliac veins
Ascending lumbar vein
L5 vein
Internal iliac veins
Iliolumbar vein
Median sacral veins
External iliac veins

Inferior vena cava

function. Pain is caused by increased pressure of blood on nerves. Affected part is unable to function properly.

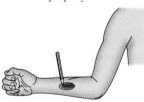

Inflammation

Inflammatory gingival enlarge-ment is caused by prolonged exposure to dental plaque. It originates as a slight ballooning of the interdental papilla and / or marginal gingiva. In early stages, a line preserving shape bulge is seen around the teeth. It progresses slowly uniting the part of the crowns. It is usually painless, unless complicated by acute infection or trauma. Occasionally, discrete, sessile or pedunculated mass may be present, which may be inter proximal or on the marginal or attached gingival. Painful ulceration may occur by the folds of the mass and adjacent gingiva. The gingiva may be deep red or bluish red in color, soft and friable in consistency, soft and shiny surface bleeds easily. Histologically, connective tissue shows preponderance of inflammatory cells. There is vascular engorgement with new capillary formation. The gingiva may be relatively firm, resilient and pink. When superimposed with infection, involved tissue appears glossy, smooth, edema-tous and bleed readily. Fetid odour may occur. Drifting of teeth occurs in long standing cases. In mouth breathers; maxillary anterior gingiva is affected. Local treatment is of value.

Inflammatory pocket wall is said to be occurred where there is presence of inflammatory fluid. Pocket wall appear red, soft, spongy, friable with the smooth and shiny surface.

Inflammatory spine pain is worst in the morning and improves with activity. Any activitiy makes it worst. Pain may come down to knees, hips and shoulder. Such lesions include sacro-iliac joint inflammation/fusion, peripheral joint arthritis etc.

Influenza starts suddenly with all signs of fever, cough and running nose like common cold. Fever is often associated with chills or rigor like malaria. Body ache is too much. Several strains of influenza have been discovered. There is no specific test to diagnose it.

Infra red relief of pain It is an effective means of relieving pain. Relief of pain is due to sedative effect on the superficial sensory nerve endings. It has been suggested that pain may be due to deposite of waste products of metabolism and an increase of blood flow removes these products. Pain due to actue inflammation is relieved by mild heating. One should note that intense heat may cause an increase in exudation of fluid into tissues increasing the pain.

Infrabony pocket / **Infracrestal pocket** / **Infralveolar pocket** is the term used where the base of the pocket is apical to the level of adjacent alveolar bone.

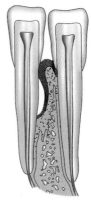
Infrabony pocket

Infrared soldering is also procedure when dental appliance is be soldered using an infrared light source. Here focused light beam is used. The light supplies the sufficient heat to bring the parts to the soldering temperature and melt the solder.

Ingot refers to cast rod of alloy.

Inhalation anesthetic agents are those drugs which are administered in the body by means of inhalation. Nitrous oxide is the gas which is constantly used with at least 20% oxygen. It requires a specific equipment to mix the gas in the specific proportion. Any drug or equipment necessary for resuscitation should be easily available in emergency.

Inhalation transmission is due to inhalation of micro-organism aerolised from a patient's blood or saliva when doctor is using high speed of ultrasonic equipment.

Inherited taste disorder dysautonomia is rare found in jews.

Affected children are usually hypotonic, easily being disturbed. There is an excessive sweat and mucus production. Such children don't have vallate and fungiform papillae. Tongue is devoid of taste receptors.

Injury to oral tissues results in tissue damage. Physical injury can affect teeth, soft tissue and bone. Chemical injury occurs due use of caustic materials. Micro-organisms can cause injury by invading oral tissue.

Inlay is a gold, porcelain, or composite custom-made filling cemented into the tooth. If it covers the tips of the teeth, it is called an onlay.

Innate/Immunity refers to any inborn resistance that is present. First time the pathogen is encountered. It does not require previous exposure and is not modified significantly by repeated exposures to the pathogen over the life of an individual.

Inoculation is introduction of micro-organism into living tissues culture media.

Inositol in 1940 Dr Wooley in America discovered that mice fed on diet deficient in inositol suffered from stunted growth and falling hair. Its high concentrations are found in muscles of heart and brain. Lack of it results in baldness. If taken with vitamin E it stimulates hair growth. Daily requirement is 10 mg.

Insertion is the point where muscle attaches to bone.

Insidious refers to coming on gradually.

Integrin mediated phase develops slowly but leads to stable long lasting molecular contacts that prevent further movement of neutrophils and cause it to flatten out against the endothelium. Once attached, neutrophils actively move themselves between endothelial cells to migrate out of the venule. Emigration and chemotaxis are facilitated in part by binding of neutrophil surface integrins to fibronectin and other components of extracellular matrix.

Integrins are a group of heterodimer proteins with alpha and beta polypeptides chains. Integrins bind a variety of ECM cells as well as non-integrin adhesion molecules such as vascular cell adhesion molecule found on stoma cell surface. They allow progenitors to bind tightly to marrow stoma and are responsible for sequestering progenitor cells in appropriate microenvironment. Contact of integrin with its ligand also transmits a signal into the integrin expressing cell, which can stimulate its growth and other activities.

Intelligence quotient refers to the relationship between intelligence and chronological age.

Intention tremor is the manifestation of cerebellar disease, the superior cerebellar peduncle .

Inter costal muscles are respiratory muscles found in between ribs.

Inter radicular means between the roots.

Inter transitional period is the period which maxillary and mandibular arches consists of sets of deciduous and permanent teeth. Between the permanent incisors and first permanent molars are the deciduous molars and canines. This phase during the mixed dentition period is relatively stable and no change occurs.

Interceptive orthodontics is phase of science and art of orthodontics employed to recognize and eliminate potential irregularities and malpositions in the developing dentofacial complex. These procedures are employed to lessen or to eliminate the severity of developing maloc-clusion either due to heredity or extremes or intrinsic factors.

Intercuspal position (ICP) refers to that position of mandible when there is maximal inter-cuspation between the maxillary and the mandibular teeth.

Intercuspation is the interlocking; a cusp-to-fossa relationship of the maxillary to mandibular teeth.

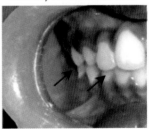

Intercuspation

Interdental eyelet wiring is a wiring technique where eyelets are constructed with a help of artery forceps, these eyelets are fitted between two teeths and push the wire on the lingual/palatal aspect as eyelets tend to get displaced. The free ends are then passed from the adjacent proximal contact, the distally placed free end wire is passed through the eyelet and then it is twisted along with the mesially placed free wire. To connect the upper and lower jaw, the wire is passed through the upper and lower eyelets and then plaited together at the lower border of the mandibular teeth.

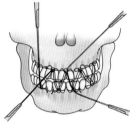

Interdental eyelet wiring

Interdental gingiva occupies the gingival embrasure, which is the interproximal space beneath the area of tooth contact. The interdental gingival can be pyramidal or have a "col" shape in the adult dentition, which is more susceptible to infection. In the primary dentition, inter-dental spacing is common. Hence saddle areas are present resulting in a well-keratinized interdental surface. This may be the reason for lower prevalence of periodontal lesions in children

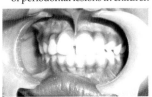

Interdental gingiva

because these areas are less vulnerable to development and progression of the inflammatory spaces.

Interdental knives are knives used in the interdental area. These are spear shaped knives that has cutting edge on both the sides of the blade that are available in double ended or single ended blades e.g. Orban knife no 1-2 and Merrifield knife no 1-4.

Interference/ Supracontact refers to any contact in ICP or other movements, that prevents the remaining occlusal surfaces to achieve stable occlusion.

Interlabial gap is the vertical distance between the upper and lower lip ranges between 0 and 3 mm.

Intermaxillary fixation (IMF) is a method where the immobilization is achieved by the help of intermaxillary wiring, a clinical union of bone can be expected with in four weeks and without using general anesthesia.

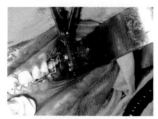

Intermaxillary fixation

Intermittent fever refers to a fever that is present only for several hours during the day.

Internal bevel incision is the incision used in periodontal surgeries. It is the incision from which flap is reflected to expose the underlying bone and root. It starts from the designated area on the gingiva and is directed to the area at or near the crest of the bone.

Internal resorption is an insidious process when the afflicted pulp is completely symptom free. Symptoms of internal resorption depend primarily on whether the process had broken through the external tooth surface. The pulp that erodes through the root surface may give vague pain on mastication. Percussion may be of little value. Pulpectomy is the only treatment for internal

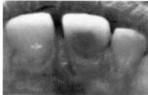

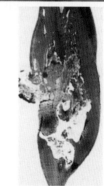

Clinical of histological view of internal resorption

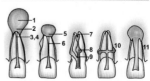

Patterns of internal resorption

resorption. No early symptoms are present. Generally only one tooth is affected. On radiograph involved tooth shows a round or oval radiolucent area in central portion of tooth. If tooth is not treated, complete perforation may take place.

Interneuron are nerves that conduct impulses from sensory neurons to motor neurons.

Interoceptors are the pain receptors which are located within the body cavities, there serve involuntary bodily function below conscious levels, e.g. Free nerve endings: perception of visceral pain and other sensation. Pacinian corpuscles gives perception of pressure.

Interpret is to offer an explanation.

Interproximal is the space present between two adjacent surfaces.

Interradicular fibers occurs in a multirooted tooth as they fan out from the cementum of the tooth in to the furcation area.

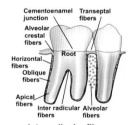

Interradicular fibres

Interstitial brain edema occurs during acute hydrocephalus due to sudden or persistently high intraventricular CSF pressure, the ependyma gets damaged and CSF escapes to the periventricular white matter interstitial space known as interstitial edema. Fluid spreads along angles of lateral ventricle.

Intervertebral disk rupture produces gradual or sudden low backache with or without sciatica. Pain radiates to legs. Pain is increased by coughing, spasm. Reflexes are decreased on affected side. Patient leans towards the affected side.

Intestinal tuberculosis is a disease involving caecum, mesenteric glands and peritoneum are generally involved. Miliary TB is the primary lesion. Common presenting symptoms are abdominal pain, malabsorption, diarrhea, low grade fever and loss of appetite. Ulcers are circular and may cause obstruction. Mantoux test may be positive. Ascites is exudative in nature with raised protein and plenty of leucocytes. Treatment is with INH, rifampicin, pyrazinamide and streptomycin for 3 months and INH and rifampicm for another 9 months.

Intracerebral hemorrhage is also called apoplexy. Most commonly seen in individuals over 50 years of age. Intracerebral hemorrhage may develop in any blood vessel, but usual source of bleeding is from arteries. Two major sources of intracerebral hemorrhage are ruptured arterial aneurysms and hypertensive vascular disease. Rupture occurs with sudden increase in local pressure. Clinically most cases of intracerebral hemorrhage occurs while patients are engaged in normal activities like heavy lifting, factors categorized as physical stress and that are associated with elevation of blood pressure.

Both anxiety and pain are associated with significant increase in heart rate and blood pressure of patient making development of a hemorrhagic CVA more likely.

Intra ligamentary anesthesia refers to the administration of anesthetic agent in to the ligament. Some people find an inferior dental block unpleasant due to tongue and lip being made numb. So injection is given directly down the gingival crevices. It immediately anesthetize the tooth. Special syringe/cartridge and needle are required for administrating anesthesia. Gingiva should be healthy for such type of L-A.

Intractable pain is when pain unresponsive to usual methods of pain management.

Intradermal nevus is congenital development of tumor like malformation of the skin/mucus membrane. Function of nevus cells is to produce melanin. These are commonly known as mole of dark brown color. It is slightly raised. Intraoral lesions are commonly seen over hard palate or gingival. These grow slowly. Under microscope nevus reveals cluster of nevus cells

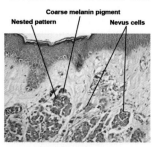

Coarse melanin pigment
Nested pattern   Nevus cells

Intradermal nevus

confined within connective tissue. No mitotic activity is seen. These generally don't require any treatment.

Intramembranous ossification is a physiological process of bone formation where bone is formed directly in membranous tissue.

Intraocular pressure means pressure within eye.

Intraoral is inside your mouth.

Intravenous anesthetics is simpler and leads to rapid pleasant induction. Recovery is swift without nausea and vomiting and there is lack of pulmonary irritation. I.V. anesthesia can be used for induction of anesthesia as a solid agent for very short procedure. It should not be used for maintenance of anesthesia. Extra venous injection may produce local necrosis. Overdose and too rapid injections are its cautions.

Intravenous sedation is a method where drug is introduced through I.V. method. It can be given to reduce anxiety in an over anxious patient. This may be insufficient for certain restorative and minor surgical procedure. Intravenous diazepam is commonly used. It is injected into a bigger vein to avoid thrombophlebitis. Dizepam produces muscle relaxation and also a dry mouth.

Intrusion is the term given to displacement of tooth in an apical direction.

Invagination is to enclose within.

Invasiveness refers to the extent and degree of involvement. Benign tumors are generally confined to a fibrous capsule or one well circumscribed. Capsule is formed by atrophy of cells at the periphery of expansile growth. Malignant tumors don't respect normal anatomical boundaries. In some malignant tumors invasion is seen only under microscope.

Investment material is a special gypsum product that is able to withstand extreme heat.

Iodine deficiency - T_3 and T_4 production decrease because iodine is necessary for the synthesis of these thyroid hormones. Low plasma levels of T_3 and T_4 cause the secretion of TSH. A persistent secretion of TSH causes the thyroid gland to enlarge, producing a goiter.

Iodine forms thyroid hormone. Its deficiency results in goiter. One third iodine of whole body lies in thyroid. An ovary also contains more of iodine. Whole blood contain 3 to 30 microgram. It is constituent of thyroxin, an active principle of thyroid gland. It plays an important role in energy metabolism and in growth of body. Adult body contains 50 mg of iodine. Cabbage, cauliflower and radish are goitrogenic not allowing food iodine make available to body.

Iodine-tincture is used as tincture of iodine since 1839. Like chlorine it is a powerful bactericide and a fungicide. It is used as sterilization of skin prior to surgery. Weak iodine solution contains 2.5% iodine and 2.5% potassium iodine in an alcoholic solution. Local toxicity is very slow. Some patient may show hypersensitivity. Weak solution is used as counter irritant in traumatic periodontitis.

Iodophore are complexes of iodine and surface active agents such as non-ionic detergents, quaternary compounds and macromolecules. The iodine is held in a loose combination and about 70-80% may be available when the solution is diluted. Iodophores are non-toxic, non-irritating, non-staining and miscible with water in all proportions. They do not produce sensitivity and are therefore used in prophylaxis.

Ion is an electrically charged particle at atom that gains or loses an electron.

Ionizing radiation is a radiation that is capable of producing ions including electromagnetic radiation.

Ionophor is the process of introducing a drug through the dental enamel by use of an electrical current; often used in the treatment of dentin hypersensitivity.

Iron deficiency anemia is a chronic microcytic hypochromic type of anemia and exists most commonly. It may cause pale skin and generalized weakness. Some may develop splitting and cracking of hair. Palpitation, dizziness and sensitivity to cold may develop. It occurs due to: inadequate absorption of iron and excessive loss of iron. Oral Manifestations include pallor of oral mucosa and gingiva. atrophic mucositis, loss of tongue papillae, glossitis and angular chelitis. Total RBC count is low. Stool should be examined for occult blood. Ferrous sulphate in sufficient quantity helps.

Iron in pregnancy Total of 300 mg of iron is needed for the growth of fetus, 70 mg for placenta and 500 mg for the synthesis of hemoglobin with increased blood volume. Iron accumulates at the rate of 0.5 mg/daily in first trimester. It may increase 3 to 4 mg/day in second and third trimester. This extra iron need cannot be met through diet so it has to be supplied from outside.

Iron is needed for formation of blood and is absorbed in the upper portion of duodenum. When hemoglobin level is short, absorption is high otherwise it is low. Total iron in body is 3-4 gm and daily requirement is 20 mg. Idiopathic hemochromatosis results in excessive iron absorption. Deficiency of iron result is anemia.

Irreversible Index is an index that measures conditions that will not change. Irreversible index scores cannot decrease in value on subsequent examinations. Eg: An Index that measures dental caries.

Irreversible pulpitis is an inflammation of the pulp and reached a point when no treatment is feasible.

Irrigation is the technique of using a solution to wash out your mouth.

Irrigation syringe is a blunt-tipped syringe used to irrigate the surgical site with sterile saline solution.

Irritable bowel synodrome is principally a motility disorder of intestine due to response to cholecystokinin after food. First group has abdominal pain and constipation, second group has watery diarrhea without pain, and third group has both. Some go to 3-4 times in morning to clear their bowel. In some bloating heart burn and palpitation develops.

Ischemic stroke 80% strokes are ischemic. In severe case ischemic cell death may cause infarction. T1A results from brief occlusion of an artery with restoration before irreversible damage occurs. Symptoms include monocular loss of vision and contralateral weakness. Symptoms develop within a few seconds. Loss of consciousness is very rare and signs are focal causative factor may be atheroma and thrombosis.

Isograft is a graft harvested from an identical twin. There is no rejection of this graft.

Isokinetic is an exercise in which the muscle generates force against a variable resistance and the speed of movement is maintained by a present controlled device.

Isometric exercise in which the muscle generates force but there is no observable movement. It is like pushing a wall. In other words it is the generation of force by a muscle under conditions in which the muscle length remains constant.

Isotonic – Exercise in which muscle generates force against constant resistance and movement result.

Isotonic solution is the one that has the same concentration as the solution to which it is compared.

Isotope are two or more forms of a chemical element which have different mass numbers because their nuclei contain different numbers of neurons. Radioactive isotopes are widely used as tracers.

J **Jacket crown** is used for front teeth which are too mutilated to be restored by ordinary filling. Such cases have extensive caries, fractured crown and discoloration. Outer coating of natural crown is removed to leave a stump of dentine on which artificial crown fits like a jacket.

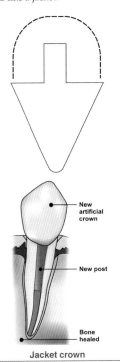

New artificial crown

New post

Bone healed

Jacket crown

Jackscrew is a small device generally used for expansion of maxilla and mandible. It is used as a removable appliance to perform interceptive orthodontic procedure. The device can be placed in anterolateral position or in midline to achieve minor tooth movements.

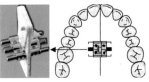

Jack screw

Jacksonian epilepsy is a neuro-logical disorder that includes the convulsions seen only in one area of the body.

Jadassohn–Lewandowsky syndrome is recognized by congenital gross thickening of finger and toe nails. Leuko-keratosis is also seen. Nail lesion is noted just after birth with a horny brownish material at nail bed. Oral leukokeratosis affects dorsum of tongue which becomes thickened and grayish white. Histologically these are similar to white sponge nevus. Frequent oral aphthous ulceration may develop.

Jaundice is a yellow pigmentation of skin and sclera of eye due to formation of excessive bilirubin. Bilirubin is formed from hemo-globin when the old RBC's are broken down by spleen. There are three types of jaundice i.e. hepatocellular jaundice, obstru-ctive jaundice and hemolytic jaundice.

Jaw is a common name for the maxilla and mandible.

Jaw thrust is the maneuver used to obtain the airway.

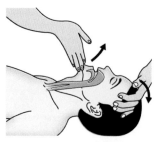

Jaw thrust manuever

Joint refers to that part of the body where the meeting of two bones occurs in order to establish movement.

Junctional epithelium is collar like band of stratified squamous nonkeratinized epithelium which is formed by the merger of oral epithelium and reduced enamel epithelium (REE) during the tooth eruption. Internally it is attached to the tooth by the means of epithelial attachment or internal basal lamina and externally it is attached to the gingival connective tissue by the means of external basal lamina.

Juvenile periodontitis/Localized juvenile periodontitis (LJP)/ Early onset periodontitis (EOP)/ Localized aggressive periodontitis

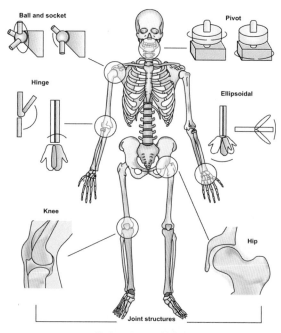

Various types of joint

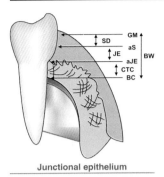

Junctional epithelium

was the term given by Chaput in 1967 and Butler in 1969 and can be defined as a disease of periodontium occurring in an otherwise healthy adolescent which is characterised by rapid loss of alveolar bone characterized by migration and loosening of the teeth in the presence or absence of either secondary epithelial proliferation and pocket formation or secondary gingival disease. Rapid periodontal destruction of selected teeth occurs at an early age. It involves severe periodontal destruction with an onset around puberty. The localized form (JP) occurs in otherwise healthy individuals with destruction classically localized and around the first permanent molars and incisors, and not involving more than two other teeth generalized juvenile periodontitis (GJP) also occurs in otherwise healthy individuals but involves more than 14 teeth that is being generalized to an area or the entire dentition.

Juvenile rheumatoid arthritis is a condition that involves joints, connective tissue and viscera. Peak incidence is 1-4 years. Child develops fever, lymphadenopathy, hepatosplenomegaly, abdominal pain and pleura pericarditis. Any form of arthritis in younger age for more than 3-4 months with subcutaneous nodules, symmetric joint involvement, morning stiffness and osteoporosis without erosions are diagnostic. Aspirin is the drug of choice.

J

Kala azar is characterized by fever, hepatic and splenic enlargement. Fever is having double daily remission. There is dusky pigmentation which is noted on feet, hands and abdomen. There will be generalized enlargement of glands. Blood shows leucopenia and Leishman – Donovan bodies. Specific complement fixation test will become positive.

Kaolin is a fine powder used in pharmacy in ointments and coating pills.

Kaposi's sarcoma is a malignant neoplasm arising from endothelial cells of capillaries. With AIDS lesions are multicentric. It affects skin, lymph nodes, bone and viscera. It develops after age of 50. Tumor shows multiple capillaries. Inflammatory cell infiltration is common. Homosexuals are affected more easily. It has 3 stages. *Patch stage* – It is the initial stage having red, pink or purple. These develop over oral mucosa. *Plaque stage* – Patch converts into plaque. Lesion is large and raised. *Nodular stage* – There develops multiple nodular lesions on the skin. Being multicentric surgery is not feasible. Radiotherapy and chemotherapy is given.

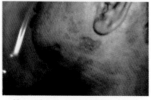

Kaposi sarcoma (patch stage) affecting skin

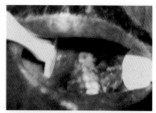

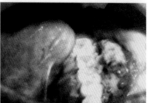

Kaposi sarcoma (nodular stage)

Kawasaki's disease occurs in children there is development of persistent fever, oral mucositis, occular and cutaneous lesions. Lingual papillae swells.

Keloid is a painless and progressive enlargement of scar. Itching is a prominent manifestation. Area in front of sternum face and neck are commonly involved. It is reddish and elevated from surface. It is firm and irregular with claw like processes invading healthy skin.

Keratoacanthoma is a fast growing neoplasm that resembles squamous carcinoma. Lesion is an elevated umbilicated lesion with a depressed central core. It measures 1.0 to 1.5 cm in diameter. It starts as a small, firm nodule and within 2 months develops to a full size. It may heal spontaneously. The size of the lesion will vary from 1 cm to several cm. There will be a central keratin filled crater. Many suspect a viral cause. Surgical excision is the treatment.

Keratomalacia consists of softening of entire thickness of part or whole process is rapid one and may lead to necrosis, ulceration and destruction of eye ball.

Keratosis follicularis is a gemodermatosis transmitted as autosomal dominant characteristic. It is manifestated during childhood. Skin lesions appear as small, papules which are red. When macerated, they produce foul smelling masses. Oral lesions develop as minute, whitish, papules most commonly found on gingiva and tongue. In less severely affected cases intraoral lesions are keratotic and papular. It is referred as warty dyskeretoma. In severe cases dermal inflammatory exudates and a tendency to cobblestone changes is seen. Some persons may develop psychological problem and mental disability.

Kerosene poisoning can occur due to consumption of kerasene instead of water. There may be burning pain in the throat and feeling of warmth. A smell of kerosene oil in the vomited matter is characteristic. Patient develops cough and become drowsy. Face may be pale or cyanosed. Pulse is feeble and respratory rate may increase, convulsions may be seen in some children. Bronchopneumonia may be developed.

Ketamine is related to arycyclo alkylamines which produces dissociative anesthesia. Patient loses consciousness rapidly but with only slight depression of normal reflexes. Analgesia and amnesia are marked but there is poor muscular relaxation. Dreams and hallucinations are common. Recovery period is slow. Analgesic effect, remains for hours.

Ketoacidosis is mostly found as a complication of diabetes mellitus. Low blood pH is caused by the presence of an abnormally large number of ketone bodies produced when fats are converted to form of glucose to be used for cellular respiration.

Kinesics means body language.

Kirkland curette is a heavy surgical curette often required during the surgical procedures for the removal of granulation tissue, fibrous interdental tissue and tenacious subgingival deposits.

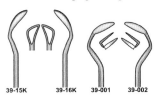

39-15K   39-16K   39-001   39-002

Kirkland curretts

Kirkland knives/periodontal knives/ Gingivectomy knives is a representative of knives commonly used as Gingivectomy. They are available either as single ended or double ended instruments. The entire periphery of kidney shaped knive is the cutting edge of the instrument.

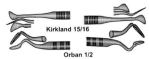

Kirkland 15/16

Orban 1/2

Kirkland knives

Kramer curette number 1, 2 and 3 are heavy surgical curette often required during the surgical procedures for the removal of granulation tissue, fibrous interdental tissue and tenacious subgingival deposits.

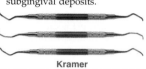

Kramer

Krushkal – Wallis test is the non parametric version of one way analysis of variance.

Kyphosis is an excessive backward curvature of spine. It results in lump or a more gradually rounded back. It may be a result of osteoporosis, fracture of vertebra or tuberculosis.

K

L

Labial is relating to the lip; another name for the facial surface of anterior teeth (next to the lip).

Labioversion refers to abnormal protrusion of maxillary incisors towards the lips.

Lacrimal gland refers to the gland that produces tears, located in upper lateral portion of orbit.

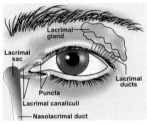

Lacrimal system

Lactational mastitis refers to infection of breast of nursing mother caused by introduction of infection into breast through cracked nipple. Patient develops pain in breast, chills and fever. Condition may be treated by antibiotics, hot and wet dressings

Lactobacilli are gram positive, non spore–forming rods that generally grow best under micro aerophilic conditions. Isolation and enumeration of oral lactobacilli have been facilitated by use of selective agar medium which suppresses the growth of other oral organisms by its low pH (5.4).

Lactose intolerance is an intestinal condition that causes symptoms like cramping, abdominal distension and gas problem. There is an absence of body enzyme lactase which breaks down lactose into glucose and galactose. In this condition lactose descends directly to the large intestine where intestinal bacteria break it down into acid and gas causing discomfort.

Lag screws are used for rigid immobilization where the thread of the screw engages only in the inner plate of bone. The hole is drilled in the outer cortex and is slightly of a larger diameter than the threaded part. Once tightened, the head of the screw engages in the outer plate and the fracture is compressed.

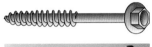

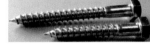

Lag screw

Lamina propria is a layer of connective tissue that lies just under the epithelium of the mucous membrane.

Laminate veneer is porcelain, or composite covering which is bonded to restore discolored, or damaged teeth.

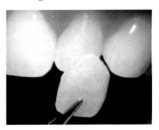

Veneers

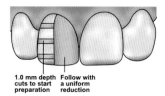

1.0 mm depth cuts to start preparation | Follow with a uniform reduction

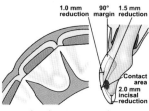

1.0 mm reduction | 90° margin | 1.5 mm reduction

Contact area
2.0 mm incisal reduction

Laminate preparation

Landau reflex can be elicited by suspending the neonate in the prone position by putting a hand under the abdomen. The normal response consists of extension of head, trunk and hips. When the head is flexed the trunk and hips also flex.

Langhan's giant cell are big. These have large number of nuclei. Nuclei are vesicular. Nuclear arrangement is in the form of horse shoe. Cytoplasm is in abundant. Mostly are seen in tuberculosis.

Laparoscopy is the visualization of pelvic and abdominal viscera and can be done without major injury to abdominal wall. It can be done by using a fibreoptic, telescope illuminated by a light source.

Laryngitis refers to the inflammation of larynx result due to abnormal use of vocal cord. Excessive smoke may also cause laryngitis. Rest to the voice is helpful. Symptoms will clear in few days. Carcinoma of larynx produces hoarseness of voice.

Laryngospasm is evidenced by high pitched inspirations and dyspnea. It is caused by partial or complete spasm or the vocal cords. In complete spasm breath sounds may be absent and abdominal heaving becomes prominent.

Larynx is a hollow tube with a flap of epiglottis protecting the airway from ingestion of food material. Highly mobile vocal cords function in phonation. Larynx is divided into supraglottis, glottis and sub glottis. Only the true vocal cords are covered by non keratinised squamous epithelium.

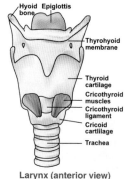

Hyoid bone
Epiglottis
Thyrohyoid membrane
Thyroid cartilage
Cricothyroid muscles
Cricothyroid ligament
Cricoid cartilage
Trachea

Larynx (anterior view)

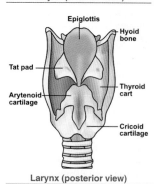

Epiglottis
Hyoid bone
Tat pad
Arytenoid cartilage
Thyroid cart
Cricoid cartilage

Larynx (posterior view)

Laser (Light Amplification by Stimulated Emission of Radiation).

Laser burns are the burns caused by lasers, basically thermal burns where laser energy is used for other purposes like hair removal, resurfacing, vascular, pigmented lesions and heat released is dissipated into the normal skin leading to skin burns. The damage to the skin will depend upon the energy released by the laser, therefore these can be superficial burns which are more common or deep dermal when the energy used is very high which take a long time to heal. Therefore wet gauze should be kept in surrounding skin thus isolating the treatment field as in resurfacing and treating pigmented or vascular lesions. In case of hair removal cold air blast is needed to be given along with the laser beam to nullify the effects of heat.

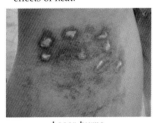
Laser burns

Laser welding means where the heat for welding is supplied by focused beam of light generated by a laser. Laser light can be focused on small regions and can apply high energy in a very short period of time. There is very little heating of total appliance except at the point of application.

Late adolescence is a period of transition as the young person (adult) consolidates his identity and comes to grips with his future.

Late shift occurs where child lack the primate spaces and thus the erupting permanent molars are unable to move forward to establish class I relationship in these cases when the deciduous second molars exfoliate, the permanent first molar drift medially utilizing the leeway space. This occurs in the late mixed dentition period and is thus called late shift.

Latent refers to concealed, not open.

Latent image is the invisible image produced when film is exposed to X-rays. It remains invisible until film is exposed.

Lateral fossa is a smooth depressed area of maxilla located between the canine and lateral incisor. It appears radiolucent.

Lateral means towards the outside or away from midline.

Lateral periodontal abscess develops in pre exiting periodontal pocket. Bacteria multiply in the depth of the pocket causing irritation. Cortical plate may be destroyed. Abscess resembles an abscess elsewhere. Abscess has to be drained out. Extraction of tooth is advised only in advanced cases.

Lateral periodontal cyst is a well recognized type of developmental odontogenic cyst. It develops chiefly in adults. No particular sign and symptoms appear and lesion is discovered accidently. Surgical excision is to be done without removing the tooth.

L

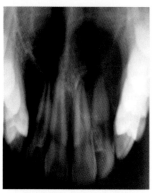

Lateral periodontal cyst

Lateral pterygoid plate is a wing shaped bony projection of sphenoid bone located distal to the maxillary tuberosity region.

Lateral sulci are the prominent grooves between the deciduous canine and the deciduous first molar segments.

Laterotrusion refers to movement of mandible laterally to the right or left from ICP.

Laterotrusive side refers to the side of either dental arch corresponding to the side of the mandible moving away from midline.

Le fort I fracture refers to the horizontal fracture above the level of nasal floor. The fracture line runs backward from the lateral margins of the anterior nasal aperture, it also passes along the lateral wall of the nose and lower third of nasal septum to coincide with lateral fracture behind the tuberosity.

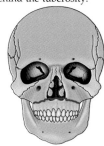

Le fort I

Auricular tubercle

Mandibular fossa particular part

Tympanic plate

Tegmem tympani

Spine of sphenoid

Foramen spinosum

Foramen ovale

Lateral pterygoid plate

Pyramidal process (tubercle) of palatine bone

Hamulus

Infratemporal crest

Inferior orbital fissure

Spheno-palatine ford (Pterygo-palatine foss

Posterior superior alveolar foramina

Tuberosity of maxilla

Lateral pterygoid

Le fort II fractures refer to those fractures which run from the middle area of the nasal bones on both the sides, crossing the frontal process and into the medial wall of each orbit.

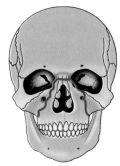

Le fort II

Le fort III fracture refer to those fractures which run from near the frontonasal suture transversely backwards, parallel with the base of the skull and involves considerable depth of ethmoidal bone including the cribriform plate, as it crosses the orbit, it involves optic foramen and inferior orbital fissure, from the

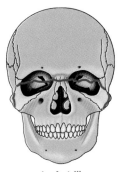

Le fort III

base of inferior orbital fissure, the fracture extends into two directions; backwards across the pterygomaxillary fissure and laterally across the lateral wall of orbit.

Lead poisoning occurs as professional hazard. It may cause serious G.I.T. disturbances. Peripheral neuritis also develops. Encephalitis may also occur. X-ray may show deposition of lead on bones. Lead line on tooth occurs. Gray/bluish black line of sulphide pigmentation is seen over gingiva. It is more diffuse than bismuth. Excessive salivation and metallic taste develops.

Lean tissue mass includes muscle other body tissues, body fluids and bone usually calculated as total body mass minus fat mass.

Ledges are the plateau like bony margins caused by resorption of bony thick plates.

Leiomyoma is a benign neoplasm of smooth muscle cells. Majority of these cases are found on posterior portion of tongue. Palate and buccal mucosa may also be involved. These grow slowly and are painless pedunculated mass. Mass does not ulcerates and maintains the normal color. Sub mucosal nodules may be seen. These are firm and yellow in color. Lesion can be multi nodular. These are composed of spindle shaped smooth muscle cells. Surgical excision including surrounding normal tissue is practiced. After surgery it does not recur nor transform into malignancy (*see* Figure on page 268).

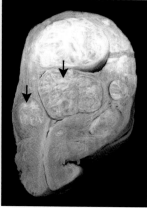

Leiomyoma in hyaline changes

Leiomyomas of uterus

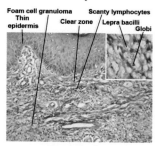

Lepromatous leprosy

Leiomyosarcoma is a malignant tumor of smooth muscle origin. It is rare in oral cavity. The cheek and floor of mouth are the common sites. It looks like leiomyoma except number of mitosis. Patient may hardly survive for 3-5 year.

Lepromatous leprosy is characterized by macules, nodules and papules the features of skin lesions. Lesions are multiple and bilaterally symmetrical. There is loss of outer eyebrows, thickened and corrugated skin of face and forehead. Skin biopsy, ear lobe clipping and nasal smear examination helps.

Leprosy is a chronic granulomatous infection caused by an acid fast bacillus. Mycobacterium lepra causes granulomatous infection of skin and peripheral nerves. Incubation period is 3 to 5 year. Clinically it can be classified into lepromatous leprosy and tuberculoid leprosy. Onset is insidious. To start a small area of impaired sensation or numbness is developed. There is lack of sweating and lack of hair in involved area surrounding cutaneous nerve is thickened. Oral lesions consist of tumor like masses called lepromas developing on lip, tongue and hard palate. Gingiva may enlarge and teeth may become loose. Long term chemotherapy is suggested.

Leptin is a body fat signaling hormone like protein secreted in blood stream. It is transported to satiety center in the hypothalamus. There is blunts the appetite when calorie intake is sufficient to maintain ideal fat store.

Lesion refers to any wound or local degeneration. It broadly include wounds, sores and any other damage or injury due to disease.

Lethargy means sleepiness.

Letterer Siwe disease is an acute, often fulminating histiocytic disorder. Patient will have constant low grade spiking fever with malaise and irritability. Oral lesions are ulcerative with gingival hyperplasia. Prognosis in letterer siwe disease is extremely poor.

Leukemia is a malignant disease with increased proliferation of WBC's at the cost of other cells. It is more common in younger age groups. Some may be of immature form. Myeloid leukemia involves granulocyte series. Lymphoid leukemia involves lymphocytic series and monocytic leukemia involves monocytic series. Each one of them may be acute, subacute or chronic. Exact cause is not known. But exposure of high doses of radiation therapy, phenyl butazone, Chloramphenicol may lead to it. Some families have more incidence of leukemia. These have been classified into acute and chronic. Generally either children or old people are affected. Persistent fever of unknown origin, spontaneous bleeding from gingiva, Multiple large ulcers may develop on mucosa, Candidiasis, histoplasmosis and HSV infections are common in leukemic patients, Teeth may start loosening, alveolar destruction may take place, Leukemic cell infiltration may cause atypical dental pain, There may be prolonged bleeding after extraction.

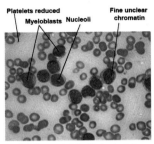

Acute myeloblastic leukemia

Platelets reduced — Myeloblasts — Nucleoli — Fine unclear chromatin

Leukoederma is a white lesion of oral cavity which clinically resembles early leukoplakia. It varies from film-like layer to greyish white cast with a coarsely wrinkled surface. It is more prominent in bicuspid to occlusal line. Etiology is not known. Intraorally, the buccal mucosa retains its normal softness and flexibility. It exhibits a greyish white folded opalescent appearance. Leukoplakia is more common to develop. Since it is a variant of normal mucosa it does not require any treatment.

Leukoplakia is a premalignant condition. It occurs as a white patch over mucus membrane of lip, hard and soft palate, floor of mouth and gingiva. Patches of leukoplakia may vary from non palpable to thick white translucent indurated lesion. These may

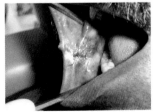

Toluidene blue uptake changes indicative of carcinomatous changes

be fissured or papillomatous. It may be localized or diffuse and is of 3 types. Homogeneous leukoplakia is a localized lesion. If extensive it is of consistent pattern. It may be wrinkled or papillomatous. Verrucous leukoplakia is an oral white lesion in which surface is broken up by multiple papillary projections. Nodular granular is hairy mixed white and red lesion. In it lesions are scattered over an atrophic patch of mucosa. Leukoplakia can be developed on any part of oral cavity but is more common on buccal mucosa and gingiva. 50% lesions affect cheeks. Tobacco, alcohol, mechanical irritants are causative factors. If floor of mouth is involved then chances of transforming into malignancy are more. Microscopically one finds cellular dysplasia. Benign leukoplakia shows hyperkeratosis and chronic inflammatory cell infiltration. Cytological study is of little importance. Topically applied Toludine blue shows the areas which are more likely to show carcinomatous changes Biopsy is to be done from that area. Surgical excision done with or without grafting remains the standard treatment for leukoplakia.

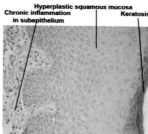

Chronic inflammation in subepithelium — Hyperplastic squamous mucosa — Keratosis

Histological section of leukoplakia

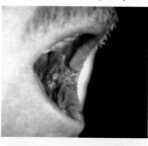

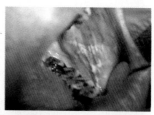

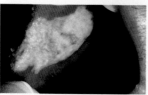

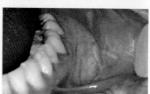

Leukoplakia involving buccal mucosa, angle of the mouth and buccal vestibule

Leukostasis syndrome is a condition where WBC count may go up to one lac per cu/mm. Person may develop headache and stroke like symptoms. Many patients may be asymptomatic. Spleen may be enlarged hugely. Unexplained leukocytosis, basophilia and thrombocytosis may be present. Bone marrow is hypercellular with markedly increased granulocyte precursor specially metamyelocytes and myelocytes.

Levator anguli oris is a facial muscle that arises from canine fossa just below infra orbital foramen and is inserted over angle of mouth. Its action is to raise angle of mouth and produces nasolabial furrow.

Levator labii superioris arises from lateral surface of zygomatic bone and passes down ward and medially into muscular substance of upper lip. It elevates the upper lip and produces nasolabial furrow.

LI (Labrale Inferius) is the median point in the lower margin of the lower membranous lip.

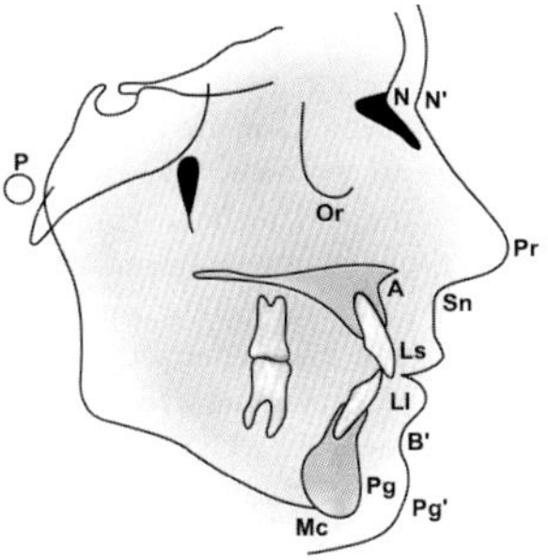

Labrale inferius

Lichen planus is a common dermatosis developing on mucus membrane which appears as small, angular, flat topped papules only a few millimetres in diameter. Papules are sharply demarcated. Center of papule may be slightly umbilicated. Its surface is covered by greyish white line known as wickhane's

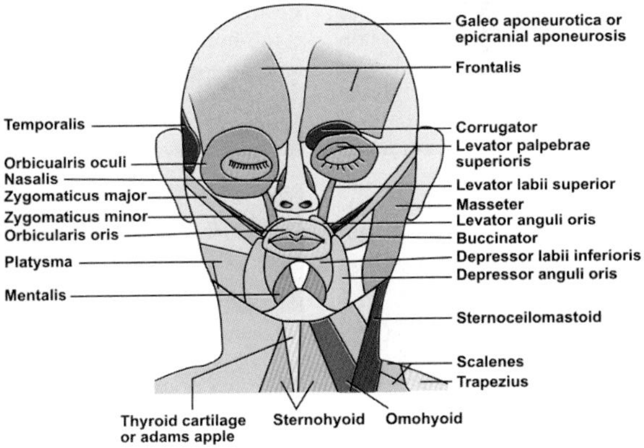

Facial muscles

striae. Face generally remains uninvolved. Early symptom is pruritis causing severe itching. Causative factor of lichen planus is immunologically induced degeneration of basal layer of epithelium. There are three basic types of erosions, keratosis, erosions and bulla formation. Psychogenic problems play an etiological role. During deep emotional problems remissions and exacerbations are seen. It may be associated with diabetes. Generally it is a bullous form of disease and a painless lesion, the reticular form is slightly elevated, fine, whitish line. Lines are fine radiating of lacing in nature cheeks and tongue are generally affected. In the popular form lesion is less than 1 mm in size. It is whitish elevated lesion. Bullous lichen planus is rare. It presents coexisting bullous pemphigoid. Atrophic lichen planus is inflamed area covered by red, thinned epithelium. Erosive lesion is a complicated atrophic process when thin epithelium is ulcerated. Main histological features of lichen planus are Areas of hyper-parakeratosis, Liquefaction degeneration, dense epithelial band of lymphocyte damage of basal cell layer is the diagnostic point. The lesions of oral lichen planus appears, regresses and reappear in unpredictable fashion. Lesions are too diffuse to remove surgically and may transform into malignancy. Antihistamine rinses and corticosteroids are useful. In resistant cases intra lesional injections of trimcinolne acetonide are useful. Retinoids may be given in addition.

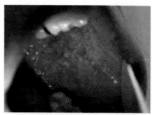

Lichen planus of bucal mucosa

Lichenoid drug reactions are white patches identical clinically to lichen planus and are caused by a mucosal reaction to certain drugs. Drugs include phenothiazines, dental amalgams and dental composites, non steroidal anti-inflammatory drugs and anti-hypertensive.

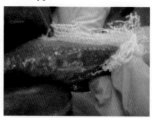

Lichenoid reaction on the lateral border of tongue

Life expectancy is the average number of years lived by an individual or group born in the same period.

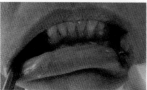

Lichen planus of labial vestibule

Ligatures are fine wires or elastic bands used to tie or ligate the arch wire to the brackets.

Light is necessary for efficient vision. Poor light causes fatigue and loss of efficiency. An illumination of 15-20 foot candles is accepted as a basic minimum for satisfactory vision. In dental surgery 100% light should be directed towards the area of surgery i.e. interest.

Light activated denture base material is used to fabricate dentures with light activation. Advantage of it is reduced polymerization shrinkage, possible better fit than conventional base material and not much of equipment is required. But disadvantage is an increased elastic deformation during mastication.

Light cure system are those system that require light exposure for the setting to occur. Light cure materials such as durofill or pekafill need exposure to bright light for setting. A special lamp is used and it makes a material set in about a minute. No mixing is required. Just a thin layer of composite is needed to fill a shallow cavity and one application of curing light is needed.

Lightening injuries have variable affects. It may not always be fatal but patient may fall unconscious and stop breathing. However, these patients withstand prolong periods of apnoea and respond very well to immediate CPR. Burn markings are characteristic for lightening injuries. There is a spidery pattern of skin burns which is caused by the currents passage along pathway of skin dampness where the resistance is the lowest.

Lightning is degradation of high molecular weight complex organic molecules that reflect specific wave length of light responsible for the color of the stain into lower molecular weight and less complex molecules that reflect less light is called lightning.

Lignocaine is a local anesthetic agent and was introduced in 1948. It diffuses rapidly and onset is rapid. It produces anesthesia within 2-3 minutes. It is easily absorbed from mucus membrane. It is an effective surface anesthetic. It is more potent than pilocaine. It is available in spray form and also a cream in concentration of 5%. Saliva can washout its effects.

Limb placement reflex is said to have occurred when the front of the leg below the knee, or the arm below the elbow is brought into contact with the edge of the table, the child lifts the limbs over the edge.

Limbic system is also known as emotional brain. It is a collection of various small regious of brain that act together to produce emotions (*see* Figure on page 252).

Lime is an disinfecting agent. It is used in the form of fresh quick lime or 10-20% aqueous suspension of milk of lime. Faeces and urine can be disinfected by mixing 10-20% aqueous suspension.

Linea alba is a white line extending antero posteriorly on buccal mucosa along occlusal plane.

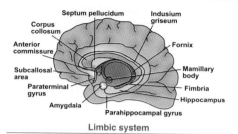

Septum pellucidum
Corpus collosum
Anterior commissure
Subcallosal area
Paraterminal gyrus
Amygdala
Indusium griseum
Fornix
Mamillary body
Fimbria
Hippocampus
Parahippocampal gyrus

Limbic system

Linear epitopes when all the amino acids or sugar residues that form an epitope are positioned in linear sequence. Not affected by heat, denaturation.

Lines of Cleavage and surgery – In certain regions of the body, collagen fibers tend to orient more in one direction than another. Lines of cleavage (tension lines) in the skin indicate the predominant direction of underlying collagen fibers. The lines are especially evident on the palmer surfaces of the fingers, where they are arranged parallel to the long axis of the digits. An incision running parallel to the collagen fibers will heal with only a fine scar. An incision made across the rows of fibers disrupts the collagen, and the wound tends to gap open and heal in a broad, thick scar.

Lingual refers to the surface of a tooth nearest the tongue; relating to the tongue.

Lingual thyroid nodules, the remnants follicle of thyroid tissues are found in base of tongue. It is a benign condition during puberty. It lies in mid of tongue. It appears deeply situated having a smooth surface. It has a color

of mucosa. If size is 2 to 3 cms it may result in dysphagia, dysphonia and hemorrhoage with pain.

Lingual tonsils are accumulations of lymphoid tissue on the root of the tongue. They may extend as far back as epiglottis and laterally through palatine tonsil.

Lingual varicosities are prominent purplish blue spots. These are usually observed on the ventral and lateral surfaces of tongue. Clinically red to purple dilated vessels or clusters are seen. It has no relation with jugular venous pressure or obstruction to portal venous system. These are generally seen in old age.

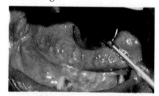

Lingual varicosities

Lining mucosa is present in non masticatory regions such as floor of mouth, central surface of tongue, soft palate, cheeks, lips and alveolar mucosa. It is not attached to bone.

Lip biting and lip sucking is an oral habit that sometimes appears after forced discontinuation of thumb or digit sucking. Lip biting most often involves the lower lip which is turned inwards and pressure is exerted on the lingual surfaces of the maxillary anteriors. Clinically it may appear as proclined upper anteriors and retroclined, hypertrophic and redundant lower lip or a cracked lip.

Lipemia is the presence of abnormally high concentrations of lipids in blood.

Lipoid proteinosis is a condition occurring due to disturbance in mucopolysacchrides metabolism. These produce yellowish hay nodules of size 0.5 cm. Such lesions may develop on eyelid. In oral mucosa yellowish papular plaques develop. Lips become thick. Painful parotitis may occur repeatedly. No specific treatment is available.

Lipolysis is a metabolic break down of fats for energy.

Lipoma is a slow growing tumor of adipose tissue. It is composed of mature fat cells. Cheek, tongue, floor of mouth and salivary glands are frequently involved. It is a single, lobulated painless lesion attached by peduncle. Epithelium is thin showing blood vessels. It is composed of mature fat cell with varying collagen strands. These are yellowish in color with smooth surface. There is no surrounding capsule. Simple surgical excision helps. Recurrence is uncommon.

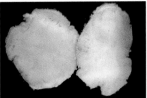

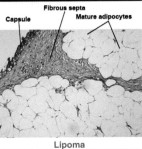

Lipoma

Liposarcoma is not a common malignant mesenchymal neoplasm. It is a slow, silent growth, submucosal or deep in location. Lesion is firm, lobulated suggestive of cyst. It may be myxoid type, round cell type and plemorphic type.

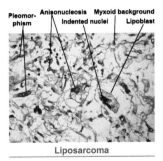

Liposarcoma

Lipostrophy is the breakdown of subcutaneous fat at the site of repeated insulin injection.

Lipping is the term given to the bulging of bone contour due to peripheral buttressing bone formation.

Liquid sterilant is a solution used for the purpose of sterilization. Instruments are immersed in a Glutraldehyde solution for 10 hours or more for sterilization.

Lisinopril is an angiotensin converting Enzyme (ACE) inhibitor that is used to treat hypertension.

Listerine is an essential oil or phenol mouthwashes used for more than a century. Phenol as an antiseptic made a breakthrough in 1867 under John Lister. Phenolic compounds used alone, or combined with mouth rinses and throat lozenges have proved to be safe. The action of phenols depends upon the concentration and contact time. Composition includes menthol 0.04%, thymol 0.06%, eucalyptol 0.09%, benzoic acid 0.015 %, ethyl alcohol 6-26%. Listerine is contraindicated for those patients on metronidazole/tinidazole as it contains alcohol.

Liver abscess is commonly caused by E.Coli. It is slow growing with fever. Pain may be a complaint. Jaundice, tenderness in right upper abdomen with leucocytosis is commonly noted. Cephalosporin and metronidazole helps but abscess larger than 5 cm may require drainage.

Loading dose is the larger dose of a drug given initially to control the disease effectively.

Lobar pneumonia is a localized infection of terminal air spaces. The usual homogeneous lung opacification is limited by fissure and affected lobes retain normal volume and show air bronchograms. Streptococcus and penumococii causes typical lobar pneumonia. Consolidation may not spread uniformly in lobe.

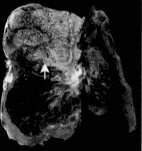

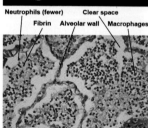

Lobar pneumonia

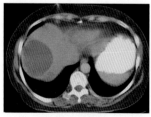

Liver abscess

Lobe refers to center of tooth formation.

Local anesthetic infiltration is a method of administrating local anesthesia that is given over apex of tooth to be anesthetized. Needle is inserted below the mucous membrane. Infiltration applies to nerve endings while nerve block is done to trunk of nerve. It is effective for all upper teeth.

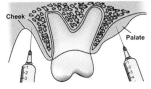

Local infiltration maxilla

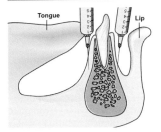

Local infiltration mandible

Local dental anesthesia is a procedure widely used in dental practice to paralyz sensory nerve endings by producing tissue ischemia, application of cold or putting pressure on nerve trunks. Local anesthetics are thought to act by stabilizing the cell membrane. These prevent inward movement of sodium ions. Most local agents are tertiary amines. Lignocaine and procaine are good agents.

Local muscle soreness is a local condition with a local cause. It is a lowered pain threshold due to strain, injury, infection of inflammation. Some pain is thought to result from accumulation of metabolites after excessive use. Both ischemia and hyperaemia are believed to relate to paingenesis.

Localized diffuse gingivitis is the one which extends from the margin to the mucobuccal fold but is limited to a particular area.

Localized enamel hypoplasia is a type of hypoplasia occasionally seen. Only a single tooth is involved, most commonly one of the permanent maxillary incisors or a maxillary or mandibular premolar. There may be any degree of hypoplasia, ranging from a mild, brownish discoloration of the enamel to a severe, pitting and irregularity of the tooth crown.

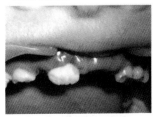

Local enamel hypoplasia

Localized gingivitis is said to occur where the inflammation is confined to a single tooth or a particular area.

Localized marginal gingivitis is confined to one or more areas of the marginal gingiva.

Localized papillary gingivitis is confined to one or more interdental spaces in a particular area.

Localized periodontitis is said to have occurred when less than thirty percent of the areas assessed in mouth demonstrate the bone loss and loss of attachment.

Localized scratch dermatitis is a chronic, superficial pruritis inflammation of the skin with dry scaling. There will be pigmented lichenified plaques with oval and irregular shapes. There is a strong psychogenic component. Outer zone of patch may have brownish discrete papules and a central zone. The involved skin will be red, moist and hyper pigmented. Diagnosis is mostly clinical. Topical corticosteroids are most useful. Zinc oxide paste can be locally applied.

Location of dental plaque Plaque is a combination of bacteria, bacterial products and saliva. Supragingival plaque is formed above gum line and consist of different bacteria sublingual plaque is formed below gum line. Plaque is adhered to teeth by a sticky polysaccharide produced by bacteria specially streptococcus mutans.

Logo therapy refers to spiritually, essentially oriented therapy that seeks to achieve healing and health through meaning.

Longitudinal study is measurement of same person or a group at regular intervals, over a period of time.

Loose tongue is also known as frenum insufficiency. Patient mostly has been operated for tongue tie. Tongue becomes loose and difficult to control. Dysarthria is present and signs of airway obstruction take place during sleep.

Loosely adherent subgingival plaque is an unattached bacterial plaque found adjacent to the gingival epithelium or pocket lumen.

Lorazepam is a drug belonging to a group of barbiturates and is 4 times more potent than diazepam. Half life is 12 hours. Onset of action is 30-60 minutes. Psychomotor impairment is seen for 12 hours. 2 mg orally of it is equivalent of 10 mg oral diazepam. 5 mg dose of it may cause disorientation.

Loss of tooth is referred to extracted tooth and not replaced artificially. In such condition opposing tooth becomes useless and it has nothing to bite. It loses its beneficial effect of cleaning and mastication. If several teeth are missing mastication will be affected to produce malnutrition. Loss of one tooth can result in plaque accumulation and in caries in at least six other teeth.

Low blood pressure refers to inadequate intravascular pressure to maintain oxygen requirement of body's tissues. It may be drug induced. Normal blood pressure varies typically a reading below 90/60 mm Hg or a drop of 30 mm Hg from base line is considered low BP. Dehydration and hemorrhage may result it.

Low testosterone levels presents as disturbed sleep pattern, loss of sensitivity of erogenous zones, cold and shriveled penis. Person starts gaining weight which is difficult to loose it. Seminal volume will be reduced with reduced facial hari growth.

Low voltage electrical burns are the electrical burns that are caused by low voltage (240 AC) domestic appliances. Though more common than the high voltage burns they may be deceptive in appearance as they may penetrate deeply. They are very commonly seen in infants crawling on the floor or in children who take the electrical wires into their mouth and chew them. They suffer severe damage to the lips, tongue and mouth and though the legion may be small the reactive edema may interfere with breathing and may require tracheostomy.

Lower lip prominence is the most prominent point of the lower lip (Li) should be 2 ± 1 mm anterior to Sn – pog' line.

Ls (Labrale Superius) is a point indicating the mucocutaneous border of the upper lip.

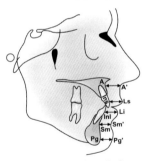

Ls (Labrale Superius)

Ludwig's angina is a cellulitis of submaxillary submandibular space and floor of the mouth. In Ludwig's angina submandibular and submaxillary spaces are involved. Second and third molars are involved. There is difficulty in swallowing with varying degrees of trismus. There develops swelling of mouth. Structures in floor or mouth are swollen and tongue is pushed up and back. Laryngeal edema may be present. Swelling is firm, painful and diffuse. Person is not able to swallow or eat. Cavernous sinus thrombosis and result in subsequent meningitis. Antibiotics are useful.

Lumbar puncture is procedure, where a hollow needle is inserted into subarachnoid space between $L_3 - L_4$ to avoid spinal cord. A sample of CSF is withdrawn and examined under microscope to rule out pathologies.

Lumbar stenosis vertebral canal space inside the ring is greatest when all the rings line up on top of each other. These vertebrae lines up best when you stoop forward. Space gets smaller when you stand up and smallest when you bend backwards. Arthritis or injury makes it further smaller. People with lumbar stenosis feel better when their spine is bent forward.

Lupus erythromatosus is a skin condition. There may be a genetic predisposition. There occur many remissions and exacerbations. Superficial painful ulceration may occur with crusting or bleeding. Margins of lesions are not demarcated. Often white straie radiate out from margins. Central healing results in central scarring.

Lupus milliaries disseminates faciei develop dark red to brown acneiform papules. These are non tender brownish red papules. There is no tendency to form pustule. No foreign material or remnants of microbes can be detected.

Luting is a mixing consistency of cement which is used for bonding or cementing two unlike substances together.

Lymph node performs biological filtration of lymph on its way to circulatory system. These are the part of body network, which filters antigen from tissue fluid and lymph during its passage from the periphery to the thoracic duct. These are located at branches of lymphatic vessels. Human lymph nodes 1-25 mm in diameter and round or kidney shaped. Indentation is present on the concave surface, where efferent blood vessels leave the node. Lymphatic afferent vessels enter through the convex surface. They have a collagenous capsule, radial trabaculae, B-cell rich cortex, T-cell rich paracortex and a central medulla with T-cell, B-cell and plasma cells. Para cortex are rich in inter digitating cells, APC, large quantity of MHC class II antigen. Medulla-cords separated by large sinuses where scavenger phagocyte cells along sinuses remove antigen form lymph. Cortex-primary and secondary follicles/ stimulated with germinal centers contain dendritic APCs and some macrophages. Involved with development of B cell response and B cell memory.

Lymphadenopathy is a condition occuring due to enlargement of lymph node. In a lymph node the B lymphocytes and T lymphocytes occupy the lymphoid follicles and paracortical areas. Lymph node enlargement occurs due to increase in number and size of lymphoid follicles, proliferation of macrophages or infiltration by abnormal cells. Enlargement of lymph nodes more than 1 cm is always pathological. Supra auricular, supra clavicular mesenteric glands and mediastinal nodes are always pathological. Lymphadenopathy may be localized or generalized.

Lymphangioma is a benign neoplasm due to proliferation of lymphatic vessels. It can be a simple lymphangioma, cavernous lymphangioma, cellular and systemic lymphangioma most of lesions are present at birth. They are similar to hemangioma except the fact that these vessels are filled with clear, protein rich fluid containing a few cells. Lymphangioma may occur in the skin mucus membrane of head and neck region. These may vary in size. Lesion is composed of numerous cytically dilated cavernous, lymphatic spaces many of which contain lymph. In the neck it is known as cystic hygroma. Mostly tongue is involved. . These are not having clear cut outline. Deeper lesions appear as diffuse nodules. These are painless, nodules or vesicle like lesions over oral mucosa.

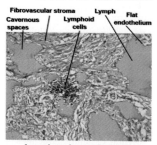

Lymphangioma of tongue

Color of lesion is lighter than surrounding mucosa. On palpation 'crepitation' sound is produced. Lymphangioma of tongue produces macroglossia. Surgical excision is the treatment of choice. It is radio resistant.

Lymphangitis is the inflammation of lymph vessels with pain in limb, pyrexia and toxaemia. Pain is throbbing or burning in nature. Pain is felt along with vessel. Superficial lymphatics of upper or lower limb are affected. Overlying skin may have edema. Regional lymph nodes are painful and enlarged. It is frequently accompanied by streptococcal or staphylococcal infection mostly in distal arm of leg. Malaise, sweating, chills and fever of 37.5 to 40°c is noted. Regional lymph nodes are enlarged and tender. Lymphangitis acute phase is seen in pyogenic infections mostly due to streptococci or other pyogenic microorganism. Skin becomes red and there is edema and tenderness over area. It may totally recover without any sequlae. In the process of healing the lymphatic may become fibrosed.

Lymphedema is anything that obstructs the lymphatic vessel causing edema of upper or lower extremities. It involves dorsal surfaces of hands and fingers or the feet and toes. Erythema is pitting initially and becomes browny and non pitting. With time ulceration, stasis and pigmentation may develop. If it persists it stimulates an overgrowth of fibrous tissue and has a brawny consistency and does not pit on pressure.

Lymphocytes are the primary white blood cells involved in immune response. These cells recognize and respond to an antigen. Lymphocytes are derived from stem cell which is located in bone marrow. These constitute 20 to 25% white cells. Two main types of lymphocytes are called B-lymphocytes and T-lymphocytes.

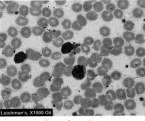
Leishman's, X1000 Oil
Lymphocytes

Lymphoepithelial cyst appears as a small, asymptomatic, well circular and elevated nodule on floor of mouth. It may be of a few mm in size. Lesion consists of a cavity lined by stratified squamous epithelium. Lumen of cyst contains lymphocytes and amorphous coagulum. Treatment includes local surgical excision. It seldom recurs.

Lymphokines are the products of lymphocytes. They have different functions. They can help monocytes to be changed in macrophages. They encourage macrophages to remain in area of injury to destroy foreign cells.

Lymphoproliferative disorders are characterized by monoclonal proliferation and accumulation of malignant lymphocytes. These include lymphoblastic leukemia, chronic lymphocytic leukemia, and Non Hodgkin's lymphoma.

Lysis is the destruction of cells resulting from damage to the plasma membrane.

Lysosomal storage syndrome includes development of childhood gingival enlargement, widened alveolar ridges and widely spaced teeth. Certain viscera's are enlarged.

Lysosome is a membrane-bound organelle visible by electron microscopy that contains acid hydrolases capable of breaking down macromolecules. Lysosome has diameters ranging from 50 nm to 1 m. A single membrane consisting of a phospholipid bilayer that undergoes selective fusion with other membranous organelles, an ATP driven h+ pump in the membrane, which acidifies the lysosomal matrix to ph 4.5–5.5, hydrolases in the inner matrix that are active at acidic ph and breakdown carbohydrates, lipids, and proteins.

L

Macrodontia is a developmental anomaly where one or more teeth are physically larger than normal. This term should not be used when normal sized teeth are crowded with in a small jaw. In such cases, the term *Relative macrodontia* is more appropriate. Regional / localized Macrodontia is occasionally seen on the affected side of the mouth in patients with Hemifacial hypertrophy. Macrodontia of single tooth is seen, but is rare. Rhizomegaly / radiculomegaly are an uncommon type of Macrodontia in which the root/roots of a tooth are considerably longer than normal. This condition is observed commonly in mandibular canines. It is associated with pituitary gigantism. Macrodontia of single tooth is not very common.

Macroglobulinemia is a variant of multiple myeloma. It develops in old age. Person develops weakness, lymphadenopathy and enlargement of liver. Hemorrhage from nasal cavity and oral cavity develops. Oral ulcers on tongue, buccal mucosa and gingiva are seen. There is no specific treatment.

Macroglossia refers to enlarged tongue. Congenital macroglossia is due to over development of tongue musculature. Secondary macroglossia may be due to diffuse lymphangioma or hemangioma. It is found in acromegaly too. There is no particular treatment of it.

Macrognathia refers to abnormally large jaw. It may be associated with acromegaly and Paget's disease. Some cases follow hereditary pattern. Prognathic patient forms long rami with less steep angle with body of mandible. There will be increased height of ramus, increased Gonial angle, decreased maxillary length, prominent chin button and varying soft tissue contours. Surgical correction is possible.

Macrolides are broad-spectrum antibiotics to which resistance develops rapidly. They inhibit protein synthesis by binding to the ribosome and are bacteriostatic at usual doses but bactericidal in high doses.

Macrophages are the monocytes that have left the blood stream, entered the tissues, and differentiated into various subpopulations. Many are found in close proximity to blood vessels. They are active in endocytosis and phagocytosis. Because of their mobility and phagocytic activity, they are able to act as scavengers, removing extravasated red blood cells, dead cells and foreign bodies from the tissue.

Magill intubation forceps is used to grasp the objects which have fallen into back of the patient's throat.

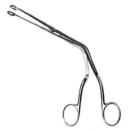

Magills intubation forceps

Magnesia core material is compatible with the high expansion porcelains normally bounded to metals.

Magnesium is the essential trace element. Human body contains 2000 mEq of magnesium. Half of it is in bones and half in soft tissues. Highest concentration is in liver and striated muscles. Daily intake is 36-48 mg. Nuts, peas, beans fruits and fish are rich sources. Plasma magnesium ranges from 1.5-2 mEq/L.

Magnetic resonance imaging (MRI) is an advanced diagnostic aid and has the great advantage over CT that the patient is not subject to radiation. Anatomical details are very well shown. Very good pictures of spinal cord and lumbar roots are seen. Different pictures can be obtained by varying the repetition time and radio frequency signal (TR) T1W1 images better anatomical details and T2W1 gives better patho-logical findings.

Mahler's theory (1933) categorizes the early childhood object relation to understand personality development. The period of childhood is classified into three stages: Normal autistic phase, Normal symbiotic phase, Separa-tion individualization phase.

Maize is a stable diet of poor class Indians. It is rich in carbohydrate and fat but is poor in essential amino acid tryptophan. Due to constant use of it may lead to pellagra. Mixing of milk, egg or wheat flour will help. Yellow maize is rich in carotenoid pigment.

Malaise refers to any vague feeling of illness, uneasiness or discom-fort.

Malaria is a type of fever occurring with rigors. It has 3 stages: Cold stage, hot stage, sweating stage. Cold stage lasts 15 minutes to 2 hours and is followed by hot stage in which fever may go very high. On an average hot stage lasts for 4 – 8 hours. It is followed by sweating stage which lasts for 1 to 4 hours. Patient may have fever, vomiting and excessive thirst. Patient feels exhausted. In malignant malaria fever may be accompanied by severe headache, diarrhea and toxaemia. There may be successive bouts of fever followed by severe cachexia. Splenic enlargement will be there (*see* Figure on page 283).

Malformation is a primary structural defect that results from a localized error in morpho-genesis e.g. peg shaped.

Malignant hypertension is a condition where patient may be normotensive or hypertensive. Both kidneys show flea bitten appearance. In acute form kidney may be swollen and pin point hemorrhages may be seen. Hypertension may result in episodes of unconsciousness or convulsions. Urine shows marked proteinuria and hematuria.

Malignant hyperthermia is a rapid onset of extremely high fever with muscle rigidity.

Malignant large intestine is a problem of rich society. Excessive fat and deficient fibre are the causative factor. Dietary fat enhances bile acid synthesis and level of sterol in intestine. Colonic bacteria convert this sterol into secondary acids which are thought to be carcinogens.

Malignant lymphoma is a neoplastic proliferative process.

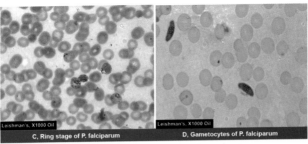

Leishman's, X1000 Oil	Leishman's, X1000 Oil
C, Ring stage of P. falciparum	D, Gametocytes of P. falciparum

Malarial Parasite (P. falciparum) in blood film

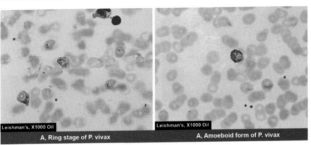

Leishman's, X1000 Oil	Leishman's, X1000 Oil
A, Ring stage of P. vivax	A, Amoeboid form of P. vivax

Malarial Parasite (P. Vivax) in blood film

M

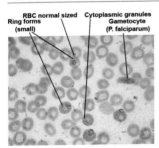

RBC normal sized   Cytoplasmic granules
Ring forms   Gametocyte
(small)   (P. falciparum)

Malarial Parasite

Lymphopoeitic portion of R.E. system, lymphomas and leukemias of lymphocytes and histocytes are identical.

Malignant melanoma develops from melanocytes of skin or mucous membrane. Although the role of melanocytes is to protect skin against development of skin cancer, but the cancer arising from the protective cell is most malignant tumor. Sunlight appears to play an important role in producing it. Commonest sites involved are hard palate and gingiva. Most of the lesions are pigmented and are dark brown in color. It starts as macular pigmented focal lesions. Initially it grows very fast into large, painful diffuse mass. Surface ulceration is very common. Small satellite lesions may develop at periphery. There is wide spread of tumor cells in lung, liver, bone and brain. Radical surgery and prophylactic neck dissection is advised. Still survival chances are bleak.

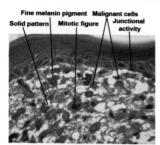

Malignant melanoma

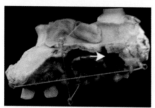

Malignant melanoma of palate

Malignant oral tumors may present as ulcers. Tobacco and alcohol consumption may cause squamous cell carcinoma. Oral epithelial dysplasia and lichen planus are the predisposing factors. These become painful when infected. Swollen non tender glands in neck may be seen. Loosening of teeth in carcinoma of gingiva is seen. Ulcer develops on tongue, floor of mouth and buccal mucosa. Shape may be round crescent or irregular. Edges are raised, rolled and everted. Base is indurated and fixed. Floor is granular and ragged.

Malignant salivary gland tumor incidence is much low. Peripheral malignant salivary gland tumors can occur anywhere in lining of oral cavity but seldom in gingiva. Central variety is still rare.

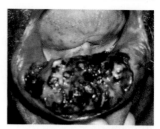

Malignant oral ulcer of labial sulcus

It generally develops between the age group 40-70 years of age. It grows slowly. When tumor infiltrates bone it produces radiolucency.

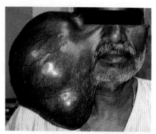

Malignant tumor of parotid salivary gland

Malignant Schwannoma arises from nerve sheath cell. Some may develop from neurofibromatosis. Complaint may be of a mass, while some may develop pain. Radiographs will show diffuse radiolucency characteristic of malignant infiltrating neoplasm. It can be treated by surgery and by radiation.

Malingerer is the one who pretends to be sick or in pain for a motive.

Malocclusion is any deviation from the ideal positioning of the teeth or jaws.

Mamelons are small elevations of enamel present on the incisors as they erupt.

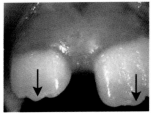

Mamelons

Mandible refers to the lower jaw.

Mammary duct ectasia is a dilation of collecting ducts in subareolar region. It is a disease of at or about menophase. Dilated ducts are bluish in color about 3 -5 mm.

Mandibular fracture amounts to 20% of all fractures of face condyle and angles are two most commonly fracture sites. Multiple fractures do take place.

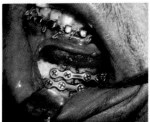

Clinical view of mandibular fracture

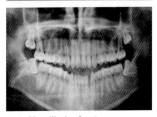

Mandibular fracture opg

Mandibular prognathism can be appreciated where a line perpendicular to the constructed horizontal is dropped from glabella. The distance of soft-tissue pogonion from this vertical line is measured. Average distance of Pog' is 0 ± 4 mm clinically mandible is placed forword than maxilla and face appears concave from side profile.

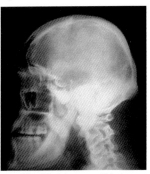

Mandibular prognathism

Mandibular subperiosteal implant is a metal frame implants that are surgically placed on top of the mandibular ridge.

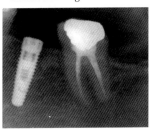

Mandibular suboeriosteal implant

Mania is an abnormal psychological state of mind with over-excitement and elevation of mood.

Mannitol is an osmotic agent that is freely filterable at the glomerular level. It is not reabsorbed by renal tubules. It has high diuretic potential so when given early in course of acute renal failure it tends to flush out cellular debris and prevent tubular cast formation. Initial test dose is 12.5 to 25 gm over 3.5 minutes. Repeat after 1-2 hours. It is used in head injury. Mannitol is also an artificial sweetener occurring in seaweed, this alcohol is metabolized very slowly by oral microbes and therefore thought to have less cariogenic effect. It is used in toothpaste, mouth rinses and as a dusting agent in chewing gum.

Marasmus is a disease occurring due to protein energy malnutrition or due to general starvation. It arises from inadequate calorie intake. There is a failure to gain weight followed by loss of weight until emaciation results. Skin becomes wrinkled due to loose subcutaneous fat. Face becomes shrunken and wizened like a monkey. Abdomen may be distended. There may be associated vitamin deficiency.

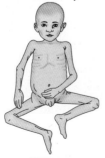

Marasmus

Marginal gingiva also known as unattached gingiva is the terminal edge of gingiva which surrounds the teeth in a collar like fashion. It also includes the gingival crevice or the sulcus and a free gingival margin. The free gingival margin is thicker and rounded around the primary teeth than in the permanent teeth, due to the morphological characteristics such as the cervical bulge and the underlying construction at the cementogingival junction, in contrast to the knife-edge margin seen in permanent dentition.

Marginal gingivitis is said to occur where the marginal gingiva is inflamed.

Margination is the process by which Neutrophils adhere to vessel wall and is divided into three phases: Selectin mediated phase, activation phase/chemoattractant and Integrin mediated phase.

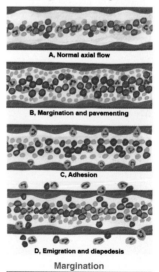

A, Normal axial flow

B, Margination and pavementing

C, Adhesion

D, Emigration and diapedesis

Margination

Maryland bridges are the one that replaces just one or two front teeth Pontic has a porcelain bonded facing. The metal backing has wring like flanges resting against palatal surface of abutments. These are bonded directly to their acid etched enamel.

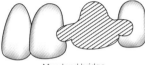
Maryland bridge

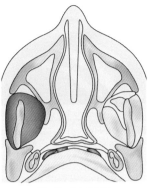
Masticator space

MASER (Microwave Amplification by Stimulated Emission of Radiation).

Mastication is conditioned reflex, learned initially by irregular and poorly coordinated, chewing movements. The TMJ and periodontal ligament of the erupting dentition establishes a stabilized chewing pattern. It is also the first stage of digestion occurring in mouth. Food is broken up into pieces and mixed with saliva. Tongue helps to roll the mixture of food and saliva into a semi liquid ball to be swallowed Teeth helps in chewing food. Mastication means chewing.

Masticator space refers to the space existing between the masseter muscle, pterygoid muscle, tendon of insertion of temporalis muscle, ramus of the mandible and the posterior part of the body of the mandible. Infection results in swelling of face, trismus and pain.

Masticatory pain is a pain that is induced by jaw movements which could be of deep somatic origin rather than neurogenic pain. Pain may be severe but trigering by superficial touch and slight movement. Masticatory pain is not arrested by mandibular local anesthetic block.

Mastoid condyle is the marked prominence of bone located posterior and inferior to the temporomandibular joint.

Mat foil is a combination of mat gold and gold foil in which a layer of gold is sandwiched between layers of gold foil. Mat foil has rapid filling properties and is suited for the use as an internal filling material in a cavity. It adapts well to the cavity wall and disadvantage is the bridging and surface pits are difficult to prevent. Mat gold is no softer than pure gold.

Materia Alba is the soft accumulation of bacteria and tissue cells that lack organized structure of plaque which can be easily displaced.

Matrix band is a stainless steel strip fabricated into a loop to fit around the prepared tooth and does not need a retainer.

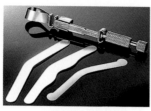

Matrix band

Matrix metalloproteinase are a family of metal binding proteinases synthesized by connective tissues cells and also by hemopoietic cells including monocytes and macrophages, keratinocytes, endothelial cells etc. They are usually secreted as a proenzyme form requiring extracellular activation. Metalloproteinase's can synergistically digest all the macromolecules of tissue matrices, although they are not necessarily produced together in any specific situations. Major sub groups of MMPS are -> Interstitial collagenases (MMP1, 8 and 13), Gelatinases (MMP 2 and 9), Stromelysins (MMP 3, 10, and 11), Membrane bound group (MMP14, 15, 16 and 17), Matrilysin (MMP 7) and metalloelastase (MMP 12).

Maturation is the qualitative change or aging.

Maxilla means the upper jaw.

Maxillary antrolithiosis may occur at any age. Sometimes it is marked by pain, sinusitis and foul discharge. It is a complete or partial calcific encrustation of an antral foreign body. It has to be removed surgically.

Maxillary arch is also known as upper jaw. The teeth present in position in the alveolar process of maxillae.

Maxillary nerve is one of the three divisions of trigeminal nerve. It is entirely sensory in function supplies the skin of middle part of face, nasal cavity and side of nose, lower eyelid, upper lip and mucus membrane of nasopharynx, soft palate, tonsil, maxillary gingiva and teeth.

Maxillary prognathism can be described as a line perpendicular to the constructed horizontal is dropped from glabella. The distance of subnasale from this vertical line should be 6 ± 3 mm.

Maxillary tuberosity is a rounded prominence of bone that extends posterior to the third molar region. It appears radiopaque on X-ray.

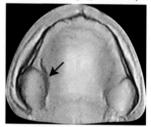

Maxilla tuberosity

Mc'means soft tissue menton i.e. Lowest point on the contour of the soft-tissue chin.

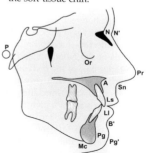

Soft tissue menton Mc

Mean is the sum of observations divided by the number of observations.

Meaningful habits are habits that have a psychological bearing.

Measles is contagious, viral disease of children. Incubation period is 8-10 days and child develops fever, cough, lacrimation and eruptive lesions of skin/mucosa. These appear as macule/papule which enlarge and coalesce. Oral lesions develop 2-3 days earlier of cutaneous rash. Intraoral lesions are known as Koplik's spot. These spots occur on buccal mucosa and are small, irregularly shaped appearing as bluish white specks surrounded by bright red margin.

Mechanical antidotes are those drugs that inactive poisons by mechanical action. Finally powdered charcoal in a dose of 4-8 gram acts mechanically by absorbing and retaining within its pores organic and to a less degree of mineral poison. One gram of charcoal absorbs about 500 mg of strychnine.

Meckel's syndrome presents as a midline clefting of tongue is a feature of this syndrome. Tongue is also thrown into multiple nodular or papillomatous projections.

Medial means relating to the middle or medial plane.

Median is the middle score of a ranked distribution.

Median palatal cyst arises from epithelium along the line of fusion of palatal process of maxilla. It lies in midline of hard palate. It requires surgical removal and curettage.

Median Rhomboid Glossitis is a congenital anomaly occuring due to failure of tuberculum impar to withdraw before fusion of 2 hours of tongue hence a structure devoid of papillae lies in between them. It is seen as an ovoid or rhomboid shaped reddish patch on dorsum of tongue anterior to circum vallate papillae. It is flat but slightly raised area.

Medical ethics are the special rules and regulations from the point of view of morality which a medical man should obey its violation is not an offence legally but is disgraceful and shameful from the point of view of profession.

Medical history refers to the history of any medical condition or any recent hospitalizations.

Medication is the use of medicine.

Medication order also known as prescription is the name and directions for giving a drug.

Medico legal autopsy is done to determine the identity of a person, to know the cause and time of death. It is also helpful in case of mutilated or skeletal remains to recognize the sex of it.

Mediotrusive side refers to the side of either dental arch corresponding to the side of the mandible moving towards the midline.

Medulloblastoma is the commonest variety of primitive neuroectodermal tumor. It amounts 25% of child tumors usual location is inferior portion of cerebellar vermis.

Mega dose is an amount at least 10 times greater than RDA. In mega doses, vitamins act as drugs.

Megadontia refer macrodontia

Megalodontia refer macrodontia

Melanin is a non – hemoglobin – derived brown pigment which is responsible for the normal pigmentation of skin, hair, gingiva and the rest of the oral mucous membrane. It is generally present in all individual and is very prominent in black individuals.

Melanocytes are the dendritic cells present in the basal and the spinous layer of gingival epithelium. They are mainly responsible for the production of a pigment called melanin which consequently attributes to the darker pigmented gingiva.

Melasma is a facial hypopigmentation seen commonly in pregnancy. There will be blotchy macules involving cheeks, temples and forehead. Sunlight increases the pigmentation while at the end of pregnancy it dissolves out. It may also develop during the use of oral contraceptive.

Melatonin is an important hormone produced by pineal gland believed to regulate onset of puberty and menstrual cycle.

Memory cell are the cells that remain in reserve in lymph nodes until their ability to secrete antibodies is needed.

Menarche is the beginning of menstrual function or it is the first menstruation which marks the onset of puberty in the female. It usually occurs between the age of 11 to 16 years.

Meningeal carcinomatosis refers to a condition where diffuse infiltration of meninges occurs in 8% of patients with advanced malignancy. Lesions such as lymphoma, melanoma and adenocarcinoma of breast are noted. Seizures and cranial nerve palsy are noted.

Meningioma is a tumor of arachoid cell of meninges. These are well circumscribed extra axial lesions that causes symptoms due to mass effect on under lying structures. These are completely resectable. Calcification in these is sufficient to make it radio opaque. On CT (Computed Tomography) these are seen as well defined hyperdense solid mass.

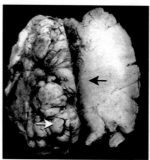

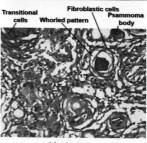

Meningioma

Meningitis is a condition occuring due to infection of meninges, brain stem and spinal cord covered by 3 membranes from within outwards, pia mater, arachnoid and dura mater. Organisms can enter meninges from without by penetrating wounds, from extension from brain abscess and through blood stream. One develops fever, diffuse headache, vomiting, and neck stiffness and in children convulsions may be developed.

Menopause is the period during which menstruation ceases and female reproductive cycle comes to an end. Contrary to certain fears sexual desire and enjoyment are maintained.

Mental health is not mere absence of mental illness. Mental health is a state of balance between the individual and surrounding world, a state of harmony between oneself and others, coexistence between realties of self and that of other people and that of the environment.

Mental nerve is the branch of inferior alveolar nerve which exits in mandible through its foramen. It innervates chin and mucus membrane of lower lip.

Mentalis is conical muscle present at the side of frenulum of lower lip. It raises and protrudes the lower lip and wrinkles the skin of chin.

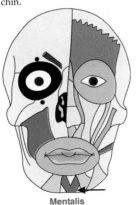

Mentalis

Mentalis space refers to the space existing in the region of mental symphysis, where the mental muscle, depressor muscle of the lower lip and the angle of the mouth are attached. Infection to this area results in the large swelling of the chin.

Meprobamate is a common propanediol derivative used in treatment of anxiety and tension. It acts as muscle relaxant too, but is less potential than diazepines. It reduces muscle tone but can cause tolerance and physical dependence. It produces sleep, ataxia and hypotension.

Mercury alloy ratio is the ratio of amongst of mercury to be mixed with an amalgam alloy.

Mercury	Hg	50%
Silver	Ag	35%
Tin	Sn	13%
Copper	Cu	0-3%
Zinc	Zn	0-1%

Mercury is a metal, component of amalgam fillings.

Mercury poisoning occurs due to fatal dose of 3-5 grams of mercuric chloride and fatal period is 3-5 days. Symptoms include metallic taste in mouth with a feeling of constriction and chocking in throat. It is followed by burning sensation. Mucus membrane becomes white and swollen. Vomits may contain mucous with blood. Stools become watery with mucus and blood. As treatment B.A.L. 300 mgm 1 M at once followed by 150 mgm during next 12 hours.

Mercury toxicity may be acute or chronic. It develops gastric disturbances, excitability, headache and mental depression. Patient may develop fine tremor.

M

Nephritis is common. There is a increased flow of saliva. Salivary glands may be swollen. Tongue may be swollen and painful. Loosening of teeth may occur. Treatment is supportive only.

Mercy killing is a painless killing of that person who has outlived his utility and is suffering from a disease which is incurable and painful. It has no legal sanction.

Merrifield's Z angle is an angle formed by the intersection of Frankfort horizontal (FH) and a line connecting the soft-tissue chin (Pog') and the most protrusive lip point of upper or lower lip. Average value, 80 degree (± 9).

Mesh size is a numerical grading of particle size. larger numbers e.g. 320 denote fine particles and smaller numbers denote coarse particles.

Mesial is the surface of the tooth nearest the midline of the dental arch. Mesial is toward the midline.

Mesial step terminal plane is a type of relationship where the distal surface of the lower second deciduous molar is more mesial than that of the upper. Thus the permanent molar erupts directly into 'Angles' Class I occlusion. This type of mesial step terminal plane must commonly occur due to the early forward growth of the mandible. If the differential growth of the mandible in a forward growth persists it can lead to Angles Class III molar relation and if the forward mandibular growth is minimal it can establish a Class I molar relationship.

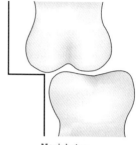

Mesial step

Mesiodens is the most common supernumerary tooth located between maxillary central incisors near the midline. Also refer supernumerary teeth.

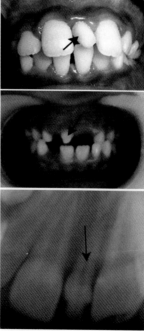

Mesiodens

Meta analysis in it research results across several different studies are synthesized in a quantitive way.

Metabolic acidosis occurs due to loss of alkalies from the kidney. In mild case it may be asymptomatic while in severe case patient may develop hyperpnea. Cardinal clinical findings include hyperventilation. There will be increased depth and respiration frequency. Lips will become dry and parched tongue may be present especially in diabetic acidosis. Acidosis depresses cardiac response to catecholamines. It reduces red cells. Anorexia and fatigue are common. Confusion and stupor may occur. In acute renal failure organic acid retention cause fall in plasma bicarbonate by 1-2 mEq/L/day. Patient may have circulatory shock.

Metabolic alkalosis develops due to loss of acids from kidneys or stomach. It has raised plasma bicarbonate and pH. There is mild rise in $PaCO_2$. Urine pH below 7. Urine chloride less than 10 mE/Q1L. There may be tetany, apathy and confusion.

Metal ceramic crowns are the type of crowns where the dental porcelain can be bonded to variety of metal alloys. These alloys fall into three categories: precious metal alloys, semi-precious metal alloys and base metal alloys. The advantages of these crowns are strength, minimal palatal reduction, adaptability; wherein the disadvantages includes aesthetics, strength, loss of tooth substance and the cost.

Metal is a crystalline material that consists of positively charged ions in an ordered closely packed arrangement and bonded with a cloud of free electrons.

Metalizing is a coating of impression material with a powdered metal to make it electrically conductive.

Metallic stains due to drugs are generalized unlike other stains and may affect all the surfaces of the tooth, these drugs enter the plaque substance and impart its color to plaque and calculus e.g. consumption of iron will give rise to black or brown stains, manganese will give rise to black stains.

Metallic stains due to industries occur mastly on the cervical third of the anterior teeth are primarily affected by the inhalation of metallic dust through mouth bringing them in contact with teeth, these metals along with bacterial plaque impart their color to the plaque present which occasionally may penetrate the tooth substance and give rise to endogenous stains. Copper will give bluish green stains, nickel will give green stain, and cadmium will give yellow or golden brown stains.

Metamerism is the change in color matching of two objects under light source is called Metamerism. Two objects that are marched under one light source but not under other light source forms metameric pair.

Metaplasia is conversion of one type of differentiated tissue into another type of differentiated tissue. Metaplasia can be of epithelial or connective tissue type. Metaplasia of columnar to squamous epithelium occurs in respiratory mucosa.

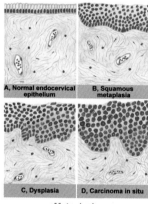

A, Normal endocervical epithelium

B, Squamous metaplasia

C, Dysplasia

D, Carcinoma in situ

Metaplasia

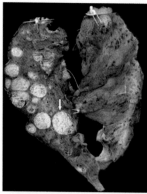

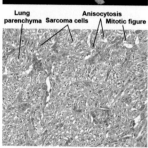

Lung parenchyma   Sarcoma cells   Anisocytosis   Mitotic figure

Metastatic sarcoma of lung

M

Metastasis is a spread of tumor from one site of organ to another with no direct continuity with the main or primary tumor mass. Tumor thus formed is a secondary deposit. Metastatic spread can occur through lymphatic channels, blood vessels. Metastatic spread is the hall mark of malignant neoplasm. Benign tumors never metastasize.

Metastasis melanomatous nodes patient is a young person between 20 to 30 years. Lymph nodes are firm, massive but not tender. These are mobile in early stage but later become fixed.

Metastatic calcification is the deposition of calcium in normal viable tissue due to hypercalcemia. It is due to hyperparathyroidism, vitamin D intoxication and osteolytic bone secondaries. Gastric mucosa, lungs, blood vessels and kidneys are involved. Deposition is around the tubules in kidney.

Metastatic carcinomatous nodes are the solitary or multiple nodes involved. It is hard but not tender. To start these are mobile and fixed. It may macerate or fungate. Primary lesion may be known.

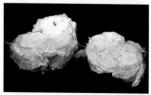

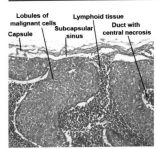

Metastatic carcinoma of
lymph nodes

Metastatic liver neoplasm Metastatic tumors are much more common. Cancer of breast, stomach, pancreas, kidney, and uterus are most to metastasize. Weight loss, anorexia and fatigue are the common complaints. CT scan is a better tool to diagnose it. Survival is 3 months to 3 years.

Metastatic tumors of jaw are formed by cells that have been transported from the primary tumor to site not connected to original tumor. These are not frequent and may be asymptomatic. If mandibular nerve is involved there may be paresthesia of lip or chin. Teeth may become loose. Expansion of jaw is a constant finding. Mandible is affected more than maxilla. On X-ray these produce metastatic lesion. Diffuse destruction may lead to pathological fracture. Prognosis is not good.

Metastatic vertebral tumor causes low back pain. Typically pain begins abruptly with cramping muscular pain. Pain is worst during night and is not relieved by rest.

Methadone was discovered in 1940 in Germany and produces mild analgesia. It is well absorbed form G.I.T. Its effective oral dose is 5-15 mg depending on severity of pain. Side effects are less common.

Methohexltone is two and half times more potent drug as thiopentone. It is prepared by mixing the powder in sterile distilled water. Average induction dose is 1.0 to 1.5 mg/kg body weight. It is the best anesthetic induction agent. It can be best used singly for extraction of tooth. If it is injected extravenously it may cause necrosis and ulcer formation.

Metronidazole is a gram negative antimicrobial that is active against wide range of micro-organism specially trichomonads. It is used in ulcerative gingivitis. It is well tolerated when given orally except some G.I.T. upsets.

Micro abrasion is a drill-free technique using an instrument resembling a tiny sand blaster that delivers tiny aluminium oxide particles to the surface of teeth.

Microangiopathy is the abnormalities in the structure and function of blood vessel.

Microdontia is a developmental anomaly where the teeth are physically smaller than usual. Widely spaced normal sized teeth may appear small within the jaws that are larger than normal and is termed as relative microdontia. But this in true sense represents macrognathia, not microdontia. If all the teeth in both the normal sized arches are smaller than normal it is referred to as generalized microdontia. True generalized microdontia is seen in pituitary dwarfism, Down's syndrome. Isolated microdontia/ microdontia involving one or two teeth are far more common than

M

generalized types. Most commonly affected teeth are maxillary, lateral incisor or maxillary third molars. Maxillary lateral incisors typically appear peg shaped crown.

Microfilled composite resins Conventional resins are 500 times greater than that of particles in microfilled resin. Some pulpal protection is necessary under deep cavities.

Micrognathia means a small jaw. Either a maxilla or mandible may be affected. True micrognathia may be congenital or acquired. In case of maxilla deformity is of middle third of face retracted. Congenital micrognathia is difficult to explain. Acquired type is due to disturbance of temporomandibular joint. There is severe retrusion of chin, steep mandibular angel and deficient chin button.

Micron 0.001 mm or 0.00004 inch. 1/1000 millimetres.

Microshock low voltage but high amperage electricity.

Microstomia is a condition where patient present with an abnormally small opening of mouth associated with functional disability. Shape of opening is circular and it appears as if patient is whistling. It may be congenital or may develop after burns.

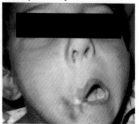

Microstomia

Microwave diathermy is a therapy where microwaves penetrate more deeply than infrared rays but don't pass through the tissues in any appreciable density. This is not suitable for treatment of deeply placed structures than short wave diathermy. Average depth of penetration is 3 cm. These are effectively absorbed by water so there is an appreciable heating of tissues having rich blood supply. It is very good in traumatic and inflammatory lesions. So it is useful in trauma and rheumatic condition. Skin must be dry because water is heated rapidly. Wet dressings should be avoided.

Mid sagittal plane is also known as midline vertical plane that divides the body into two equal left and right halves.

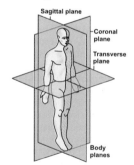

Various body planes

Middle cerebral artery ischemia is the largest branch of internal carotid artery and supplies the lateral surfaces of frontal, parietal and temporal lobes. Complete occlusion results in contralateral sensory loss, motor weakness with positive Babinski sign of upper motor neurone lesion.

Middle superior nerve is a branch of infraorbital nerve within the infra orbital canal, provides sensory innervations to maxillary premolars, periodontal tissue facial soft tissue and bone.

Midline is the imaginary line through the middle of an object which divides it into two equal parts.

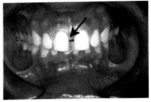

Mid line diastema

Miescher's syndrome is manifested as diffuse swelling of lip. Scaling, fissuring, vesicle or pustule formation of vermillion border may take place.

Migraine is a familial disorder characterized by recurrent paroxysmal attacks of headache it is one of the most disabling disease. Often there is a strong family history. It is a paroxysmal unilateral headache, preceded by visual and sensory phenomena. It may be accompanied by nausea and vomiting. It is due to vasospasm in extra and intra cranial arteries. It starts just after waking up. Visual aura is common. It may be hemianopic field defect and transient blindness. Sensory aura includes tingling, numbness and pins and needles in corner of mouth. Treatment is disappointing.

Migraine without aura is of an abrupt onset. Nausea and vomiting are common. It is strongly familial. Headache may awaken patient from sleep. Photophobia and homophobia are common. In status migrainous hospitalization may be needed.

Migratory glossitis is also known as wondering rash of tongue of unknown etiology. Emotional stress may result in it. It shows multiple areas of desquamation of filiform papillae in an irregular pattern. Central portion looks inflamed, while borders are outlined by thin yellowish white line. Area of desquamation heals and appear at other location. It gives an idea of migration. Condition may remain for months. Since the etiology is unknown treatment is empirical.

Mikulicz's disease shows both inflammatory and neoplastic characteristics. There is enlargement of parotid or sub maxillary gland. There may be fever, loose tooth and oral infection. Mass may increase or decrease in size.

Military tuberculosis lung is due to hematogenous spread of infection. X-ray may show small, discrete nodules 1-2 mm. in diameter distributed throughout both lungs. These nodules may enlarge and coalesce (*see* Figure on page 300).

Milk is a complete and ideal food and is a balanced diet. It contains 3.5% proteins. Carbohydrates are in form of milk sugar. Human milk contains more sugar than cow's milk. It is a poor source of vitamin C and does not contain vitamin E. It is a good source of calcium but is a poor source of iron. Fat is in the form of glycerides in emulsified form.

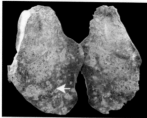

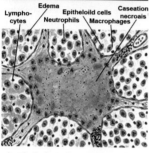

Lympho- | Edema | Epitheloild cells | Caseation necroais
cytes | Neutrophils | Macrophages

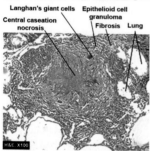

Langhan's giant cells | Epithelioid cell granuloma
Central caseation nocrosis | Fibrosis | Lung

H&E. X100

MIlitary tuberculosis of lung

Mineral elements are the trace elements found in body. There are 24 minerals. About 4-6% of body weight is made up of mineral elements. Bones and teeth store these. These maintain acid base balance, control of water balance, contraction of muscles and clotting of blood. This helps in formation of bone and teeth formation.

Mini bladed curettes are the modification of extended shank or after five curettes. They are half the size of standard Gracey curettes; they have shorter blades which allow easier insertion and adaptation into deep pockets, furcation areas, developmental grooves etc.

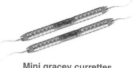

Mini gracey currettes

Mini plates were introduced by champy et al in 1978 customized for mandibular fractures. They were initially available in stainless steel which has now been replaced by titanium. These non compression mini plates are confined to outer cortex allowing the fixation of plates both sub apically and the lower border. After healing these plates can be left in vicinity permanently without causing any trouble.

Minor oral surgery instruments include scalpal, periosteal elevator, tissue retractor, kilner cheek retractor and Austin retractor.

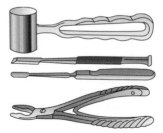

Bone instruments: Mallet, Bone chisel, Bone file, Bone forceps

Minor salivary gland are found deep to the mucosa of the upper and lower lip, cheeks, undersurface of the tongue, soft palate, dorsal surface of the tongue and lateral parts of hard palate behind the first premolar. These small glands have short ducts which open directly onto the surface of the mucosa by multitude of openings.

Mismatched blood transfusion refer where patient of a particular group has been transfused another group of blood. Person develops fever with rigor. There develop pain with rigor in pericardium area. B.P. falls and pulse goes high. Skin becomes cold and clammy with cyanosis. Urine becomes scanty.

Mitotic activity is a process of cell division. It determines the response of a cell to radiation.

Mitotic figures are seen in any proliferative tissue including benign tumors. A high mitotic index is not diagnostic of malignancy. Abnormal mitotic figures such as triploid and tetra polar mitoses occur exclusively in malignant lesion.

Mitral regurgitation – occurs when left atrial pressure rises rapidly leading to pulmonary edema. When chronic, left atrium enlarges, exertional dyspnea and fatigue progresses. Mitral regurgitation may predispose to infective endocarditis. There will be pan systolic murmur maximal at apex radiating to axilla.

Mitral stenosis –There will be dyspnea, orthopnea and paroxysmal nocturnal dyspnea. Prominent mitral first sound, opening snap and apical diastolic crescendo. ECG shows left atrial abnormality.

Mixed dentition is a type of dentition that contains both the dentition as this is the transient phase where there is exchange of primary dentition to permanent dentition. It is also known as transitional dentition.

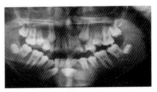
Mixed dentition opg

Mixing tip is used with an authmix impression system.

Mm Hg – Millimeters of mercury a unit measuring pressure.

Mode is the most frequently occurring score within a distribution.

Moderate bone loss of 10 to 33% measured on a dental radiograph.

Moderate interproximal lesion extends greater than halfway through the thickness of enamel, but does not involve the dentero enamel junction (DEJ). A moderate lesion is seen in enamel only.

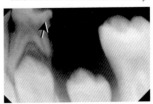
Moderate proximal caries

Moderate periodontitis is said to have occurred when the periodontal destruction is 3 to 4 mm of clinical attachment.

Moderate pulpalgia may start spontaneously from such a simple act as that of lying down. Hot food or drink excites the pain. Warm water will not relieve the pain and cold water sometimes makes it worse. The pain is a true toothache. Pain is of nagging or of boring type. Pain to start is localized and later becomes diffuse or referred to another area. Pain does not resolve once the irritant is removed.

Modified DMFT Index was introduced by Joseph Z Anaise in 1983. The DMFT index Klein and Palmer is one of the simplest and most commonly used indices in epidemiologic dental health status based on the number of decayed, missing and filled teeth. The index however does not provide an accurate description of previous dental care nor does it provide information regarding the severity of the carious attack or the indicated treatment. Thus, a modification of the DMFT index was developed. The modification of DMFT index involved a division of the 'D' component into four separate categories. With the addition of these categories, the index remains simple, and yet provides description of one's previous dental experience. It further shows the extents of dental services needed by the population, which can be interpreted in terms of treatment hours and costs. Basically, this modified DMFT index involves the same operation procedures applied to the common DMFT index. The only difference is the scoring criteria for 'D' component of the index. In this modified DMF index, the 'D' component is divided into 4 separate categories.

Modified pen grasp ensures the greatest control in performing intraoral procedures. The thumb, index and the middle finger is used to hold the instrument as a pen is held. This grasp enhances control because it enables the clinician to roll the instrument in precise degrees, also it enhances tactile sensitivity.

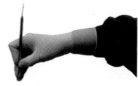

Modified pen grasp

Modulus of elasticity is a measure of materials stiffness. Stiffness is an important issue when selecting restorative materials because large deflections are undesirable. To withstand forces of mastication material should have high modulus of elasticity.

Moist heat sterilization denatures and coagulates the protein of microbe. It is highly efficient due to latent heat of vaporization present in moist heat. Portable steam sterilizers are being used.

Molar forceps are the surgical instruments to perform extraction. These have pointed blades to fit the bifurcation of molar roots. Upper molar forceps have one pointed blade to fit the bifurcation of buccal roots and a rounded blade to fit the single palatal root. Lower molar forceps have two identical blades. Left and right lower molars are extracted with it (*see* **Figure on page 303**).

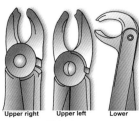

Upper right   Upper left   Lower
Molar forceps

Molar is the posterior most teeth of the oral cavity. They have large occlusal table and play a major role in chewing. There are first, second and third molars; these are the sixth, seventh and eighth teeth from the center of the mouth, respectively. Third molars are also known as wisdom tooth.

Molecular death means death of an individual cells or tissues of body. It takes sometime after the somatic death. The period between somatic death and cell death is rarely more than 3-4 hours. Signs of molecular death include loss of elasticity of skin, changes in eyes, cooling of body, flaccidity and lately rigor mortis.

Moller's Index is a system that was developed by Moller I.J and Poulsen S in 1964 is a standardized system for diagnosing, recording and analyzing dental caries data. The basis for the development of this system was to make available a system which could be used in many different situations. The advantages of the system seems to be its flexibility in meeting the varying needs of different types of clinical studies on dental caries.

Molluscum contagiosum is due to infection with a large DNA virus, a member of pox virus group. It causes small umbilicated 1-3 mm in diameter lesion which may express cheesy core on pressure. It is more common in children. Multiple, discrete elevated nodules occur on face and trunk. Disease appears to be spread by autoinoculation. Oral lesions occur on lips, tongue and buccal mucosa, surgical excision may be required.

Monellin is 3000 times sweeter than sucrose. It is extracted from an African berry. Like Aspartame, it is a protein–derived sweetener.

Monocytes are the largest normal cell in blood. Nucleus may be round, kidney shaped, oval or lobulated. Cytoplasm is slightly grey. Chromatin is arranged in fine strands with sharply defined margins. It is also of same size as that of Neutrophils, i.e. 10 mm diameter but they are conventionally known as macrophages when they leave the blood as they began to differentiate and grow larger in size up to 22 mm diameter. They are best suited for communicating with lymphocytes and other surrounding cells.

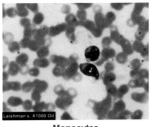

Leishman's X1000 Oil

Monocytes

Monomorphic adenoma is a benign encapsulated salivary gland. These are composed of uniform pattern of epithelial cells.

These have no connective tissue like component. These are treated surgically.

Moral values are standards of conduct and are influenced by family, religion, culture and society.

Morbidity is sickness/illness.

Morgue is the area where dead bodies are temporarily held or examined.

Morning sickness develops in early pregnancy. Nausea and vomiting is seen. It may be due to hypoglycaemia.

Moro reflex is any sudden movement of the neck initiates the reflex. This can be elicited by pulling the baby to a sitting position from the supine and suddenly let the head fall back to a short distance. This reflex consists of a rapid abduction and extension of the arm with the opening of hands. This gives an indication of muscle tone. The response may be asymmetrical if muscle tone is unequal on the two sides, or if there is a weakness of an arm or an injury to the clavicle. This reflex usually disappears in 2 to 3 months.

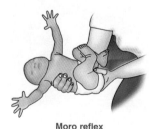

Moro reflex

Morphine is an opioid drug that was first isolated in 1903 by Serturner. It is derived from papaver somniferu. It chiefly affects CNS and bowels. 5-10 mg I.V. reduces pain within 20-30 minutes. There develop a feeling of drowsiness and euphoria. It is effective against all types of pain but not very effective in sharp intermittent pain. It depresses respiration. Cough reflex is also depressed and death is due to respiratory failure. Itching and urticaria may also develop. It develops tolerance and physical/psychical dependence. Heroin is more effective than morphine.

Morphology is the science that deals with form and structure without reference of function.

Mortal Pulpotomy Ideally, a non-vital tooth should be treated by pulpectomy and root canal filling. However, pulpectomy of a primary molar is often impracticable and a two-stage pulpotomy technique is therefore more commonly used. Necrotic coronal pulp is first removed and the infected radicular pulp is treated with a strong antiseptic solution, which is applied on a cotton pellet and sealed in the pulp chamber for 10-12 weeks. Beech wood creosote is usually used (Hobson 1970) 52 but formocresol (Droter 1963) or camphorated monochlorophenol may also be used. Beech wood creosote is a mixture of cresol, glycol and other phenols, which is less irritant to the tissue than phenol itself.

Mortality means death.

Moss hypothesis according to moss states that the "bone" does not regulate its own growth. The genetic and epigenetic determines of matrix, are, muscle, nerve glands, teeth, neurocranial fossa, and nasal, orbital, oral, and pharyngeal cavities. This is primary while the growth of the skeletal unit is secondary. However, although the functional matrix principle describes what happens during growth, it does not account for how it happens. Functional matrices, which can be further, divided in to capsular and perosteal matrices have the primary control for the growth of cranio-facial structures. Bone responds to the matrices in a passive manner and doesn't have any primary growth potential.

Motor neuron transmits nerve impulses from brain and spinal cord to muscles and glandular epithelial tissue.

Mottled enamel was described first by F. McKay in 1916. Ingestion of fluoride containing drinking water during the formation of tooth leads to it. Severity of it increases with increasing amount of fluoride. Above the level of 0.9 to 1.0 ppm fluoride may cause it. Mild changes manifest by white opaque areas. Moderate and severe change shows pitting and brownish staining. Fracture enamel may be seen. Bleaching of affected teeth gives cosmetic relief.

Mottling fluoride is endemic in areas where fluorides in drinking water exceeds 2 ppm. It has a geographical distribution and permanent teeth are affected. Mottling of deciduous teeth is rare. Mottled teeth are less susceptible to caries. Mottling ranges from paper white patches to opaque, brown, pitted and brittle enamel.

Mould is a cavity into which molten metal is cast.

Mouth breathing is an oral habit where mouth has been attributed as a possible etiologic factor for malocclusion. The mode of respiration influences the position of the jaw, the tongue and to a lesser extent the head. Mouth breathing can result in altered jaw and tongue posture, which could alter the oro-facial equilibrium thereby leading to malocclusion. It can be obstructive, habitual or anatomic in nature. Classified into a. Obstructive, b. Habitual, c. Anatomic.

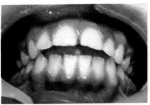

Mouth breathing and tongue thrust

Mouth guard is a removable appliance used to protect teeth from injury during sports.

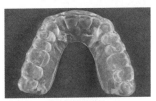

Mouth guard

Mouth rinse reduces the number of intraoral microbes by as much as 50 percent. There is an element of mechanical removal and reduction due to antiseptic too. Chlorhexidine is commonly used.

M

Mucin is a secretion of mucus cell a polysaccharide protein which when combined with water forms a lubricating solution.

Mucocele is a clinical term used to describe swelling caused by pooling of saliva at the site of damage or obstruction. It is generally of traumatic origin. It is of 2 types (i) extravasation of mucocele or (ii) retention mucocele. It generally occurs on lower lip palate, cheek and tongue. Lesions may be fairly deep in tissue. Superficial lesion is a raised circumscribed vesicle Mucus extravasation type is common mucocele and is caused by laceration. Mucus retention type is due to obstruction resulting in cyst formation. Mucoceles show flattened epithelial lining. Treatment includes excision.

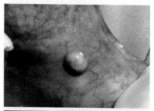

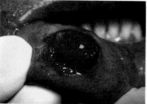

Mucocele of buccal mucosa and labia mucosa

Mucocutaneous lymph node syndrome is a self limiting febrile illness. Etiology is not known.

Clinical features include fever for 5-7 days, bilateral conjunctivitis, and peripheral edema. Acute non purulent swelling consist of cervical lymph nodes of 1.5 cms. Majority of cases are self limiting.

Mucoepidermoid tumor is an unusual type of malignant salivary gland neoplasm with varying degree of aggressiveness. Tumor generally involves parotid gland. It is similar to pleomorphic adenoma, it is a slow growing, painless swelling, it has cystic feeling, X-ray will show unilocular or multilocular radiolucent areas in jaw, parotid tumor shows relatively, focal nodular swelling, swelling is mobile, facial nerve paralysis may develop, low grade tumor shows fluctuation, but high grade tumors are fixed to the adjacent areas, in a few cases tumor may be fast growing with ulceration, hemorrhage and paresthesia.

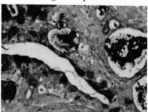

Mucoepidermoid cancer

Mucogingival surgery is the term given to describe the surgical procedures that were performed for the correction of relationship between the gingiva and oral mucous membrane with the reference to specific problems associated with attached gingiva, shallow vestibules and frenum involving marginal gingiva.

Mucomycosis is caused by an infection with a saprophytic fungus. Fungus is generally non pathogenic. It occurs normally in soil or as a mould on decaying food. There is development of ulcerative lesions. Denudation of underlying bones may develop. Negative cultures don't rule out the disease. Microscopically necrosis may be seen. Fungus invades arteries resulting in thrombosis and ischemia. Fungus may spread from oral and nasal area to brain causing death. In oral cavity it results in ulceration of palate resulting necrosis. Ulcers may develop on gingiva, lip and alveolar ridge. Treatment includes surgical debridement of an infected area with Amphotericin – B for 3 months.

Mucoperiosteum is the soft oral tissue covering the bone that consists of mucosa and the periosteum.

Mucosa is the thin, outer pink or red membrane lining the inside of the oral cavity.

Mucositis is the direct cytotoxic action of chemotherapeutic agents on the oral mucosa resulting in atrophy or thinning of oral mucosa, erythema and ulceration.

Mucous membrane pemphigoid is an autoimmune disease affecting eye, skin and oral mucosa. Symptoms include painful, blood filled blisters which rupture to form ulcer. Rupture bullae is having well defined margins. Floor is having an inflamed base.

Mulberry molar is a developmental anomaly of teeth that is suggestive of congenital syphilis. Buccal and lingual surfaces are normal but occlusal surfaces looks like mulberry.

Multilocular cyst is the most frequently encountered entity in jaws. It is always of soap bubble type. It is a true cyst of jaws. Small cyst is usually asymptomatic. It increases slowly and may cause displacement of teeth. Root can be resorbed. If the overlying bone becomes thin it may produce crackling sound. Later covering plate may be destroyed. It may contain thin, straw colored fluid.

Multilocular lesion is the one which extends beyond the confines of one distinct area and is defined as many lobes. Odontogenic keratocysts is an example of multi ocular lesion.

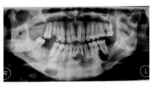
Multiple odontogenic keratocysts

Multilocular radiolucencies are produced by multiple adjacent frequently coalescing and overlapping compartments in bone. Mostly these occur in maxilla. The term soap bubble, honeycombs and tennis racket are frequently used.

Multiple endocrine neoplasias are also known as MEN syndrome. It is inherited as an autosomal dominant. The lesion involves certain endocrine glands. They produce bumpy lips. Anterior 1/3rd of tongue is involved. These appear as tortuous masses of nerve fibres.

M

Multiple fractures refer to the fractures occurring at various sites resulting from single injury. The most common one is caused by the fall on the midpoint of chin resulting in fractures of symphysis and both the condyle.

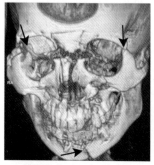

Multiple fracture (panfacial)

Multiple myeloma develops from bone marrow resembling to plasma cell. IL-6 is the major myeloma growth and C-reactive protein is a peripheral marker of 1L-6. It develops in elderly age group. Pain is the early feature. Back pain, anemia and bone pain are common. Any movement increases pain. Pain is due to osteoclastic lesion. Collapse of vertebra or of a long bone is due to lytic lesion. Pathological fracture is common. Bence Jones proteinuria develops along with unexplained weakness, fatigue, osteoporosis. Ramus angle and molar region of mandible are the commonest sites involved. X-ray will show multiple sharply punched out areas. Size may vary from a few mm. to 1 cm. There is no peripheral bone reaction. It infiltrates bone and soft tissue.

Bones anywhere in the body can be affected. Deep bone pain is the early feature. Pain increases with movement. Numbness of chin and lips may develop. Jaw swelling and pain may be confused with toothache. Jaw swelling, crackling or pathological fracture may develop. Extraction of teeth results in severe hemorrhage. Radiographs will show numerous punched out areas of radiolucency with peripheral bone reaction. Chemotherapy is given but disease is fatal.

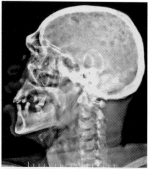
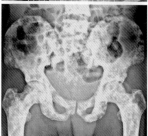

Multiple myeloma of skull and hip bone showing multiple punched out areas

Multiple organ failure is the condition in which two or more organ system gradually cease to function.

Mumps is an acute contagious viral infection. There is unilateral or bilateral swelling of parotid glands. Submaxillary and sublingual glands may be involved. Incubation period is 2-3 weeks. Disease is preceded by chill, fever, pain below ear. Later on swelling becomes firm and rubbery. Complications include, orchitis, pancreatitis and Otitis. Orchitis is unilateral and serum amylase level is increased.

Mumps-vaccine is highly effective live attenuated vaccine is available for prevention of mumps. Single dose 0.5 ml. I.M. produces detectable antibodies in 95% cases. It should not be given to pregnant women or in severely ill patient.

Muscle relaxants are neuromuscular blocking agents producing their effect by interfering with the excitatory action of acetylcholine at the motor end plate. These provide paralysis of voluntary muscles during clinical anesthesia. These are of two types, (i) non depolarizing neuromuscular blocking agents and (ii) depolarizing neuromuscular blocking agents.

Muscle splinting pain is defined as rigidity of muscles occurring as a means of avoiding pain caused by movement of a part. Muscle splinting is involuntary contraction that tends to immobilize the part. At rest a splinted muscle relaxes. Splinting of masticatory muscles occurs as a protective mechanism to limit excessive functioning of TM joint.

Muscle strain causes mild to severe pain with movement. The reduction of movement may cause muscle weakness and atrophy.

Muscular contact position (MCP) refers to that position of mandible where the mandible is lifted into contact from resting position.

Musculoskeletal pain is non-inflammatory in origin. It results from muscles spasm, it is reactive, and it is protective. Muscles splinting is a temporary protective mechanism. Such splinting serves to rest the muscle until the symptoms disappear.

Mutism is a total inability to speak. It may be seen without any organic disease of CNS. It may be psychogenic in origin.

Mycobacterium leprae – Humans are the only hosts. These reside in skin and nerves. Prolonged contact is required for transmission. It is aerobic, acid fast bacilli. These are not alcohol fast and no known toxins. Leprosy bacillus causes slow progressive chronic disease affecting skin and nerves.

Mycobacterium tuberculosis is responsible for tuberculosis (TB) and is found in infected humans mainly in lungs. Spread is by droplet. It is acid and alcohol fast, slender, beaded bacilli. Ziehl – Nelson stain is required to see them.

Myeloblast is round and large, about 14 to 18 micro mm in diameter. Nucleus is very fine of the cell. Nuclear chromatin is very fine and two to five nucleoli are present. Cytoplasm is basophilic.

Myeloid is pertaining to bone marrow.

M

Mylohyoid ridge is a linear prominence of bone located on internal surface of mandible appearing radiopaque.

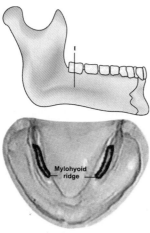

Mylohyoid ridge

Mylohyoid ridge

Myocardial infarction is an area of ischemic necrosis of myocardium caused by insufficient blood supply due to coronary artery occlusion.

Myoclonic seizures are sudden brief bilaterally synchronus muscle contractions of face and trunk without loss of unconsciousness. Although idiopathic it is seen in association with uraemia and hepatic failure.

Myoclonus is a brief, involuntary random muscle contractions occurring with rest in response to sensory stimuli. It may involve as single motor unit or group of units. Sudden brief lapses of contractions known as negative myoclonus. Myoclonic jerks may be focal, segmental or generalized. Etiogically myoclonus can be classified as physiologic myoclonus, essential myoclonus, epileptic myoclonus and symptomatic myoclonus.

Myoepithelioma is an uncommon salivary gland tumor. Parotid gland is mostly involved and palate is the common intraoral site to be involving tumor has to be removed surgically.

Myofacial pain comes from muscles and surrounding soft tissues. Injury or overuse results in painful muscle spasm and may last long after an injury or muscle overuse. Muscles become short and tender. Pressing trigger point causes increased pain. Physical therapy and stretching exercises help.

Myofunctional appliance is defined as loose fitting or passive appliance, which harness natural forces of the oro-facial musculature transmitted to the teeth and alveolar medium through the medium of the appliance.

Myopathy is any disease or abnormal condition of muscle tissue.

Myosin is an actin accessory protein that functions as a molecular motor. There are several isoforms of myosin, and muscle and non-muscle forms have slightly divergent amino acid sequences. It is composed of two heavy chains and four light chains.

Myositis ossificans is the formation of bone within a muscle which is contused.

Myotonic appliances are functional appliances that depend on the muscle mass for their action.

M

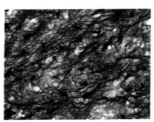
Myxoma

Myxoma resembles primitive mesenchyme and is true neoplasm. Oral submucosal area, salivary gland and jaw bones are commonly affected. It is a slow growing invasive tumour that sometime reaches large dimensions. Jaw is distended. X-ray will shows a soap bubble appearance. Being locally aggressive radical surgery is advised.

M

N is the Nasion the most anterior point of the nasofrontal suture in the median plane. (On radiograph) and clinically. N′ is the soft tissue nasion the point of greatest concavity in the midline between the forehead and the nose.

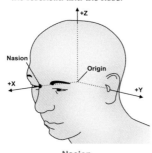

Nasion

Nails are thin plates of stratified squamous epithelial cells. It contains a very hard form of keratin. These are found on the distal ends of fingers and toes. It has free edge, nail body and nail root. Extent of nail growth is represented by half moon shaped lanula.

Nalgonda technique (named after the village in India where the method is pioneered) is a deflouridation technique based on chemical reaction where raw water is mixed with adequate lime and alum. The amount of lime depends upon the alkanity of the raw water. If the raw water has adequate alkalinity the lime addition is not required. Alum solution is added after the addition of lime stirred gently for 10 minutes and the flocs formed are allowed to settle. This process of floc formation and setting requires an hour.

Nance method is similar to the Tweeds technique and involves the extraction of the deciduous first molar followed by the extraction of the first premolars and the deciduous canine.

Napkin holder is a standard item available in different styles used to secure a dental napkin around a patient's neck.

Narcolepsy sleep may occur in inappropriate situations during conversation or meals. There develops a rapid sleep of poor quality. One develops hallucinations and sleep paralysis.

Nasal glioma is tumor like lesion in nose in children. It presents as a rounded projection in the nose. Microscopically it is made up mature glial tissue.

Nasal polyp may be unilateral or bilateral and can be divided into non allergic and allergic. Non allergic polyps consist of an edematous fibrous stroma. Variable infiltrate of lymphocytes, plasma cells and neutrophils are seen.

Nasal reflex is the stimulation of the face or nasal cavity with water or local irritants, produces apnea (stops breathing) in neonates – this leads to bradycardia and lowering of the cardiac output.

Nasofacial angle is formed by the intersection of a line drawn from glabella to soft-tissue pogonion with a line drawn along the axis of the radix of the nose. Average values are 30 to 35°.

Nasolabial angle is formed by the intersection of a columella tangent and an upper lip tangent. Normal ranges from 90 – 110°.

Nasomental angle is constructed by a line drawn along the axis of the radix and a line drawn from the tip of the nose to soft tissue pogonion (e-line) normal=120-132.

Nasopalatine nerve is the nerve which leaves the pterygopalatine ganglion and passes forward and downward entering the oral cavity through incisive foramen. It provides sensory innervations to the bone and lingual soft tissues in the premaxilla.

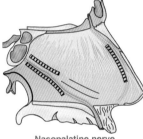

Nasopalatine nerve

Nasopharyngeal carcinoma symptoms include pain, restricted movements of jaw and ear complaints. There may be nasal stiffness, nosebleed and neck mass. Treatment requires radiation along with chemo-therapy.

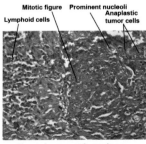

Mitotic figure Prominent nucleoli
Lymphoid cells Anaplastic tumor cells

Nasopharyngeal carcinoma

Nasopharynx lies behind the nasal cavities and in the widest part of pharynx. During swallowing, the nasopharynx is closed below by the soft palate and at other times it is of free communication with oropharynx. Ostia of auditory tubes are in lateral walls.

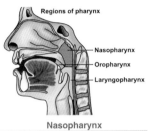

Regions of pharynx
Nasopharynx
Oropharynx
Laryngopharynx

Nasopharynx

Natural markers are the persistence of certain developmental features of bone, which are used as natural markers. Trabaculae, nutrient canals and line of arrested growth can be used for reference to study deposition, resorption and remodelling.

Nd: YAG lasers as a solid active medium, a crystal of yttrium – aluminium – garnet doped with neodymium. Fiberoptically delivered in a free running pulsed mode, most often in contact with the tissue. First laser designed exclusively for dentistry. Emission wavelength is 1064 nm. Highly absorbed by pigmented tissue and is about 10,000 times more absorbed by water than an Argon laser. Common clinical applications are for cutting and coagulation of dental soft tissues with good hemostatic capability.

Neck-tongue syndrome is characterized by unilateral upper nuchal or occipital pain with or without numbness in these areas. There is simultaneous numbness of tongue on the same side.

Necrosis means the tissue death within the living.

Necrotic pulp refer to the dead or devitalized tooth. There are no true symptoms of complete pulp necrosis for the simple reason that pulp is destroyed along with its sensory nerves. Many cases of pulp necrosis are discovered because of discoloration of crown. This applies primarily to anterior teeth. The radiography may be helpful if a periapical lesion exists for its presence and usually indicates associated pulp death. On radiograph necrotic pulp may exhibit only slight periapical change. The tooth with a necrotic pulp may also be slightly painful to percussion.

Necrotic tissue is a non living tissue.

Necrotizing sialometaplasia is a benign inflammatory reaction of salivary gland tissue with unknown etiology. Acinar necrosis is fairly typical of coagulation. It develops due to infarction of tissues fourth decade of life is mostly affected. Lesion generally presents as an ulcer. Most cases occur in palate. It is a painful lesion; mucus secreting glands produces ulceration with rolled borders. Ulcers measures 2-3 cm in diameter. At the base a few grey granular lobules are present. Some patients may complaint of numbness or a burning type pain in that area. Biopsy will not show any sign of malignancy. Debridement will serve the purpose and the lesions will heal automatically within 1-2 months. There are no chances of recurrence.

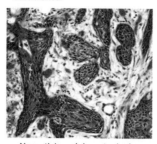

Necrotizing sialometaplasia

Necrotizing ulcerative gingivitis (NUG) is an inflammatory destructive disease of the gingiva. NUG mostly occurs as an acute condition but mostly undergoes a diminution in severity, leading to a subacute stage. It is generally of sudden onset, clinically it appears as punched out lesions, with a crater like depressions involving the papillary gingiva which subsequently involves the marginal gingiva as well, and spontaneous bleeding on slightest provocation is also noted. The lesion is extremely sensitive and patient may complain of pain which gets intensified on eating spicy food. Patient also complains of metallic foul taste and oral malodour.

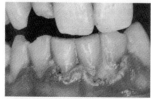

Necrotizing ulcerative gingivitis

Necrotizing ulcerative periodontitis (NUP) is considered to be an extension of necrotizing ulcerative gingivitis in to the periodontal structures leading to attachment and bone loss. The clinical pictures of NUP includes necrosis and ulceration of interdental papilla, gingiva appears erythematous, presence of oral malodour in addition to fever, malaise and lymphadenopathy. Stress, smoking and poor dietary nutrition are considered to be the main causative factors.

Needle holders are instruments which are beneficial during the suturing of flap or the tissue at the desired position.

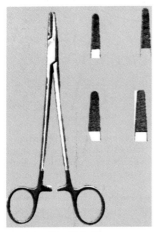

Needle holder

Negative reinforcement involves removal of unpleasant stimulus following a response, e.g., if the parent gives into the temper tantrums thrown by the child, he reinforces this behavior.

Neonatal palatal cyst appear as small, white, raised nodules. Size may go up to 2 to 3 mm in diameter. These are true cysts lined by stratified squamous epithelium. They heal automatically and don't require treatment.

Neonatal seizures occur in first 4 months of life. These may be focal or multifocal, clonic or focal tonic or generalized myoclonic.

Neoplasia is an abnormal mass of tissue, the growth of which exceeds and is uncoordinated with that of normal tissues. Neoplasia means the process of new growth. Neoplasm's which progress and results in death of organisms are termed cancerous. Not all neoplasms are malignant. Those with a favorable clinical course and complete recovery are termed benign neoplasm.

Neoplasm is uncontrolled growths due to irregular growth of its cells. The new growth comprised of abnormal collection of cells, the growth of which exceeds and is irregular A malignant tumor arising from epithelial tissue is known as carcinoma, from gland is known as adenoma, from cartilaginous tumor it is called as 'chondroma'.

Nephroblastoma is an embryonic tumor derived from primitive renal epithelial and mesenchymal components. Abdominal mass is the commonest complaint with hematuria and hypertension. Tumor is single, large circumscribed mass is firm usually solid. Tumor may become huge 500-2500 grams.

Nerve block is a procedure done to block the nerve conduction by

N

administration of local anesthetic agent. It is a one where several teeth in one quadrant or where local infiltration is not workable/useful. Nerve block is done in soft tissue before it enters the jaw to reach the teeth. Pain sensations from every part supplied by nerve are blocked. Inferior dental block is commonly done.

Nerve impulse is a signal that carry information along the nerves.

Nerve is a composite of multiple neurons, where as neuron is a single nerve cell. Nerve contains many fibers bundled together with blood vessels and wrapped in connective tissue. Nerves are located outside the CNS.

Nerve root compression occurs when nerves which transmit pain impulses are compressed in spinal cord/roots, one feels unpleasant, burning pain often accompanied by painful sensations. Some features are due to direct nerve irritation and others are due to ischemia. Pain due to compression of peripheral nerve is referred to skin from which it receives sensory fibres. Root pain radiates throughout the dermatome of root concerned.

Nerve supply of lower teeth Branches of mandibular nerve supply lower teeth.

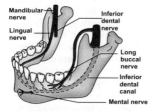

Nerve supply of mandibular teeth

Neuralgia trigeminal is a condition where pain is associated with trigeminal nerve. Pain generally affects one side of face around eye, over cheek or into jaw and teeth. Pain is excruciating and is triggered by touching a specific area of the face, talk or chew the food.

Neurilemmoma originats in the schwann cells. It is a slowly growing lesion of long duration. The lesion is painless. In mandible it is located as central lesion. There may be destruction of bone and extension of cortex. It requires surgical excision.

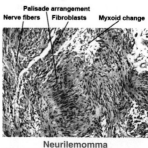

Neurilemomma

Neurofibroma arises from perineural fibroblasts. It is a dominant hereditary condition with overgrowth of nerve sheath.

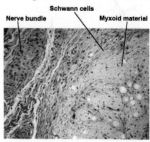

Myxoid changes in neurofibroma

These present as small and asymptomatic. These are submucosal with multi lobulated surface and are painless. On skin these are soft and firm, freely mobile nodules. Nodular lesions vary in size and number varies widely. Radiographically it is well demarcated unilocular or multilocular radiolucent areas are seen.

Neurofibromatosis has a hereditary impact and occurs in 2 forms i.e. in one form numerous sessile or pedunculated, elevated nodules of variable size are scattered. In second form deeper, more diffuse lesions of greater proportions are developed known as 'elephantiasis neuromatosa'. Transformation into malignancy is known. On buccal mucosa discrete, non nucleated nodules, of mucus colour are noted. Tongue may be enlarged. There is no satisfactory treatment.

Neurofilaments are those filaments that are found in neuron, axons that accounts for the strength and rigidity of the axon.

Neurogenic pain may indicate a disease process affecting a particular nerve fibre.

Neurogenic sarcoma is a malignant tumor of Schwann cells. It has a poor prognosis. These are rapidly growing and painful. It is an exophytic mass. Lips may be anesthetized. Expansion of mandible occurs. Lesions don't move and are fixed to underlying tissue. Nuclei are often pleomorphic and hyper chromatic. Neoplastic cells spread along the affected nerve.

Neuron is a nerve cell.

Neuropathic ulcer occurs where patient may be having some neurological problem. Ulcer may be single or multiple. It is generally on pressure point. Edge is punched out, pale and hard. There is purulent offensive discharge. Base is non tender.

Neuropathy is any abnormal condition characterized by inflammation and degeneration of peripheral nerves.

Neurotoxin – Tetanus, diphtheria and botulinium toxins are all neurotoxins and act via neuronal pathways.

Neurotransmitters are chemicals by which neurons communicate.

Neutral atom is an atom that has an equal number of protons and electrons.

Neutral crest cells are the one which arise from ectoderm along the lateral margins of neural plate and migrate extensively to form dental papilla.

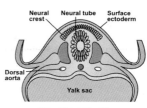

Neural crest cells

Neutrophils are the predominant leukocyte in the blood accounting for about two-third of all the blood leukocytes. As neutrophils do not need to differentiate they are best suited for rapid responses. Neutrophil has a size of 10 micro millimeter in diameter. Neutrophils are also known as polymorphonuclear leukocytes and microphage.

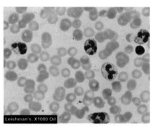

Neutrophils

Nevoid basal cell carcinoma syndrome manifests as jaw cysts, facies, calcification, bifid ribs and skin lesions. Multiple pink to brown papules appear on face. In 50% cases pitting of soles and palms is seen.

New attachment is the process of embedding the new periodontal ligament fibers into newly formed cementum and attachment of gingival epithelium to the tooth surface which was denuded by the disease.

Newton is a force required to give a mass of one kilogram in acceleration of one meter per second.

Niacin can be formed from essential amino acid tryptophan. In human 1 mg niacin is formed from 60 mg dietary tryptophan. In body it is converted into nicotinamide which is a component of coenzyme needed for carbohydrate metabolism. Liver, ground nut, pulses and fish are good source of it. Milling may remove most of it. Recommended daily requirement is 6.6 mg/1000 calories.

Nickel-titanium wires are the wires that is used for orthodontic treatment. It has weight percentage of 55% nickel and 45% titanium. Nickel titanium alloys with shape memory behavior activated at body temperature have been introduced. It has excellent spring back in bending particularly for super elastic and shape memory alloys. Super elastic alloys can be heat treated by clinician.

Nicotine poisoning Nicotine is easily absorbed from the mucous membrane of the mouth when smoke is held in oral cavity for 2 seconds. About 70% of it is absorbed. During deep inhalation about 90% of it is absorbed. Nicotine as such is one of the most fatal and rapidly acting poisons. It can even penetrate through the intact skin. Fatal dose of nicotine is 60 mg for an adult but even 4 mg may cause alarming symptoms in non habitual person. At the rate of one packet a day of 20 cigarette smoker inhales 100 mg of nicotine a week which in a single dose will kill the person as quickly as bullet.

NIDR monograph the national caries program of the national institute of dental research has published a monograph, preventing tooth decay, to assist dentists, dental hygienists, public health administrators, school officials, and teachers implementing self-applied fluoride programs in schools. The monograph was prepared by the staff at the national caries program of the NIDR and describes in detail the methodology, strategy, and estimated cost of materials, addresses of suppliers, sample order forms, and checklists to ensure the success of such a program. It is highly recommended for public health officials and school personnel.

Nidus refers to the point of origin.

Night blindness refers to the reduced vision in the dimlight. Retinol is essential component of pigment rhodopsin (visual purple) on which vision in dim light depends. Hence lack of retinol may result in impairment of dark adaptation.

Night guard is a removable acrylic appliance to minimize the effects of grinding (bruxism) and TMJ associated problems.

Night terrors can be confused with nocturnal disorder of seizures due to frontal lobe epilepsy. Night terrors are likely to cause the child to sit up and scream. Involuntary motor components are unusual.

Nitrogen balance refers to a balance between the input and output of nitrogen. Negative protein balance exist when output is greater than input as in fever, starvation etc. During growth and pregnancy protein need increases so is defined as a positive protein balance.

Nitrous oxide is a colourless, slightly sweetish gas with no odour. It is heavier than air. It has low solubility in blood and does not combine with hemoglobin. It has low anesthetic potency which limits its use as a sole anesthetic agents. Current limit recommended for all brief anesthetic procedures is 65% N_2O/35% O_2 at sea level. Its side effect includes mild depression of myocardial contractility. Recovery from nitrous oxide is quick. It does not produce muscle relaxation and it readily crosses the placenta.

Noble metal is resistant to oxidation includes gold, platinum, and palladium.

Nocturia is night time urination.

Nodular goiter is nodular on palpation. If it is present in more than 10% of an area it indicates that condition is endemic. Iodine deficiency is the main cause.

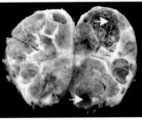

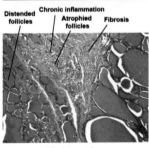

Distended follicles | Chronic inflammation | Atrophied follicles | Fibrosis

Nodular goiter

Nodular hyperplasia prostate is an overgrowth of prostatic glandular and fibromusclular elements. Enlarged prostate weighs more than 40 grams. Nodules show slit like spaces containing milky fluid. Nodular hyperplasia causes elongation, compression and tortuosity of posterior urethra. It may lead to retention of urine and cystitis.

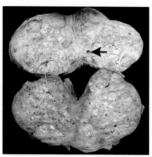

Intraglandular epithelial hyperplasia
Convolutions   Corpora   Fibromuscular
                amylacea   stroma

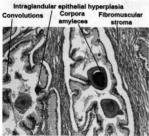

Nodular hyperplasia prostate

Noise is an unwanted sound. Noise has been described as wrong sound, in the wrong place at the wrong time. Noise pollution is the cacophony of sounds leading to health hazard.

Noma is rapidly spreading gangrene of oral and facial tissue in physically weak person localized to orofacial region. Tissue necrosis progresses after infection with anaerobic bacteria. It starts as a small ulcer of gingival mucosa. It may spread to jaws and cheeks. It starts around fixed bridge or crown. Commencement of gangrene is seen as blackening of skin. Smell is very foul. Mortality rate is higher. Broad spectrum antibiotics help.

Non - specific plaque hypothesis was given by Walter Loesche in 1976 was given by according to this hypothesis, periodontal disease results from the elaboration of noxious products by the entire plaque flora. When only small amount of plaque are present, the noxious products are neutralized by the host. Periodontal disease was believed to result from an accumulation of plaque over time in conjunction with a decrease host response and increase host susceptibility of age. All plaque was thought to be alike and equally capable of causing disease.

Non-compression small plates are the small conventional orthopedic plates which were previously used for fixing mandibular fractures. These appear larger than the recently designed mini plates and offer no other advantage except compression to the fracture due to larger dimensions as compared to mini plates.

Non-critical instruments are those which does'nt come into contact with body fluids and have low risk of transmitting infection. These can be put in low level disinfectants detergents or simple washing will serve. These include jars, cavity liners etc.

Non-displaced flaps are the ones, when the flap is returned and sutured in its original position.

Non-experimental research in which there is no manipulation of an independent variable.

Non- Hodgkin's lymphoma is a heterogeneous group of neoplasm that arise from a monoclonal cell of lymphoid

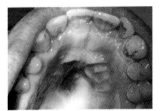

Non-Hodgkin's Lymphoma
of the Palate

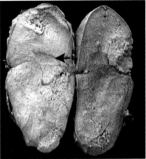

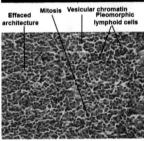

Non-Hodgkin's lymphoma

origin. These involve lymph nodes and lymphoid organs, extra nodal organs and tissues. Patient of any age can be affected. Abdominal and Mediastinal lymphadenopathy, fever, night sweats and loss of weight is seen. The cell type may be well differentiated lymphocyte, poorly differentiated lymphocyte, mixed lymphocyte, diffuse histiocytes or lymphoblastic. Malignant cells may replace the node in a diffuse pattern. Mediastinal node involvement is common and enlargement of liver may develop. Multiple lymph nodes are firm and rubbery. Non-Hodgkin's lymphoma is also noted in AIDS patients. Oral lesion is fast growing, painful and firm. There may be ulceration and bleeding. Swelling of gingiva and palate are common. In nodular pattern neoplastic cells aggregate so that cluster of cells are seen, while diffuse pattern is seen as monotonous distribution of cells. Floating teeth in radiolucent area may be seen. There will be diffuse, large, irregular areas of radiolucency with expansion and destruction. Biopsy of lymph glands gives an accurate diagnosis. Aggressive chemo therapy followed by radiotherapy helps.

Non-parametric test are the statistical tests that don't rest on assumption related to the distribution of populations from which samples are taken.

Non-productive cough is a noisy cough and forceful expulsion of air from the lungs that does not yield sputum or blood. Coughing is an protective mechanism of clearing air way.

Non-screen film is an extraoral film which does not require the use of screen for exposure.

Non-union refers to the fracture that is only not united but will not also unite by itself. Non union also includes the condition of fibrous union. It may occur due to infection, inadequate immobilization or unsatisfactory apposition of bone.

Non-vital pulpotomy refer mortal pulpotomy.

Non-compulsive habits are habits that are easily learned and dropped as the child matures.

Non-pressure habits are those habits that do not apply a direct force on the teeth or its supporting structures, e.g. mouth breathing.

Nonspastic myofacial pain is where there is no muscle spasm and pain is the only complaint. There is no muscular dysfunction. Palpable trigger may elicit acute pain at the trigger site when manipulated and may overshadow the referred pain momentarily.

Normal aging is a biological, sociological or psychological process, that is inevitable and occur as the result of maturation or passage of time.

Nuclei poisoning is the inactivation of nuclei of crystallization by the deposition of foreign material on their surface.

Nummular dermatitis is a chronic dermatitis with inflamed, coin shaped vesicular, crusted scaling and pruritic lesions. The discoid lesions start as pruritic patches of vesicles and papules that later ooze serum and form crusts. Lesions are widespread. No satisfactory treatment is available. Oral antibiotics are given empirically. Oral corticosteroids with ultraviolet may be required.

Nursing bottle syndrome occurs in babies on bottle feeding containing more of sugar. It results in multiple numbers of caries in many teeth mostly the upper one.

Nystatin is an antifungal drug that acts by causing loss of potassium ion from pathogenic fungi. It is used in candida infections of mouth and to be applied locally.

N

O

Oblique fibers extends from cementum in a coronal direction obliquely to the bone

Oblique ridge is a linear elevation that transverses a surface.

Obstructive mouth breathing is usually a result of nasal obstruction such as nasal polyps, nasal tumors, chronic nasal inflammatory conditions, obstructive adenoids, and deviated nasal septum.

Obstructive sleep apnoea is a sleep related upper airway collapse leading to frequent apnoeas with sleep fragmentation. Obesity, alcohol and other sedative may result it.

Obstructive voiding symptoms – hesitancy is a delay in the initiation of micturation. Decreased forced of stream results from the high resistance the bladder faces and is often associated with decrease in calibre of stream. Post void dribbling may be due to benign prostatic hyperplasia.

Obtunding material is that reduces irritation or has a soothing effect on tissue.

Occipital lobe tumor causes contralateral hemianopia with sparing of macular vision. Dominant hemispheric lesions produce visual aganosias. Agnosia is loss of recognition of object. Visual ataxia is seen with extensive bilateral occipital lesion.

Occipital neuralgia is pain in the distribution of sensory branches of cervical plexus in neck. Trauma, neoplasm or infection is the most important cause.

Occlude is to bring together.

Occlusal equilibration is the removal of all occlusal interfaces on the teeth.

Occlusal guard see night guard.

Occlusal plane is the imaginary surface on which upper and lower teeth meet.

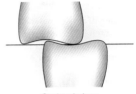

Occlusal plane

Occlusal projection is a mandibular topographic a type of occlusal projection used to examine the anterior teeth of mandible. Occlusal projection maxillary topographic is an occlusal projection used to examine the palate and anterior teeth of maxilla.

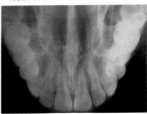

Occlusal projection

Occlusal refers to the chewing surface of teeth.

Occlusal rims are the wax spaces used during fabrication of removal prosthesis to determine the jaw relationship for missing teeth (*see* Figure on page 324).

Occlusal sealants are defined as the application and mechanical

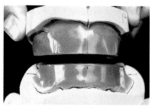

Occlusal rims

bonding of a resin material to an acid etched enamel surface thereby sealing existing pits and fissures from the oral environment.

Occlusal splints if pain and dysfunction persist following treatment of muscles of mastication splint to cover maxilla should be used. It is made of acrylic. It has to be used for long term.

Occlusal surfaces are the chewing surfaces of posterior teeth.

Occlusal trauma results from excessive force placed on a normal dentition, i.e. grinding and clenching of teeth. If left uncontrolled, occlusal trauma may result in rapid attachment loss and bone destruction.

Occlusion is the relationship of the teeth in a closed position in both the maxillary and mandibular arch.

Occulo-dento-osseous dysplasia is characterized by microophthalmus, iridal anomalies, bony anomalies of the digits and syndactyly, with enamel hypoplasia. The teeth show large multifocal hypoplastic defects and pitting yielding a moth-eaten pattern radiographically.

Occulomotor nerve is a cranial nerve number three. It is a motor nerve and lifts upper eye lid, turns eyeball upward downward and medially. It constrict pupil and accommodates eye. This nerve emerges from the anterior aspect of midbrain medial to cerebral peduncle. It enters the orbit through the superior orbital fissure.

Occupational exposure refers to the contact with blood or other infectious materials involving skin, eye or mucus membrane those results due to normal procedures done by dental professional.

Odontoblast layer of pulpitis is present immediately subjacent to the predentin, mainly composed

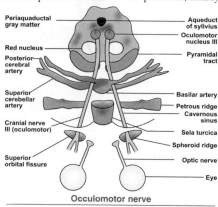

Periaquaductal gray matter
Red nucleus
Posterior cerebral artery
Superior cerebellar artery
Cranial nerve III (oculomotor)
Superior orbital fissure

Aqueduct of sylivius
Oculomotor nucleus III
Pyramidal tract
Basilar artery
Petrous ridge
Cavernous sinus
Sela turcica
Spheroid ridge
Optic nerve
Eye

Occulomotor nerve

of the cell bodies of the dentin forming odontoblasts. Actually it is composed of the cell bodies of odontoblasts along with capillaries, nerve fibres and dendritic cells. In the coronal portion of a young pulp the odontoblasts assume a tall columnar form. The tight packing together of these tall, slender cells produces the appearance of a palisade. The odontoblasts vary in height; consequently their nuclei are not at the same level.

Odontoclasia is a circular hypoplastic zone or line of primary enamel, which is susceptible to dental caries. The condition was first described in 1927 as a certain type of rampant caries among Hawaiian children.

Odontogenic cysts are defined as pathological epithelium lined cavity containing fluid or semi solid material.

Odontogenic fibrosarcoma is malignant counterpart of fibroma. It occurs more frequently in children and young adults. On X-ray it produces expansile multilocular radiolucency. Treatment is surgical excision.

Odontogenic keratocysts may develop at any age. Peak incident lies in 2nd and 3rd decade of life. Mandible is affected more. There is no characteristic clinical manifestation of keratocysts. Pain, soft tissue swelling and expansion of bone may be seen. Lesion may displace tooth.

O

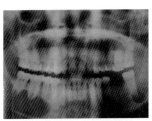

Odontogenic keratocyst

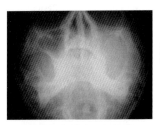

Odontogenic keratocyst

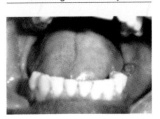

Odontogenic keratocyst

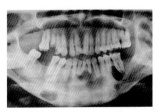

Multiple odontogenic keratocysts

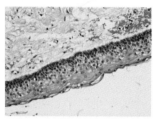

Histological slide of high power OKC

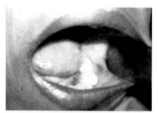

Odontogenic myxoma intraoral view

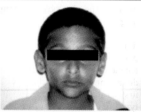

Odontogenic myxoma showing facial asymmetry

Odontogenic myxoma is a benign tumor of bone developing only in jaws. It contains myxomatous tissue. It develops from mesenchymal portion of tooth germ. It is a central lesion of jaws. It is made up of loosely arranged spindle shaped and stellate cells. Intracellular substance is mucoid. X-ray may show unilocular cyst like radiolucency, Pericoronal radiolucency and a mixed radiolucent radiopaque image. Tennis racket appearance is very common. Very few tumours cross the midline. It generally develops between the age group of 25-35 years. Tumor develops slowly as painless expansion of jaw. Rarely there may be numbness of lips. Tumor may cause facial asymmetry. Sometimes it may perforate the cortices. Skin over tumor looks normal.

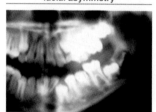

Odontogenic myxoma OPG

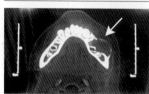

Odontogenic myxoma showing jaw expansion

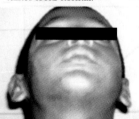

Odontogenic myxoma extraoral view

Odontoma has on odontogenic origin. Etiology is unknown. It may be inherited or may be due to mutant gene. It can be discovered at any age. Mostly it affects anterior maxilla. It is clinically asymptomatic. These are situated between the roots of teeth. It appears as calcified mass surrounded by a narrow radiolucent periphery. Ghost cells are present. Surgical removal helps and there is no recurrence.

Oedema is the swelling of tissue due to excessive fluid accumulation out side the cells.

Oedipus complex is said to have that young boys have a natural tendency to be attached to the mother and they consider their father as enemy. Hence they strive to imitate their father to gain the affection of the mother. Freud also described oedipal complex as a desire to have sexual relation with the mother. Name oedipal complex is derived from Greek mythology. Oedipus is king, unwittingly slew his father and married his mother. The little boy adopts his father's manners, attitude, thinking that by becoming like his father he can win his mother's sexual love.

Oil plants contain an abundance of natural oils which are having healing properties. Low levels of important fatty acids in diet may cause dry, flaky complex, weak nails and dull hair. Oils are good source of vitamin a, d, e and k. Many natural oils also contain lecithin which has water retention properties. It delays ageing by slowing down wrinkles.

Olfactory nerve is a nerve of small and cranial nerve number one. It originates as the central process of olfactory receptor nerve cells in mucus membrane of nose. It is a sensory nerve.

Oligodontia is a congenitally missing six or more teeth.

Oligomer is a polymer made up of two, three or four monomer units.

Omega-3 reduces the chances of blood cells and platelets to form blood clots. It reduces LDL and increases HDL. It decreases production of triglycerides.

Omission refer to removal of the pleasant response after a particular response e.g., if the child misbehaves during dental procedure. If a favorite toy is taken away for short time resulting in the omission of the undesirable behavior.

Oncology is the science of neoplastic growth.

Onlay is a laboratory processed restoration made of metal, porcelain or acrylic that replaces one or more of cusps of a tooth.

Opacifiers are the white oxides added to decrease the transparency of the porcelain, usually tin oxide or titanium dioxide.

Open bite is said to have occurred when jaws are closed, the mandibular anterior tooth don't contact the lingual surfaces of the maxillary anterior tooth. It then refers to increased distance between the two arches.

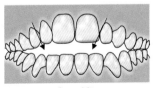

Open bite

Open chain exercise is the exercise in which the distal segment of the extremity does not bear weight.

Operant conditioning is significant extension of classical conditionings. Individual response is changed as result of reinforcement or extinction of previous responses. Hence satisfactory outcome will be repeated while unsatisfactory outcomes will diminish infrequency. According to this theory, the consequence of behavior itself acts as a stimulus and affects future behavior. Since the behavior acts upon the environment called operant. Skinner described four basic types of operant conditioning distinguished by the type of consequence.

Operational research is the application of scientific methods of investigations to the study of human organizations and services. Its aim is to develop new knowledge. It is a team work job and involves several workers.

Ophthalmodynamometry is a technique measuring pressure in the retinal artery by applying a simple instrument to the globe of eye. It helps in diagnosing occlusion of the internal carotid artery. Pressure in retinal artery is reduced.

Opium poisoning refers to when solid opium is being swallowed it takes ½ to 1 hour before symptoms appears. In case of morphine these appear within a few minutes. In liquid form it is quicker to act.

Opposing teeth are the teeth that are located in the opposite arch of the crown or bridge restoration onto the tooth preparation.

Opposite arch finger rest is a type of rest which can be established

tooth surfaces of the opposite arch.

Optic disc is the area in the retina where the optic nerve fibres exit and there are no rods and cones.

Optic nerve is a cranial nerve two, a nerve of sight is about 1.6 inches long. It leaves orbital cavity passing through optic canal. It is a sensory nerve. The nerve on both sides now joins one another to form optic chiasma. Here the nerve fibres that arise from medial side of retina cross the midline and enter the optic tract of the opposite side while the fibres from the temporal side reach the optic tract of the same side.

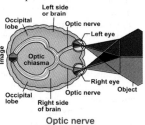

Optic nerve

Optical caries monitor is an instrument, which quantifies incipient smooth surface lesions. It has been seen that *in vitro* lesions reflect much more light than sound enamel.

Optical pyrometer is a device to measure temperature by matching the color of an electrically heated wire to the color of the surface being tested; current required is calibrated against temperature.

Oral cavity refers to the mouth cavity.

Oral drive theory given by Sears and Wise (1982) suggested that the strength of the oral drive is in part a function of how long a child continues to feed by sucking. Thus, sucking is the result of prolongation of nursing and not the frustration of weaning.

Oral habits are learned patterns of muscular contraction (Mathewson 1982).

Oral health promoter is a person who explains disease, causes, home care techniques.

Oral Health Status Index (OHSI) is an index developed by Marcus M., Koch A.L. and Gershen, J.A. in 1980. This index measure included the three components of the dmft (decayed, missing and filled teeth) and 15 other variable such as temporomandibular dysfunction, degree of periodontal disease and tumors. To calculate this measure for a population, a prior planning is needed to develop an examination protocol that includes all appropriate measurements. In a modified oral health index, "Marcus, Koch and Gershen" (1983, 1985 used weights for bone loss, missing free ends and decayed/fractured and replaced teeth. This modified index is easier to use in epidemiological setting but its various components still need to be part of the planned protocol.

Oral herpangina is characterized by sore throat, dysphagia, and stiff neck with loss of appetite. There develops small papulovesicular lesions about 1-2 mm in diameter with a grayish surface surrounded by red areola in palate. Disease lasts for 4-5 days.

Oral hygiene consists of keeping the teeth clean and free of food debris. It prevents accumulation and persistence of plaque which leads to dental disease. Tooth brush is an effective tool. Eating raw, firm and fibrous food/fruits as apples, pears and carrots also help to clean the teeth.

Oral hygiene index given by John C. Greene and Jack R. Vermillian introduced the oral hygiene index, while they were developing a plan to study variations in gingival inflammation in relation to the degree of mental retardation in children, as it became apparent that it would be necessary to separate out the effects of variations in oral cleanliness. In 1960, the "oral hygiene index" (OHI) was introduced a "sensitive, simple method for assessing group or individual oral hygiene quantitatively". The oral hygiene index requires the user to make more decisions and to spend more time in arriving the result. Therefore, an effort was made to develop another equally sensitive index which would reduce both the number of decisions and time required. This index was named the "simplified oral hygiene index" (OHI -S). The OHI and OHI-S were developed primarily to serve as systematic approaches to quantitating the oral cleanliness variable in population studies.

Oral indices (George P. Barnes et al) are essentially sets of values, usually numerical with maximum and minimum limits, used to describe variables of specific conditions on a graduated scale, which use the same criteria and method to compare a specific variable in individuals, samples or populations with that same variable as is found in other individuals, samples or populations.

Oral irrigation is to direct stream of water or therapeutic agent over the teeth, gingival tissues or into a periodontal pocket. It removes the debris and reduces pathogens.

Oral is pertaining to mouth.

Oral malodor is a generic descriptor for foul smells emanating from the mouth which encompasses ozostomia, stomatodysodia, halitosis (either pathological and physiological, fetor oris or fetor ex ore). The latter term denotes local or systemic production of malodor.

Oral manifestation is a sign of disease in oral cavity.

Oral mucosa is the lining of the oral cavity of mucus membrane composed of connective tissue covered with stratified squamous epithelium. It serves to protect these organs and to receive and transmit stimuli from the environment.

Oral pathology is concerned with the nature of diseases affecting oral structure. Doctor is known as oral pathologist.

Oral polio vaccine was discovered by Sabin in 1957. It contains an attenuated virus (type 1, 2 and 3) grown in primary monkey kidney or human, diploid cell culture. Three doses are given at the interval of one month. It induces both Humoral and intestinal immunity. It is cheaper and effective. It should not be given in acute infection.

Oral screen is a functional appliance that produces effect by redirecting the pressure of the muscular and soft tissue curtain of the cheeks and lips. It is also used to counteract deficiencies in lip posture and function and to prevent oral respiration when anterior and posterior oral seals are inadequate. It prevents child from placing the thumb or finger into the oral cavity during sleeping hours. It is also used to control tongue thrusting.

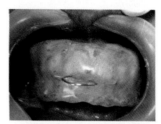

Oral vestibular screen

Oral sub mucous fibrosis (OSMF) is a precancerous condition and is a slow growing disease in which fibrous bands are formed. Etiology is not known. There is a burning sensation of mouth when one consumes spicy food. Vesicles and later ulceration may develop. Salivation increases. Oral epithelium is atrophic. Systemic corticosteroids and local tropical hydrocortisone helps (*see* Figure on page 331).

Orange and red stains appear at cervical third, occurs more frequently on anteriors than compared to posterior covering both facial and lingual surfaces of anterior teeth. These stains are generally caused by chromogenic bacteria.

Orange stain a light thin material of brick red orange color is seen on teeth. Its cause is not known. This stain is due to pigment producing micro-organism. Stain is easily removed.

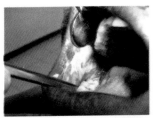

Oral sub mucous fibrosis (OSMF)
of buccal mucosa

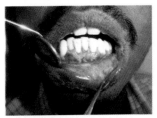

OSMF of labial mucoa

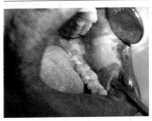

OSMF of buccal mucosa

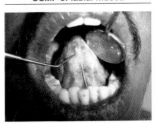

OSMF involving ventral surface of
the tongue

Order of use is the sequence in which dentist uses series of instruments.

Organogenesis is the formation of organs from the primary germ layer of an embryo.

Orgasm is the climax of sexual excitement and pleasure during which ejaculation of semen occurs in male, vaginal contractions in females lasting less than a minute. Orgasm is sudden release of sexual tension during which both experience a series of contractions 6-15 in number, each lasting less than a second.

Origin is the point where muscle attaches to bone. It usually refers to the proximal attachment of the muscle.

Orofacial dyskinesia results from extra pyramidal disorder or a complication of phenothiazines therapy. It generally develops after the age of 60. There develops involuntary, dystonic movements of facial, oral and cervical musculature. There may be lip smacking, lip licking or protrusion of lip.

Orofacial pain is the pain associated with structures of oral cavity.

Orthodontics is defined as the study of growth and development of the jaws and face particularly and the body generally, as influencing the position of the teeth; the study and action and reaction of internal and external influences on the development; and the prevention and correction of arrested and perverted development.

Orthopnea is the ability to breathe easily only in upright position.

Orthoses is any device which when in contact with the body improves the function of that part.

Orthostatic hypotension is a common cause of vasomotor

O

syncope especially in elderly, diabetics or autonomic neuropathy. A greater than normal decline of 20 m.m. Hg in blood pressure is seen immediately upon arising from supine to standing position.

Orthostatic syncope occurs within seconds or minutes of assuming upright posture. Patients are vulnerable on rising and after meals. It differs from vasovagal syncope in that skin may be warm, pulse rate unchanged and sweating absent.

Osseointegration is a direct structural and functional connection between ordered, living bone and the surface of a load carrying implant or it can also be described as relationship between endosseous implants and bone where the bone is in intimate contact with implant but no ultrastructural contact is seen between the two.

Osseous craters are the concavities in the crest of the interdental bone confined within the facial and the lingual walls.

Osseous pains are due to infection or injury. Such pains are more stable than myogenous pain.

Acute septic osteitic usually is designated osteomyelitis. Pain is of throbbing quality. It induces necrosis by pressure against the unyielding walls. When cortex is penetrated pain intensity decreases. When confinement is released by rupture or surgical drainage pain intensity drops fast.

Ossifying fibroma are frequently found in paranasal sinuses especially antrum. These produce large densely calcified masses.

Osteoarthritis is an old age degenerative joint disease without systemic manifestation. Disease may be primary in interphalangeal joins. Secondary may be post traumatic. Bones X-ray may show subchondral sclerosis, cortical buttressing, trabecular hypertrophy, osteophyte, cysts and collapse. Erosive osteoarthritis occurs in menopausal women. Pain is worse on activity and is relieved on rest.

Osteoblasts are bone forming cells located on bone surfaces and helps in the growth and development of teeth and bones.

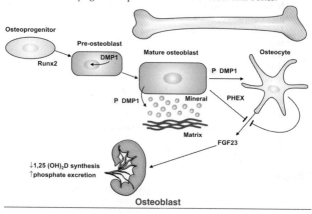

Osteoblast

Osteochondroma is a bony exostosis projecting from external surface of bone having a hyaline lined cartilaginous cap. These are found in childhood and are asymptomatic. There develops hard, painless mass near a joint of a long tubular bone. Cartilaginous cap shows irregularity and spotty calcifications. These projects away from joint. When cap becomes more than 2 cm malignant transformation may take place.

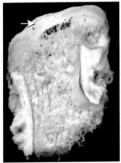

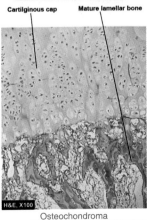

Cartilginous cap   Mature lamellar bone

H&E, X100

Osteochondroma

Osteoclastoma are brown tumors visible as distinct geographic radiolucencies. These are central, slightly expansile and septated looking like a destructive neoplasm. Mandible is mostly involved. These are markers of primary hyperparathyroidism. MRI may show fluid – fluid level.

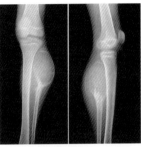

Osteoclastic   Vascular spaces
giant cells   Stromal cells

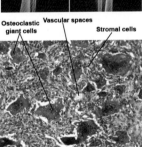

Osteoclastoma

Osteoclasts are bone removing multinucleated cells which help remodel bone.

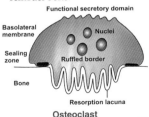

Functional secretory domain

Basolateral membrane   Nuclei

Sealing zone   Ruffled border

Bone

Resorption lacuna

Osteoclast

O

Osteoconduction is the formation of bone by osteoblasts occurring from the margins of the defect on the bone graft material. These bone graft material facilitate bone formation by bridging the gap between the existing bone and a distant location which is otherwise not possible.

Osteocyte is a mature bone cell responsible for maintaining bone tissue.

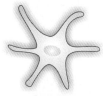

Osteocyte

Osteogenesis imperfecta is a serious disease of unknown etiology. Disease is visual at birth. Bones are fragile and porous. Fractures occur while child learns walking. It develops due to defective matrix formation and lack of mineralization. Fetal collagen is not able to transform into mature collagen. There are 4 types. Two are autosomal recessive and rests two are autosomal dominant type. Moderate and deforming type – these are associated with deciduous teeth and blue sclera. Child may have abnormal shape of skull, joint dislocations and defective heart valve. Mild not deforming type – patient otherwise is clinically normal. Person has blue sclera and dentinogenesis imperfecta. Neonatal lethal type – it is a serious form of disease. There are multiple fractures of bone. Severe non lethal type – patient develops fracture with slight trauma. Fractures heel early but deformity remains.

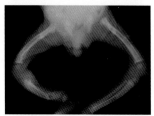

Osteogenesis imperfecta with multiple, healing fractures

Osteogenic sarcoma is a primary malignant tumor of bone. Patient is young between the age of 10-20 years. Pain and swelling are presenting features. Long bones are targets. Alkaline phosphatase enzyme will be raised. Metastasis to lung is through hematogenous route. Periosteal new bone formation occurs and is highly irregular. Sun ray appearance is characteristic. Osteogenic sarcoma of mandible is also noted.

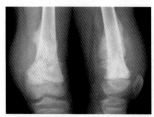

Osteroasarcoma

Osteoid osteoma is a benign tumor of bone. It rarely develops after the age of 30. Pain is severe. Radiographs will show small round radiolucent area surrounded by a rim of sclerotic bone.

Lesion is seldom larger than 1 cm. It consists of central nidus of compact osteoid tissue with calcification. Surgical excision is the treatment of choice.

Osteoinduction is a process where new bone formation occurs through the stimulation of osteoprogenitor from the defect that differentiates into osteoblasts

Osteoinducutive material is a material which causes the conversion of mesenchymal cells preferentially to bone progenitor cells.

Osteoma is a benign neoplasm. There is proliferation of cancellous bone in an endosteal or periosteum. It is not a common oral lesion. It shows a circumscribed swelling on jaw. It is not painful. Lesion is not capsulated and has to be removed surgically.

Osteomalacia is the counterpart of rickets in adults, commonly seen in women with pardah and menopausal females. Skeletal pain is usually present and persistent and ranges from backache to severe pain. Bone tenderness and muscular weakness are often present. Patient may find it difficult to climb stairs or getting out of chair. A waddling gait is not unusual. Osteoporosis which is atrophy of bone occurs and is due to defective formation of bone matrix. Bones becomes soft. X-ray shows severe asymmetric deformities of all stress bearing bones. Histological findings are non specific. Cortical bone becomes thin. Bone tenderness and muscular weakness are often present.

Osteopetrosis is a rare hereditary bone disease. There is lack of resorption of normal primitive osteochondrous tissue. Patient dies early. There may be severe anemia. Liver and spleen are enlarged with palpable lymph glands. Leukemia and sarcoma are common sequelae. All bones are of homogeneous increased density. There may be bones within a bone. Ilium shows dense curved lines paralleling to iliac crest. Skull changes include calvarial and basilar thickening and sclerosis.

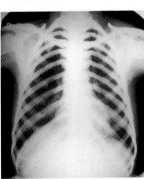

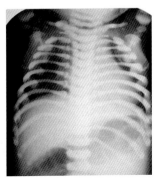

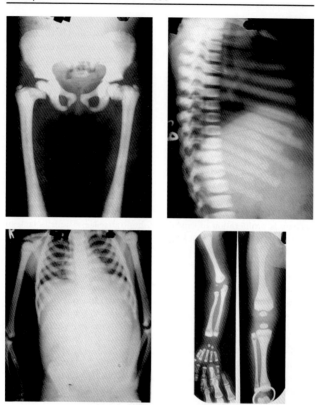

Osteopetrosis

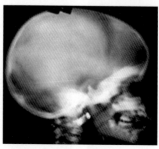

Osteopetrosis skull

Osteopoikilosis is characterized by small, round or ovoid radio opacities in juxta articular region. More of males are affected and are asymptomatic. Lesions are foci of bone which have failed to become cancellous. On X-ray lesions are symmetric of 1 to 8 mm in size these are uniformly dense.

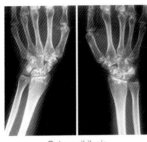

Osteopoikilosis

Osteoporotic compression fracture can occurs even during coughing or lifting a bag simply. On X-ray anterior wedge is most commonly seen in thoracic vertebra and biconcave end plate fracture in lumbar arc. Pain is so severe that person has to be admitted. Bracing is important to ambulate such patients.

Osteosarcoma is a very common neoplasm arising from bone. According to the site tumor has been divided into periosteal sarcoma, medullary osteosar-coma and parosteal osteosarcoma, soft tissue osteosarcoma. Maxilla is affected more than mandible. It s a fast growing and develops as painful swelling of jaw, Expansion and distortion of cortical plates may takes place. Severe deformity of face leads to the displacement of teeth. Overlying skin becomes red and inflamed. Ulceration, hemorrhage and pathological fracture takes place. In osteolytic type it presents irregular, radiolucent areas giving rise to a moth eaten appearance. Expansion, destruction and perforation of cortical plates are noted. Teeth are displaced in position. Osteosarcoma develops

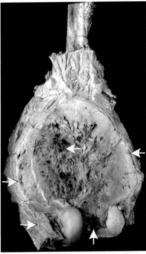

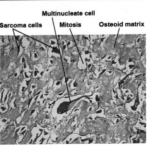

Multinucleate cell
Sarcoma cells   Mitosis   Osteoid matrix

Osteosarcoma

between the age of 10-15 years. Males are more affected. Pain and swelling are early features. It may produce facile deformity. Teeth may become loose. It contains proliferation of atypical osteoblasts and less differentiated precursors. Radiograph shows excessive bone production. In some, spicules of new bone may be seen. In jaws, cortical plates may show sclerosis. Destruction is also noted.

Osteosclerosis is a common cause of deafness and onset is in third decade. The stapedial foot palate develops fibrous fixation and the foot plate is later replaced by sclerotic bone.

Outcome research is an analysis of clinical practice as it actually occurs for the purpose of determining effectiveness of clinical methods by the researcher.

Over bite is the amount of vertical overlap between the maxillary and mandibular incisors. The relationship can be described either in millimeters or more often as a percentage of how many upper central incisors over lap the crowns of the lower incisors. The overbite in the primary dentition normally varies between 10% and 40% when the incisor edges of the incisors are at the same level the condition is described as edge to edge or zero overbite.

Over dentures is a fabricated removable prosthetic appliance attached to the abutment cylinders. It is the one which is fitted on top of standing teeth or retained roots. Advantage of it is the presence of natural roots remaining in alveolar bone. As long as any roots remain there hardly any loss of alveolar bone takes place. Where there are no remaining roots implants can be used to support an over denture.

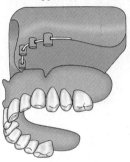

Overdentures

Over infusion is over transfusion may be of blood or saline. Respiration becomes shallow and rapid. Patient feels uncomfortable in lying supine. Neck veins are congested. There may be slight pitting edema. Crepts may be present on independent parts of body. Patient may develop dieresis.

Over jet is the horizontal relationship or the distance between the most protruded maxillary central incisor and the opposing mandibular central incisor. The relationship is expressed in millimeters. If the maxillary incisors are lingual to

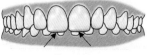

Over bite

the mandibular incisors the relationship is described as an under jet. The normal range of over jet in primary dentition varies between 0 and 4 mm. In the same study by foster the over jet was ideal in 28% of the cases and excessive in 72% of the children. Again the presence of excessive over jet was attributed to the effects of the oral habits.

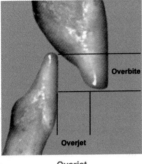

Overjet

Over use is the chronic injury by repetitive stress.

Oviducts refer to fallopian tubes.

Oxidation is a chemical reaction that occurs when processing solutions are exposed to air. It is a chemical breakdown causing decreased concentration of solution strength.

Oxidized cellulose is gauze treated with nitrogen dioxide. On moistening the gauze adheres to the bleeding tissue and readily produces a clot.

Oxygen is a molecule composed of two oxygen molecules. Air we breathe contains about 21% oxygen. It is essential for life. Oxygen we breathe is used by cells to extract or liberate the energy from food we eat.

Oxygen therapy is an administration of oxygen gas to individuals suffering from hypoxia.

Oxyphill adenoma is a benign tumor occurring in parotid gland in elderly age group. It is composed of polygonal cells with mitochondria in eosinophilic granular cytoplasm. Centrally placed nuclei are uniform, small and round. Salivary enlargement is a result of benign epithelial metaplasia.

Oxytalan fibres are made up of two immature forms of elastin, oxytalan and eluanin. These fibers run parallel to the root surface in a vertical direction, bend and attach themselves to the cementum in the apical one third of the tooth.

O

P Pachyonchia congenital is rare and inherited as autosomal dominant characteristic. It also refers to oral leukokeratosis as well as striking nail changes and develop shortly after birth. There is congenital gross thickening of finger and toe nails as they become thick and hardened with brownish material at nail bed. Corneal dystrophy, thickening of tympanic membrane and mental retardation are reported. Dorsum of tongue becomes thickened and greyish white. Cheeks may also be involved on occasion. Hyperkeratotic calluses of palms and soles may develop. Oral lesions include focal or generalized white, opaque thickening of mucosa. Angular cheliosis also develop. Frequent oral aphthous ulceration may be seen. There is no treatment available.

Packed RBCs transfusion helps in raising hematocrit. Each unit of 300 ml consists of 200 ml of RBCs. One unit of packed RBCs will raise the hematocrit by 4%.

Paget's disease is a disease of middle age. Most of patients are asymptomatic. There will be pain with multiple fractures. Milkman's syndrome are local areas of demineralization with in the bone. Pseudo-fractures may also be seen. Spinal cord and nerve root compression may be seen.

Pain is a symptom in completely subjective sense. It is a complex experience that includes a sensory – discriminatory component. Pain is accompanied by the most widespread reactions and can

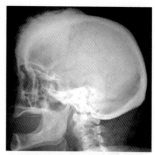
Paget's disease

sometimes be said truly to involve the whole being. The experience of pain is a subjective, private sensation, which can be described only imperfectly to others. Whereas it is possible to share other sensations, for example, listening, testing or touching with reasonable certainty of the same experience as another person but this is not possible with pain. Pain also includes the reactions elicited by the stimulus. For instance, some of the reactions to a noxious stimulus include pain. Startle response, muscle reflex, vocalization, sweating, and increase in heart rate, in addition to blood pressure and behavioral changes takes place. Therefore pain is a neuroscience characterized by 1.The more sensory nerves that supply a region of body, the more acute the sensibility in the area. 2. The higher the ratio of motor nerves to muscles, the greater the possible control finesse.

Pain threshold is that point at which sufficient pain transmitting neurochemical reach the brain to cause discomfort. Pain threshold is the amount of stimulus which produces a sensation of pain.

Palatal papillomatosis is an unusual condition involving mucosa of the palate. It develops in edentulous patient with denture. Lesion presents with numerous red, oedematous papillary projections. It may involve whole of hard palate. Each papilla is 1 to 2 mm in diameter. No specific therapy is available.

Palatal surface is the surface of the maxillary teeth nearest the palate.

Palate soft is the posterior most portion of roof of mouth separating the mouth and pharynx.

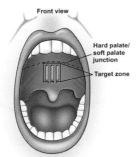

Palate soft

Palatine tonsils are paired masses of lymphoid tissue lying in lateral wall of pharynx and form part of Waldeyer's ring. Reactive lymphoid hyperplasia can result in their enlargement. It then produces difficulty in breathing.

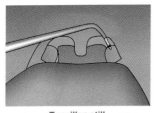

Tonsillen still

Palladium cobalt alloys contains 88% palladium and 4 to 5% cobalt by weight. It has a higher coefficient of thermal expansion which is useful with certain porcelains. Disadvantage is of formation of dark oxide at margins.

Palladium copper alloys were introduced in 1982. It contains 70 to 80% palladium a little gold, 15% copper and 9% gallium. There is no change of color problem. It generally doesn't melt easily so casting becomes difficult.

Palladium-silver alloy usually include 50 to 60% palladium with most of the balance being silver. It has good corrosion resistance. The disadvantage is that color changes to green.

Palliative refers to relief of pain but not a cure.

Pallor usually indicates anemia but may be a sign of low cardiac output.

Palm down rest are the type of extraoral rest which can be established by resting the front surfaces of the middle and fourth finger on the skin overlying the lateral aspect of the mandible on the left side of the face.

P

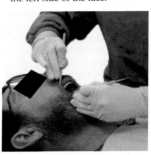

Palm down

Palm up rest are the type of extra-oral rest which can be established by resting the back of the middle and fourth finger on the skin overlying the lateral aspect of the mandible on the right side of the face.

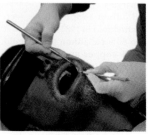

Palm up rest

Palmer's notation is an identification system for teeth; widely used to designate individual teeth amongst orthodontists. Each of the four quadrants is given its own tooth bracket made up of a vertical line and a horizontal line. This system is a shorthand diagram of the teeth as if the patient's teeth were being viewed from the outside. The teeth in the right quadrant would have the vertical midline bracket to the right of the tooth numbers or letters, just as when looking at the patient-the midline is to the right of the teeth in the right quadrant.

Palpate is to examine and explore by touching.

Panic disorder many patients with panic disorder have existing symptoms of depression with suicidal tendency. Person will develop chest pain, dyspnea, and palpitation. Sweating and trembling develops. Person develops fear of dying.

Panophthalmitis is a condition where there is development of intense pain, fever, malaise and complete loss of vision. Lids are oedematous. There is chemosis of conjunctiva. Person develops proptosis and limitation of eye movements. Anterior chamber is full of pus.

Panoramic radiographs are an X-ray film to obtain the wide view of upper and lower jaw and their associated structures. These are useful for viewing larger areas of maxilla or mandible on single film. These don't give minor details such as to detect inter-proximal bone loss or other fine changes.

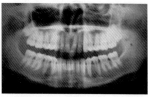

OPG

Panorex refer panaromic radio-graphs.

Pantothenic acid was discovered in the year 1940. This vitamin is widely distributed in animals and vegetable foods. No specific deficiency. This vitamin losses 15-50%, on heating drying and cooking. Milling of wheat causes 50% loss of it.

Papillary gingivitis involves the inflammation of papillary gingiva and often extends into the adjacent portion of the gingival margin.

Papilloma is a common benign neoplasm arising from epithelial tissue. There develops an exophytic papillary growth of stratified squamous epithelium. They appear as a small finger like projections giving a cauliflower like shape of surface squamous epithelium and may be caused by human papilloma virus (HPV-6, HPV-11). It is a slow growing, small, painless. Size varies from a few mm. to 1 cm. It is pedunculated, ovoid swelling white in color. Multiple papilloma of oral cavity is known as papillomatosis. It is not a premalignant condition surgical excision along with base is advised. Recurrence is very rarely seen.

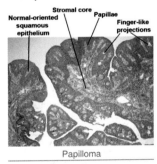

Papilloma

Papilloma of tongue is an exophytic growth where patient present with a warty swelling of tongue of long duration. Mostly it is present on dorsum of tongue. It is pedunculated, mobile and soft in touch.

Papilloma of ureters may be single or multiple, small, papillary and branching pattern. Mitosis is absent and basal polarity is retained. These can recur.

Papillon - lefevre syndrome is characterized by hyperkeratotic skin lesion, severe periodontal destruction and calcification of the dura, the cutaneous and the dural changes generally occurs before the age of 4 years. Premature loss of primary and permanent dentitions and ectopic calcifications, the syndrome is inherited and appears to follow an autosomal recessive pattern. Parents are not affected and may occur in siblings; males and females are equally affected. The syndrome is an autosomal recessive trait with a prevalence of about 1-4 per million of the population Rapid and progressive periodontal destruction affects the primary dentition with an onset at about 2 years. Exfoliation of all primary teeth is usually before the permanent successors erupt and patients may be mid to late teens.

Para amino salicylic acid is an antimetabolite of the tuberculosis bacteria. It has a weak effect.

Paracetamol is an NSAID and is more widely used as anti pyretic and anti analgesic drug. Phenacetin has a disadvantage of creating papillary necrosis and methhemoglobinemia. Paracetamol also may produce fatal hepatic necrosis. It has very minimal anti-inflammatory effect. One gram daily is a safer dose.

Parachute reflex appears about 6-9 months. This reflex is elicited by lowering the newborn in ventral suspension for a short distance. Normal reflex includes extension of arms, limbs and fingers. In children with cerebral palsy, the reflex may be absent or abnormal (*see* Figure on page 344).

Paraffin Wax – Wax bath are available in many sizes. The melted wax needs to be maintained at temperature

P

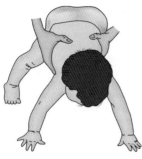

Parachute reflex

40 to 44° C. It is the most convenient way of applying conducted heat to the extremities. Wax gives off heat slowly due to its low thermal conductivity. It has a sedative effect on the sensory nerve endings.

Parahemophilia is a rare hemorrhagic disorder. It is inherited as an autosomal recessive trait. Excessive epistaxis and menorrhagia is common. Intraocular hemorrhage or hemorrhage into CNS has been reported. Spontaneous gingival bleeding occurs with no specific treatment available.

Paramyxovirus are large pleomorphic enveloped RNA viruses. These are responsible for measles, mumps para influenza and respiratory pneumonitis and bronchiolitis.

Parasitic theory was described in 1843 by Erdl described filamentous parasites in the "surface membrane" of teeth. Shortly thereafter Ficinus, a Dresden physician observed filamentous microorganisms, which he called denticulate in material taken from carious activities. He implied that these bacteria caused decomposition of the enamel and then the dentin. Neither Erdl nor Ficinus explained how these organisms destroyed tooth structure.

Paraviruses are icosahedral viruses with single stranded DNA.

Parching is a process of puffing wheat, rice and maize. Material is suddenly heated. Water escapes by puffing out the grain. Murmure and popcorn are well known parched products. This way starch becomes more digestible.

Parkinsonism is a clinical syndrome of bradykinesia, rigidity, tremor at rest and loss of postural reflexes. Bradykinesia is the diagnostic feature. There is difficulty in initiating voluntary movement. Expression is staring with drooling of saliva, hypophonia, micrographia. Gait is short and suffling with lack of arm swing. Patient is unable to perform rapid, repetitive movement. It is difficult for him to change posture in bed or rise from a chair. Tendon reflexes are normal.

Parotid gland is the largest of the three paired salivary gland. It is a bilobular serous gland overlying the masseter muscle. It extends upward to the level of the auditory canal and downward to the lower border of the mandible. Posteriorly it overlaps the sternomastoid muscles and anteriorly extends into the buccal pad of fat where it gives off its excretory duct. The salivary secretions are serous in nature and discharged into the oral cavity via the Stensen's duct.

This duct emerges part from the anterior aspect of the gland crosses the masseter, pierces the buccinator muscle and opens in the vestibule of mouth opposite to the first molar tooth. The duct is about 5 cm long and 3 mm internal diameter.

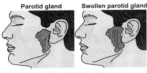

Parotid gland

Partial anodontia/Hypodontia is the congenital absence of one or more teeth. Many cases of hypodontia appear to be genetically controlled. Environment also influences the final outcome or in some cases may be responsible completely for the lack of tooth formation. For example trauma, infection, radiation, chemotherapy, endocrine disturbances and severe intrauterine disturbances have been associated with missing teeth.

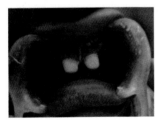

Partial anodontia

Partial seizures are simple seizure, contraction of muscles in one part of body without loss of consciousness. Each contraction is caused by discharge of neurons in contralateral motor cortex when neuronal discharge is from sensory cortex. Paresthesias hallucinations and psychic symptoms appear. Partial seizures involve a specific region of the brain. Focal seizures remain localized, in which paroxysmal neuronal activity is limited to one part of cerebrum. The individual's consciousness and awareness usually is somewhat disturbed and variable degree of amnesia may be evident. Partial seizures have highest incidence of a detectable cortical lesion. Focal seizure can turn into a generalized seizure in which case individual looses consciousness. Generalized seizures are clinically more dangerous in the dental office due to their greater potential for injury and post seizure complication.

Partial thickness flap refers to the flap that includes only the layer of epithelium and a layer of underlying connective tissue. The bone remains covered by the layer of connective tissue including the periosteum. Also known as split thickness/mucosal flap.

Partial thromboplastin time (PTT) measures the effectiveness of clot formation. This test is performed measuring the time it takes for a clot to form after the addition of a Kaolin, a surface activating factor and a cephalin a substitute platelet factor to plasma. Normal PTT is 25-40 seconds. Greater than 50 seconds may cause severe bleeding. It is used to monitor heparin therapy.

Pascal is a metric unit of pressure. 1 MPa (megapascal) is = 1 MN/m^2.

Passive eruption describes the process by which teeth continue to erupt into the mouth as tooth structure is lost to attrition and wear.

Passive immunity is the one where the antibodies produced another person is used to protect against infectious disease. It can be natural or acquired. Natural passive immunity develops when antibodies from a mother passes through the placenta to the developing fetus. These antibodies protect a child till his immune system matures. While passive immunity can be acquired through an injection of antibodies against a micro-organism to which person has not developed antibodies. This type of immunity is short lived but acts immediately.

Passive modalities are therapeutic techniques that don't require the patient's active participation.

Paste is a vehicle that contains a drug.

Patent ductus arteriosus (PDA) is a congenital heart disease. There are no symptoms unless left ventricular failure or pulmonary hypertension develops. Heart may be slightly enlarged. Pulse pressure is wide and diastolic pressure is low. Continuous rough machinery murmur accentuated in late systole at the time of S2 is heard at left first and second interspace. Thrills are common.

Pathogen refers to a microorganism capable of causing disease.

Pathologic grief is the condition in which a person cannot tolerate a grief.

Pathological fractures are the fractures resulting due to underlying pathology and not due to any type of trauma e.g. fracture occurring due to osteomyelitis.

Pathological tooth migration refers to the tooth displacement that occurs due to imbalance among the factors that maintain physiologic tooth position is disturbed by the periodontal disease.

Pathology is the study of abnormal (diseased) tissue conditions.

Pathosis refers to disease entity.

Pattern theory replaced the summation theory where by the pattern of neural impulses set up by the noxious stimuli were considered important.

Pattern Growth pattern is a set of constraints operating to preserve the integration of parts under varying conditions or through time. The interaction throughout the life between hereditary and environment determines the expression of patterns. The two aspects of normal growth pattern are: cephalocaudal gradient of growth and Scammon's growth curve.

Peak aerobic power is the maximum power output or peak oxygen intake that a person can attain safely when performing a large muscle activity as on treadmill.

Pediatric dentistry (AAPD-1985) also known as pedodontics and as dentistry for adolescents and children is the area of dentistry concerned with preventive and therapeutic oral health care for children from birth through adolescent. It also includes special care for special patients beyond the age of adolescent who demonstrate mental, physical and emotional problems.

Pediatric dentistry (AAPD-1999) is an age defined speciality that provides both primary and comprehensive preventive and therapeutic oral health care for infants and children through adolescence, including those with special health care needs.

Pediatric dentistry is concerned with the preventive and therapeutic oral healthcare of children from birth to adolescence.

Pediatrics is related to child.

Pedicle graft is the graft that remains attached to its donor site.

Pellagra is a nutritional disease occurring due to the deficiency of niacin, among poor pesant fed on maize. Greater part of niacin in maize is not available. More over principal protein of maize, zein is deficient in essential amino acid tryptophan, the alternative source of niacin. It may develop 6-8 weeks of deficiency of niacin. Pellagra has been called the disease of three D's dermatitis, diarrhea and dementia.

Pellicle is a thin deposit which may form shortly after eruption on the exposed surface of teeth, i.e. it is the first step in plaque formation; a clear, thin covering containing proteins and lipids (fats) found in saliva It is fully formed in 30 minutes and reaches its mature thickness of 0.1 to 0.6 microns within a day. It is free of bacteria. Brown pigment is due to presence of tannins in the pellicle. Acquired pellicles are composed of mucoprotenis containing lipid material.

Pemphigoid is the term that generally refers to the number of cutaneous, immune – mediated, subepithelial bullous diseases that are characterized by the separation of basement membrane.

Pemphigus erythematosus is a condition where there is occurrence of bullae and vesicles concomittent with the appearance of crusted patches. There may be fever and malaise. Even death may occur.

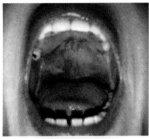

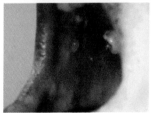

Pemphigoid

Pemphigus foliaceus is early bullous lesions rapidly ruptures and leaves masses of flakes or scales.

Pemphigus is a serious chronic skin disease with vesicle and bullae of different sizes. Etiology is still unknown. It is of many types such as pemphigus vulgaris, pemphigus vegetans, pemphigus foliciceus and pemphigus erythematosus (*see* **Figure** on page 348).

P

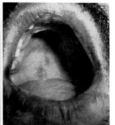

Phemphigus involving medial
canthus of the eye

Pemphigus involving
palatal mucosa

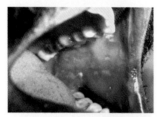
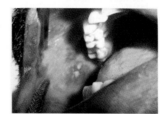

Pemphigus involving buccal mucosa

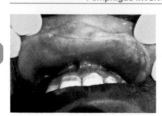
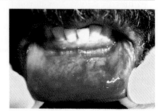

Pemphigus involving labial mucosa

Pemphigus Vegetans is a benign variant of pemphigus vulgaris. The fungoid masses are covered by purulent exudates. It shows inflamed border. It is of 2 types. Neumann type is more common. Early lesions presents as large with denuded areas, while Hallopeau type is less aggressive and appear as pustules in the initial stage. These are followed by verrucous, hyperkeratotic vegeta-

tions. Gingival lesions appear as lace like ulcers. Base is of granular/cobblestone appearance.

Pemphigus Vulgaris is an auto immune disease. It is characterized by rapid appearance of vesicles and bullae. These lesions contain a thin watery fluid. Classically lesion may appear as a thin walled bulla arising from mucosa. Bulla breaks rapidly and continues to extend peripherally. Pressure to an apparently normal surface will result in formation of a new lesion. On breaking of bullae, ulcers may appear shallow. A thin layer of epithelium peels away in an irregular manner leaving the denuded base. Edges of lesions continue to extend.

Penetration coefficient is the combination of properties of viscosity, surface tension and contact angle which promotes rapid capillary penetration.

Penicillin is an antibiotic that contains a beta - lactam ring and inhibits the formation of peptido-glycan cross-links in bacterial cell walls (especially in Gram-positive organisms). This weakens the cell wall and water enters the cell by osmosis, causing cells to burst. Penicillin is bactericidal but can act only on dividing cells and is not toxic to animal cells, which have no cell wall.

PENS stands for percutaneous electric nerve stimulation. It is a pain management technique involving a combination of acupuncture needles and trans-cutaneous nerve stimulation.

Pentazocine produces analgesic drug with no potential abuse. It produces CNS analgesia, sedation and respiratory depression. Euphoria is not much. Some may feel nightmares and hallucina-tions. 30 mg I.V. of it is effective as 10 mg of morphine. It is more potent than morphine. It causes addiction.

Penthane is halogenated either and was synthesized liquid. It is kept in opaque bottles to retard decomposition. It has a fruity odour. It is neither explosive nor flammable. It is the most potent of inhalation anesthetic drug. It is used with nitrous oxide /oxygen to produce any desired depth of anesthesia.

Pepsinogen is a component of gastric juice that is converted into pepsin by HCL.

Peptic ulcer applies to mucosal ulceration near the acid bearing regions of gastrointestinal tract. Most ulcers develop in the stomach or proximal duodenum. It may run in families. Smokers and anxiety prone personalities are more prone to it. Emotional stress, disprins and other pain killers may cause it.

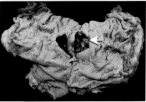

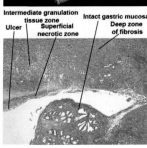

Peptic ulcer stomach

Perforated ulcer may be caused by non steroidal anti-inflammatory drug. Spillage of gastric content may cause severe peritonitis. There may be abdominal pain of sudden onset, nausea and vomiting. There will be hypovlemia, hypotension and fever with tachycardia.

Perforation refers to an opening on a tooth or other oral structure.

Periapical abscess is a suppurative process of dental periapical region. It may also develop due to traumatic injury. Tooth is extruded and becomes painful. Regional lymph glands are enlarged and fever develops. On X-ray slight thickening of membrane is seen. Radiolucent area at apex is noted. Drainage if fails extraction of tooth is the remedy.

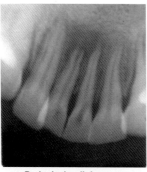

Periapical radiolucency

Periapical cemental dysplasia is a condition of unknown etiology. The lesion develops near the periodontal ligament around the apex of tooth and usually in a mandibular incisor area. It is discovered accidently during routine X-ray.

Periapical granuloma is a lesion, a localized mass of granulation tissue around the apex of a non vital tooth appears radiolucent. It is the most common squel of pulpitis. Due to infection a localized mass of granulation tissue is formed. There will be sensitivity to percussion and a

mild pain on biting or chewing. Many cases may be asymptomatic. On X-ray one can note thickening of periodontal ligament. Periapical granuloma appears as radiolucent area. It is a slow growing lesion.

Periapical means around the apex of teeth.

Periapical radiograph is an intraoral film that shows the entire tooth and surrounding anatomy.

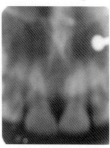

IOPA

Pericarditis is a condition where acute rheumatic carditis serofibrinous pericarditis is often seen. Both layers of pericardium are thickened covered with thin fibrin giving bread and butter appearance. Chest pain is the most common presenting symptom. Pain increases in supine posture and is reduced in sitting posture. Person will develop dyspnea, fever, fatigue, abdominal pain and syncope. Pericardial rub is best heard over the left sternal border and is increased by sitting up and leaning forward. Healing produces fibrosis and adhesion between two layers.

Pericoronitis generally refers to inflammation of the gingiva in

P

relation to the crown of an unerupted tooth. It generally occurs in a partially erupted or impacted third molar. The space present between the overlying flap and the erupting tooth provides an excellent environment for the accumulation of food debris and nurturing of oral microorganisms which leads to infection and ultimately inflammation. The patient may have erythematous, edematous and suppurative type of lesion that is quite sensitive to pain along with radiating pain to nearby areas. There might be some amount of swelling at the angle of the mouth along with local lymphadenopathy of the affected side.

Perilymph is a watery fluid that fills the bony labyrinth of the ear.

Period prevalence is less commonly used method of prevalence. It measures frequency of all current cases existing during a definite period of time. It includes caries arising before, extending into the year as well as those cases arising during the year.

Periodontal abscess is a localized purulent infection within the tissue adjacent to the periodontal pocket that may lead to destruction of PDL and alveolus bone. It appears as an avid lunation of the gingiva along the lateral aspect of root. Gingiva appears red and edematous pus can be expressed from gingival sulphurs by digital pressure.

Periodontal flap refers to the section of gingiva or mucosa that is surgically separated from the underlying tissue to access the bone and root surfaces.

Periodontal ligament is the connective tissue structure that surrounds the root and connects it with the bone. It is continuous with the connective tissue of the gingiva and communications with the narrow spaces through vascular channels in the bone.

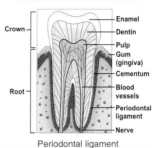

Periodontal ligament

Periodontal means around tooth.

Periodontal surgery is defined as a surgical procedure performed to correct or eliminate anatomic, developmental or traumatic deformities of the gingiva or alveolar mucosa.

Periodontal pocket can be defined as pathologically deepened gingival sulcus exceeding 3 mm It occurs due to the destruction of supporting periodontal tissue.

Periodontal probes are the instruments that are used to locate and measure the pockets as well as to determine their course on individual tooth surface. The probe is a tapered rod like instrument, calibrated in mm with a round and a blunt tip. These probes are thin and the handle allows easy insertion in to the pocket. Nabers probe is the best for evaluating the furcation areas.

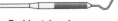

Peridontal probe

Periodontal scaling and root planing is the removal of plaque and calculus from the root surface using periodontal scaling instruments.

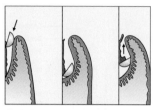

Periodontal scaling and root planing

Periodontal screening and recording (PSR) system is a device which is specially designed for faster screening and recording of the periodontal status of the patient. It uses a specially designed probe which has a ball tip of 0.5 mm and is color coded from 3.5 – 5.5 mm.

Periodontics is a branch of dentistry that is concerned with the diagnosis and treatment of disease of the supporting and surrounding tissues of tooth. Specialist is known as periodontist.

Periodontitis means inflammation of periodontium. Initially it starts as a simple marginal gingivitis as a reaction to calculus or plaque. There will be tiny ulceration of crevicular epithelium. Gingiva becomes more inflamed and swollen. Calculus may be present. Gingiva bleeds easily. Foul halitosis may be present. Teeth become mobile and dull on percussion. X-ray will show blunting of alveolar crest. If there is no excessive bone loss, the tooth can be saved.

Periodontium is the structure that surrounds and supports the teeth. Periodontium attaches the tooth to its bony housing. These are tissues that invest and support the teeth such as gingiva and alveolar bone. It provides resistance to forces of mastication, speech and deglutition. It defends against external noxious stimuli.

Periodontoblastic space is a fluid-filled space located between the dentinal tubule and the cell-wall of the cytoplasmic part of the odontoblastic process. This interstitial fluid continues beyond the cytoplasmic part of the process and extends the full length of the tubule, surrounding remnants of the odontoblastic processes found in peripheral circumpulpal dentin. It plays an important role when tissue changes occur within the primary dentin.

Perioral dermatitis is an inflammatory disorder of facial skin of unknown cause in which papules and pustules are seen around mouth. There may be a clear zone around lip. There is no persistent erytherma.

Periosteal elevator is a surgical instrument which is essentially used to reflect and move away the periosteum, once the incision is given, in order to expose the bone.

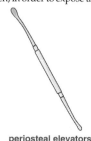

periosteal elevators

Periosteal suture is used to hold the apically displaced partial thickness flap.

Periosteum can be described as tissue covering the outer surface of the bone. Periosteum consist inner layer which has osteoblasts surrounded by osteoprogenitor cells which has the potential to develop in to osteoblasts and an outer layer which is rich in blood vessels and nerves.

Periotemp probe refers to the type of diagnostic probe that helps in detecting early inflammatory changes in the gingiva by detecting temperature rise. The probe detects pocket temperature difference of 0.1 degrees from the reference subgingival temperature.

Peripheral buttressing bone formation is the process of compensatory bone formation occurring on the external surface in an attempt to buttress bony trabaculae which is weakened by bone resorption.

Peripheral giant cell granuloma arises interdentally or from the gingival margin usually on labial surface or alveolar process anterior to molars. Size ranges from 0.5 to 1.5 cm in diameter. It is seen as fusiform swelling. The growth may be sessile or pedunculated. It may vary in appearance from smooth regularly outshined mass to an irregularly shaped, multi-liberated mass with protuberantes and surface indentations. It is usually painless unless painful ulceration occurs. It may be plain or spongy in consistency and color varies from pink to deep red or purplish red. Ulceration is less common. It contains non capsulated mass.

Capillaries are numerous. Radiograph may show superficial destruction of alveolar margin. Surgical excision is needed.

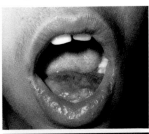

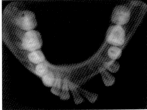

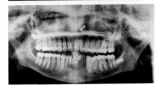

Peripheral giant cell granuloma

Peripheral nervous system includes nerves connecting the brain and spinal cord to other parts of body.

Peripheral neuritis occurs as a result of inflammatory reaction along a nerve trunk. Mucocutaneous lesions are not seen. Sensory and motor symptoms may be present.

Peripheral neuropathy is a complication mostly occurring in diabetes. Neuron is the term for nerve. Nerves that go to your arms, legs, hands, feet are called peripheral nerves. Pathos means suffering. Many diseases diabetes, thyroid, rheumatoid and kidney disease can cause damage to peripheral nerves. Damage causes tingling, numbness, burning and pain. There are no medicines to improve the nerve function in peripheral neuropathy. Aerobic exercises can reduce the unpleasant feeling.

Peripheral odontogenic fibroma is a rare lesion. These are slow growing often present for number of years. These are solid firmly attached gingival mass. Some lesions may contain a calcified stalk. Mature fibrous connective tissue stroma is present.

Peripheral ossifying fibroma is more common in younger age group. It is a well demarcated mass on gingiva. It has sessile or pedunculated base. It is slightly redden. Surface may be ulcerated. Several forms of calcification develop. Lesion may be surgically excised.

Peripheral vertigo is generally asymptomatic with prominent nausea and recent upper respiratory tract infection, ototoxic drugs or Meniere's disease. Neurological examination may be normal. Nystagmus is horizontal or rotary.

Periradicular is around the root of a tooth.

Peristalsis is a wavelike, rhythmic contraction of the stomach and intestine that move food material along the G.I. Tract.

Peritonsillar abscess are infections may come from tonsillar crypt or supratonsillar fossa. There may be pain, difficulties in swallo-wing, sore throat and fever. Cervical glands will be enlarged and possible trismus may develop. Tongue is coated with marked halitosis. Oropharynx may be narrowed.

Perleche – There develop multiple ulcers at angles of mouth with burning sensation. Person is in habit of licking angles of mouth with burning sensations. In old age there may be mild leakage of saliva, ulcers are superficial.

Permanent alopecia is a full thickness burn, completely destroy the dermis and epidermis leaving translucent alopecia. Scarring or keloid formation leads to permanent alopecia.

Permanent dentition is the second dentition which replaces the complete set of primary dentition, this dentition consist of 32 teeth i.e. 8 incisors, 4 canines, 8 premolars, 12 molars.

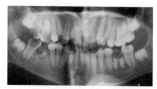

Permanent dentition opg

Pernicious anemia is due to impaired RBC maturation due to lack of B12, it is a chronic, progressive, megaloblastic anemia of adults. It shows large RBC'S with hypochlorhydria, generalized weakness, anorexia, weight loss and dyspnea. Skin becomes smooth, dry and yellow, Neurological symptoms include tingling sensation in hand and feet, Depression and irritability is seen in a few people.

Oral manifestations include beefy red tongue, areas of patchy ulceration may be noted. Tongue may be fissured or lobulated. In some cases, it may become bald. A few patients may develop macular lesions in entire mucosa and may develop burning sensation. There may be hyper pigmentation of oral mucosa.

Pertusis is a disease of infants and preschool children below the age of 5 years. Infants below 6 months have the highest involvement nasopharyngeal and bronchial secretions can spread it. It has three stages. Catarrhal stage lasts 10 days, paroxysmal stage lasts 2-4 weeks and convalescent stage lasts for 6-8 weeks. Complications include bronchitis, bronchopneumonia and bronchiectasis.

Pesso file is a long shank bur used in endodontic treatment.

Petechiae is a capillary hemorrhage appearing red initially turning brown in a few days. Petechiae secondary to platelet deficiency or aggression disorders are usually not limited to oral mucosa.

Pethidine is a synthetic derivative of piperidine. It was discovered in 1939. Its actions are similar to morphine. Its primary action is on central nervais system and smooth muscle. Somatic and visceral pain is relieved together. It has anticholinergic properties also hence it is used for visceral pain also. Analgesia is achieved in 15 minutes after intake and lasts for 5 hours. 100 mg of pethidine analgesia is equivalent to 10 mg of morphine. It may produce drug abuse and dependence as there is a euphoric effect. It depresses respiration and does not slow rate of respiration. It is not very effective spasmogenic. It does not alter the size of pupil.

Petit mal seizures can be described as sudden cessation of conscious activity or loss of postural control. Individual looks blank for a few seconds. Person quickly regains his consciousness. Incidence decreases with age and seldom seen beyond 30 years of age. These seizures tend to occur shortly after awakening or during periods of inactivity. Clinically, consists of a brief lapse of consciousness, normally lasting from 5-10 seconds and only rarely beyond 30 seconds. Individuals exhibit no movement during the episode. EEG shows symmetrical 3 Hz spike and wave discharge throughout the brain during attack.

Petrovic's hypothesis (Servo system) explains the primary cartilage in which growth occurs by differentiation of chondroblasts. It can be modified with factors which effect the direction only and not the amount of growth. Secondary cartilage has a direct cell multiplication effect but more importantly indirect affects also a play important role. e.g. it explains the mode of action of the functional appliances directed at the condyle and the upper arch acts as a mould into which the lower arch adjusts itself in such a way that optimal occlusion is established.

Peutz – Jegher's syndrome There is an oral pigmentation. Multiple, focal, melanotic brown macules are concentrated on lips. Macules may go up to 3-5 cms in size. Anterior tongue may be involved. Histologically these show basilar melanogenesis without melanocytic proliferation.

Phantom limb pain occurs after amputation of a limb. Sensation may be felt for several months as that part is still intact. Pain is unpleasant and of intolerable nature.

Phantom pains occur in orofacial area. These pains are felt in missing structures as if still present. Edentulous areas are frequent sites of such pain. Some form of memory pattern remains present.

Pharmacokinetics deals with the study of drug in the body.

Pharmacology refers to study of drugs.

Pharyngeal (branchial) arches, consist of bars of mesenchymal tissue separating from each other by pharyngeal pouches. Clefts, initially give the head and neck their typical appearance, postnatal, the appearance of teeth and paranasal sinuses provides the face with its own personal characteristics. Each arch contains its own artery, nerve, muscles element and cartilage bar, or skeletal element. Endoderm of pharyngeal pouches gives rise to a number of endocrine glands and part of the middle ear.

Pharynx tongue pushes food from mouth into pharynx popularly known as throat. Pharynx is involved in swallowing. It is a reflex action known as deglutition. Three parts of it are called nasopharynx, oropharynx and laryngopharynx.

Phenol compounds are used as disinfectants. Lipophilic viruses are susceptible but spores are resistant. If applied locally it has a depolarized local anesthetic action. It may be used in alkaline phenol mouthwash containing 3% liquified phenol.

Phenotype is the viable expression of the hereditary constitution of an organism.

Phenyl butazone is an anti analgesic, anti-inflammatory drug used for the treatment of rheumatoid arthritis. It can produce bone marrow depression and gastrointestinal effects. These can produce oral ulcer hence should be avoided in dental diseases.

Phenytoin gingival enlargement is an abnormal enlargement of gingiva due to use of phenytoin drug. Phenytoin (5–Diphenylephentain) has been used to control seizures. Phenytoin selectively deposes the Mater carter of the CNS and stabilizes manual excitation by blocking or interfacing with Ca^{+2} influx across cell membrane. The clinical onset of gingival overgrowth is reported after 1 month of use of the drug. This reaches its maximum by 12 to 18 months.

Phenytoin is a drug that is widely used in all epilepsies except petit mal epilepsy. It does not produce CNS depression. It limits the convulsions activity. Their side effect includes behavioral changes and megaloblastic anemia. Ataxia and diplopia are commonly seen. It may develop gingivitis.

Phenytoin gingivitis overgrowth involves inter dental papillae which becomes bulbous and overlap the teeth. Typically gingiva is firm and becomes orange in color.

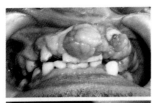
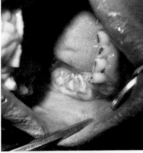
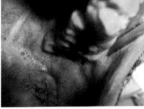

Phenytoin induced hyperplasia

Pheumothorax is an accumulation of air in the pleural space causing collapse of the lung.

Phosphorescent re-emission or tissue fluorescence is a photo chemical interaction which may be used as a diagnostic method to detect light reactive substances in tissue.

Phosphorus Eighty five percent of it is present in bones in combination with calcium. It is essential for most metabolic processes. Phosphorus depletion can occur from prolonged and excessive intake of aluminium hydroxide, antacid which binds dietary phosphate in the gut. Features include anorexia, malaise and weakness.

Photo ablation is a photo thermal interaction which refers to the removal of tissue by vaporization and superheating of tissue fluids, coagulation and hemostasis.

Photo plasmolysis describes how tissue is removed through the formation of electrically charged ions and particles that exist in a semi-gaseous, high-energy state.

Photo sensitization is sometimes an enhanced response of skin to U.V. irradiation. The agent responsible is usually a chemical present in skin which absorbs U.V. and transfers the energy to adjacent tissue molecules in a photochemical reaction.

Photo-acoustic interactions, which involve the removal of tissue with shock wave generation.

Photo-disassociation is the breaking apart of structures by laser light.

Photodynamic therapy is a photo chemical interaction which is the therapeutic use of lasers to induce reactions in tissues for the treatment of pathologic conditions.

Photopyrolysis is a photo thermal interaction which means burning away of tissues.

Phycomycosis is of two types superficial and visceral. The only clinical manifestation of the disease is the appearance of a reddish black nasal turbinate. Infection of head organisms are characterized by classical syndrome of uncontrolled diabetes, cellulitis and meningo-encephalitis.

Physical activity is an activity of any type which induces an increase over resting expenditure. It may be planned sport or unplanned domestic work.

Physician (According to WHO) is a person who, have been regularly admitted to a medical school duly recognized in the country has successfully completed the prescribed courses of studies in medicine and has acquired the requisite qualification to be legally licensed to practice medicine using independent judgement to promote community and individual health.

Physiologic occlusion is said to be present where there are no signs of disease and is not indicative of any type of treatment.

Physiologic tongue thrust comprises of the normal tongue thrust swallow of infancy.

Physiological saline solution is 0.9% sodium chloride solution which exerts an osmotic pressure equal to that of blood. It is compatible with blood.

Pigmented mole is a congenital developmental tumor like malformation of skin and mucus membrane. It is a superficial lesion of nevus cells. These may be congenital or acquired. Acquired have been classified as compound nevus, junctional nevus, spindle cell nevus and blue nevus. Treatment is not possible mole being multiple in number.

Pindborg tumor develops in middle age; mandible is more affected than maxilla. This tumor is very similar to ameloblastoma. Radiographically it appears as either a diffuse or a well circumscribed unilocular radiolucent area. Bony trabaculae may be irregular. Calcified flecks are distributed throughout the lesion, enucleation has to be done.

Pineal tumors are most common during childhood and produce precocious puberty in males. Tumor may compress aqueduct of sylvius to produce hydrocephalus and headache.

Pit and fissure caries are those originating in the pits and fissures found on the lingual surface of maxillary anterior teeth and on the buccal, lingual and occlusal surfaces of the posterior teeth.

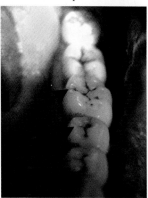
Pit and fissure caries

Pit and fissure sealant is a material mainly composed of fluid resin that is applied to posterior occlusal surfaces of caries prone teeth to seal pits and fissures from bacterial action. Principal monomer used is Bis GMA. It may be lightly filled with ceramic filler particles to improve wear resistance.

Pit is defined as a small pinpoint depression located at the junction of developmental grooves or at terminals of those grooves. The central pit describes a landmark in the central fossa of the molars where developmental grooves join.

Pituitary tumors compress optic chiasma producing bitemporal hemianopia, optic atrophy and diabetes insipidus. Secretary tumors includes cushings disease, gigantism or acromegaly.

Pityriasis rosea is an unknown skin eruption of unknown etiology. There are superficial light red macules or papules. Lesions may accompany headache, low grade fever and enlargement of lymph glands. Disease occurs seasonally. Lesions occur only on buccal mucosa. These are asymptomatic and require no treatment.

Placebo effect is positive response from non medicine part.

Planing refers to smoothening of root to remove infective and necrotic tooth substance.

Plantar fasciitis Planta is the Latin word for bottom of your foot. It is a tough band of tissue giving support to the arch of foot. Prolonged standing, excess activity may cause band tight causing pain. This pain is worst in the early morning and improves with continued walking. It is treated with anti-inflammatory medication.

Plaque is a sticky film that accumulated on teeth. It is a highly variable entity resulting from the colonization and growth of microorganisms on the surfaces of the teeth and oral soft tissues and consisting of a number of microbial species embedded in an extracellular matrix. It sticks to tooth surface and has to be removed. With food it provides nourishment for bacteria. Plaque grows thicker and results in caries and periodontal disease.

Plasma cell gingivitis is considered to be allergic response or hypersensitivity reaction to some component of chewing gum, dentifrice or diet. It is also known as atypical gingivitis plasma cell gingivostomatitis or plasma cell granuloma' (localized form). C/F: More common in young females. There is intense hyperaemia and edema of free and attached gingiva. It is sharply demarcated from alveolar mucosa that appears red soft and friable with fissuring of commissars. Patient complains of burning recreations and is sensitive to dentifrices and legibly seasoned foods.

Plasmacytoma is a solitary bone tumor and biopsy shows plasma cell histology. There is an absence of myeloma cells. Anemia is not present. Clinical features are similar to multiple myeloma i.e. pain, swelling and pathological fracture. Surgical excision followed by radiotherapy suits the patients.

Plaster of Paris is a gypsum product, used to make models of teeth. It is a dry form and is commonly used for immobiliza-tion of fractures. The plaster sets in a given shape. Conversion is irreversible. It can be used as a slab or a cast. Plaster slab covers only a part of the circumference of limb. It is used for soft tissue injuries and for reinforcing plaster casts. Plaster cast covers whole of a circumference of a limb.

Plastic instruments are blunt double end instruments having round or flat ends and are used for inserting fillings. One can manipulate linings with it.

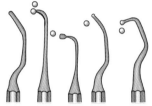

Plastic instruments, (a) Flat plastic; (b) Ball ended burnisher; (c) Pluggers

Plasticizer is a small molecule that when added to a polymer lowers its glass transition temperature and increases the rate at which solvents penetrate the polymer.

Platinized gold foil is prepared as gold foil except that a layer of platinum is sandwiched between two layers of gold and hammered. Platinum makes 15% of the alloy. It increases the hardness of the alloy. Disadvantage is that it makes finishing more time consuming.

Plax is a pre brushing mouth rinse containing sodium benzoate and other nontoxic surfactants. It contains 7.5% alcohol. It reduces bacterial plaque.

Pleomorphic adenoma is a benign mixed tumor of gland. It can occur at any age. It accounts for more than 50% neoplasm of parotid gland. It is a slow growing, well delineated, exophytic growth. Neoplasm is solitary but in some cases there may be multiple recurrent lesions. Neoplasm is rubbery and painless. Overlying mucosa may remain intact. In lip, pleomorphic adenoma presents small, painless, well defined, movable nodular lesion. Clinical features includes well circumscribed, lobulated, globular mass surrounded by capsule. Cut surface is not smooth and shows cystic and hemorrhagic areas. There may be intermittent growth. It is not fixed to deeper structures. Size may or may not reach beyond 2 cms. Surgical excision is the line of treatment.

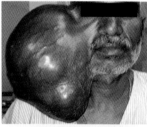

Pleomorphic adenoma

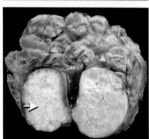

Salivary tissue at periphery   Pseudocartilage
         Capsule   Islands   polygonal
                                tumor cells

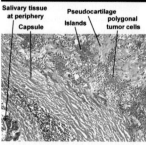

Pleomorphic adenoma salivary gland

Plummer – Vinson syndrome is iron deficiency anemia developing due to chronic loss, inadequate dietary iron intake, faulty iron absorption or increased requirement for iron. It may develop at any age. One can notice cracks and fissures at corners of mouth, smooth red painful tongue with atrophy of filliform papillae. Koilnychia develops and nails become brittle. Anemia responds well to iron therapy and a high protein diet.

Plunging ranula is a slow growing swelling in the floor of mouth as well as in one of the submandibular region below the angle of mandible. Cross fluctuation is present between oral and cervical swelling.

Pneumoconiosis may lead to mild chronic obstructive disease. Rare cases go into 'Progressive Massive Fibrosis'. In it large rubbery nodules of black fibrosis and dust are formed. Lesion develops as a radiating lesion around the bronchioles.

Pneumonitis is an inflammation of lung tissue caused by infective agent. Majority are caused by virus but bacteria and fungus may also cause it. Viral pneumonia causes mild cough, sometime productive, mild fever and dyspnoea. Symptoms of bacterial pneumonia are more marked. Patient looks ill, fever and chest pain develops. X-ray chest helps in diagnosis. Antibiotics such as erythromycin are helpful.

Pocketing it is a characteristic feature of periodontitis. Pockets round the teeth provide a protected environment in which bacteria can grow freely. These also favor growth of anerobes.

Pog, Soft-tissue pogonion is the most prominent or anterior point on the chin in the midsagittal plane.

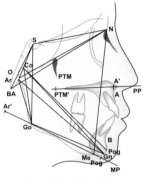
Ref points and planes

Point angle is an angle in cavity formation formed by junction of 3 walls.

Point prevalence is number of all current cases (old and new) of a disease at one point in time relation to a defined population. Point prevalent can be made specific for age, sex and other relevant factors.

Poison is any substance which when induced by any route in particular produces ill health, disease or death.

Poisson's ratio is the ratio of transverse contraction per unit dimension to elongation per unit length.

Poliomyelitis is the disease where the causative agent is poliovirus which has three serotypes 1.2 and 3. Most out breaks are due to type I virus. In a cold environment virus can survive for 4 months, faeces for 6 months. Cases are most infectious 7 to 10 days before and after onset of symptoms.

Incubation period is 7-14 days. In paralytic polio of 1% cases virus invades CNS and causes varying degrees of asymmetrical flaccid paralysis. Fever with paralysis is highly suggestive of polio. There may be signs of neck and back muscles. Paralysis is descending starting from hip to come down to knees. Paralysis reaches its maximum within 4 days. There is no specific treatment. Proper vaccination helps in prevention.

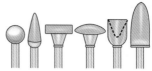

Polishing instruments (a) Huey mandrel; (b) Moor mandrel; (c) Pinhead mandrel; (d) Polishing brushes; (e) Abrasive rubber cups and discs for Huey mandrel; (f) Mounted fine abrasives

Polishing instruments are those instruments that are designed to perform the polishing and finishing action once the whole procedure is completed; it is mostly used with hand piece. Finishing burs and stones are used for smoothing cavity margins.

Polishing is a dental procedure that removes stain, plaque and acquired pellicle by using an abrasive polishing paste in a rubber cup attached to a slow-speed handpiece. It is a prophylactic procedure and is indicated when there are surface irregularities serving as plaque trap due to roughness of surface.

Polishing strip is an abrasive material placed on a length of plastic. It is used to smooth and polish the interproximal areas of composite restoration.

Polishing instruments These generally comprise fine abrasive stones, wheels, discs and strips. These are mostly used with a hand piece.

Polyacid-modified composite resins contain calcium aluminium fluorosilicate glass filler and polyacid components. They contain either or both essential components of a GIC, but are not water based and therefore no acid–base reaction can occur. As such, they cannot strictly be described as GICs. They set by resin photo polymerization. The acid–base reaction occurs in the intra-oral moisture and allows fluoride release from the material.

Polyarteritis nodosa is a non infective necrotizing vasculitis involving the small and medium sized muscular arteries of any organ. Nodular indurations and focal dilatations may be seen in course of affected arteries.

Polychromatic X-ray beam is a beam containing many different wavelengths of varying intensities.

Polycystic kidney is the most common inherited disorder. There is enlargement of both kidneys due to focal cystic dilatation of tubules. There may be accompanied hepatic cyst and mitral valve prolapsed. Grossly kidneys are huge but maintain shape. Cysts contain clear yellow fluid to gelatinous red or brown material in case of hemorrhage. Infantile polycystic kidney is rare.

Polycythemia is a condition where there is an abnormal increase in number of circulating all blood cells. It is manifested as headache, dizziness, tinnitus, visual disturbances and mental confusion. Skin is flushed or reddened. Spleen is enlarged. Gastric belching is common. Oral mucosa becomes deep purplish red. Cyanosis in a few cases may be present. Submucosal petechiae are also common. RBC count may go above 10000,000 cells per cubic millimeter. Bleeding and clotting time remains normal. Oral mucosa becomes deep red to purple and gingiva can be edematous. Gingiva may bleed easily. There can be excessive bleeding after oral surgical procedures. Total blood volume rises and blood viscosity increases. Platelet count is increased. Serum uric acid level goes up very high. Complications may lead to myocardial and cerebral infarctions. Patients may develop thrombophlebitis. Over production of uric acid produces gout. Acute leukemia is the terminal stage of Polycythemia. No specific treatment is available.

Polymyositis Dermatomyositis is an acute or chronic inflammatory disease of muscle and skin that may occur at any age.

Polyneuropathy is carcinomatous and myelomatous polyneuropathy that develops even before detection of primary tumor. Presenting features include motor weakness, muscle atrophy and sensory loss in limbs.

Polyols are artificial sweeteners. The most commonly known polyols namely sorbitol, mannitol and xylitol have the same caloric content as sucrose although less

sweetners. Products sweetened by polyols have been described as sugar-free.

Polyphyodont is possessing a several sets of teeth during a lifespan.

Polysaccharide is a large carbohydrate polymer formed by linking many monosaccharide's in a sequence.

Polysulfide was the first rubber impression material developed. It has many useful properties such as accuracy of detail. Lead dioxide is the catalyst giving strong odour and results in staining of clothes.

Pontic is an artificial tooth. It is the component of a bridge that replaces the missing teeth.

Population at risk is also known as defined risk and is crucial in epidemiological studies. It provides the denominator for calculating rates which are essential to measure the frequency of disease and study its distribution and determinants.

Porcelain is tooth-colored sand like material; much like enamel in appearance.

Porcelain jacket crowns are the oldest type of tooth colored crown. It consists of an even layer of porcelain of 1-2 mm thick covering the entire crown. Conventional dental porcelain is more like a glass than what is used for domestic purposes. It is relatively brittle and can be broken easily before cementation. It has following advantages i.e. aesthetics, brittleness, dimensional stability, economical and resistance to plaque accumulation. disadvantages includes the marginal fit and compromise of tooth substance (*see* **Figure** on page 364).

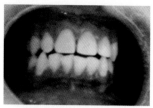

Porcelain jacket crowns

Porcelain veneer - ultra-thin shells of ceramic material bonded to the front of the tooth.

Porokeratosis here the plaques are surrounded by raised border of epidermal proliferation. Plaques are produced by mutant clones of epidermal cells. On sections oral lesions show characteristic cornoid lamella.

Porosity is a state in which there are voids in a solid.

Porous bones are said to have occurred when adults achieve peak bone thickness around the age 20-30 years. After middle age bones become thin and brittle. X-ray may show wider, thin trabaculation known as osteoporosis.

Portal hypertension is said to have occurred where portal vein pressure is more than 30 mm or 5 mm Hg above inferior vena cava. It may be caused by portal vein occlusion. Cirrhosis and veno occlusive disease may predispose it. It may produce oesophageal varices and hemorrhoids.

Positioner is a soft plastic appliance used immediately after the fixed orthodontic appliances are removed.

Positive health implies the notion of complete and perfect functioning of body and mind.

Positive pressure oxygen is an essential part of an emergency set up. If the patient collapses and breathing is reduced oxygen is to be used. Patient breathes a higher concentration of oxygen.

Post canal pluggers are spreaders having a long, tapered smooth point used to condense the filling against the canal walls and obliterate the gaps.

Positive reinforcement occurs if a pleasant consequence follows the response e.g., a child rewarded for good behavior following dental treatment.

Post crown is generally used when root has been filled. Natural crown is cut off and a post is fitted down the root canal. Artificial crown is made on this post. Post may be gold casting or of stainless steel.

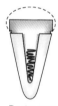

Post crown

Post canal reamers these resemble wood drills used for enlarging root canals so that a filling can be inserted. Length of all is same with increasing range of widths. Each reamer is numbered. These are rotated with hands. Reamers are also available for use in low speed hand pieces.

Post herpetic neuralgia can be manifested by pain in the distribution of affected area. In younger patients pain generally revolves within a few weeks but in older people pain may continue for years. Even powerful analgesics fail.

Post is an endodontic pin which can be made with different materials such as metal or carbon and placed in the root canal. Its function usually is to provide support for a grossly decayed tooth. It is available in prefabricated form but can be customised also according to the morphology of the canal.

Post syncope phase, the patient may demonstrate pallor, nausea and weakness and sweating which can last from a few minutes to several hours.

Post traumatic neuralgia has the unremitting, bright burning pain which suggests painful neuritis. It may be accompanied with neuritic manifestation. Neuritic pain is interrupted by paroxysms of typical neuralgic pain.

Post tussive tongue ulcer occurs where the child having whooping cough presents with an ulcer of tongue. It is situated on the under surface near frenulum linguae. It is round and edge is sloping. Yellowish or greyish slough is present at floor. It is soft in consistence and regional lymph glands are not enlarged.

Posterior bridge Bridges replacing back teeth usually have full veneer crowns on abutment teeth.

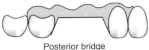

Posterior bridge

Posterior cerebral artery occlusion arises from basilar artery and supplies occipital lobe. On occlusion visual cortex is affected.

When thalamus is affected contralateral sensory loss may develop.

Posterior cranial base length (S-A) the magnitude of posterior cranial base length depends on posterior face height and the position of the fossa. Short posterior cranial bases occur in vertical growth patterns and skeletal open bites and gives poor prognosis for functional appliances therapy.

Posterior superior nerve is a nerve that descends from the main trunk of the maxillary nerve just before it enters the infraorbital canal; the branch provides sensory innervations to the pulpal, gingival and osseous tissues.

Posterior teeth are the back teeth i.e. premolars and molars.

Post-eruptive phase takes place after the teeth are functioning to maintain the position of the erupted tooth in occlusion while the jaws are continuing to grow and compensate for occlusal and proximal tooth wear.

P

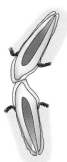

Post-eruptive phase

Postmortem caloricity occurs where body instead of coming down to normal temperature after death shows a rise of temperature which persists for an hour or so. It is due to action of micro-organisms in living body. It may happen in tetanus, cholera, rheumatic fever, abscess and strychnine poisoning.

Postmortem eye changes there will be loss of lusture in the eyes. One will notice loss of papillary, corneal and conjuctival reflexes. Cornea becomes opaque, hazy or cloudy. It becomes soft and pits on pressure. Shape of pupil may change from roundness to oval.

Postmortem finding of mercury poisoning – Post mortem will show erosion in mouth and esophagus. The mucous membrane of stomach becomes salty gray with multiple cracks and fissures. Kidneys are found enlarged and deeply congested with minute hemorrhagic spots. Liver and heart show fatty degeneration.

Postmortem findings of carbon monoxide poisoning – Body surface especially lips and fingers appear to be bright red or cherry color. Irregular patches of bright red color are found over anterior surface of body. Blood becomes fluid and bright red. Lungs are oedematous. Petechial hemorrhages are seen on brain and meninges.

Postmortem lividity is a reliable sign of death and gives information about the position of the body at the time of death. It helps to estimate the time since death and its color may suggest the cause of death.

Postnatal history refer to the history of a newborn child that includes the type of feed child is taking, vaccination or immunization status or any type of deleterious habit.

Postprandial is following a meal.

Postural Hypotension is also known as orthostatic hypotension a leading cause of transient loss of consciousness. Postural hypotension is defined as disorder of autonomic nervous system in which syncope occurs when patient assumes upright position.

Potassium is present mostly intracellular. Diet generally contains 2 to 4 gram of potassium daily. Requirement is more during active growth. About 90% of excreted from body goes out through kidney. Death in potassium deficiency may result from respiration or cardiac failure.

Potency is the strength of a drug in terms of tis ability to have a particular result.

Pott's disease is the most common manifestation of bone and joint infection by tuberculous bacilli. Tuberculous bacilli reach the spine by blood route. Lesions are rarely detected within six months of onset of symptoms. Symptoms include dull growing pain, anorexia and low grade fever. It may start involving in the intervertebral disc producing narrowing of disc space. Anterior collapse results in kyphosis.

Powdered gold – It consists of small appropriate particles blended with an organic indicator, compressed into small spheres and wrapped in gold foil. Powdered gold has greater mass than gold foil. It can be used both internally and on surface. Because of density it fills cavity rapidly. It may be overlaid with gold foil.

Poxviruses are the largest viruses to infect humans or animals. Small pox was the example of it.

P-Pronasale is the most prominent or anterior point of the nose (tip of the nose).

Pre-eclampsia and eclampsia is a complication of pregnancy characterized by hypertension, edema and proteinuria. Seizures may begin. There will be swelling of hands, face and legs. Headache and visual disturbance with altered mental status will be there. Petechial and bruising may be noted.

Pre-functional eruptive phase starts with initiation of root formation and made by teeth to move from its position within bone of the jaw to its functional position in occlusion. Has an intraosseous and extraosseous compartment. It has four stages: root formation, movement, penetration, occlusal contact.

Preanesthetic medication is given prior to anesthesia in order to alleviate anxiety, to enhance narcotic effect of general anesthetic agent and to minimize undesirable side effects of general anesthesia. Benzodiazepines are commonly used. Usual regime is to begin tranquillizing drug the day before the dental operation and continue a day after. Hypnotics are good to ensure a good night's sleep prior to dental surgery.

Pre syncope is a condition where patient in sitting position complains of a feeling of warmth in neck and face, loses color (pale or ashen gray skin color). Patient may feel nauseous. Blood pressure at this time is at baseline level or lower, whereas heart rate increases and presyncope continues, yawning, increased depth of respiration and coldness in hands and feet are noted.

Precordial pulsations are a parasternal lift usually indicates right ventricular hypertrophy, pulmonary hypertension or left atrial enlargement.

Predentin (dentinoid) is a narrow band of uncalcified predential matrix. It is 20-25 mm in width. It is situated between the odontoblast layer and the mineralized dentin. It signifies a lag period in the mineralization of the dentin matrix. It is always present as long as odontoblasts are present. It is equal to osteoid in composition.

Predictive theory that is used to make predictions based on relationship between variable.

Predictive validity is the ability of a measurement made at one point in time to predict future status.

Pre-eruption bulge is a bulge present in the gingiva before the eruption of the crown in to the oral cavity. The bulge is firm, slightly blanched due to the pressure of the erupting tooth and conforms to the contour of underlying crown.

Pre-eruptive phase is a phase of tooth eruption where all movements of primary and permanent formation to the time of crown completion end with early initiation of root formation.

Pre-eruptive phase

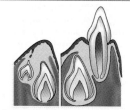

Pre-eruptive phase-bodily movement

Pre-eruptive-eccentric movement

Pregnancy associated enlargement may be marginal or gingival or may occur as a single or multiple tumors like masses. Enlargement is mainly related to elevated hormonal level during pregnancy which not only increases vascular permeability but also after the sub gingival microform with a predominance of p. intermediate.

Pregnancy epulis is a soft swelling on the gum which bleeds easily and may be painful on ulceration. Onset is usually at the end of third month. It is reddish purple colored swelling on the gum more frequently seen in anterior region. It usually regresses after birth of a child.

Pregnancy gingivitis becomes more severe in pregnancy. Inflammatory erythema and edema becomes more severe.

Pregnancy Granuloma is a hyperactive inflammatory response due to bacterial plaque mediated by systematic condition, it usually occurs during the 1st and 3rd trimester of pregnancy. It usually appears as a mushroom like flattened spherical mass that protrudes from the gingival margin or inter-proximal space and attached by a sessile or pedunculated base. It tends to expand laterally and pressure from tongue and cheek predestined its flattened appearance. It is usually seen at upper anterior teeth. The granuloma appears dusky red or magenta in color (Rasberry Like Appearance) with numerous deep red, pinpoint markings and a smooth, glistening surface. It has a semi firm consistency, but may be soft and friable, it does not innate the underlying bone. It bleeds spontaneously on mild provocation. It is usually painless, but painful ulceration many occur if it interferes with occasion.

Premature death is the death during the period when otherwise a person would have alive in normal course.

Premaxilla is the intermaxillary bone situated in front of maxilla proper.

Pre-Medication is the medication needs to be taken before treatment.

Premolars are the two-cusped teeth immediately in front of molars.

Prenatal history generally refers to the maternal history during pregnancy, which can be linked with present condition e.g. enamel hypoplasia, intrinsic stains of fluoride or tetracycline.

Presbyopia is impaired vision due to loss of elasticity of lens especially in old age.

Pressure habits are those habits which apply pressure on the oral soft tissues and hard tissues, thus having deleterious effect on the dentition and the oral structures. These include sucking habits like lip sucking, finger sucking, and thumb sucking.

Pressure is the force applied to a surface as a force per unit area.

Pressure syringe is an instrument with a trigger mechanism that delivers a measured dose of anesthetic solution and allows to express more easily the solution despite tissue resistance.

Pressure ulcer is caused by excessive non relieved pressure. In animals a pressure of 60 mm Hg of pressure applied to skin for 1 hour may produce muscle degeneration/tissue necrosis. When patient lies on hospital bed pressure can range from 100-150 mm Hg. Muscle tissue is more sensitive to ischemia than overlying skin. Hence necrotic tissue is usually wider and deeper. Treatment includes relief of pressure with special cushions, beds and nutritional support.

Pressure welding is a form of welding in which weld is made by pressure.

Prevalence is the number of disease cases in a population at a given time.

Prevalence refers to the total number of all cases who have an attribute or disease at a particular time or during particular period divided by population at risk of having the attribute or disease at this point in time or midway through the period. Prevalence refers specifically all current cases (old and new) existing at as given point in time or over a period of time in a given population.

Preventive a procedure performed to aid in preventing decay and/or gum disease.

Preventive dentistry is that branch of dental practice that deals with the establishment and maintenance of an oral environment conducive for the prevention of a sound and healthy stomatognathic system. The rationale is to promote optimal health of the oral tissues and to prevent damage of any sort.

Preventive orthodontics is the action taken to preserve the integrity of what appears to be normal at a specific time. This includes early correction of carious lesions, particularly proximal caries, early recognition and elimination of oral habits, using space maintainers in case of early loss of deciduous tooth.

Prilocaine was introduced in 1963. It is equally effective as Lignocaine. It contains slight vasoconstriction properties whereas Lignocaine does not. It is available in 4% solution without added vasoconstrictor.

Primary complex consists of three lesions (i) Ghon's focus (ii) caseous tuberculosis and (iii) chain of tubercles along with the lymphatic pathway between Ghon's' focus and mediastinum.

The bacilli are inhaled into the alveoli where they are ingested by macrophages. Epitheloid cells are the hallmark of tuberculosis.

Primary dentition is the first dentition which occurs in the oral cavity. It consist of twenty teeth i.e. 8 incisors, 4 canines and 8 molars, which are exfoliated or shed naturally and replaced by permanent dentition.

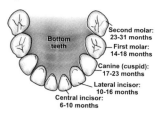

Second molar: 23-31 months
First molar: 14-18 months
Canine (cuspid): 17-23 months
Lateral incisor: 10-16 months
Central incisor: 6-10 months
Bottom teeth

Primary dentition

Primary displacement is the process of physical carry taking place in conjunction with a bones own enlargement.

Primary herpetic gingivostomatitis is caused by Herpes Simplex Virus I and II. There is abrupt onset of fever, malaise and lymphadenopathy of cervical chain of glands. Vesicles rupture soon forming painful ulcers. Lesions are highly infectious, gingiva is erythematous, ulcerated and enlarged. Lesions resolve automatically within 10-14 days.

Primary lymphoid organs are thymus for the T cells, bone marrow for the B cells.These are the major sites of lymphopoiesis. Lymphocytes differentiate from lymphoid stem cells, proliferate and mature into functional cells. Lymphocytes acquire them repertoire of specific antigenic receptors in order to cope with the antigenic challenge the individual receives during life. Learn to discriminate between self-antigens, which are tolerated and non-self antigens, which are not tolerated.

Primary lymphoma of bone develops rarely in jaws but mandible is affected more. Oral mucosal lesion is ulcerated. Teeth become loose, maxilla may be expanded, X-ray shows radiolucency of alveolar bone. In some cases periosteal reaction may be seen. Biopsy confirms the tumor. Radical surgical excision is helpful.

Primary neuritic leprosy Disease presents with nerve thickening and loss of sensation without any skin patches and skin smear examination is negative. Histological examination of the involved nerve shows many L. Laprae with infiltration by lymphocytes and histiocytes.

Primary pain is the source of hyper excitability that in turn produces secondary or referred pain. It is mostly deep somatic of visceral origin. More continuous, more severe, longer the duration more chances of secondary pains to occur. Referred pains occur most frequently in structures innervated by same branch that mediates the primary pain.

Primary parathyroidism is due to adenoma of one of the four parathyroid glands. Pathological fracture may be the first sign. Cyst of jaw may be seen. Generalized osteoporosis develops. Lobulated lesion of mandible is to be differentiated from ameloblastoma. Small cystic areas may be seen in calvarium. Jaw may give ground glass appearance. Excision of parathyroid tumor will treat the patient.

Primary prevention is the intervention of disease before it develops.

Primary prevention includes techniques, designed to prevent the onset of disease, reverse the initial stages of disease. It includes arrest of a disease before treatment is needed.

Primary syphilis The characteristic primary lesion of syphilis is called 'chancre' and is a solitary, painless, indurated, ulcerated or eroded lesion. To start it develops as a dull red macule which becomes eroded. Regional lymph nodes are enlarged, painless and are rubbery.

Primary teeth are also known as the baby teeth or the primary dentition.

Primary trauma from occlusion is said to have occurred if trauma from occlusion is the prime etiologic factor in periodontal destruction e.g. high filling, faulty prosthetic appliance, drifting and orthodontic movement which are functionally unacceptable.

Primate spacing is the normal physiological spacing present between primary anterior teeth.

Primer is a solution applied to the acid etched surface of tooth. It acts as a wetting agent. It enhances the adhesive quality of bond agent.

Primordial cyst develops through cystic degeneration and liquefaction of stellate reticulum. It may be associated with a retained erupted deciduous tooth. Unless infected it is not painful. On X-ray it is seen as round or ovoid well demarcated radiolucent lesion. It will show as a sclerotic border. Wall of cyst is made up of parallel bundles of collagen fibers. Surgical removal is the remedy.

Principal fibers are the most important element of the periodontal ligament which are collagenous in nature and are organized in the form of bundles.

Pro vitamins are not vitamins themselves but capable of conversion into vitamins in course of digestion. Carotenes are pro vitamins of vitamin A and to some extent at least, the amino acid tryptophan can be converted to niacin.

Probes Small occlusal cavities are found with a blunt pointed instruments called probe. Mesical and distal cavities can be found with a special double ended probe called briault probe.

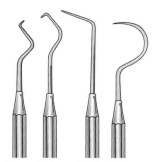

Probes (a) Ends of Briault probe; (b) Right angle probe; (c) Sickle probe

Prodrome is an early symptom of a disease.

Prodrug is the drug that undergoes metabolism in the body generally in liver.

Productive cough is produced when the active respiratory efforts expel the excessive tracheobronchial secretions. Commonly it results from infections. About 100 ml of mucous is produced in the tracheobronchial tree on daily basis. It is treated by antibiotics, steam inhalations and the drugs which cause softening of sputum.

Professional misconducts can be described as unethical acts which should not be practised ideally. These include to issue certificate which are untrue, misleading or improper. One should not employ an unqualified assistant. You are not permitted to canvass directly or indirectly to promote practice or keeping touts to improve your clientage. One should not disclose the secrets of patients. Improper relations with patients of opposite sex are not allowed.

Professional responsibility is the obligation to fulfill specific requirement to maintain expertise and knowledge associated with profession.

Prognosis is a prediction of a course, duration and outcome of a disease once the disease is present. The prognosis can be described in various forms such as excellent prognosis, good prognosis, fair prognosis, poor prognosis, questionable prognosis and hopeless prognosis.

Prolactin is called lactogenic hormone. It promotes milk production in women. Its target organ is breast. If the lactating mother continues to breast feed hormone level remains high.

Prolonged anesthesia is a condition where patient experiences numbness for many hours or days following a local anaesthetic injection. It may result due to irritation to the nerve after injection of a contaminated anaesthetic agent. The ensuing edema places pressure on the nerve. Persistent anesthesia also results from trauma to the nerve sheath.

Promyelocyte is larger than Myeloblast. Chromatin is coarser but nucleoli are present. Cytoplasm is basophilic with a small number of prominent large red granules.

Propanidid Epontal is a yellowish oily viscous liquid. It is a derivative of eugenol. It is less potent and is available for injection in 5% solution dose varies from 5-7 mg per kg body weight. It brings rapid unconsciousness and maintains anesthesia for 2-3 minutes. There becomes a transient fall of BP for 2-3 minutes. Its period of narcotic activity is short.

Prophy - see prophylaxis.

Prophy paste is an abrasive agent usually made from floor of pumice that is used to remove plaque and polish the tooth.

Prophylaxis is a general meaning to clean the teeth, also known as a prophy. Prophylaxis is a procedure designed to prevent the onset of disease.

Propionic acid is an NSAIDS and Ibuprofen is the main drug. These are better tolerated as compared to other NSAIDS like phenyl butazone. It is better tolerated than aspirin in terms of G.I.T. disturbances. It is one of safest drug. Its half life is of 2 hours similar to paracetamol. Abdominal dyspepsia may be a side effect.

Proprioreceptor are those receptors located in muscles, tendons and joints. These allow body to recognize the position of the body. Proprioreceptor are also the pain receptors involved in automatic functioning and perceive movement, pressure and position free nerve endings, deep somatic pain and other sensations.

Propronolol is a widely used beta receptor antagonist. It blocks all beta adrenergic receptors. It reduces heart rate and cardiac output. The force of myocardial contraction and blood pressure are reduced. Response of heart to exercise and exertion is diminished. It is used in angina, cardiac arrhythmias and hypertension. It can also be used in hyperthyroidism.

Prosopagnosia is a agnosia for faces. It has an acute onset and is due to involvement of cerebral artery. He cannot recognize face but recognizes person from voice and movements. Prosopagnosia which persists beyond a month is due to bilateral lesions at the level of lingual and fusiform gyri.

Prostaglandin E2 (PGE2) is a vasoactive eicosanoid produced by monocytes and fibroblasts, induces bone resorption and matrix metalloproteinase secretion. Evidence that prostaglandin could mediate bone resorption was first reported by Klein and Raisz in 1970 and a role for prostaglandin in periodontal bone loss soon followed (Goldhaber 1971) Prostaglandin E2 exhibits a broad range of pro inflammatory effects. It contributes to the flare and wheal effects by inducing vasodilatation and increasing capillary permeability, and these effects are enhanced by synergism with other inflammatory mediators. Prostaglandins sensitize nociceptors to different types of stimuli, thus lowering their pain thresholds to all types of stimulation. Prostaglandin E increases the response of slowly adapting Admethane receptors to non-noxious stimuli.

Prosthesis is a replacement of a missing body part.

Prosthetic instruments include plaster knife, wax knife and Lecron carver.

Prosthodontics is concerned with restoration of natural teeth and contiguous oral and maxillofacial tissues with artificial substitute. Specialist is known as prosthodontist.

Protamine Zinc insulin is a result of combination of protamine and insulin. Addition of zinc produces depression of blood sugar. Little effect is observed for 3-4 hours and takes 12 hours before the maximum activity is produced. It may be active even 24 hours after injection.

Proteins means necessary for life because vital parts of nucleus and protoplasm are made up of proteins only. One sixth of body weight is made up of proteins. Proteins contain 16% nitrogen. Daily requirement is 1 gm per kilo gram of body weight.

Proteolysis-chelation theory According to this theory, decalcification is mediated by a variety of complexing agents, such as acid anions, amines, amino acids, peptides polyphosphates, and carbohydrate derivatives. Oral karatinolytic bacteria are thought to be involved in the process. Differences in the keratin content of the enamel in children with high caries and low caries experience are considered important. It should be noted that only a small fraction of the protein of enamel bears any resemblance to the keratin of hair. Schatz and Martin challenged the chemoparasitic theory advocated the proteolysis – Chelation theory and stated that acid may prevent tooth decay by interfering with growth and activity of proteolytic bacteria.

Proteolytic theory –According to this theory, the organic component is most vulnerable and is attacked by hydrolytic enzymes of microorganisms, this precedes the loss of the inorganic phase. Gottlieb (1944) maintained that the initial action was due to proteolytic enzymes attacking the lamellae, rod sheaths, tufts and walls of the dentinal tubules. He suggested that a coccus, probably staphylococcus aureus, was involved because of the yellow pigmentation that he considered pathgnomonic of dental caries. Frisbie (1944) also described caries as a proteolytic process involving depolymerization and liquefaction of the organic matrix of enamel. The less soluble inorganic salts could then be freed from their "organic bond" favoring their solution, by acidogenic bacteria that secondarily penetrate along widening paths. Pincus (1949) contended that proteolytic organisms first attacked the protein elements, such as the dental cuticle and then destroyed the prism sheaths. The loosened prisms would then fall out mechanically. He also suggested that sulfatases of gram-negative bacilli hydrolyzed "mucoitin sulfate" of enamel or chondroitin sulphate of dentin and produced sulfuric acid. The released sulfuric acid could combine with the calcium of the mineral phase. It should be noted that the composition of the organic components of enamel does not resemble that of connective tissue and an abundance of sulphated polysaccharides has not been demonstrated. The Pincus' theory remains, therefore, without experimental support.

Prothrombin time measures the patient's ability to form a clot. It is performed by measuring the time it takes for a clot to form when calcium and a tissue factor are added to plasma. It is between 11 and 16 seconds. Prolonged prothrombin time is associated with post operative bleeding.

Proton is a positively charged particle.

Protrusion refers to the movement of the mandible anteriorly from ICP.

Provisional – Temporary.

Provisional diagnosis refers to the term where the diagnosis is based on clinical impression without any investigations. *Provisional prognosis* is that stage where it allows the clinician to start with the best available treatment that has questionable prognosis and at the same time hope for the favorable response which may shift the balance and help in controlling the disease.

Provitamins are vitamin related compounds that can be converted to active vitamins in body such as tryptophan can be converted to vitamin niacin, carotene to Vitamin A and cholesterol to Vitamin D.

Proximal Caries–susceptible zone. This region extends from the contact point down to the height of the free gingival margin. It increases with the recession of the alveolar bone and gingival tissues.

Proximal half crown is a ¾ crown that is rotated 90°, and distal rather than buccal surface left intact. It can be a retainer on a tilted mandibular FPD abutment. This design can be used only in mouth with excellent hygiene and low incidence of inter proximal caries. It is contra indicated if there is blemish on distal surface.

Proximal is the nearest point of attachment.

Proximal surface is the surface of the tooth adjacent to the next tooth.

Pseudo cysts are that cyst that doesn't have epithelial lining and hence are not true cysts.

Pseudo pocket refer gingival pocket.

Pseudomembrane is a membranous layer of exudates. It contains precipitated fibrin, organisms, necrotic cells produced by an inflammatory reaction on the surface of tissue.

Psoriasis is characterized by thick elevated, scaling, erythromatous plaque. There develops small, sharply delineated, dry papules, each covered by silvery scales like mica. On removal of these scales bleeding points may be seen. Cutaneous lesions are painless. Papules enlarge and become raised. New lesions slowly arise over weeks/months. Oral mucosa is rarely involved but lips may be involved. On treatment may subside for sometime then may reappear. Long term cortisone is used.

Psuedomembranous candidiasis is also known as thrush. It is an acute infection but may persist intermittently for months using corticosteroids topically or aerosol in HIV infected individuals. It has white membrane on the surface of oral mucosa, tongue and elsewhere. Confluent plaques can be scrapped leaving a raw erythematous bleeding base. White patches consist of necrotic material and desquamated epithelium.

Psychoanalytical theory According to this theory oral habits are the product of pleasure, child derives from stimulation of oral erogenous zone. The pleasure derived may be sexual or escape from a painful situation, as in case of infant who sucks when he is hungry. The habit is associated with pleasurable stimuli early in life but is not discarded at the usual time due to some underlying psychological disturbance. Proponents of this theory reason that if the habit is taken away from such an emotionally disturbed child, the child may substitute an even less desirable one in its place. One of the concepts of thumb-sucking that is brought about by the psychoanalytic theory is that humans possess a biologic sucking drive. This concept is supported by the observation of intrauterine sucking and by the neonatal reflex of rooting and placing, as described by Benjamin (1967). In the rooting reflex, if a well defined area around the mouth is touched by an object opens the mouth. The placing reflex is the sucking activity that occurs with the object making contact with the infant's mouth.

Psychodynamics is psychoanalysis. It includes motivations, perception and emotions.

Psychogenic headache occurs in neurotic, hyptochondrical or hysterical individual. The character is like a sense of pressure or like a tight constricting band.

Psychogenic malodor The halitosis may be attributable to a form of delusion of mono-symptomatic hypochondriasis (self-halitosis; halitophobia). Such patients rarely wish to visit a psychological specialist because they fail to recognize their own psychological condition and may have latent psychosomatic tendencies.

Psychogenic pain is a psychic and emotional states influencing pain perception and its expression. These patients are emotionally disturbed and are very common in young women. Such pain can continue for days together.

Psychological dependence is characterized by intense craving and compulsive perpetuation of abuse to repeat the desire of the drug. But not necessarily everybody taking the drugs may be an addict or drug dependent.

Psychology is the science dealing with human nature, function and phenomenon of his soul.

Psychophysiological is a measurement of physiological process in an effort to draw conclusions about psychological states.

Psychosexual theory Sigmond Freud in the year 1905 was the originator at psychoanalytical approach. He thought that personality development, is a result of satisfaction of a sex. He categorized it into different psychosexual stages. At each stage sexual energy is integrated in a particular part called erogenous zone. Two categories in concept of Freudian theory first describe level of consciousness (or) awareness; the second function component is personality. He proposed 3 basic psychic structures for personality of individual. There are three level of consciousness they are: 1. Conscious- part of personality, of which is aware of thought feelings for basic activities. 2. Preconscious-part of personality of which individual is not aware at the moment however able to recollect into awareness without great difficulty. 3. Unconscious-part of personality of which individual is unaware, which generally cannot brought into awareness without the help of assistant.

Psychosocial theory In Erickson's view "Psychosocial development proceeds by critical steps – 'critical' are characteristics of turning points, of moments of decision between progression integration and retardation. Each stage represents a "psychosocial crisis" which is influenced by social environment. Chronological ages are associated with Erickson's developmental stages as in physical development, the chronological age varies among individuals but developmental stage remains constant. Unlike Freud, Erickson emphasis the conscious self as much as unconscious instincts.

Psychosomatic is pertaining to mind body relationship.

Pterygium is a triangular fold of conjunctiva encroaching the cornea in the horizontal meridian. It may come from single or both sides of conjunctiva. It may be thick, fleshy and vascular associated with opaque spots in the cornea.

Pterygomaxillary fissure is a cleft that separates the lateral pterygoid plate and maxilla.

Puberty is the period between the ages of 12-15 years in girls and between 13-16 years in boys. During which secondary sexual characteristics develop and become expressed.

Public health is defined as 'the organized application of local, state, national and international resources to achieve 'Health for all' i.e. attainment by all people of the world by the year 2000 'of a level of health that will permit them to lead a socially and economically productive life.

Puddings are customary in formal dinners being served as the finishing item. In the process of eating food one loses certain amount of energy. To compensate lost energy it easily absorbs readymade glucose/fructose/levulose. That is why after 15 minutes of taking puddings one feels energetic.

Pulmonary hypertension is the counter part in the lungs of systemic hypertension. There is hyperplasia of medial coat of vessels. Second feature is ventricular hypertrophy.

Pulmonary infarction is an infarct, an area of coagulation necrosis produced by a sudden cut off of arterial supply but in the lungs there may be vascular occlusion without infarction and there may be infarction without vascular occlusion. The infarct is always a red infarct because of dual blood supply. It is a wedge or pyramid shaped.

Pulp calcification may be discrete as pulp stones or diffuse calcification. Diffuse calcification is seen in the canals of teeth known as calcific degeneration. It is an amorphous, unorganised linear strand.

Pulp canal is a portion of pulp cavity located in root area. The constricted opening at root apex is known as apical foramen through which nutrient and nerve supply enter.

Pulp capping is a procedure done when vital pulp is exposed, either root filling or pulp otomy is done to conserve the tooth. It cannot be done immediately so pulp capping is a valuable temporary measure. The exposed part is covered with calcium hydroxide paste and cavity paste. Cavity is filled with temporary cement.

Pulp chamber is the largest enlarged portion of pulp cavity found in coronal portion of tooth and has pulpal norms. It is the portion of the pulp in the crown of the tooth.

Pulp horn is the portion of the pulp chamber that extends towards the cusp.

Pulp is a delicate connective tissue of mesenchymal origin found in central portion of a tooth surrounded by dentin. It is composed of blood vessels, connective tissue, special dentin formation cells called odonto-blasts. Composition includes cells, intercellular substance, and tissue fluid. Cells are the fibroblast, histocytes, undifferentiated mesenchymal cells and odontoblasts. Zones of the Pulp - Odontoblastic zone – outermost layer, Cell free zone, Cell rich zone. Functions of the Pulp is formative, sensory, nutritive, and defensive.

Pulp tissue is the soft (not calcified) tissue in the pulp chamber; composed of blood vessels and nerves.

Pulp-Dentin complex is the close relationship between odonto-blasts and dentin, sometimes referred to as the pulp-dentin complex, is one of the several reasons why dentin and pulp should be considered as a functional entity. Not only do the two tissues have a common embryonic origin, but they also remain in an intimate relationship throughout the life of the vital tooth. Anything that affects dentin will affect the pulp and vice-versa. In other words, pulp lives for the dentin and the dentin lives by the grace of the pulp.

Pulpectomy is the removal of the whole pulp inside a tooth.

Pulpitis irreversible is an inflam-mation of the dental pulp in which pulp will not recover and will require endodontic treatment.

Pulpotomy "amputation of the af-fected or infected coronal portion of the dental pulp preserving the vitality and function of all or part of remaining radicular pulp" (AAPD 1996).

Pulpotomy can be defined as procedures involving removal of vital, partially inflamed coronal pulp tissue and placing a dresser over the amputated pulp stumps and then place the final restoration". (DB **Prosthetic instruments:** These include plaster knife, wax knife and Lecron carver. Kennedy 1986).

Pulpotomy is complete removal of the coronal portion of the dental pulp followed by placement of a suitable dressing or medicament that will promote healing and preserve the vitality of the tooth" (Finn 1995).

Pulse is produced by the force imparted to arterial blood each time the left ventricle contracts and expels blood into aorta. Pulse travels to wrist taking 0.1 to 0.2 seconds after the contraction. Pulse wave depends on the stroke volume, the force of expulsion and rigidity of blood vessels.

Pulseless disease also known as Takayasu's disease is rare of unknown cause. In branches of aorta stenosis, occlusion and aneurysms may occur. Early disease is accompanied by fever, myalgias, arthralgias and pain over involved artery. There may be syncope, dizziness, stroke, angina and claudication.

Pulses alternans when the left ventricle is severely diseased, it characteristically develops alternate strong and weak beats.

Pulses are the rich source of proteins. Price wise the proteins of pulses are cheaper than proteins of animal origin per unit. Hence pulses are known as poor man's meat. Pulses contain 20-25% of protein. Pulse proteins are class II proteins. It contains fair amount of calcium and iron. Pulses are rich in lysine but poor in methionine. If taken with wheat rotis, it compensates. During sprouting concentration of vitamin C increases.

Pumice is a ground volcanic ash used for polishing.

Punched out papillae is a cratered papillae characteristic of acute necrotizing ulcerative gingivitis.

Punctate resembles or marked with dots/points.

Punishment involves introduction of an aversive stimulus into a situation to decrease the undesirable behavior, e.g., use of parental rake in correction of tongue.

Purple lesions are some vascular lesions appearing blue while some may appear purple. Purple color is due to basic bluish color being modified by normal pink mucosa. Purple vascular lesions are bullae while purple lesions resulting from deposition of pigments are usually nodules or tumors.

Purpura is a reddish blue or purplish discoloration of skin or mucosa resulting from deficiency in blood platelets or increase in capillary fragility. It results in oozing of blood from gingiva. Petechiae and echymoses may be present. It is the extravasations of small amount of blood into mucous membrane. It generally develops in young adults. Bleeding spots on skin or mucosal surfaces, epistaxis, hematuria and hematemesis are common. Intracranial hemorrhage may produce hemiplegia. Bleeding in joints may limit its movements. Spleen

is not enlarged. Gingival bleeding and palatal ecchymosis is seen, Bleeding in temporomandibular joint result in pain, Trismus may develop. Muscle bleeding may result in closing and opening of mouth. Steroid therapy and repeated transfusions help.

Putrefaction starts immediately after death at cellular level. It is due to action of many enzymes. Chief destructive bacterial agent is Clostridium Welchi which causes marked hemolysis. First sign is greenish discoloration of skin over caecum where the content of bowel is more fluid and full of bacteria putrefaction starts above 10° C and optimum at 21° C to 38° C. Organs containing water decomposes early. Fat and flabby bodies decompose early.

Pyelitis is more commonly known as pyelonephritis. There may be high fever and acute severe rigor. Several bouts of fever may come in a day. There will be frequency, urgency and burning in micturation. Pain may be radiated to lumbar region. Kidney area becomes tender. Urine will show pus cells. RBC's and albumin. E.coli is the causative factor.

Pyknodysostosis is transmitted by an autosomal recessive trait with increased bone density, dwarfism and skeletal fragility. Patient is short statured. Dentition is anomalous and palate is high and arched. Hands and feet are stubby and finger clubbing is noted Osteosclerosis is most prominent in long bones. Facial bones and sinuses are hypoplastic. Mandibular hypoplasia with an obtuse angle results in receding jaw.

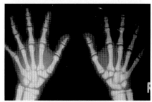

Pyknodysostosis showing dense bones, wide open sutures and absent angle of mandible

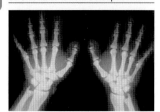

Pyknodysostosis with sclerotic bones and hypoplastic distal phalanges, which differentiates it from osteopetrosis

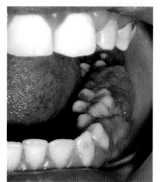

Pyknodysostosis with symmetrical increase in density of bones and typical hypoplastic distal phalanges

Pyogenic granuloma is a tumor like non specific conditioned enlargement in repose to minor plasma. It is usually seen on gingiva, but may also arise from lips, tongue and buccal mucosa. Lesion varies from a discrete spherical tumor like mass to a flattened, keloid like enlargement with a broad base. It is usually bright red or purple in color with a friable or fruits consistency. It bleeds on slight promulgation. Surface may show ulceration and purulent exudates may be present. It is painless. Surgical excision is the treatment.

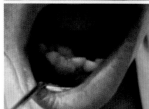

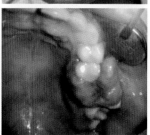

Pyogenic granuloma

Pyorrhea is a purulent discharge of pus.

Pyostomatitis vegetans is an uncommon inflammatory disease. There develops large number of broad based papillary projections with tiny abscesses. Tongue is involved more. Buccal mucosa gives a cobble stone appearance.

Pyraxolones is a most potent NSAID but the adverse effects are serious. It may cause agranulocytosis. It relieves pain of rheumatoid arthritis. It has unusual sodium retaining power hence has to be avoided in hypertension and renal disease.

Pyridoxine Vitamin B6 was discovered by Gyorgyi in 1936. Vitamin exists in three forms pyridoxine, pyridoxal and pyridoxamine. It plays a vital role of metabolism in amino acids. Liver, meat, fish, whole cereals are rich source of it. Treatment with INH and oral contraceptives may cause its deficiency. If diet is containing 100 gm of protein the requirement is 1.25 mg. its deficiency may cause glossitis, dizziness and vomiting. Morning sickness of pregnancy also responds to it. Daily requirement depends upon consumption of total quantity of protein. Oral manifestations include angular chelitis, glossitis, stomatitis, and atrophy of papillae on dorsum of tongue.

Pyrogen is a substance or agent producing fever.

P

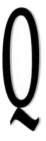

Q-sort is a survey research technique in which respondents generate is forced to choice ranking of many alternatives.

Quadrant denotes one of four equal sections in the mouth. The upper right, upper left, lower right or the lower left.

Quadriplegia means paralysis of all the four limbs and trunks. It is the resultant of spinal cord disease or fracture. There will be clumsiness of leg movements or unsteadiness of gait and other walking problems. Quadriplegia is due to cervical cord lesion. The ipsilateral lesion is involved first, followed in sequence by weakness of ipsilateral leg, the contralateral leg and finally the contralateral arm. Peripheral neuropathy produces symmetrical distal muscle weakness (*see* Figure on page 383).

Qualitative research is a research paradigm based in part on assumption of multiple constructed realities. There is independence of investigator and participant, time and context dependency information.

Quantitative light induced fluorescence is the technique used for caries detection. The use of fluorescence for the detection of caries dates back 1929, when Benedict observed normal teeth fluoresce under ultraviolet illumination. He suggested that fluorescence might be useful in the determination of dental caries when monochromatic light is used at 350 nm, 410 nm and 530 nm. Additionally, he noted a difference in fluorescence between sound and caries enamel. In the carious lesions the emission spectra shifts to more than 540 nm or the red range of the electromagnetic spectrum. The largest difference between the carious and non-carious spectra is found at 600 nm. He stated that when the enamel is illuminated with light in the blue-green range, the observable fluorescence occurs in the green-yellow range.

Quartan fever is said to have occured when two days intervene between consecutive attacks of fever.

Quasi experimental is a form of experimental research characterized by non random assignment of subjects to groups or repeated treatments to the same group.

Questionnaire is a written self report instrument used in survey research.

Quotidian fever is said to have occured when a paroxysm of intermittent fever occurs daily.

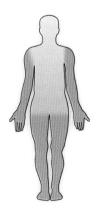

Quadriplegia

All four limbs are
involved

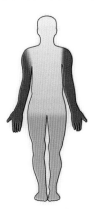

Diplegia

All four limbs are
involved. Both legs are
more severely affected
than the arms

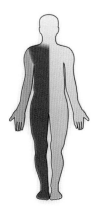

Hemiplegia

One side of the body
is affected. The arm is
usually more involved
than the leg

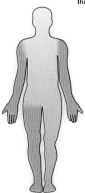

Triplegia

Three limbs are
involved, usually both
arms and a leg

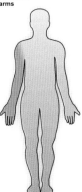

Monoplegia

Only one limb is
affected, usually
an arm

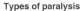

Types of paralysis

Rabies encephalitis is a disease that spreads along peripheral nerves to reach CNS (central nervous system). One may develop severe anxiety, speech and psychomotor over activity. Dysphagia and spasm of throat muscles may take place. Coma follows and death is due in 4-7 days.

Radiation is the emission and propagation of energy through space or material in the form of waves or stream of particles.

Radiation scatter is a form of secondary radiation, resulting from an X-ray beam that has been deflected from the path.

Radicular atrophy of pulp teeth are symptomless and respond normally to vacuolated spaces. Odontoblasts start disappearing. It may result due to improper fixation of tooth and pulp after extraction.

Radicular dentin dysplasia is inherited as autosomal dominant trait. It is characterized by teeth with normal crowns and abnormal tooth-roots. Radiograph will show partial lack of pulp chambers and root canals. Color of tooth is normal. Roots are short. Pulp chamber of permanent teeth are not obliterated.

Radio isotopes of certain elements or compounds when injected in to tissue get incorporated in the developing bone and act as *in vivo* markers. The radioisotopes can later be detected by tracking down the radioactivity they emit.

Radio surgery is a surgical technique that uses radio waves to produce a pressure less, bloodless incision.

Radiograph refers to an X-ray picture.

Ramford Index teeth are those six index teeth that are often used when evaluating periodontal health i.e. maxillary right first molar, left central incisor, left first premolar, mandibular left first molar, right central incisor and right first premolar. These teeth are used in clinical trial research as a representative sample of entire dentition.

Rampant means spreading unchecked.

Randomization is a statistical procedure by which the participants are allocated into groups called study and control groups. It is an attempt to eliminate the vias. It is a 'high' point of control trial.

Randomized clinical trial is a clinical research in which subjects are randomly assigned to treatment and control groups.

Ranula is a special type of mucocele which occurs on floor of the mouth from trauma of submandibular or sublingual gland. It is slowly enlarging painless mass on one side of the floor. A lesion is deep seated and mucosa over it is normal. Some prefer to excise entire sublingual gland.

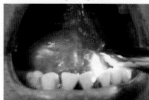
Ranula showing transillumination

Rape is an unlawful sexual intercourse by a man with his own wife under the age of 15 years or any other women under the age of 16 years or above that age against her will or when her consent has been taken by putting her in fear of death or hurt or when the man knows that he is not her actual husband as the lady believes.

Raphe is a union of soft tissue.

Rapid cell growth refers to most malignant type of cell or tumors that grow in rapid and invasive fashion, while benign tumors grow in a slow, expansile manner. Most neoplasms arise from a single stem cells.

Recession is the exposure of root surface by an apical shift in the position of the gingiva. The recession may be of two types: one, which is clinically apparent and other, the hidden one, which can be determined only by the insertion of probe. Recession may also be localized to one tooth or a group of teeth.

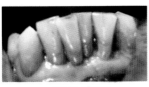

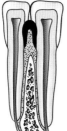

Clinical and line diagram showing gingival recession

Recovery period is the illness that subsided has and patient returns to health during this period.

Recurrent aphthous stomatitis (RAS) refers to the condition where there is development of painful, recurring solitary or multiple recurring ulcers confined to oral mucosa with no other signs of disease. These have been classified as recurrent aphthous minor and major. These ulcers begin as a single or multiple superficial erosion covered by gray membrane. It is well circumscribed by erythematous halo. Lesions are very painful and patient is not able to eat. In one outbreak number of ulcer may go up to 100. Size may vary from 2-3 mm Size of the minor ulcers is less than 1 cm. These ulcers heal without scar formation. They may start after trauma, menstruation or contact with certain foods. Within hours a small white papule forms, ulcerates and gradually enlarges over the period of next 72 hours. Lesions are round, symmetric and shallow. Multiple lesions are present. Lesions heal slowly and leave scars.

R

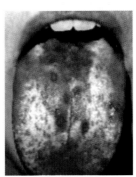

Stomatitis

Recurrent gingivitis can be described as the recurrence of disease after it has been eliminated.

Recurrent herpes simplex is a viral infection where there is a prodromal period of tingling or burning. Edema is followed by clusters of small vesicles of 1 to 3 mm. Bigger lesions may cause discomfort. Large, frequent, painful or disfiguring lesions require consultation. Oral acyclovir is effective.

Red blood cells carry hemoglobin and has a life span of 120 days. The cell is flexible, biconcave disc. Majority are of disc form and minority are bowl shaped, normocytic are of normal size and normochromic are having normal amount of hemoglobin. RBCs carry oxygen from lungs to the tissues and return in venous blood with carbon dioxide to lungs. Lack of RBCs count may result in anemia.

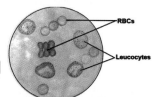

RBCs and pus cells in urine

Red-green color blindness is said to have occured when a single group of color receptive cones is missing from the eye. The person is unable to distinguish some colors from others or when person is lacking either red or green types of cones, person is known as red green color blind.

Reduction of a fracture means the restoration of a functional alignment of the bony fragments.

Referred pain is generally described when there is a close segmental relationship between the primary initiating pain and secondary effects of noxious stimulus. Most secondary symptoms occur in structures innervated by the same major nerve that mediates the primary pain. Sensory effects resulting in referred pain and secondary hyperalgesias. (e.g. angina pectoris radiates to the top of the left shoulder). The exact mechanism is unclear but appears to depend on convergence of afferent inputs on to central neurons from both the source and the referred sites, in addition to central summation (*see* **Figure on page 387**).

Reflex sympathetic dystrophy is a minor form of causalgia involving face/mouth. It has all the features of autonomic reflex pain. It may follow trauma, surgery or infection. It is a dull, persistent, diffusely located burning symptom. It is arrested by a diagnostic analgesic block of the stellate ganglion.

Refractory periodontitis has been defined as those patients who are unresponsive to any type of treatment provided.

Refractory refers to a heat resisting material i.e. capable of resisting high temperature.

Regeneration is the growth and differentiation of new cells to form new tissues or parts of the body.

Regional odontodysplasia affects more of maxillary teeth. Etiology is unknown. There is either a delay or a total failure in eruption. Shape is irregular with defective mineralization. Tooth assumes a ghost appearance. There is

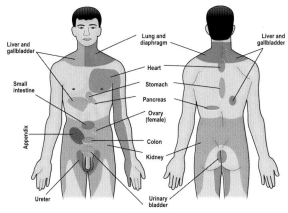

Liver and gallbladder

Small intestine

Appendix

Ureter

Lung and diaphragm

Heart

Stomach

Pancreas

Ovary (female)

Colon

Kidney

Urinary bladder

Liver and gallbladder

Referred painregions

marked reduction in dentin. Reduced enamel shows many irregular calcified bodies.

Regulation of body temperature is maintained at 98° F. Hypothalamus controls it. Three structures within skin assist in body temperature, blood vessels, sweat glands and muscle contraction.

Rehabilitation is the combined and co-ordinated use of medical, social, educational and vocational measure for training and retraining the individual to the highest possible level of functional ability. It includes all measures to reduce the effect of disability.

Reiter's syndrome is a clinical tetrad of non specific uretheritis, conjunctivitis, uveitis, mucocutaneous lesions and arthritis. Arthritis is asymmetric and involves weight bearing joints. It is totally confined to man between 20-30 years. Oral lesions are painless, red, elevated areas with a white border on buccal

mucosa, lips and gingiva. The palatal lesions appear as small, bright red pupuric spots. Antibiotics and corticosteroids help. Disease may undergo spontaneous remission.

Relative humidity is the percentage of moisture present in the air, complete saturation being taken as 100. Greater the relative humidity nearer is the air to saturation. If relative humidity is more than 65% in a room, person feel sticky and uncomfortable. Better ventilation lowers down the humidity.

Relative polycythemia is a condition occurring due to decreased plasma volume and not to increase in RBCs. It can be caused by diuretic use, diarrhea and excessive sweating.

Remittent fever, is said to have occured when daily fluctuation of fever is said to have occured varies more than 2° C.

Remodelling is the major pathway of bony changes in shape, resistance to forces, repair of wounds and calcium and phosphate homeostasis in body.

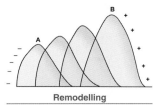

Remodelling

Remodelling of callus is always over abundance of newbone produced to strengthen the healing site because it may contain a dead bone also. These fragments are slowly resorbed and replaced by mature type of bone. External callus is remodelled to give a shape.

Removable functional appliances are the myofunctional appliances that can be removed and inserted into the mouth by patient themselves e.g. activator and bionator.

Removable habit breakers are a passive removable appliance that consist of a crib and is anchored to the oral cavity by means of

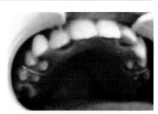

Removable appliance

Renal amyloidosis refers to a condition where kidneys become white and enlarged. They have smooth surface and widened pale cortex. Microscopically amyloid deposits are seen in glomeruli appearing in meningeal region. Deposits obliterate capillary lumen. Amyloidal deposits are also seen in blood vessels.

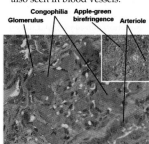

Amyloidosis kidney

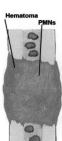
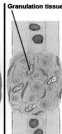
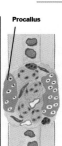
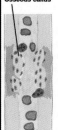
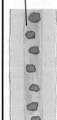

Remodelling of callus

Renal artery stenosis is produced by atherosclerotic occlusive disease. It may cause renovascular hypertension and ischemic nephropathy.

Renal calculi may be of various types. Pain travels from ribs to vertebral angle to flank. Pain may excruciate if it is horny and travels down the ureters. When stones are in renal pelvis it causes constant dull pain. 70-75% of renal stone are purely calcium oxalate or calcium oxalate + calcium phosphate. 15% of calculi consist of magnesium ammonium phosphate. 10% stones are of uric acid. Stones may be present with or without symptoms but when these pass down to ureters may produce renal colic. There develop hematuria. Urinary infection causes dysuria. About 60% small stones pass spontaneously.

Renal cell carcinoma is usually solitary, unilateral tumor. It is seen at upper pole in elderly age group. These are solitary, unilateral tumors, a golden yellow circumscribed mass. Large areas of hemorrhage, necrosis and cystic changes give variegated appearance. It spreads by blood stream.

Renal cortical adenoma is small 0.5 to 3 cm grey or greyish yellow nodule in cortex. There may be scars of atherosclerosis. Microscopically these show clear cells. Cells show uniform nuclei and no mitosis. Less than 3 cms are benign.

Renal cortical necrosis is of 2 types i.e. Diffuse of patchy. Diffuse bilateral cortical necrosis with sparing of medulla is very uncommon. When present it is an evidence of renal failure. Renal cortical necrosis may be seen in gram negative endotoxic shock and hemolytic uremic syndrome. In some lesion may be patchy. Patient may develop sudden oliguria, anuria or hematuria.

Renal edema in acute glomerulonephritis is due to retention of sodium and water due to fall in glomerular filtration rate. Distribution of edema is in loose tissues, face and around the eyes. Fluid is transudate.

Renal hamartomas are often bilateral. It shows mixture of irregular fibrous and fatty tissue blood vessels and smooth muscle cells. It may be associated with fibroma's and lipomas.

Renal transplant is an accepted modality of treatment of chronic renal failure and end stage renal disease. In order to suppress the rejection, immunosuppression with a single or combination of drugs is achieved.

Renal tuberculosis is common in India. Patient develops urinary symptoms and abacterial pyuric recurrent cystitis I.V.P. will show irregularity, cavitation, calcification and diminished renal function. Demonstration of tubercle bacilli is the most specific test. It results from hematogenous seeding of renal cortex to form small caseous foci and spread to medulla. Eventually loss of function with hydronephrosis develops.

Repair is the process which restores the continuity of the disease and re-establishes a normal tissue.

Reproductive system in male's includes testes, prostate and seminal vesicle while in females it includes ovaries, fallopian tubes, uterus and vagina.

Research hypothesis is a statement that makes predictions about the expected outcome of study, contrast and null hypothesis.

Reserpine is a rauwolfia alkaloids. It blocks postganglionic sympathetic nerve endings. It reduces peripheral sympathetic tone. Its central effect reduces anxiety. It is used as hypotensive agent. Long term use in females may cause carcinoma of breast.

Residual volume is the volume of air in the lungs which cannot be expelled.

Resilience is the energy needed to deform a material to the proportional limit.

Resin-modified glass ionomers (RMGIs) resin-modified glass ionomers were developed to overcome the problems of moisture sensitivity and low initial mechanical strength of GICs. They consist of a GIC with an added resin system that allows light setting followed by the acid–base reaction of the glass ionomer. This occurs within the light-polymerized resin framework. The resin increases fracture strength and wear resistance. Adhesion is enhanced by the use of enamel and dentine-conditioning agents before placement.

Resorb is to dissolve into the tissue.

Resorption of teeth in addition to deciduous teeth the roots of permanent teeth may also undergo resorption. External resorption may be due to periapical inflammation, reimplantation of teeth, tumors or cysts, impaction of teeth and idiopathic. Resorption of primary dentition is physiological in nature where as resorption of permanent dention is pathological in nature.

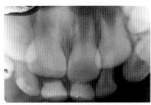

Resorption

Respiratory acidosis occurs due to depression of carbon dioxide washout. It may be caused by depression of respiratory center by drugs; patient may develop anorexia, confusion, mental disturbance. $PaCO_2$ is elevated and ph is decreased. HCO_3 is increased.

Respiratory exchange ratio is the ratio of oxygen uptake to CO_2 output at rest and during exercise.

Resting plaque refers to plaque 2 - 2.5 hours after the last intake of dietary carbohydrate as opposed to starved "plaque" which has not been exposed to carbohydrate for 8 - 12 hours. Resting plaque ph is usually between 6 and 7 whereas the starved plaque ph is normally between 7 and 8. A large range of plaque pH values seem to be compatible with oral health, but due to the multifactorial nature of dental caries, what may be healthy for one individual may be unhealthy for another. Resting plaque contains relatively high concentrations of acetate compared with lactate. The predominant amino acids are glutamate and proline, with ammonia also found at significant level. The presence of elevated levels of acetate is due to the accumulation of end products of amino acid breakdown as well as those of carbohydrate metabolism. These metabolic products are present at much higher concentrations than in saliva.

Resting Lymphocytes Ig is expressed on cell surfaces when they serve as membrane bound receptors for specific antigen. It may express tens of thousands of membrane Ig. Also known as virgin and B-Lymphocytes.

Restoration is any replacement for lost tooth structure or teeth i.e. bridges, fillings, crowns and implants.

Restorative dentistry is a branch of dentistry that deals with the process of restoring missing, damaged or diseased teeth to normal form and function.

Resuscitation is bringing back to life.

Retained infantile swallowing is a swallowing pattern that is seen due to persistent presence of this swallowing reflect ever after arrival of permanents teeth. The tongue lies between the teeth in front and on both sides, particularly noticeable are the contractions of the buccinator muscle. In expressive faces the 7th cranial nerve muscles are not being used for the delicate purpose of facial expression. Modification often occurs between the tongue tip and palate because of the in adequately occlusal contact.

Retainer is a removable appliance used to maintain teeth in a given position. Retainer can be of 2 types functional and non functional.

Retention cyst of maxillary sinus are mostly asymptomatic and are found on radiography jaw. Discomfort on maxilla/cheek may be present. Upper lip may become numb. Pain and soreness of head and face may be present. X-ray shows well defined radiopacity which is well defined. These cysts may persist or disappear automatically.

Retention grooves are the markings in the surface of the tooth that enhance placement and retention of restoration.

Retinal migraine manifests as episodes of unilateral transient visual disturbance such as prolonged visual blackout and brainstem symptoms such as vertigo, double vision and loss of consciousness. Headache and vomiting are usual.

Retro fill amalgam is the sealing of apex of tooth with amalgam following an apicoectomy.

Retro viruses are large, spherical enveloped RNA tumor viruses. These are having unique enzyme, genome and mode of replication.

Retrocuspid papilla is a small, elevated nodule located on lingual mucosa of mandibular cuspid. It is a soft, well circumscribed, sessile, mucosal nodule. It is bilateral and is common in children. It regresses with age and does not require any treatment.

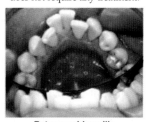

Retrocuspid papilla

Retrograde amnesia refers to failure to remember up to the time of injury.

Retrograde pulpitis is a condition where the bacterial and the inflammatory products of periodontitis gain access to the pulp via the accessory canals, dentinal tubules or apical foramina. The reverse effects of necrotic pulp on periodontal tissue is known as retrograde pulpitis.

Retrusion refers to movement of the mandible posteriorly from ICP (Intercuspal position).

Reverse smoking is seen in coastal communities of India. It causes increased frequency of oral lesions.

Reverse three – quarter crown is used on mandibular molars to preserve on intact lingual surface. It is useful on FPD (Fixed partial dentures) abutments with severe lingual inclination, preventing destruction of large quantities of tooth structure that could occur if a full veneer crown were used. The grooves at linguo proximal line angles are pointed of an occlusal offset on buccal slope of lingual cusps. This preparation closely resembles a maxillary three fourth crown preparation because axial surface of non penetration cusp is uncovered.

Reversed architecture is a bony defect produced by the loss of interdental bone that includes facial and lingual plates, reversing the normal architecture

Reversible index is a index that measures conditions that can be changed. Reversible index scores can increase or decrease on subsequent examinations, e.g.

Indices that measures periodontal conditions.

Rh classification – Rh factor is an antigen located on the surface of RBC. If an RBC contains Rh factor the blood is said to be Rh positive and if RBC lacks Rh factor it is said to be Rh negative.

Rhabdomyoma is a benign neoplasm of striated muscles. Tongue and floor of mouth are usually involved. It is a slow growing. It is well circumscribed painless mass. Lesion is often deep seated. It is a well circumscribed tumor of unknown duration. Tumor is composed of large, round cells with eosinophilic cytoplasm. Floor of mouth may develop it. Most of tumors develop from childhood. Tongue and palate are usually affected. It is a rapidly growing lesion. It causes swelling, pain and extensive tissue damage. These are fixed, ulcerated and hard. It has a poor prognosis even after surgery, chemotherapy followed by radiotherapy.

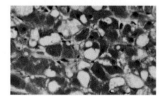

Rhabdomyoma

Rheumatoid arthritis is a chronic recurrent systemic inflammatory disease primarily involving the joints. Begin in small joints of hands and feet and progress in centripetal and symmetric fashion. Its exact cause is not known. Onset is insidious with pain, swelling and stiffness of joint. Usually proximal interphalageal joints are involved. It is polyarticular and symmetrical. It presents exacerbations and remissions. T.M. Joint is not commonly involved. Person develops fever, loss of weight and fatigue. Movement of jaw causes stiffness. Clicking and snapping is not common. It is also associated with vasculitis, skin and muscle atrophy, subcutaneous nodules, lymphadenopathy, splenomegaly and leucopenia. Hemorrhagic infarcts in nail fold and finger pulp are due to vasculitis. Over years ankylosis may develop. Malocclusion develops. Rh factor is positive in 75% of cases. There is no specific treatment. Cortisone helps. In severe cases condylectomy may be needed to regain movement.

Rheumatoid nodule occurs in 25% of cases. It is generally present as subcutaneous or intracutaneous nodule. These are discrete, firm, non tender swellings on extensor surfaces of fore arm. Wrist and ankle are also involved. Some nodules may even break.

Rhinophyma is also known as potato nose. There is painless and slowly growing swelling of nose of insidious onset. It may develop due to longstanding rosacea but may develop as a complication of acne also. There develops irregular thickening of nose. Distal part of nose swells and becomes irregular with many shallow pits. Swelling is of bluish red color and a few dilated capillaries are seen. Hypertrophy of nose leads to lobulated and purplish vessels. Face, cheeks and fore head may be affected.

Rhinosporidiosis is caused by rhinosporidium seeberi, a fungus. Skin lesions are like wart with peduncle. Oral lesions are soft, red polypoid growth of a tumor like nature which spread to the pharynx. Lesion bleeds easily. There is no specific treatment.

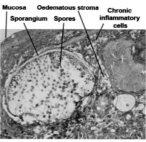

Rhinosporidiosis of nose

Riboflavin is a yellow green fluorescent compound soluble in water. It is soluble in water being part of vitamin B complex and is decomposed by heat and on exposure to light. Liver, meat, milk, eggs are good source of it. Cereals don't remain rich source as milling of grains remove it. Daily dose is 1.7 mg in adult man. Deficiency of it affects eyes and nerves. Lips are cracked at corner of mouth and tongue gets swollen. Therapeutic dose is 5 mg.

Rickets is the disease occurring in children due to the deficiency of vitamin D. The infant with rickets often receiving sufficient calories may appear well nourished but will be restless, fretful and pale with flabby muscles. Sweating of head is common. Abdomen distends. Development of child is delayed and teeth erupt late. Infant becomes prone to develop respiratory disease. In some cases knock knee and bow legs are seen.

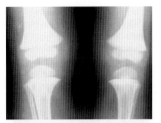

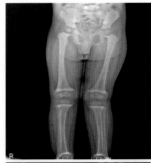

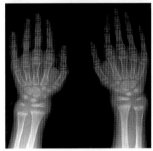

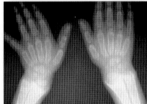

Rickets before treatment shows cupping and fraying

Ridge is a linear elevation.

Rifampicin is a drug used against tuberculosis. It is metabolized in liver and excreted in bile. Urine is stained red.

Rigidity refers to increased muscle tone.

Rigor mortis starts after a gap of two hours. Once body becomes stiff it remains for 20 hours. It first appears in involuntary muscles of the heart and then spreads to the voluntary group of muscles. It develops due to coagulation of muscle plasma and formation of lactic acid. It develops early in feeble, fatigued and exhausted muscles in warm and moist air.

Ringworm lesion is a fungal infection. Lesions are red, annular round, scaling which develops suddenly. Ringworm lesion may be single or if multiple may not be symmetrical. Acute infective disorder may be confused with psoriasis.

Risk factors when present, increases the likelihood that an individual will get a disease. These factors include environmental, behavioral and biologic factors.

Risk indicators are probable risk factors that has been identified in cross – sectional studies but not confirmed by longitudinal studies

Risk is the probability, that an individual will get a specific disease in a given period of time. The risk of developing a particular disease varies from an individual to individual.

Rodent ulcer occurs due to basal cell carcinoma. It is over face near the medial canthus of eye. It is a large, irregular having a well defined, raised and beaded eye. It is indurated. Regional lymph nodes are not enlarged.

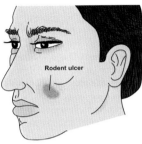

Rodent ulcer

Roentgen is the traditional unit of exposure for X-rays, the quantity of X-radiation that produces an electrical charge of 2.58×10^{-4}.

Romon syndrome patient develops gingival and alveolar enlargement and micro ophthalmia. Cornea becomes cloudy. Hypopigmentation results with athetosis. Mental retardation is rare.

Rongeur forcep is a nipper like instrument to trim alveolar bone.

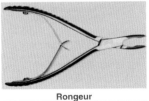

Rongeur

Root amputation is to remove one or more roots of a tooth.

Root canal files are hand instruments resembling reamers and made in standard length but in different width. Their job is to smooth and clean the walls of enlarged root canals and remove debris. After inserting in canal they are used in up and down filing action against canal wall. These are used in increasing sizes.

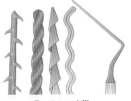

Root canal file

Root canal pluggers are the endodontic hand instruments that have a long tapered smooth point. Their aim is to fill any gap that is existing. They have a long handle with a small head.

Root canal obtruation is to remove inflamed or dead pulp from a tooth and replace it with a insert, sterile, non irritant, insoluble root canal filling. It is generally done in two stages. First is to prepare the canal and second to insert the root filling. In first stage pulp is removed then canal is enlarged and cleaned to prepare a dry, smooth empty canal tapering from pulp chamber to apex. Then temporary filling is done to cover entrance of empty root canal. In second stage temporary filling is removed and if canal is clean and dry it is filled to seal off the entire canal to within a millimeters of an apex.

Root canal reamers are hard as well as rotary instrument used to enlarge the root canal. These are having set length but different width. Each one is numbered to indicate its size. First small reamer is inserted with hand rotation

R

with successively wider reamers until canal becomes large enough for filling.

Root canal therapy (RCT) is a clinical procedure used to save an abscessed tooth in which the pulp chamber is cleaned out, disinfected, and filled with a permanent filling.

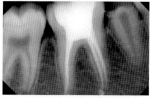

Root canal therapy (RCT)

Root caries index is the epidemiological index that is best choice for evaluating caries prevalence in the senior population of the community. Old generation is more prone to root caries.

Root forceps have blades with rounded ends. There are different patterns available. Different angles are made with handle. Lower root forceps are used for all lower teeth, straight forceps for upper incisors and canine. Read forceps for premolars and molar, bayonet forceps for upper premolars and molars.

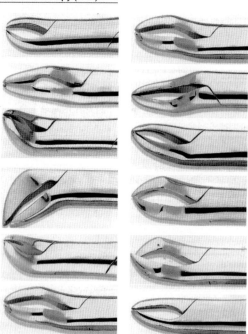

Root forceps

Root picks are surgical probes used to remove root fragments which may break away from tooth during extraction. Various shapes and sizes are available.

Rootless teeth are very short and conical. Pulp chambers are obliterated by multiple nodules.

Root planing stroke is a moderate to light stroke used for planing or final smoothening of root surface or the removal of plaque embedded calculus and altered cementum from the roots of teeth.

Root trunk is that portion of the root that is not bifurcated or trifurcated.

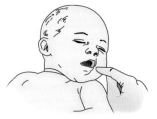

Rooting reflex

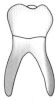

Root trunk

Rooting reflex and sucking reflex is a reflex when the full term infant sucks vigorously, when the breast is brought into contact with the infants cheeks, he/she seeks the nipple. Stimulation of the upper and lower lip produced movements of the lip and tongue in the direction of the stimulus. Rooting reflex is weak, not synchronized with swallowing at 28 weeks of gestation. It is stronger and well synchronized at 32 week of intrauterine life.

Rotary scrub method of tooth brushing is a method of tooth brushing in which circular strokes are used.

Rotatary paste fillers are engine instruments for inserting pastes

into root canal. These consists of spiral wire fitting into hand piece. It propels the required material to the full length of root canal.

Rothera's test – 10 ml of urine is saturated with an excess of ammonium sulphate crystals, 3 drops of strong freshly prepared sodium nitroprusside and 2 ml of strong ammonia solutions are added. A deep permanganate color is produced by acetone and acetoacetic acid. Positive test confirms presence of ketone bodies.

Rubber cups are the polishing instruments which consist of a rubber shell with or without webbed configurations in the hollow interior. They are placed in handpiece with a special prophylaxis angle.

Rubber dam punch is used to punch holes in the rubber dam to be placed over tooth.

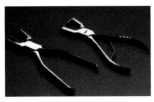

Rubber dampunch

Rubella is also known as German measles. It is caused by RNA virus of togavirus family. Child of 3 to 10 years in mostly affected. It is transmitted directly. Incubation period is 2 to 3 weeks. 50% patients are asymptomatic. There develops low grade fever and lymphadenopathy. Rash is an inconstant feature.

Rule of 5 is the simplest method for calculation of TBSA (total body surface area) is to subtract 1% from head and neck and adding 1% to lower limb for every year after 1 year of age. This charting technique has been described by *Lund and Browder Rule of 5* has also been used though infrequently. According to this rule, the body is divided into 20 areas of 5 % each by dividing the body into coronal and sagittal planes.

Rule of nine is a frequently used method to determine the extent of burn injury. The body is divided into 11 areas of 9% each to help estimate the amount of skin surface burned in an adult.

Rutherford syndrome has congenitally enlarged gingiva, delayed tooth eruption and superior corneal opacities that have curtain like appearence patient may be mental retarded, aggressive behavior along with dentigerous cysts.

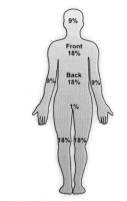

Rule of nine for body areas

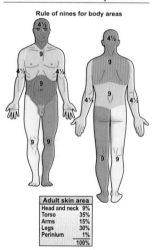

Rule of nines for body areas

Adult skin area	
Head and neck	9%
Torso	35%
Arms	15%
Legs	30%
Perinium	1%
	100%

Rule of 9

S

S refers to sella, the midpoint of hypophyseal fossa.

Saccharine is an artificial sweetener that is 500-600 times sweeter than sucrose, is stable in aqueous solution and is compatible with most food and drug ingredients. Its major disadvantage is its metallic aftertaste.

Sacro iliac strain is a hip joint pain that may radiate to buttock, hip and lateral aspect of thigh. There may be tenderness over symphysis pubis and person may limp.

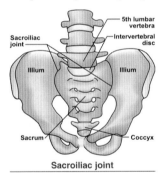

Sacroiliac joint

Saddle angle (N-S-A): is the angle formed by joining these three points providing a parameter for assessment of the relationship between anterior and posterior lateral cranial bases. Thus a large saddle angle usually signifies a posterior condylar position and a mandible that is posteriorly positioned with respect to the cranial base and maxilla.

Safe period is the period of menstrual cycle when conception is least likely to result from intercourse without use of contraceptive device.

Sagittal plane is an imaginary longitudinal vertical plane that divides the mouth into two halves left and right.

Salad is a roughage and best to start a meal with fresh raw salad. Common vegetables used for salad are salad leaves, onions, cucumber, green chillies, carrots and turnip. All these contain minerals and vitamin C. On cooking these nutrients are being lost hence should be used in raw form but before consumption these should be properly washed in fresh water. Most of these contain cellulose which is not digested but does not allow constipation to develop. Salad is having negative calorific value.

Salicylate is the widely used analgesic and was first used in medicine by Dreser in 1899. It is an antipyretic, analgesic and anti inflammatory drug. Pain is relieved by peripheral and central nervous system effect. It inhibits the synthesis of prostaglandins which occur in inflamed tissue. It reduces the sensitization of pain receptors to local stimuli. Antipyretic effect only occurs when temperature is above normal. It dissipates body heat also. It should not be used in cases of G.I.T. Ulcer/acidity. It may cause microscopic hemorrhage. It may result in skin rashes, urticaria and angioedema.

Saliva is the glandular secretion, which constantly bathes the teeth and the oral mucosa. It is constituted by the secretions of the three paired major salivary glands, the parotid, submandibular sublingual, the minor salivary glands and the gingival fluid. Saliva is armed with various defense mechanisms, such as the immunological, enzymatic and other organic and inorganic defense system. In addition, saliva has the ability to protect the mucosa against mechanical insults and to promote its healing via the activity of the epidermal growth factors. The involvement of the oral tissues in diverse functions as mastication and deglutition of food, taste sensations, speech and initial digestion of carbohydrates would not be possible without salivary secretions. The interface between saliva and oral tissues is the site of many dynamic reactions, which affect the integrity of both the soft and hard tissues of the mouth. Saliva constitutes one of the main natural defense systems of the oral cavity. Salivary organic, inorganic and physical factors are indispensable for the control of different oral microorganisms and its product for the maintenance of homeostasis in the oral environment. The challenges to homeostasis are met with a variety of host defense mechanisms. Several protective barriers exist for the soft tissues of the oral cavity. Bacterial penetration of the oral mucosa is first impeded by the salivary barrier. This barrier confronts the bacteria with a variety of antibody and innate immune components (e.g., mucin, lactoferin, lysosome, lactoperoxidase) that can mediate protective effects in several ways.

Saliva ejector is connected to a low velocity vacuum to remove saliva from the patients mouth during a dental procedure.

Salivary amylase is a digestive enzyme found in saliva that begins chemical digestion of carbohydrates.

Salivary duct stones are the calcareous concentrations in salivary duct. There is severe pain just before during and after meals. There is no free flow of saliva. Swelling is due to obstruction of saliva. Occasionally stone present may not show any symptoms. Stone may measure from a few mm to a cm. Small calculi may be sometimes removed manually, bigger stones require surgery.

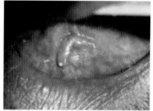
Salivary duct stone

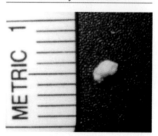
Salivary stone

Salivary hypofunction results due to three main causes, dehydration, damage of salivary glands or interference with the neural transmission.

Salt and milk fluoridation is a method of providing systemic fluoride by adding fluoride to salt i.e. by spraying a concentrated solution of NAF2 or KF on salt on a conveyor belt, another method is by adding premixed granules of caf2 and Po$_4$ to salt. Salt fluoridation first started in Switzerland in 1955 and subsequent tests revealed a 20-25% decrease in caries experienced by using salt with 90 ppm of F. In 1967 Muhlensen found that 300 mg f/kg salt yielding 1.5 mg, Zeigler (1956) first explored that possibility of fluoridating milk. In 1959, Inamura (Japan) reported a 33.3% caries reduction in school children served daily with milk containing 2.5 mg F. In India since there is no central milk supply regulating this method caries prevention would be a daunting task. Moreover, socio-economic religious and ethnic factors affect the quantity of milk consumed.

Salt restricted diet normal consumption of 5 gm daily in salt restricted diet only 2 gram of it is permitted. Sodium restricted diets are advised in congestive cardiac failure. In renal disease it reduces edema while in toxaemia of pregnancy it prevents fluid retention. During act and cortisone therapy also it has to be avoided. Person should avoid all salted and canned vegetables, pickles, salted butter, cheese and salted nuts.

Sampling distribution is a distribution of sample formed by drawing repeated sample from the same population.

Sanguinarine is an herbal root extract of the plant Sanguinria Canadensis; it is a mixture of benzophenanthridine alkaloids. Evidence from studies Loesche (1976), Southard et al (1984), and walker (1990) supports the claim of its antibacterial properties, anti-plaque effects, and anti-inflammatory activity. Sanguinary can reduce the acid producing ability and affect the adherence of bacteria. Since it contains alcohol (11.5%), it may produce a burning sensation and is contraindicated with the use of Metronidazole / Tinidazole.

Sarcoid sialadenitis in 5% cases parotid is involved in 3rd or 4th decade. There is bilateral, firm, painless enlargement. Decreased or absent salivation is present. Biopsy helps in diagnosis. Treatment is symptomatic. Corticosteroids are effective.

Sarcoidosis is a chronic glaucomatous disease which involves lymph nodes, lungs, speech, seen in 2nd and 3rd decade of life and more in blacks. It is a disease of unknown cause. It generally affects hilar lymphadenopathy pulmonary infiltration and skin. Symptoms are not severe enough to cause an alarm. Mild malaise and cough may be clinical features. Oral manifestations are sarcoid granuloma, Sarcoid gingivitis, gingival tissues are hyperplastic with a granular appearance. They are red in color and bleed on probing. There is painless enlargement. Lesions of lips are manifested as small, popular nodules or plaques on palate and buccal mucosa. Lesions are bleb like. Kviem-siltzbach test is an important aid. Histopathologically, connective tissue shows, non caseating whores of epithelial cells and multinucleated foreign body type giant cells with peripheral mononuclear cells. In some cases, severe and rapid periodontal destruction can occur.

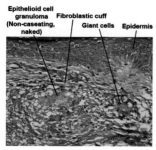

Epithelioid cell granuloma (Non-caseating, naked) Fibroblastic cuff Giant cells Epidermis

Sarcoidosis of skin

Satiety centers stimulation of lateral hypothalamus causes to eat voraciously while stimulation of ventromedial nuclei of hypothalamus causes complete satiety and person will refuse to eat.

Scabies is caused by sarcopties scabie. Transmission is by direct personal contact or through linen, towels, etc. The most frequent areas involved are interdigital folds, penis, scrotum and hypothenal eminence on genitalia. Lesions are firm of 5 m.m. Red nodules are noted. Intense pruritus is worse at night. 1% gamma benzene hydrochloride is effective to skin for 12-24 hours. Re application is required after 5-7 days to kill newly hatched nits. Antihistamines may be given if itching is more.

Scalds are moist heat injuries produced by application to the body of a liquid at or near boiling point or by steam. Scalds are not as severe as burns and produce hyperaemia or vesiculation.

Scaling is the process of removal of plaque and calculus from the crown and root surfaces of the teeth. Curettes and scalers are used for this purpose.

Scaling stroke is a powerful stroke which can be used in a pull motion to remove hard and tenacious calculus.

Scammon's growth curve explains that different tissue systems of the body grow at different times and rate. The four important tissue systems that show characteristic growth pattern are: lymphoid, neural, general and genital. As the graph indicates, the growth of neural tissue is nearly complete by 6 to 7 years of age. General body tissue including muscle, bone and viscera shape curve with a definite slow rate of growth, during childhood. There is acceleration during puberty. Lymphoid tissue proliferates far beyond adult amount in late childhood and then undergoes involution. At the same time, the growth of genital tissue is rapid (*see* Figure on page 402).

Scarlet fever is caused by streptococcal organisms of beta hemolytic type producing erythrogenic toxin. It looks like tonsillitis. Number of different strains of streptococci produces the disease. Incubation period is 3-5 days. Oral manifestation is 'stomatitis scarlantina, mucosa of palate is congested and throat becomes red. Tonsils are swollen. Tongue becomes strawberry. Tongue shows coating, papillae become edematous with small red knobs. Later tip of tongue becomes clean and then lateral borders follow. At last tongue becomes smooth and glistening. No reliable prevention is feasible.

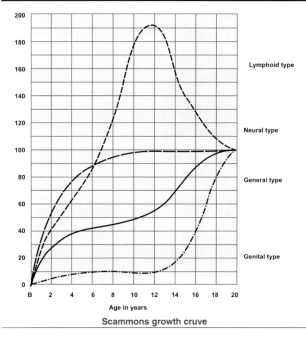

Scammons growth cruve

Scheffe test multiple comparison procedure.

Schistosomiasis is caused by schistosomiasis hematobium; cercariae are the infective stage of parasite. Adult worm reside in portal vein and in bladder venous plexuses. Hemorrhage can occur due to erosion of blood vessels. Urticaria, fever anaphylactic reaction may be seen. Bladder wall is calcified.

School water fluoridation is an alternative therapy in community water fluoridation. The recommended concentration is 4-5 ppm. It is shown to reduce caries experienced by 40%. The disadvantage is that children start receiving the advantage of fluorides only when they start school.

Schwannoma is a slowly enlarging lesion that is derived from Schwann cells. Intraorally, dorsum of tongue is most favoured location. Buccal mucosa floor of mouth, gingiva, and lips can also be involved. It is painless, nodule of different size. Sometime small, lobulated, firm growth may occur in gingiva. It has a true capsule. Surgical excision is the line of treatment (*see* Figure on page 404).

Schwartz periotrievers are the set of two double ended, highly magnetized instruments that are designed for retrieval of periodontal instrument from the deep periodontal pockets and the furcation areas.

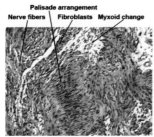

Schwannoma (Neurilemmoma)

Scientific misconduct is fabrication, calsification and other defilations from accepted practice in carrying out of reporting results from research.

Scissors and nippers are the surgical instruments which are used for removing tissues, trimming of flaps, enlarging the incisions and for removing muscle attachments.

Scleroderma/progressive systemic sclerosis is a disease of unknown cause characterized by an increased collagen deposition in skin.

Sclerotic bone is a well defined radio opacity seen below the apices of vital non carious teeth.

Sclerotic cemental masses are multiple, symmetric lesions producing pain and localized expansion.

Scope of Pedodontics refers to the range of activities or range of therapeutic treatment to be considered in a pediatric dental practice.

Scot Sanchis method is used for estimation of fluoride in water. This fluoride estimation test is based on the reaction between the fluoride and the red zirconium alizarin. The fluoride forms a colorless complex ion (Zr f6) and liberates free alizarin sulphuric acid, which is yellow in acid solution. As the amount of fluoride increases, the color produced varies from yellow to red. The fluoride level in the test material is determined by comparing the color thus produced with the standards.

Scott's hypothesis (cartilaginous theory) cartilage grows actively, bone later replaces it. Thus cartilage has innate growth potential. Transplantation and extripation experiments prove that some innate potential is evident though results are equivocal. e.g. mandibular growth has been explained that the condyle act as diaphysis of a long bone with growth occurring at both ends. Recent studies have proven that growth at the condyle is mostly reactive and not of primary nature and maxillary growth can be explained due to translation of nasomaxillary complex as a unit.

Scratched film is a film handling error. A scratched film is showing white lines from which emulsion has been removed by a sharp object.

Scrotal tongue also known as fissured tongue. It shows many small furrows on dorsal surface. It is a painless condition unless infected material is lodged in fissures.

Scurvy is a condition that occurs due to long term deficiency of vitamin C. Children between the age of 4 and 18 months are affected. Bleeding gums and hematuria may be presenting symptom. Cartilage cells don't proliferate at normal rate. Radiographs will show osteopenia, white line of Frankel, Winberger sign and Pelken's spur.

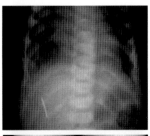

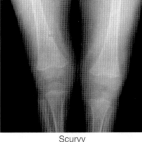

Scurvy

Se is the midpoint of the line connecting the posterior clinical process and anterior opening of the sella turcica.

Sealant is the application of a clear resin over the biting surfaces of teeth to prevent decay.

Sebaceous cysts of breast are not uncommon in skin covering breast. These can develop at periphery of areola. These can become quite large, tender and inflamed and are difficult to treat. Incision and drainage is needed.

Sebaceous glands are associated with hair follicles. These secrete an oily substance called sebum. Sebum lubricates and helps water proof hair and skin. Sebum inhibits the growth of bacteria on surface of skin. It inhibits the growth of bacteria.

Seborrhoeic dermatitis is an inflammatory scaling disease of scalp and face in general. Composition of sebum remains normal. Onset in adults in gradual and dermatitis is apparent only as dry. There may be diffuse greasy scaling of scalp. Marginal blephritis and dry yellow crusts and conjuctival irritation may be present. It does not cause hair loss. Seborrhoeic dermatitis is common at all ages. Flexures of face are mostly involved. Rash is red and scaly, a few papules and pustules may develop.

Second branchial arch gives rise to the cartilage of the second or hyoid arch (Reicherts cartilage) appearing at the 45th – 48th days. Reichert's cartilage attaches to the basicranial optic capsule, where it is grooved by the facial nerve. It provides the remaining cartilaginous circumference to the labyrinthine and tympanic segments of the facial canal. The muscles of the hyoid arch subdivide and migrate extensively to form the stapedius, the stylohyoid, posterior belly of digastric, the mimetic muscle of the face and levator velipalatine muscle. All of these are innervated by the seventh cranial or facial nerve, serving the second arch. The path of migration of these muscles is traced out in the adult by the distribution of branches of facial nerve. The special sensory component of is nerve for taste, known as Chorda

S

tympani nerve, invades the first arch as a pretrematic nerve and thus comes to supply the mucosa of the anterior two thirds of the tongue. The artery of this arch forms the stapedial artery which disappears during the fetal period leaving the foramen in the stapes. The Stapedial artery, derived from the second aortic arch, is significant in the development of the stapes ear ossicles. The Stapedial blastoma grows around the stapedial arch forming a ring around the centrally placed artery. The mid portion of the stapedial artery involutes, leaving the foramen in the stapes. Stapedial arterial branches persists, to become part of the internal carotid artery proximally and the external carotid artery distally.

Second degree burns are those which involve epidermis and varying depths of dermis. These have been further divided into superficial and deep second degree burns (*see* Figure).

Second pharyngeal pouch the ventral portion of this pouch is obliterated by the developing tongue. The dorsal portion of this pouch persists in an attenuated form as the tonsillar fossa, the endodermal lining of which covers the underlying mesodermal lymphatic tissue to form the palatine tonsil.

Second transitional period is characterized by the replacement of the deciduous molars and canines by the premolars and the permanent canines respectively. The combined mesiodistal width of the permanent canines and premolars is usually less than that

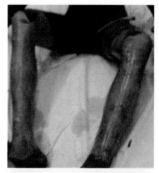

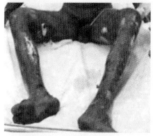

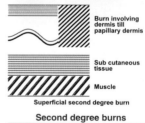

Burn involving dermis till papillary dermis

Sub cutaneous tissue

Muscle

Superficial second degree burn

Second degree burns

of the deciduous canines and molars. The surplus space is called leeway space of Nance. The amount of leeway space is greater in the mandibular arch than in the maxillary arch. It is about 1.8 mm (0.9 mm on each side of the arch) in the maxillary arch and about 3.4 mm (1.7 mm on each side of the arch) in the mandibular arch. This excess space available after the exchange of the deciduous molars and canines is utilized for mesial drift of the mandibular molars to establish Class I molar relation.

Secondary dentin refers to a dentine that is formed after the deposition of primary dentin. Physiologically it happens in old age. Pathologically it results from abnormal irritation. It develops due to dental caries, abrasion, attrition and erosion. Dentin forms an additional insulting layer of calcified tissue between the pulp and the pathological process. On X-ray size of pulp is decreased.

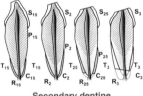

Secondary dentine

Secondary displacement is said to have occurred when movement of the bone is not directly related to its own enlargement. For example anterior direction of growth by the middle cranial fossa and the temporal lobe of the cerebrum displace the maxilla anteriorly and inferiorly.

Secondary effects are related to drug administration but not directly attributable to drug action. For example during broad spectrum antibiotic therapy super infection with Candida Albicans may cause thrush.

Secondary hyperparathyroidism can be seen in rickets, osteomalacia and chronic renal failure.

Brown tumors are less frequently seen. Calcification of arteries and soft tissue occurs.

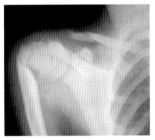

The 'rotting fence post' sign of secondary hyperparathyroidism

Secondary lymphoid organs are those that include the lymph nodes, spleen, and MALT: mucosa associated lymphoid tissue e.g. tonsils. GALT: gut associated lymphoid tissue e.g.: payers' patch. SALT: skin associated lymphoid tissue. These organs create an environment where lymphocytes can interact with each other and with antigen and disseminate the immune response once generated.

Secondary polycythemia is said to have occured when number of RBCs increases due to decreased oxygen. Decreased oxygen in blood triggers an increase in erythropoietin by kidneys which results in increase in RBCs. Pulmonary disease, high altitude and elevation of carbon monoxide may cause it.

Secondary prevention includes techniques designed to terminate disease and restore tissues to near normal function. Secondary prevention is done to diagnose the proliferation of a disease in its early stages and retard or stop the progress so that the damage is minimized and the subsequent repair is facilitated.

Secondary spacing was initially described by Baume, 1950. In closed dentitions the permanent mandibular lateral incisors emerge and the primary mandibular canines are moved laterally. Thus a space is created that cause the permanent maxillary lateral incisors to emerge into a favorable alignment.

Secondary syphilis usually appears in about 6-8 weeks after the appearance of primary chancre. It is characterized by skin and mucosal lesions. There will be generalized lymphadenopathy. Skin lesions may be macular, papular, follicular or lenticular. Coin like lesions are common on face. Areas of hyper pigmentation can be seen on soles and palms. Lymph nodes are painless, discrete and not fixed to the surroundings. With or even without treatment lesions heal in 2-4 weeks.

Secondary syphilitic oral ulcer appears in 3-12 weeks after primary lesion. Oral lesions are rarely seen without rash appearing. Ulcers are painless. Palate, tongue and lips may be affected. Shape is flat and irregular ulcer covered by grey membrane. They coalesce to form rounded areas known as mucus patches. Person will have fever and malaise. There may be skin rash on palms and ulcers are serologically positive and highly infective.

Secondary trauma from occlusion is said to have occurred when the adaptive capacity of the tissues to withstand occlusal forces is impaired due to bone loss.

Sedation refers to allaying stress, irritability, excitement or calming a person with the help of drugs.

Selected polishing refers to polishing only those teeth affected with stain and plaque.

Selectin is a class of adhesion proteins that recognize specific oligosaccharide residues displayed on cell surface glycoprotein's called mucin.

Selectin mediated phase is a phase where the neutrophils collides with vessel wall, allowing P selectin and E selectin molecules on activated endothelial cells to bind neutrophil surface mucin. L-selectin which is expressed on neutrophil, bind to its own set of target mucin on endothelial cell surface. These three types of selection establish initial adhesive contact between neutrophil and vessel wall. Selectin and mucous ligands are elongated molecules located at the tip of microvillus. Selectin bind tightly to their ligands in less than a millisecond so that even momentary contact can tether a moving neutrophil firmly to the wall. Neutrophil continues to roll or skip intermittently along vessel wall due the force of the following blood. The rolling exposes neutrophil to a diverse group of substance leucocytic chemotactic factor expressed by activated endothelium or diffuse into blood from injured tissue.

Selective anesthesia is given to know which tooth is paining. If specific tooth is involved pain will disappear on anesthesia.

Semi critical instruments are those that remain in contact of oral tissues like mirror, plastic instruments, burr etc. These should be sterilized after each use. Some may be kept in disinfective solutions for 6-10 hours.

Semicircular fibres are the group of fibres which are attached at the proximal surface of tooth below the CEJ, go around the facial or lingual margins of the tooth and attach on the other proximal surface.

Semiconductor lasers, sometimes called diode lasers, are not solid-state lasers. These electronic devices are generally very small and use low power. They may be built into larger arrays, such as the writing source in some laser printers or CD players.

Semi-longitudinal method means monitoring age-groups or sub groups at different level of development only for a period which separates one group from the next.

Senile caries are those that occur during old age. This may be due to reduction in salivary secretion or exposure of roots following gingival recession.

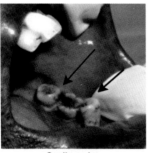
Senile caries

Senile cataract occurs due to ageing. There will be gradual impairment of vision. In immature cataract lens appears greyish, iris shadow is present. Finger counting at a short distance may be present. In mature cataract lens appears partly white and iris shadow is absent. The vision is reduced to perception of hand movement. There is no red fundal glow when examined in dark room.

Senile gait in old age looses speed and balance. Gait is slow, stiff with decrease in length of stride. Skeletal deformity and joint abnormality affects gait.

Sensory ataxia lesions occur in posterior column of spinal cord, posterior roots or peripheral nerves causes sensory ataxia. Patient clears the ground abruptly. He walks in a flexed posture. Romberger sign is positive. It is seen in subacute combined degeneration and spinal cord compression.

Sensory interaction theory contended that pain result from the interaction of both nociceptive and non-nociceptive afferent fibers on central neurons, the resulting excitatory or inhibitory interactions determining whether or not pain was perceived.

Septic arthritis of TMJ commonly results from blood borne bacterial infection. It may involve joint by direct trauma or infection may extend from infection of maxillary sinus or parotid.

Sequestrum is a piece of necrosed bone that has become separated from the surrounding as seen in chronic osteomyelitis.

Serial extraction is an interceptive orthodontic procedure usually initiated in early mixed dentition when one can recognize and anticipate potential irregularities

S

in the dentofacial complex and is corrected by a procedure that includes the planned extraction of certain deciduous teeth and later specific permanent teeth in an orderly sequence and pre-determined pattern to guide the erupting permanent teeth into a more favorable position.

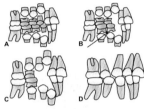

Serial extraction

Serotonin is associated with vascular pain syndromes as an algogenic agent, an important endogenous anti-nociceptive mechanism.

Setting time is the time calculated from the very beginning of mixing of the cement the formation of a hard and rigid cement.

Severe internal hemorrhage can be manifested when the patient becomes pale and restless. Patient may develop thirst and visual black outs. Skin becomes cold and moist. Pulse becomes thready and rapid. Body temperature comes down and B.P. Falls. Subcutaneous vein collapse and it becomes difficult to locate vein.

Severe periodontitis is said to have occurred when the periodontal destruction is generally considered severe when 5 mm of clinical attachment loss has occurred.

Sex drive is the primary instinctual urge of sexual gratification. It reaches its peak in late teens in males and mid thirties among females. In contrast of animals the human sex drive is less seasonal, less dependent upon an oestreous cycle, more varied in expression and aroused by a wide range of stimuli.

Sexual apathy is a negative attitude towards sexual relations, ranging from indifference to listlessness to active repulsion. Apathy is often based on distasteful or painful experiences and monotonous and unimaginative approach of the partner.

Sexual ecstasy is the peak of pleasure, excitement and euphoria experienced at the moment of orgasm.

Sexual flush is the rushing of blood during sexual excitement, especially in women. Flushing begins with rash like discoloration of lower chest and spreads to breast, rest of chest, neck, reaching a peak during the late plateau phase.

Shade card is an assortment of number coded shade samples used to match a patient's tooth coloring for an esthetic crown.

Shape memory is a property of certain wires that will permit shaping at a higher temperature, followed by deformation at a lower temperature and a return to the original shape by reheating.

Sharpey's fibers can be described as a terminal portion of principal fibers that gets inserted into cementum and bone.

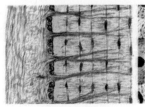

Sharpey's fibers

Shelf life is the period of time during which a compound retains its useful characteristics.

Shell teeth There is thin shell of hard dental tissue surrounding overlap pulp chamber. Pulp consists of coarse connective tissue.

Shigellosis is caused by Shigella Sonnei. Illness starts abruptly with abdominal cramps and diarrhea. Fever, chill, loss of appetite and headache develops. Patient becomes more dehydrated. Abdomen is tender. Stool culture is positive. Stool will contain red cells and leucocytes.

Shovel shaped incisors is a developmental anomaly where affected incisors demonstrate prominent lateral margins creating a hollowed lingual surface resembling shovel. Typically the thickened marginal ridges converge at the cingulum, not uncommonly there is a deep pit or dens invaginatus at this junction. Maxillary incisors are more commonly affected.

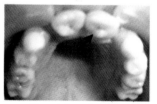

Shovel shape incisors

Shunt is to divert from one location to another.

Sialadenosis is a non neoplastic, non inflammatory enlargement of salivary gland. There develops recurrent, painless enlargement. Parotid glands are affected. There is significant elevation of salivary

potassium and decrease in sodium in saliva is seen.

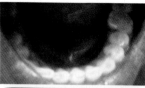

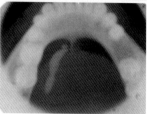

Submanidbular sialolith

Sialolithiasis results in painful intermittent swelling in area of a major salivary gland. Pain worsens while eating food. Stasis of saliva leads to infection, fibrosis and atrophy of parenchyma. Sialography remains the best method to diagnose. Acute infections secondary to stasis should be treated with antibiotics.

Sickle cell anemia is a hereditary type of chronic hemolytic anemia. It is more common in females. On dental X-rays mild to moderate osteoporosis is seen. Trabecular change is prominent in alveolar bone. Hair on end appearance of skull may develop. Outer table appears absent and diploe thickened. Hemoglobin level is decreased. No specific treatment is available except blood transfusion. One may live a normal life span.

Sickle scalers are the hand instruments used to remove plaque, supragingival calculus from the crown of the tooth. These scalers are bulky with a flat surface and two cutting edges that converge to form a pointed tip. The tip is used primarily to remove the hard deposits present on the crown.

Side effects are those unwanted effects that are due to normal pharmacological actions of drug.

Sigmoid volvulus exhibits generalized lower abdominal distension. X-ray will show a greatly distended loop of bowel. There is loss of haustral markings. On barium enema a bird's beak deformity with spiral narrowing of the upper end of lower segment is pathogomonic. Laparotomy is the ultimate answer.

Significant caries index A new index, the significant caries index was introduced by Bratthall (2000) in order to bring attention to the individuals with the highest caries values in each population under investigation. The significant caries index is calculated as follows: individuals are sorted according to their DMFT values, one third of the population with the highest caries scores is selected, and the mean DMFT for this subgroup is calculated. This value is the SCI index.

Signs are the effects of disease noticed by doctor.

Signs of abortion – signs of recent delivery are found. There will be bloody discharge from the dilated vagina. There may be excoriations or lacerations in the mucus membrane and uterus may be enlarged.

Silent primary pain may be inhibited unless is felt by patient. Thus leaves the secondary referred pain as his main complaint.

Silicate cement is mostly used even being extremely injurious filling material. It is used in restoration of proximal cavities of anterior teeth. Phosphoric acid is an injurious agent in silicate cement.

Silicon rubber is a polymer resulting from the formation of silicon – oxygen – silicon bonds.

Silver + copper amalgams are currently in clinical use because of their resistance to corrosion and their higher creep. At 5 weeks they elicited only slight response.

Silver permanent pigmentation of skin and mucus membrane is due to reduction in silver compound in tissues. Pigmentation of oral mucus membrane is diffusely dispersed in oral cavity.

Simple caries lesions are involving only one surface of the tooth.

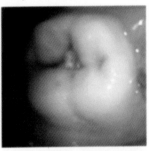

Simple caries

Simple fracture refers to the closed linear fracture.

Simple index is the index that measures the presence or absence of a condition.

Simple tongue thrust is a thrust with a malocclusion which demonstrates a well circumscribed anterior open bite and posterior teeth in a stable inter digitations. Associated with a digit habit may persist after the digit habit has subsided. Once the malocclusion is resolved, the tongue will usually change its swallow pattern and adapt to a new tooth alignment. Complex tongue thrust occurs with a teeth apart. There is generalized open bite and poor posterior occlusal fit and during swallowing, contraction of the lip, Mentalis and facial musculature, mandibular and maxillary teeth not in contact and the tongue held between the teeth. It is often associated with chronic airway problems such as mouth breathing, tonsillitis, pharyngitis or nasorespiratory distress.

Simplified fluoride mottling index (FMI) was introduced by Rahmatulla M and Rajasekhar A in 1984. The FMI is based on enamel opacities/lesions present on facial surfaces of the six upper and lower anterior teeth, which are aesthetically important. The scoring is based on a hypoplastic facial surface which may range from opaque white spots to grayish-yellow discolored surfaces. The weighting score assigned is restricted to four.

Simplified indices are those indices which measure only a representative sample of the dental apparatus. e.g. Greene and vermillion's oral hygiene index-simplified (OHI-S).

Simplified oral hygiene index (OHI-S) proposed by Greene and Vermillion in 1964 as a modification of the OHI. Assess oral cleanliness by estimating the tooth surface covered with debris or calculus. The OHI-S has two components, the simplified debris index and the simplified calculus index. The two scores may be used separately or may be combined for the OHI-S.

Single visit endodontic therapy is defined as the conservative, non surgical treatment of an endodontically involved tooth consisting of complete biomechanical preparation and obturation of the root canal system in one visit.

Sinter consolidating particles produce a more dense agglomerate without melting. It takes place during manufacture and during heating to drive off impurities.

Sintering is a densification process in which solid particles are fused together at high temperature.

Sinusitis is a generalized inflammation of paranasal sinuse's mucosa. Cause may be allergic, viral or bacterial. It causes blockage of drainage and thus retention of sinus secretion. It may be caused by extension of dental infection. Sinusitis is divided into three types: Acute sinusitis is of less than two weeks, Subacute sinusitis is up to three months, Chronic is when it exists for more than three months. Clinical features include common cold, nasal discharge, allergic rhinitis, pain and tenderness over the sinus involved. Pain may be referred to premolar and molar teeth with fever, chills and malaise. Secretions reduce air and make sinus radiopaque, mucosal thickening at floor and later on may involve whole sinus. Thickened mucosa may be uniform or polypoid, air fluid level may also be present due to accumulation of secretions. It is horizontal and straight. Chronic sinusitis may result in opacification of sinus.

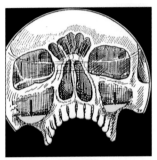

Sinustitis

Sixth branchial arch the cartilage of this arch probably forms the cricoid and aryteriod cartilages of the larynx. The mesoderm forms the intrinsic muscles of the larynx, which are supplied by the nerve of the arch, the recurrent laryngeal branch of the tenth cranial i.e. vagus nerve. The nerve of this arch passes caudal to the fourth arch artery in its recurring path from the brain to the muscles it supplies, the differing fate of the left and right fourth arch arteries, when migrating caudally into the thorax accounts for the different recurrent paths of the left and right laryngeal nerve. The right recurrent laryngeal nerve recurves around the aorta (fourth arch artery) the dorsal part of the sixth aortic artery and the entire fifth aortic artery having disappeared. The sixth arch arteries develop in part into the pulmonary arteries. The remainder disappears on the right side and forming on the left side of the temporary ductus arteriosus of the fetal circulation that becomes the ligamentum arteriosum.

Sjögren's syndrome is a triad consisting of keratoconjunctivitis sicca, xerostomia and rheumatoid arthritis. It is an autoimmune disorder of exocrine glands which may be associated with neuropathy and lymph proliferative disorder. Histological hallmark is focal lymphocytic infiltration of exocrine glands. Epstein – Barr or a type a retrovirus is the causative organism. Xerostomia is a major complaint in most patients with parotid gland enlargement. Enlargement of submandibular gland may be there. There may be symptoms of rheumatoid arthritis. Kidney involvement is noted. Generally women are affected above the age of 40. Hypofunction of salivary and lacrimal glands, dryness of mouth and eyes is seen. There will be intense lymphocytic infiltration of gland or there may be atrophy of gland. There is no satisfactory treatment.

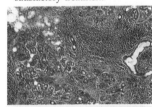

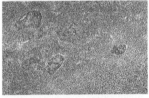

Sjögrens syndrome

Sjögren's syndrome tongue is typically red with atrophied papillae. Dorsum becomes lobulated with a cobblestone appearance. Amount of saliva is reduced.

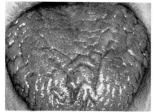

Sjögren's syndrome tongue

Skewed distribution is not symmetrical. It is with a long tail at its upper or lower end.

Skin is the outermost covering of the human body. It has two layers. An outer layer called epidermis and an inner layer is dermis. Epidermis has five layers. The stratum germianativum is the layer in which cell division takes place. New cell produce keratin and die and are pushed towards surface. Dermis is the true skin. It lies on subcutaneous tissue. Color of skin depends on amount of melanin.

Skin nasion is the point of maximum convexity between the nose and forehead.

Sleep apnea are bouts of breathing cessation during sleep due to closing of upper airway associated with obesity due to deposition of fat.

Sleep is a periodical physiological depression of function of parts of brain controlling consciousness. As sleep deepens there is a transition from normal alpha waves to a phase of bursts of more rapid wave and then development of slow random waves. It is known as non REM sleep. It has four stages. Insomnia in elderly is associated with awakenings and with a reduced proportion of paradoxical sleep. Pulse rate, B.P. and respiratory rate falls.

Sleep paralysis is a condition in which the patient when falling asleep or more often on walking find himself unable to move a muscle.

Slight periodontitis is said to have occurred when the periodontal destruction is 1 to 2 mm of clinical attachment.

S-line or Steiner line is a line drawn from soft-tissue pogonion to the midpoint of the s-shaped curve between subnasale and nasal tip. Lips lying behind this reference line are too flat and those lying anterior to it are too prominent.

Sling ligation is the suture used for flaps on one surface of the tooth that involves two interdental spaces.

Slough is a mass of dead tissue.

Slow rising pulse is an arterial pulse in aortic stenosis. The pulse is of small volume with a late systolic peak. There is a drill in carotid pulse.

SLS (superior labial sulcus) is the point of greatest concavity in the midline of the upper lip between subnasale and labrale superius.

Slurry is a mixture of pumice and water used to remove plaque and debris from crown of tooth.

Small bench top automatic autoclaves are sterlizing instruments and are very popular in dentistry. In it there is down ward displacement of air because steam enters at the top of chamber. It requires

S

136° C at 32 pound pressure for 5 minutes.

Smoke tar is a brownish liquid which is obtained when tobacco smoke is cooled or condensed. It contains polycyclic aromatic hydrocarbon compounds. Actually these are produced as a result of incomplete combustion of tobacco. When the cigarette of 85 mm length is smoked, having a butt of 30 mm. Total quantity of tobacco smoke or effluent formed is about 500 mg in weight. Tobacco tar formed is 17-40 mg by weight. Dry tobacco gives more tar than tobacco containing moisture.

Smoker's melanosis is diffuse macular melanosis of the buccal mucosa, lateral tongue, palate and floor of the mouth noted in smokers. Lesions are brown, flat and irregular/map like configuration.

Smoker's palate is a specific lesion which develops on palate in heavy cigarette, pipe and cigar smokers. Lesions are more prominent on keratinized hard palate. To start mucosa is red but later on becomes greyish white, fissured and thickened. Histologically epithelium shows acanthosis and hyper keratosis.

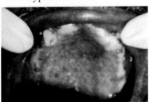
Smoker's palate

Smoker's throat there are number of constituents in tobacco smoke in sufficient concentration to produce irritation to throat. The delicate mucous membrane becomes inflamed which induces cough of a persistent nature. As long as person smokes his cough persists.

Smooth surface caries is the carious lesion located on surface other than pits and fissures classified as, smooth surface lesions. Smooth surface lesions may be further subdivided as inter-proximal, occurring on mesial or distal contact points, cervical, occurring on buccal or lingual surface near the dentine-enamel junction.

Sn (subnasale) is the point at which the columella (nasal septum) merges with the upper lip in the midsagittal plane.

SNA (sella-nasion-point A) is the angle expressing the sagittal relationship of the anterior limit of the maxillary apical base to the anterior cranial base. It is large in prognathic maxilla and small in retruded maxillas. In class ii division 1 malocclusion caused by prognathic maxilla in which SNA angle is larger than normal, the use of an activator is contraindicated. Mc Namara (1981) in his study stated that the SNA angle does not vary much among the different types of malocclusion nor does it change much with functional appliance treatment. The growth increments are small for this criterion, and the difference between growth direction and types is insignificant.

Snake venom is highly concentrated digestive juice of snake. Venom on drying forms fine needle like crystals which are easily soluble in water. Its toxic properties are due to proteolytic enzyme. Phosphatidase causes hemolysis and toxic effect on heart and circulation. There is hemorrhage from lungs due to damage of capillary endothelium. Neurotoxin produces curare like effects as well as paralysis.

SNB (sella-nasion-point B) expresses the sagittal relationship between the anterior extent of the mandibular apical base and anterior cranial base. With a prognathic mandible it is large, and with a retrognathic mandible it is small. Functional appliance treatment is indicated if the mandible is retrognathic and has a small SNB. This angle provides information only on the anteroposterior direction of the mandible, not on its morphology or growth direction. A posteriorly located mandible can be large or small, if it is small the prognosis for anterior posturing in the mixed dentition is good because a larger growth increment can usually be expected.

Snow capped teeth is a type of amelogenesis imperfecta, inherited defect in enamel matrix opposition and characterized by teeth having normal enamel thickness but low value of radiodensity and mineral content. The problem is related to the persistence of organic content in rod sheath resulting in poor calcification, low mineral content and a porous surface that becomes stained. Defect is due to altered matrix apposition (or) large amount of poorly calcified enamel matrix, which result in enamel, which is relatively soft becomes discolored. Enamel is soft and vulnerable to attrition.

Hard tissue is neither structurally weakened nor more susceptible than normal tooth structure to caries. It manifests as a white, chalky, opaque discoloration of the incisal and occlusal 3rd of the crown. The opaqueness may be solid or freckled, appears to involve only the surface of the enamel. The junction of the opaque white and translucent enamel is very sharp. The pattern of affected teeth has a distinct anteroposterior relationship and does not correlate with chronologic order of tooth development.

Social learning theory was given by Bandura in the year 1963. Social learning theory is thought to be the most complete. It is clinically useful and theoretically a sophisticated form of behavior therapy. Advantages include less reductionist, provides more explanatory concepts, encompasses a broader range of phenomena. The learning of behavior is affected by 4 principle elements. Antecedent determinants: the conditioning is affected if the person is aware of what is occurring. Consequent determinants. Person's perception and expectances (cognitive factors) determine behavior. Modelling: learning through observation eliminates the trial – error search. It is not an automatic process but requires cognitive factors and involves 4 processes which are- Attentional processes, retention processes, reproduction processes, Self – regulation: this system involves a process of self-regulation judgment and evaluation of individual's responses to his own behavior.

Socket wall can be described as dense, lamellated bone which is partially arranged in the Haversian system and partially in bundle bone.

Sodium hypochlorite is an excellent disinfectant and is bactericidal. It is corrosive to aluminium, nickel, steel and other metals. Items may be disinfected for 20 minutes. Gloves can be disinfected thoroughly by rinsing gloved hands and then rinsing with soap and water.

Sodium–our body contains 70-80 grams of it. Over 1/3rd of this amount is in skeleton. Enamel ash contains 0.3%. It plays an important role in maintenance of acid base equilibrium. When tissues are lacking potassium, sodium may substitute for it. It regulates the heart's contraction. 5 gram is the daily requirement. Heart patient should take 2 gm/daily ideally. In hot season sweat may contain 2 to 3 gm of salt per litre. Kidney is the organ to excrete it.

Sodium valporate is an anti epileptic drug controls petit mal epilepsy and psychomotor epilepsy. Patient becomes more alert. It generally doesn't produce side effects.

Soft acrylic liners – its advantages include high peel strength to acrylic denture base and high rupture strength. It has reasonable resistance to damage by cleaness. Disadvantage of it is of poor resilience and some buckle in water.

Soft drinks are carbonated drinks that exceed in food calories. A 300 ml of soft drink will contain about 140 calories. Each bottle contains about 6 teaspoon full of sugars. Most of the soft drinks contain sodium which increases the requirement of water. Sodas contain hardly any calories.

Soft lasers are thermal low energy lasers emitted at wave length, which are supposed to stimulate cellular activity.

Soft liner is a soft polymer used as a thin layer on tissue bearing surface of a denture.

Soft palate is a posterior tissue portion of the roof of the mouth.

Soft tissue cysts are commonly occurring masses in musculoskeletal system. On MRI these show uniform low and high signal on T_1 and T_2W1.

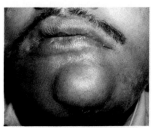
Soft tissue cysts

Soft tissue sarcoma arises from mesenchymal tissue. Many soft tissue sarcomas are poorly differentiated. These include malignant fibrous histiocytoma, liposarcoma and leiomyosarcoma. Large rheterogeneous painless mass with in a deep compartment should be regarded with a high suspicion of malignancy (*see* Figure on page 419).

Solar cheilitis can result in degeneration of tissue of lips due to sun exposure. Condition is related to the total cumulative exposure to sunlight and amount

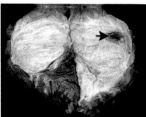

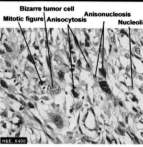

Bizarre tumor cell
Mitotic figure Anisocytosis   Anisonucleosis
                                Nucleoli

H&E, X400

Soft tissue sarcoma

of skin pigmentation. Lower lip is generally involved. Vermillion border of lip is affected and not specific treatment is required.

Soldering is a laboratory procedure done to join together with the help of solder. Larger fixed partial dentures are frequently cast in parts and later on are soldered together. Surfaces to be joined should be without contamination. A metal or alloy with lower melting point should be brought to the solder's melting temperature. Then ports and shoulder is being brought to the solder's melting temperature. If molten metal wets the solid metal it will spread between the flux and the metal part providing good contact. Solder penetrates joints by capillary action.

Solid-state lasers have lasing material distributed in a sold matrix (such as the ruby or neodymium: yttrium-aluminium garnet "Yag" lasers). The neodymium-yag laser emits infrared light at 1,064 nanometers (nm).

Soluble insulin is standardized to contain 20, 40 per ml. It is normally given at subcutaneous route and full effects come in 2-3 hours. Duration of action is 5-8 hours.

Somatic is the nerve that supplies muscles.

Somatic pain often reflects a pathological lesion in a specific organ or tissue.

Sonicare is an electric toothbrush. It vibrates at over 31,000 brush strokes per minute. Most models offer a 3 - minute timer.

Sorbitol is a sugar alcohol made from glucose. These also give 4 calories per gram as sucrose but don't promote cavities because these are not easily metabolised by bacteria in mouth. Sorbitol was isolated in 1872; sorbitol is mainly used in chewing gum. Intraoral trials have indicated that plaque pH does not drop below 5.7 after chewing sorbitol sweetened gum and the need for further studies is emphasized, more so by the fact that Smutans is known to metabolize sorbitol.

Sore mouth mucosa beneath denture may become red, smooth, swollen and granular. It is painful. Severe burning sensation is common. Condition is not due to allergy.

Soup is an appetizer that is served in the beginning of all formal dinners. It stimulates appetite. Clear soups introduce fluid to the diet. These provide sodium chloride, potassium and minerals.

Cream of soup only provides calories.

Soyabean is a protein It is three times of an egg and four times of wheat. It contains 20% fat. Except for a deficiency of cystine and methionine it is well balanced as regards amino acids are concerned. It contains trypsin inhibitor which does not allow all proteins to be utilized.

Sp reader is a long, pointed hand instrument used with lateral pressure to condense the gutta parcha points against the wall of root canal.

Space regainer is an appliance used in situation where there is premature loss of deciduous teeth resulting in the migration of adjacent teeth, into the edentulous space and interferes in the eruption of the succedaneous permanent teeth, due to inadequate space appliance used in such situation to regain the lost space due to migration and to provide space for the eruption of permanent teeth. Space regaining using springs the molars can be distalized to regain space by using removable appliances that incorporate simple finger springs.

Spacing usually exists between the deciduous teeth. These spaces are called physiological spaces or developmental spaces. The presence of spaces in the primary dentition is important for the normal development of the primary dentition. Absence of spaces in the primary dentition is an indication that crowding of teeth can occur when the larger permanent teeth erupt. The spacing is invariably seen mesial to the maxillary canines and distal to the man-

dibular canines. These physiological spaces are called leeway space of Nance.

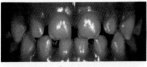
Spacing

Spasmodic dysphonia is a chronic phonatory disorder of adulthood without any obvious cause. It results from intermittent spasmodic hyper adduction of vocal folds leading to jerking, effortful strained sounds with laryngeal discomfort.

Spasmodic torticollis–when head is flexed it is known as ante collis, extended it is known as retrocollis. It may be tilted, twisted and rotated. Some may show head tremor and muscles involved are sternocleido-mastoid, trapezius and scalenus.

Spastic gait – Patient walks on a narrow base, has difficulty in bending his knees. Actually patient drags his feet. Foot is raised by tilting the pelvis and leg swings forward. It is seen in spinal cord disease.

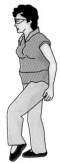
spastic gait

Specific gravity is the ratio of the mass of a material to an equal volume at 4° C.

Specific heat is the ratio of thermal capacity of a material to that of water at 15° C.

Specific plaque hypothesis (Walter Loeshe – 1976) states that only certain plaque is pathogenic and its pathogenicity depends on the presence of or increase in specific micro-organisms. According to this hypothesis plaque harboring specific bacterial pathogens results in periodontal disease. These organisms produce substances that mediate the destruction of host tissues. Acceptance of the specific plaque hypothesis was confirmed by recognition of AA comitans as pathogens in localized aggressive periodontitis. An increased risk for periodontal breakdown is observed in sites colonized by same potentially pathogenic organisms.

Specific plaque hypothesis revisited the disease is associated with specific strains of a given species. It's likely that most, if not all, recognized periodontal pathogens demonstrated difference in phenotypic properties related to their ability to cause disease i.e. genetic (molecular) basis for variability in virulence properties among pathogenic strains to cause periodontal diseases.

Specificity theory of pain was considered a specific sensation with its own anatomically distinct receptors, primary and cortical reception areas. This theory contended that only free unmyelinated nerve endings in the orofacial area were activated by noxious stimuli. More recently, the anatomical specificity of receptors has been discarded as most receptors, if sufficiently stimulated can respond to noxious irritation.

Spermatid is the cell derived from the secondary spermatocyte by fission, develops into a mature spermatozoon.

Sperms starting from puberty sperm production remains continuous throughout life. Fifty thousand are produced at every minute. It takes seventy days to mature fully. Once sperm are manufactured these move for storage and maturation to epididymis. When man becomes sexually aroused about 500 million mature sperms are moved through vas deferens. Epididymis has two degree F less temperature than body temperature.

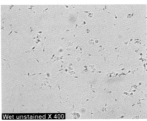
Wet unstained X 400

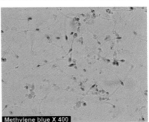
Methylene blue X 400

Spermatozoa in semen

S

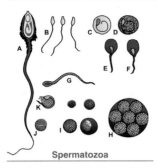

Spermatozoa

Sphygmomanometer is an instrument used in conjunction with a stethoscope to measure blood pressure. It consists of cloth cuff, a pressure bulb, a measuring gauge and a release valve. These are of two types mercury and aneroid one.

Spinal cord is a continuation of brain stem. It is a tube like structure located within the spinal cavity. It is 17 inches long and extends from foramen magnum of occipital bone to L_1 level.

Spinal cord syndrome – There is a typical type of analgesia with thermo anesthesia bilaterally in several dermatomes. It extends in a cap like fashion over arms, back and shoulder. Spastic weakness of legs may develop. When brain stem is involved facial analgesia may develop. Atrophy of tongue results in dysarthria. Person may develop dysphagia.

Spinal tuberculosis is a condition where there will be variable loss of pain and temperature sensation and motor function. It also causes spasticity, bladder incontinence and absent abdominal reflexes.

Spindle cell carcinoma is an unusual form of poorly differentiated squamous cell carcinoma consisting of spindle shaped epithelial cells. Lesion develops pain, ulceration and swelling. There is fleshy but polypoid growth pattern. Histologically tumor cells often exhibit marked nuclear hyperchromatism. There is a minimum degree of epithelial dysplasia with little or no keratin formation. This tumor is less aggressive hence wider surgical excision serve the purpose.

Spleen is a secondary lymphoid organ located in the upper left of abdomen behind stomach, close to the diaphragm. It has a collagen capsule. Histologically it contains a red pulp, where destruction of RBCs takes place along with venous sinuses and cellular chords. White pulp contains lymphoid tissue arranged around a central arteriole, periarteriolar lymphoid sheath. It is also organized into distinct 'b' cell areas and 't' cell areas or follicles. Primary unstimulated follicles and secondary stimulated follicles with germinal center contain follicular dendrite cells, phagocyte and macrophages, principally the antigen presenting cells.

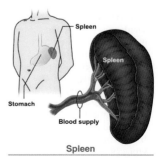

Spleen
Spleen
Stomach
Blood supply

Spleen

S

Split tooth or incomplete fracture is a tooth that is split or cracked but not yet fractured. The tooth may be uncomfortable only occasionally during mastication. Pain may be like unbearable stab. This is when there is crack in the dentin and suddenly spreads as the cusp is separated from the remainder of tooth. Pulp may remain hypersensitive for years. Most frequent complaint is of pain while biting or contracting cold fluids. If the pulp is involved in fracture any exciting agent will bring on discomfort.

Sporotrichosis is caused by sporotrichum schenckii and develops after exposure to animals. It involves skin, oral, nasal and pharyngeal mucosa. Regional lymph glands are enlarged. Lesions are healed by soft, pliable scars even though causative organism may be present. There is no specific treatment.

Spot welding is used to join orthodontic bonds and brackets and to join orthodontic wires. Work is pressed together between two copper electrodes and electric 2 to 6 v for 1/25 to 1/50 seconds at 250 to 750 ampere is employed.

Sprain is an injury limited to ligament. Sprain is a stretching injury to a muscle or its tendinous attachment. First degree sprain is a tear of only a few fibres of a ligament. There is minimal swelling and localized tenderness. In second degree sprain all the fibres of a ligament are disrupted. There is pain, swelling and inability to use the limb. In third degree sprain there is a complete tear of ligament.

Often pain is minimal. It requires immobilization of 4-6 weeks.

Spreading pain is due to development of painful muscle spasms. The secondary myogenous pain may occur some distance from the site of its mother primary pain. But its location bears/a segmental relationship to the nerve which mediates the primary pain.

Spring catarrh patient is usually a young boy who presents with marked itching in the eyes which becomes worse in summer. There develops flat cobble stone like papillae in the upper tarsal conjunctiva.

Sprouting many cereals and dals can be sprouted to advantage. The vitamin 'C' content goes up several times and contents of thiamine, riboflavin and nicotinamide are often doubled. Iron also becomes free and absorption becomes easier.

Sprue is a part of malabsorption syndrome. There develops glossitis, large pale, foul stools. The disease starts with intestinal problems. Excessive amount of fats are passed in stool. There may be severe glossitis and atrophy of filliform papillae. Painful burning sensations of tongue are common. Blood findings are similar to pernicious anaemia. Vitamin B_{12} helps. Gluten wheat and rye flour should be avoided.

Squamous acanthoma has no distinctive clinical appearance and can develop at any site of oral mucosa. It is a small, flat or elevated white or sessile or pedunculated lesion.

Squamous cell carcinoma is an intraoral white lesion and is most common to develop.

All squamous cell carcinoma don't invade and destroy bone. Carcinomas originating on or near the crest of mandibular ridge or on the posterior hard palate are the tumors to cause destruction of bone. Such tumors can be of two types peripheral or mucosal. In peripheral type patient may complain of worsening oral ulcer. Person may be alcoholic or smoking heavily. Other complaints are foul odour and taste. There may even be anesthesia of lip. While in central type patient will complain of pain and swelling. There may be anesthesia also. In peripheral type lytic effects of two types are seen. Semicircular or saucer shaped erosion into bony surface with ill defined borders. Mandibular lesion with advanced horizontal resorption is seen. Tooth may be migrated, loose and resorbed. Regional lymph glands will be enlarged. Glands will be enlarged, painless and very firm. Central squamous cell carcinoma is rare and appears as rounded radiolucency. To start border is smooth and regular, later on wall may be destroyed with ragged definitions. It may appear as extended oral leukoplakia and erythroplakia. It may be symptom less, white or red variegated patch. It is painless. Advanced lesion is fast growing irregular with large tumor mass. Ulcer has indurated borders with everted margin. Secondary infection may result in pain. It bleeds on touching. Tumor is fixed to tongue. Regional lymph nodes are tender, fixed and enlarged. Untreated case may destroy oral tissue and extend through cheek. Patient may not be able to eat food as pathological fracture of jaws may take place. Such cancer may also be present in intestine and lung. In an oral cavity itself two or more separate malignant lesions may be seen. Tongue lesions are more vascular and start bleeding even on slightest touch. Tongue may be fixed to mouth and patient may be unable to talk or swallow. Histologically lip carcinoma is well differentiated. Prognosis is good, before the metastasis occurs Radiographically bone involved shows large, irregular and ill defined radiolucent area and appears as of 'moth eaten' type. In addition to histopathology, exfoliative cytology is helpful. Toludine blue test is needed to detect dysplastic lesions.

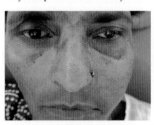
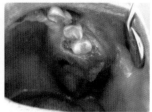

Squamous cell carcinoma of oral cavity

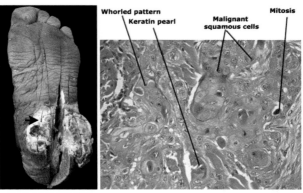

Squamous cell carcinoma foot

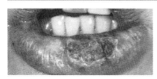

Squamous cell carcinoma

Squamous odontogenic tumors in maxilla, lesions are centered on the incisor cuspid area while in mandible lesions had a predilection for bicuspid molar area. Lesions are asymptomatic. On X-ray it looks as triangular or semicircular translucent area with or without sclerotic areas. It is made of squamous mature epithelium. Peripheral layer is flattened. Post surgery, there is no recurrence.

Stab wound is one in which depth of wound is more than length of skin. It is caused by sharp, pointed object like knife, spear, dagger etc. Edges of object may be sharp or blunt. If sharp the wound will be incised and blunt wound will be lacerated and `penetrating.

Stability of vitamins carotene is destroyed by heat in presence of air and copper. It can withstand boiling in alkaline solution. Thiamine is unstable in alkaline condition. Riboflavin is stable to air and destroyed by excessive heat and light. While nicotinic acid most stable of B-vitamins being unaffected by light, heat, air, acid or alkali. Only loses are during washing. Vitamin C is destroyed by enzyme present in leafy vegetables. Vitamin D is stable to all normal storage and processing conditions.

Stafne bone defect is a sharply defined cyst like area of radiolucency seen near the angle of mandible.

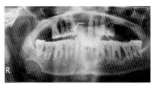

Stafney's cyst

Staggering gait is common to alcohol and barbiturate intoxication. Base is wide and steps are irregular.

Stain, extrinsic is a stain located on the outside of the tooth surface originating from external substances such as tobacco, coffee, tea or food; usually removed by polishing the teeth with an abrasive prophylaxis paste.

Stain, intrinsic is a stain originating from the ingestion of certain materials or chemical substances during tooth development, or from the presence of caries. This stain is permanent and cannot be removed.

Stainless steel is steel containing at least 12 percent chromium that forms a protective oxide coating keeping it away from corroding.

Stainless steel wire has good combination of mechanical properties and corrosion resistance in oral environment. Cost is reasonable. Modulus of elasticity ranges from about 160 to 180 gpa. The yield strength of these wires ranges from 1100 to 1500 mpa. Austenitic stainless steel alloys can be rendered susceptible to inter granular corrosion when heated to 400°C to 900°C due to formation of chromium carbides at grain boundaries.

Stainless-steel crowns are preformed extra coronal restorations that are particularly useful in the restoration of grossly broken down teeth, primary molars that have undergone pulp therapy, and hypoplastic primary or permanent teeth. They are also indicated when restoring the dentition of children at high risk of caries, particularly those having treatment under general anesthesia. SSCs are very durable restorations and should be the restoration of choice in the high-caries mouth.

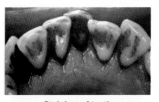

Staining of teeth

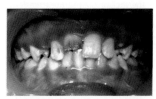

Stain occuring due to trauma

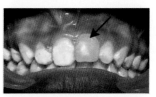

Stains occurring post composite restoration

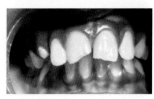

Stains occuring due to obturating material

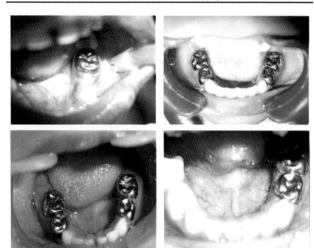

Primary stainless-steel crowns (SSC's)

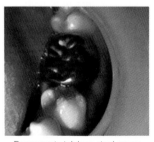

Permanent stainless-steel crown

Stammering is a disorder of articulation by repetition of sounds or syllables and by prolonged pauses in speech. Facial grimacing may accompany. It is not a result of acquired organic disease.

Stamping gait is seen in sensory ataxia. patient raises his feet very suddenly often abnormally high and then jerks forward bringing to the ground with a jerk. It is seen in tabes dorsalis.

Standard deviation is the square root of the variance expresed in units of original measure.

Standard error of measurement is a measure of absolute reliability. It represents the standard deviation of measurement errors.

Standard normal distribution is a normal distribution with a mean of 0.0 and a standard deviation of 1.0.

Staphylococcal pneumonia needs a separate description. It may cause a confluent bronchopneumonia in children. Due to appreciable tissue necrosis produces thin fluid pus. Small cystic cavities contain thin pus and air. It responds to antibiotics.

Staphylococcal scalded skin syndrome is an illness which is caused by exfoliative endotoxins produced by S. Aureus. Symptoms include rash, fever, malaise and irritability. There develops diffuse, tender, red rash with a sand paper texture. Bullae and

S

vesicles may appear and exfoliation of large sheets of epidermis is seen.

Startle reflex is similar to Moro reflex, but it is initiated by a sudden noise or any other stimulus. In this reflex, the elbows are flexed and the hands remains closed and there is a less outward and inward movement of the arms.

Starvation is when necessary food has been suddenly withheld. Feeling of hunger lasts for 36-48 hours. It is succeeded by pain in epigastrium relieved by pressure. After 4-5 days eyes appear sunken and glistening pupils are widely dilated. Cheeks become hollow. Lips become dry and cracked. Tongue becomes dry and coated with thick fur. Voice becomes weaker.

Static bone cyst is not a true cyst since it is not lined by epithelium. Hence it is known as pseudo cyst. Radiographically it is a well defined cyst like radio lucency in mandible inferior to mandibular canal. It may not require any treatment.

Static stretching is stretching a muscle in a stationary position.

Steam sterilization is a process where steam under pressure kills all bacteria, spores, fungi and viruses. Steam is produced in autoclave and is kept at temperature of 134° C for at least 3 minutes. Whole process may take 20 minutes. Steam is suitable for metal instruments, diamond and tungsten, rubber, swab, cotton and most plastics.

Stethoscope is an instrument used to amplify sound of heart and lungs.

Stevens – Johnson syndrome is a very severe bullous form of erythema multiforme with widespread involvement of skin, genitals and eyes. Suddenly patient may develop fever, photophobia and eruption of mucosa of oral cavity, skin and genitalia. Oral lesions may be so severe that mastication becomes impossible. There is no specific treatment. Sometimes cortisone helps.

Sticky wax is a brittle wax containing resin used to hold metal parts in investment of soldering. It fractures instead of deformed under stress.

Stillman's tooth brushing method is a method of tooth brushing providing gingival stimulation. Bristles are placed partly on cervical portion of tooth and partly on gingiva. Strokes are completed in each region and bush is moved to another area. Bristle ends are not directed into sulcus so can be recommended for clients with progressive recession. It is considered less traumatic to gingiva.

Stomion inferius (Stmi) is the median point in the vermilion of the lower lip.

Stomion superius (Stms) is a point indicating the mucocutaneous border of the upper lip. The most anterior point of the upper lip.

Stomach is a dilated portion of alimentary canal and has 3 functions. It stores food having a capacity of 1500 ml then it mixes the food with gastric secretion to form a semisolid chime and thirdly it regulates the rate of delivery of the chyme to small intestine. It has two openings cardiac and pyloric, two curvatures greater and lesser.

S

Stomatitis is also known as leukokeratosis. Smoker's patch develops on palate in heavy smoker. Lesions are limited to smoke area. To start with mucosa is reddened but becomes greyish white. It is thick and fissured. Histologically epithelium shows acanthosis and hyperkeratosis. There is chronic inflammation in the sub epithelial connective tissue. If smoker stops smoking changes are reversible. Lesion has no precancerous potential.

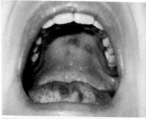

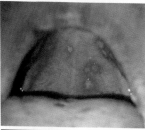

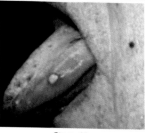

Stomatitis

Stomatitis medicamentosa is the term given to the eruptions occurring in the oral cavity due to the sensitivity of the drugs which has been consumed orally.

Stomatitis venenata also known as contact stomatitis is term given to the local reaction caused due to the use of medicament in the oral cavity e.g. aspirin burn .

Stone's index was introduced by Stone H.H, Lawton F.E, Bransby E R and Hartley H.O in 1949. The scoring is done as follows: 1- one point of one or more cavities in the same tooth detectable by sharp probe where the lesion has not penetrated through the enamel to involve the dentine. 2- Two points to one or more cavities in the same tooth where the dentine is involved, where a total of less than a quarter of the crown is estimated to have been destroyed. 3- Three points to one or more cavities in the same tooth resulting in a total destruction of more than a quarter of the crown

Stops are small, round, sterile pieces of rubber or plastic that are placed on endodontic instruments to mark the working length.

Storage phosphor screen technology this screen contains embedded phosphorus crystals that luminescence when stimulated by light at a specific wavelength. The energy released results in a latent image that is stored in the screen rather than on conventional film. No darkroom/day light loader required. No processing chemicals needed. Less image resolution. Less radiation required. The image detector is generally larger.

S

The image is immediately available. Image may be electronically transferred. Image may be enhanced. Image is easily altered. Image is easily copied. No duplicating film equipment needed. Image is large enough to be seen by patient.

Strain is defined as the deformation of the length/dimension of a dental material that results from applied stress. The stiffness of an object determines its ability to resist dimensional change or strain.

Streptococcal gingivostomatitis is a rare condition characterized by a presence of diffuse erythema of gingiva and other parts of oral mucosa, sometimes it may also appear as marginal erythema, studies indicate that group a beta-hemolytic streptococcus may be a main cause to this lesion.

Streptococcus mutans in 1924 Clarke isolated a streptococcus that predominated in many human carious lesions and that he named streptococcus mutans because of its varying morphology. Clarke noted that s.mutans adhered closely to tooth surfaces in artificially induced caries for the next 40 years; s.mutans was virtually ignored, until the 1960s when it was "rediscovered" and its prevalence in plaque confirmed. Characteristics of this group of streptococci have been described as non motile, catalase-negative, gram–positive cocci in short or medium chains. On mitis-salivarius agar they grow as highly convex to pulvinate (cushion–shaped) colonies. These colonies are opaque; the surface resembles frosted glass. These s.mutans variants also posses caries –inducing properties, and when re-isolated from infected animals they may resume the original rough colonial form.

Streptomycin is bactericidal and acts against gram positive and gram negative bacteria prevents bacterial protein synthesis. It is active against tuberculosis. In high doses toxicity is marked of eighth cranial nerve, vestibular damage is first noted. Auditory division is less vulnerable but tinnitus and deafness can occur. It is given I.M and is painful.

Stress is when an external force is applied to a specimen an internal force equal in magnitude but opposite in direction is set up. Stress = f/a where 'f' is the applied force and 'a' is the cross sectional area.

Stridor is a respiration produced by turbulent air flow through a narrow air passage. Inspiratory stridor is produced in obstructive lesions of supraglottis while expiratory stridor is produced in lesions of thoracic trachea and bronchial foreign body and tracheal stenosis. It is a noise produced by breathing when the trachea or larynx is obstructed. It is louder than wheezing.

Stroke is an abrupt loss of neurological function. It may be caused from atherosclerosis, aneurysm and malformations, decreased perfusion pressure and hemorrhage. Atherosclerosis is the most common cause of cerebral infarction. Hyper viscosity, hypercoagulability by producing cerebral venous thrombosis can impair cerebral blood flow. Smoking, diabetes mellitus, hypertension and hyperlipidemia with obesity are the predisposing factors.

Strokes are referred as the vertical or oblique movements performed during instrumentation.

Structural spinal disorder pain disc degeneration result in pain which is aggravated by activities. Staying in one position for long may also result in pain. Partial relief may be got by rest. Disc pain becomes worse with sitting, bending, lifting and straining activities. Pain is worst with extension type of activities.

Strychnine poisoning occurs due to poisonous, flat, circular disc, concave on one and convex on other side. They are 2 cm in diameter and ¼" thick. Ash gray in color have shiny surface. These are too bitter. It acts with in 5 to 10 minutes. Chocking sensation in throat and stiffness of neck, face and stretching of face start. Convulsion are first clonic and then becomes tonic.

Sturge – Webber disease is congenital disease with combination of angioma of lepto meninges over cerebral cortex with angiomatous lesion of face. Sturge – Webber syndrome person develops orofacial and meningeal angiomatosis with secondary mental deficiency. There may be seizures, hemiplegia and mild to severe enlargement of gingiva. Hyperplastic vascular gingival blanch on pressure. Bony hemangiomas and delayed tooth eruption may be noted. Convulsions may be controlled by anticonvulsant drugs.

Subarachnoid hemorrhage can be caused by rupture of a cerebral aneurysm or rupture of arteriovenous malformation. Early diagnosis and surgery has a significant future. Symptoms include worst headache of life, neck pain and back and radicular pain. Focal or generalized neurological abnormalities may be seen. Causative factors are saccular aneurysm, ruptured AV malformation and hypertension. Saccular aneurysms are congenital thin sac like protrusion from circle of wills. It develops in anterior circulation. Mycotic aneurysms occur at distal ends of cerebral vessels. Person will develop orbital pain/occipital headache. CSF study shows blood. Xanthochromia and RBC in CSF disappear after 2 weeks of blood.

Subclinical is without clinical manifestation.

Subdural hematoma There will be decreased level of consciousness involving head injury. Seizures may develop with focal neurologic symptoms. Confusion and personality change results. Pupil will dilate with hemiparesis.

Subgingival biofilm forms below the subgingival plaque residing in a more protected location is not subject to the same degree of intraoral abrasion or salivary host defense components. The main determinants limiting its growth are physical space and the innate defense system of the host. One result of subgingival plaque accumulation is a continual increase in the space available by reducing epithelial cell attachment levels and increasing pocket depth. The innate host defense system limits this spread by maintaining an intact epithelial cell barrier. GCF, although a rich source of nutrients, contains a potent array of antimicrobial activities. It contains innate components which include lysozymes, complement and a variety of vascular permeability enhancers such as Bradykinin, thrombin and fibrinogen and adaptive components including antibodies and lymphocytes.

Subgingival calculus is the one which is located below the crest of the marginal gingiva and is therefore not visible in the oral cavity. The calculus is hard, dense and frequently dark in color. Sublingual calculus are generally much harder being denser. Such calculus is less extensive, flatter and more brittle and darker in color. These are deposited at irregular intervals throughout life.

Sublingual gland produces 2-5% of total salivary volume. It lies above the mylohyoid, below the mucosa of the floor of the mouth, medial to the sublingual fossa of the mandible and lateral to the genioglossus. About 15 ducts emerge from the gland. Most of them open directly into the floor of the mouth on the summit of the sublingual fold. A few of them join the submandibular duct.

Sublingual keratosis develops as white lesion on the floor of mouth and ventral tongue. Malignant changes have been noted. It is a white soft plaque with a finely wrinkled surface. There is irregular but well defined outline. There is no associated inflammation (*see* Figure).

Sublingual plaque is a plaque that forms under the gum line.

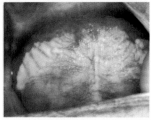

Sublingual keratosis

Sublingual space refers to the space existing below the oral mucosa in the anterior part of the floor of the mouth and contains sublingual gland, its excretory ducts, submandibular duct which is traversed by lingual nerve and hypoglossal nerve. Infection to this area raises the floor of the mouth and displaces tongue, resulting in pain and difficulty in swallowing.

Submandibular gland is a paired muco-serous gland lying in the submandibular space. The inferior surface is covered by skin, platysma, and submandibular lymph nodes. Lateral surface is related to, submandibular fossa of mandible and medial surface is related to the extrinsic muscles of tongue and mylohyoid muscle. Secretions are discharged into the

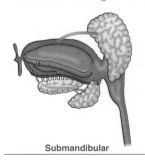

Submandibular

oral cavity through Wharton's duct which runs forward from the anterior border of the upper part, raising a fold of mucous membrane in the floor of the mouth and opens on little papilla to the side of the lingual papilla just behind the lower incisor teeth. The submandibular duct is approximately 5 cm long.

Submandibular space refers to the space existing external to the sublingual space, below the mylohyoid and hyoglossus muscle. The space contains the submandibular gland, which extends slightly above the mylohyoid muscle thus communicating with sublingual space.

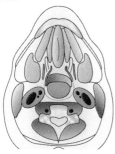

Submandibular space

Submental space refers to the space existing between the mylohyoid muscle superiorly and the platysma inferiorly, bounded posteriorly by hyoid bone and laterally by mandible. It is traversed by anterior belly of digastrics muscle. Infection results in swelling of submental region.

Submerged teeth are generally deciduous teeth specially second molar which undergoes variable degree of root absorption. It

becomes ankylosed with bone. X-ray confirms it.

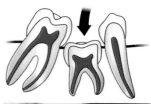

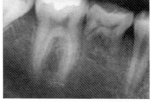

Submerged, ankylosed teeth

Subphrenic abscess intra peritoneal infection, appendicitis or perforation of G.I. Tract may result in it. Pus may track from one compartment to another compartment. General symptoms are more marked than any local symptoms. There will be unexplained fever, right upper abdominal tenderness and pain. Liver is pushed down and diaphragm is elevated. Chest movement is slowed down. Surgical drain under antibiotic cover helps.

Substance polypeptide acts as an excitatory neurotransmitter. It is released from spinal cord cells by A and C fibre afferent stimulation and excites dorsal horn neurons.

Substrate is the material being abraded.

Succedaneous is a tooth that replaces or succeeds another.

Succedaneous teeth are permanent teeth which replace or succeed the primary teeth. While permanent molars are nonsuccedaneous teeth they don't replace primary teeth.

Suckling is a specialized form of ingestion where mother's nipple is drawn deep in mouth. Everted lips form a seal lingual muscular activity generates a peustaetic wave moving posteriorly which milk the nipple and propels it toward the pharynx.

Sucralose is an artificial sweetner that is 600 times sweeter than sucrose derived from sucrose. It is claimed not to be hydrolyzed nor dechlorinated in the body.

Sucrose is a disaccharide composed of glucose + fructose i.e. table sugar.

Suicidal wounds are located inside the mouth, over temple, under chin or on left side of chest. *Fire arm* may remain grasped in cadaveric spasm. Wound is directed from below upwards. Wound is single. Due to close range of wound scorching or blackening of area is found. There will be no signs of struggle. Room may be locked from inside and farewell note may be found.

Sulcular epithelium lines the sulcus of the gingiva and can be described as thin, nonkeratinized stratified squamous epithelium which extends from the coronal limit of the junctional epithelium to border of marginal gingiva.

Sulcular fluid is the tissue fluid that seeps into the gingival sulcus through the wall of sulcus.

Sulcus is a broad depression on the chewing surfaces of your back teeth.

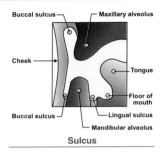

Sulcus

Sulphonamide are generally bacteriostatic rather than bactericidal. It acts by interfering with the utilization of para amino benzoic acid bacteria. In 1900 first sulphonamide para-amino-benzene-sulphomide was synthe-sized. It is extensively used in gonorrhoea. Kidney excretes it. Occasional occurrence of Agranulocytosis may develop. Mostly these are used in respiratory and urinary tract infection.

Summation theory is an alternative theory postulating that pain does not depend on specific pathways but on excessive stimulation involving all types of receptors with the resultants central neural summation or convergence of activity.

Superego is prohibition learned from environment, more from parents and authorities. Act as censor of acceptability of thoughts feeling and behavior. It is determined by regulation imposed on the child by parent's society and culture. It is internalized control produced a feeling of shame guilt. The expression of discomfort (anxiety fear) by the child is the result conflict between the three components as the psychic structure.

Superficial dermal burns are the one which involve the epidermis and the papillary dermis. These also heal on their own by epithelial growth from the abundant skin appendages but slower than epidermal burns because as we go deeper the number of epithelial cells decreases and amount of connective tissue increases. Therefore the healing in these burns is by regeneration and repair both which gives a scar. These usually heal in 14 days.

Superficial partial thickness burns refer superficial dermal burns.

Superior alveolar neuritis involves maxillary dental plexus and is the direct extension of inflammation of antral mucosa. There may be burning neuritic pain. No muscle or autonomic symptoms are present.

Superior levator labii alaque nasi arises from frontal portion of maxilla. It passes obliquely downwards and divides into two medial and lateral slips. The laterals slip raises and events the upper lip, the medial slip acts as a dilator of nostril.

Supernumerary breasts usually occur along milk line extending from nipple to the symphysis pubis. These can be seen as small spots of two to three minutes.

Supernumerary roots refer to development of increased number of roots on a tooth compared with that classically described in dental anatomy. Both deciduous and permanent can be involved. Detection of supernumerary root is critical when endodontic therapy and exodontics is under taken. Otherwise no specific treatment is required.

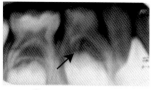

Supermumerary root

Supernumerary teeth are the extra teeth, in addition to the development of the normal 32. *Supernumerary teeth* occur more frequently in the permanent dentition. 90% of the cases occur in the maxilla with strong predilection for the anterior region. The most common region is the maxillary central incisor followed by maxillary 4th molar. Most supernumerary teeth are unilateral. Supernumerary tooth located between maxillary central incisors is termed mesiodens. Supernumerary 4th molar is called distomolar. A supernumerary tooth situated lingually or buccally to a molar is called paramolar. Supernumerary teeth are morphologically classified as either supplemental or rudimentary. Supplemental teeth duplicate the typical anatomy of posterior or anterior teeth. Rudimentary supernumerary teeth are dysmorphic and can assume conical or tuberculate form. The eruption of supernumerary teeth is variable and depends on the space available. 70% of supernumerary teeth in the anterior maxilla fail to erupt. In such situation midline diastema is common. Whenever there is a large midline diastema, radiographic evaluation to detect presence of supernumerary tooth is essential. Supernumerary teeth can also prevent eruption of adjacent teeth, displacement or rotation, crowding. Unerupted supernumerary teeth can be associated with cyst. At times they can erupt into nasal cavity as well. Meticulous clinical and radiographic examination is required to detect supernumerary teeth. Horizontal tube shift technique where two periapical radiographs are taken at different horizontal angulation is helpful in detecting the position of the unerupted teeth.

Suppurations is a purulent discharge forming in the wound cavities. Common suppuration is lung abscess, brain abscess, pyocele and perpural sepsis. Similarly common infection can also give rise rigors such as tonsil-litis, sinusitis and bronchiectasis.

Suppurative arthritis of Temporo mandibular Joint consists of spasm of masseter muscles, difficulty of opening of mouth. There can be fever, leukocytosis and general malaise. X-ray may show normal findings.

Suppurative inflammation damage to vessels is severe. Plenty of neutrophils are killed in inflammation. Dead neutrophil and degraded products, necrosed tissue with inflammation is called purulent inflammation.

Suprabony pocket pocket is the term used where the base of the pocket is coronal to the under-lying alveolar bone. It is also known as supracrestal and supra alveolar pocket.

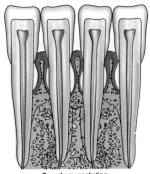

Suprabony pocketing
(horizontal bone loss)
Suprabony pocket

Supragingival biofilm forms above the gingival margin. Supragingival plaque growth, being located in contact with the oral cavity, is subject to much more intraoral abrasion which restricts its net accumulation. In addition, this biofilm is subject to flow characteristics of saliva and its host defense components. Saliva contains secretory IgA, lactoferrin, lysozymes and peroxidases that display a wide spectrum of antimicrobial activity and serve to limit both coloniza-tion and spread of the supr-agingival bacterial biofilm.

Supragingival calculus is the calculus which is present coronal to the gingival margin and is visible in the oral cavity. It is usually whitish yellow in color, clay like consistency and easily detached from the oral cavity. It mainly occurs on the lingual aspect of the lower incisors and the buccal aspect of the maxillary molars.

Supragingival is the area above the gingival margin.

Supragingival plaque is a plaque located above the gingival margin.

Surface anesthetics are the agents that anesthetize the surface of mucous membrane so that syringe needle can be inserted painlessly. It is used as spray, solution/paste. It is applied a few minutes before the injection. 5% lignocaine generally used.

Surface coat is the first coating applied to a wax pattern or the surface of mould that comes in direct contact with a cast metal.

Surface energy is an extra energy that atoms or molecules on the surface of a substance have over those in the interior. The surface energy of a liquid is referred to as surface tension expressed in erg/cm^2.

Surface tension force acting parallel to the boundary surface, generally expressed in $dynes/cm$.

Surgical chisels and hoes are the instruments used during the periodontal surgery for removing and reshaping the bone. The hoe has curved shank and blade whereas the chisel is straight shanked. The surgical hoe has flattened fishtail shaped blade with a pronounced convexity in its terminal portion. It is used for detaching pocket walls after the gingivectomy incisions. It is helpful for smoothening root and bone surfaces.

Surgical ciliated cyst of maxilla develops after surgical entry into maxillary sinus. Patient complains of nonspecific poorly localized pain and tenderness. Swelling is evident. X-ray will show radiolucent area closely related to maxillary sinus. Filling defect of cyst can be seen. Treatment includes enucleation.

Surgical crown lengthening is the process where clinical crown height of teeth can be increased by surgically repositioning the gingival margin with alveolar bone recontouring. This procedure creates longer teeth but maintains the existing vertical dimension.

Surgical files are instruments which are mainly used for smoothening of bony ledges and to remove all areas of bone.

Surgical mallet is a special nylon tipped hammer used with a surgical chisel to remove bone.

Surgical scissors are sharp bladed scissors used to trim soft tissues and cut suture material.

Surgical stent is a clear acrylic template placed over the alveolar ridge to assist in locating the proper placement for dental implants.

Surgical suction tip is a small sized evacuator tip used to remove blood and other oral fluids from the wall of root canal.

Survey is a research method based on self reported information from participants rather than observations.

Susceptible host is the one who is unable to resist infection by the pathogens. Host is in poor health and has compromised immune system.

Sutural dominance theory was put forward by Sicher and says that proliferation of sutural connective tissue causes appositional growth. Genetic factor was accepted and the membranous bones were considered as growth centers.

Suture is a joining of two bones, also stitches.

Suture instruments include dissecting forceps, needle holders, suture needle, spencer wall forceps and scissors.

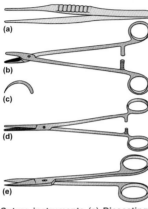

Suture instruments (a) Dissecting forceps; (b) Needle holders; (c) Suture needle; (d) Spencer Wells forceps; (e) Scissors

Suture needle is a curved needle used with suture material to close the surgical site.

Swallowing is a complex muscular act which prevents the ball of food entering nasal cavity or larynx. It is propelled by the tongue from mouth to the back of throat. From here it goes down to esophagus.

Sweat retention syndrome is an extravasation of sweat in the tissue with subsequent inflammation, keratin plug formation in sweat glands.

Sympathetic nervous system is the part of autonomic nervous system which arises in the thoracic and first three lumbar segments of spinal cord.

Symptoms of nicotine poisoning are nausea and salivation occurs quickly and is followed by pain and severe diarrhoea. Cold sweat is prominent. Headache, dizziness, disturbed hearing and vision, mental confusion are experienced. Respiration is stimulated and blood pressure may be elevated. Pupils first constrict and later on dilate.

Symptoms are effects of disease noticed by patient himself.

Synchondrosis refers to absent or minimal movements of joints. Examples include intercostals joint and a joint between diaphysis and epiphysis.

Syncope is a transient loss of consciousness without prodromal symptoms that is followed within seconds to minutes (< 30 minutes) by resumption of consciousness. Although many causes do exist, a closer examination reveals 3 factors. These factors include stress, impaired physical status, administration or ingestion of drugs. Syncope is a complicated problem frequently encountered in clinical practice. It describes a loss of consciousness, usually from a sudden decrease in cerebral blood flow. Brain can with stand only a few seconds of total interruption of blood flow without loss of consciousness. It is the most common medical emergency encountered in dental office cause may be fear, anxiety, emotional upset or pain due to reduced flow of blood to the brain. Facial skin becomes pallor and clammy. Pulse rate increases markedly, pupils dilate and depth of respiration increases.

Syndesmoses in these joint bones are held together by an intraosseous ligament. Example includes inferior tibiofibular joint and radio ulnar joint.

Synergistic acting jointly. Adding the effect of another drug.

Synovial ball and socket joint is a multiaxial joint having movements around more than 2 axes. Examples include hip and shoulder joint.

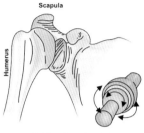

Ball and socket joint

Synovial chondromatosis contains multiple cartilaginous nodules of synovial membrane and loose calcified bodies in joints. Part of the synovium calcify and break off into the joint space.

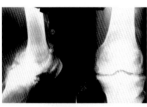

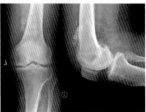

Synovial chondromatosis

Synovial condylar joint are biaxial joints and movement include flexion, extension, abduction and adduction. Examples are wrist joint, metacarpophalangeal joint atlanto-occipital and meta tarso phalangeal joint.

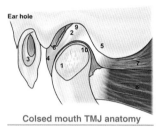

Colsed mouth TMJ anatomy

Synovial hinge joint results movement around one joint, flexion and extension. Elbow joint and interphalangeal joints are its example.

Synovial pivot joint is a uniaxial joint and rotational movement. Examples of joint includes superior and inferior radioulnar joint.

Synovial sarcoma is malignancy arising from articulate or para articular site, bursae or tendon sheath. It develops in young people. In oral cavity cheek, tongue, floor of mouth and soft palate are involved. There may be fibrosarcoma like proliferation of cells with collagen and reticulin. Early radical excision gives better results.

Synthetic phenols are compounds with broad spectrum disinfecting action.

Syphilitic oral ulcer is painless until secondarily infected. Lip or tip of tongue is affected. Size may vary from 5 mm to several cms. Edges of ulcer are raised and indurated. It is highly infectious and heals without scar. Regional lymph glands are enlarged, rubbery and discrete.

Systemic lupus erythematosis was described by Sir William Osler in 1895. He described the systemic manifestations of this chronic systemic inflammatory disease with alternating exacerbations and remissions. It is characterized by multi organ involvement including polyarthritis (poly-arthralgia, avascular bone necrosis). Skin butterfly rash, is an erythematous rash involving areas of body, chronically expo-sed to UV light, mucosal ulcera-tion, oral and genital mucosa in 15% cases. Nephritis, glomerulitis either diffuse membranous, sclerosing with small vessel vasculitis, splinter hemorrhage, periungual occlusion, finger pulp infarctions may develop.

Systemic sclerosis is a progressive fibrosis of skin and multiple organs. There is induration of skin and fixation of epidermis to the deeper subcutaneous tissue. It begins on face, hands and trunk. Skin becomes yellow, gray or ivory white waxy appearance. Tongue, soft palate and larynx are the structures involved. Tongue often becomes stiff and board like. Gingival tissues are pale and unusually firm. Lips become thin, rigid and partially fixed. Dysphagia and chocking sensa-tion also develop. There is no adequate treatment.

Systemic therapy is a treatment that reaches and affects cells through out the body.

T-cells do not express Ig but detect presence of foreign substances by way of surface protein called T Cell Receptor (TCR). TCR is a heterogeneous clan of membrane proteins on T-cells consisting of a pair of transmembrane polypeptides of alpha and beta chains. TCR share structural and functional properties with Ig and are closely related to each other in evolution. TCR are *never secreted*; hence, T cells lack the ability to strike their targets at long distance. They exert their protective effects through direct contact with a target or by influencing activity of other immune cells. They are the principal cells involved in cell-mediated immunity. T cells can detect foreign substances only in specific context; can recognize a foreign particle only if first cleaved into small peptides and displayed on the surface of second host cell 'antigen presenting cell (APC)'. Antigen presentation depends on specific protein *'Major Histocompatibility Complex (MHC)'* in surface of APC and this combination is recognized by a T cell receptor.

Tactile pertaining to touch.

Tactile sensitivity is the ability to distinguish relative degrees of roughness and smoothness on the surface of tooth.

Talons cusp (Accessory cusps/ supernumerary cusps) is a cusp like structure projecting from the cingulum of incisors. In shape it resembles an eagle's talon. It can be considered as dens evaginatus of anterior teeth. It is predomina-

tely seen on maxillary permanent lateral incisors and very rarely seen on deciduous teeth. Like dens evaginatus talon cusp is composed of enamel, dentin and pulp extension. Talon cusp is common in Chinese, Caucasians and African –Americans. Incidence of talon cusp is high in patients with Rubinstein – Taybi syndrome and Sturge-Weber syndrome.

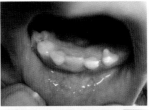
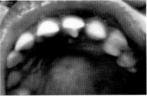
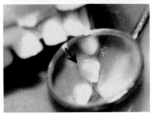

Talon cusp

Tansfixation is a type of method of achieving immobilization in dentulous as well as edentulous mandible using Kirschner wires, where 2 mm krischner wire is inserted within the medullary cavity across the fracture line.

The wire is cut off at skin entry point from where it can be withdrawn once.

Tardive dyskinesia is a repetitive uncontrolled activity of head, jaw, tongue and lips. It may occur due to long term use of phenothiazines. Symptoms include rapid repetitive movements of lips.

Tarnish is a chemical reaction between a metal and its environment that results in discoloration of the surface of metal.

Tartar see calculus.

Taste is a sensation and may be deformed in many ways. Ageusia is a complete loss of taste while hypogeusia is decreased taste for all taste stimuli. Dysguesia is a perversion of taste. Hypergeusia is an increased sensitivity for all tastes, while gustatory agnosia is a loss of ability to distinguish and identify different tastes.

Taurodontism is an enlargement of the body and pulp chamber of a multirooted tooth with apical displacement of the pulpal floor and bifurcation of the roots. Affected teeth tend to be rectangular in shape and a bull like appearance. There is increased apico-occlusal height of pulp chamber and furcation is close to the apex. The diagnosis is made from the radiographic appearance. Depending on the degree of apical displacement of the pulpal floor taurodontism can be mild, moderate or severe. If endodontic treatment is required in such tooth, the shape of the pulp chamber increases the difficulty of locating, instrumenting and obturating the pulp canals.

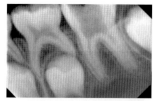
Mild taurodontism

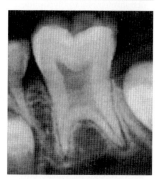
Taurodontism

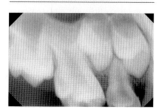
Severe taurodontism of maxillary molar

Teething is a process where the baby teeth are pushing through gums.

Temper refers to the spring character of an orthodontic wire, which is related to the mechanical properties of yielding strength and resilience.

Temporal arteritis is a rare, febrile or inflammatory disease of variable duration. Distended arteries are extremely tender on palpation. Headache, scalp hyperalgesias and painful mastication are present. It is a type of immunologic vasculitis and is a self limiting disease of many days.

Temporal lobe tumor produces expressive aphasia and impaired performance of hearing. Auditory illusions, hallucination psychomotor seizure or visual hallucination develop.

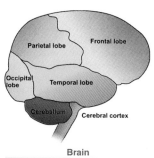

Brain

Temporary bridges are those intermittent restorations that are necessary between visits to prevent pain and space closure.

Temporary fillings are a first aid measure to relieve pain. Zinc oxide, Zinc phosphate and gutta percha are used. These are soft and soluble and will not remain for long hence are not to be used for permanent filling.

Temporomandibular disorder is a deviation from normal function which includes restricted movement of mandible, 2 mm deviation of mandible on opening, pain on palpation of masticatory muscles. There may be sound in temporomandibular

joint and pain during chewing and swallowing.

Temporomandibular dysfunction involves both muscle and joint derangements. Physical therapy and relaxation techniques are beneficial. Intraoral splints provide relief.

Temporomandibular joint (TMJ) is a synovial joint where temporo (temporal bone), mandibular (lower jaw) is the connecting hinge between the lower jaw and base of the skull.

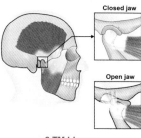

2.TMJ-Image

Temporomandibular joint arthritis occurs during periods of severe psychic stress, clenching and bruxism may become exaggerated and lead to severe mandibular joint and muscle pain. Marital problems, menopause and fatigue all may result the condition. X-ray may show evidence of bone resorption or irregularity of head of condyle or anterior slope of glenoid fossa.

TENS stands for Transcutaneous electrical nerve stimulation which has been used in the treatment of phantom limb pain; peripheral nerve injury joint pain, etc. Electrical stimulus is typically generated from a portable battery operated device. Mode of action is not very well understood. It blocks pain signals carried over to small unmyelinated 'C' fibres.

Tension headache is bilateral and diffuse. It is felt as a sense of tightness, pressure in head and band like constriction. Onset is gradual and may persist for a few days. During worry and anxiety headache is worst. These responses best to anxiolytics and antidepressants.

Teratogenesis is the development of organic defects due to certain drug used in pregnancy.

Teratoma is the neoplasm composed of multiple tissues including those which are normally not found in the organ in which it arises. It is a heterotopic collection of various forms. Benign tumors are cystic lesions. Walls of lesion are thickened. These contain hair, sebaceous material and teeth. Teeth are uncommon in malignant form of teratoma. Teeth resemble bicuspid.

Tertian fever refers to the type of fever that comes on alternate day.

Tertiary health care offers super specialized care. It is proved by regional and central level of institutions.

Tertiary prevention is a post pathogenic prevention. It includes techniques designed to replace lost tissues and rehabilitate a normal like function. It is done to prevent any further damage and maintain homeostasis.

Tertiary syphilis develops after 5-10 years of primary lesion affecting every organ of the body. It mainly affects CNS and CVS. Typical lesion is 'gumma'. It is a localized chronic granulomatous lesion having either nodular or ulcerated surface. Ulcer is a punched out ulcer having vertical walls. Base is dull, red granulomatous with irregular outline. Skin lesions leave tissue paper like scars.

Tertiary syphilitic oral ulcer is a very rarely seen after the invent of penicillin. It is known as gumma, a destructive granulomatous process. It is painless. Usually palate, tongue and tonsils are affected. Shape is round with punched out areas. Floor is depressed with a pale appearance. Edges are punched out.

Testes are located in scrotum. Testosterone is a steroid secreted on the stimulation of luteinizing hormone. It helps in maturation of sperm and is responsible for

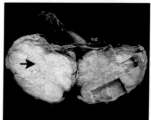

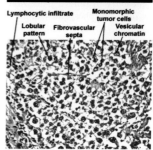

Lymphocytic infiltrate   Monomorphic tumor cells

Lobular pattern   Fibrovascular septa   Vesicular chromatin

Seminoma testis

sex characteristics. It helps in growth and development of male reproductive organs, musculoskeletal growth, growth and distribution of hair and enlargement of larynx accompanied by voice changes.

Tetanus is a disease that is caused by a gram positive, actively motile, anerobic spore bearing rod called clostridium tetani. It is found in soil and horse dung. Organism may enter through injury. Clinical features develop within 14 days. Symptoms appear once toxins fix to cell bodies of motor nerves. Incubation period is 5 to 15 weeks. Short duration indicates of serious disease. Titanic spasm follows within 24-72 hours of lock jaw. Diagnosis is clinical and does not require clinical confirmation. Convulsion becomes less frequent after 10 days and survivors recover completely by 4 weeks. There develops pain and stiffness in jaws and neck muscle. It results in dysphagia. After stimuli reflex spasm develops. Cranial tetanus paralyses 7th nerve.

Tetany is a condition that occurs due to low extracellular calcium condition developing with marked muscle cramps, twitching and convulsions.

Tetracycline is a broad spectrum antibiotic drug which forms complex with calcium and deposit on tooth. Tetracycline has a wider range of activity. Spectrum includes most species of gram positive and gram negative bacteria and spirochetes. These are absorbed slowly from GIT. Larger the dose, less of proportion is absorbed. Peak levels in blood occur after 3 hours hence 6 hour interval between two doses is sufficient. All tetracyclines are chelating agents. In fetus or growing child permanent staining of teeth may occur. The degree and color of staining varies with different tetracycline in different doses. Retardation of fetal growth is noted down when given during pregnancy.

Tetracycline pigmentation fluoresces bright yellow under ultraviolet light. Tetracycline can cross the placenta to stain the developing teeth and fetus. It is deposited along the incremental lines of dentine. Long treatment produces broader band of stain and deeper discoloration. Stain is permanent and incisors become ugly.

Tetracycline stains are endogenous stains that occured due to the use of tetracycline drug at the time of prenatal or postnatal dental development. The drug was widely used once upon a time to fight variety of infections. At that point little was known about the side effects of the drug. The antibiotic has an affinity towards the mineralized tissue and gets absorbed by the hard tissues of the body. Since the drug also has a capability to pass across the placenta and enters the fetal circulation, so when the expecting mother is administered this drug during the third trimester, the drug gets deposited in the forming bones and teeth of the fetus. Discoloration can also occur when the drug is administered to the child in infancy and early childhood.

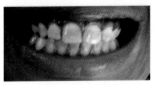

Tetracycline stains

Thalamic pain can occur due to spinal cord lesions that affects spinothalamic tracts resulting in painful limbs. Similarly a lesion of thalamus itself may cause severe pain in the contralateral face and arm/leg. Thalamic pain is intense, burning and continuous. It is felt around angle of mouth and cheek.

Thalassemia is a group of chronic hemolytic anemia. The disease is inherited as autosomal dominant trait. It produces thin, fragile erythrocytes. In this condition, there is insufficient synthesis of alpha and beta chains of hemoglobin. It is detected in first two years of life. There may be jaundice, fever with chills. Marked anemia is of micro-chronic microcytic type. WBC count is high with malaise. Bone marrow shows cellular hyper-plasia with large number of immature primitive and stem form of red cells. Spleen is enlarged. Mongoloid face is due to prominence of premaxilla. Death often occurs during puberty. Oral manifestations include spacing of anterior maxillary teeth. Pallor of oral mucosa, bimaxillary protrusion and Prominent molar bones with delayed pneumatization of sinuses develop discoloration of teeth is due to iron. Skull bones will show "hair on end"

appearance. Jaw bones may show "salt and pepper effect".

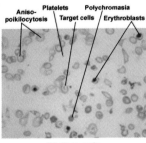

Thalassemia

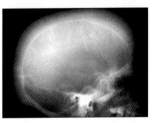

Sun ray appearance

Thelarche is faster breast development in absence of additional signs of sexual maturation. Exact cause is not known.

Theory is a paper about relation-ship specially defined concepts that describe, explain or predict some phenomenon in professio-nal discipline/action.

Therapeutic Inhalation Menthol and eucalyptus form an aromatic inhalation and this when mixed with hot water gives rise to vapors. These when inhaled sooths the inflamed mucous membrane. Steam serves the purpose of humidifying the dry mucosal secretions and facilitate their removal.

Therapeutic occlusion is said to be present where the specific interventions are designed to treat the disease.

Therapy refers to the treatment of a disease.

Thermal conductivity is a measure of speed at which heat travels per second through a given thickness of 1 cm when one side of material is maintained at a constant temperature i.e. 1° C higher than the other side. Thermal conductivity depends on the distance heat travels, area through which heat travels and the difference of temperature between source and destination.

Thermal diffusivity is a measure of heat transfer of a material in the time dependant state.

Thermogenic is a process that creates heat.

Thermometer is the device used to measure temperature.

Thermoplastic is the property of softening on heating and hardening on cooling.

Thermoset is a polymer which is not able to undergo softening upon heating.

Thiamine (Vitamin B$_1$) was the first of the Vitamin B complex discovered. Thiamine B$_1$ vitamin is water soluble and is destroyed by refining, exposure to alkalies such as baking powder. Up to 50% is lost in cooking water and 15% during baking. Toasting of bread destroys further 15% for thick slice or up to 30% for thin slice. Recommended daily intake is 0.4 mg/ 1000 Kcal or about 1.2 mg in adult man. Limited amount is synthesized by microorganisms in GIT. Normally, about 25-35 mg is stored in the body. Deficiency of it leads to accumulation of pyruvic and lactic acid in tissues and body fluids. Severe deficiency may lead to neurological and mental deficiency.

Thiazides are derivatives of sulphonamides and are used as weaker diuretics. These exert their diuretic effect by inhibiting the Na$^+$ CL$^-$ transport in early distal convoluted tubules. These cause increased loss of K$^+$ and Mg but reduce calcium excretion. These are indicated in hypertension, mild heart failure, and idiopathic hypercalciuria.

Thiopentone has lately been superseded in outpatient dental practice by short acting methohexitone. Thiopentone is freshly prepared to produce 2.5% solution by dissolving powder in sterile distilled water. Dose is 4 to 7 mg/kg body weight. It is a powerful myocardial depressant.

Third branchial arch Branchial arches are formed in the pharangeal wall due to the prolyeratring ateral plate mesoderm and migrating neural crest cell. The arches are clearly seen as bulges on the lateral aspect of the embryo and are externally separated by small cleft called branhial grooves and internally small depression called pharyngeal pouches. The cartilage of this small arch produces the greater horn and caudal part of the body of the hyoid bone. The remainder of the cartilage disappears. The mesoderm forms the stylopharyngeal muscle, inerveted by the IXth nerve glossopharyngeal supplying the arch. The mucosa of the posterior third of the tongue is derived from this arch, which accounts for its sensory innervations by the glossopharyngeal nerve. The artery of this arch contributes to the common carotid and part of the internal carotid arteries. Neural crest tissue in the third arch forms the carotid body which first appears as a mesenchymal condensation around the third aortic arch artery. This chemoreceptor body thus derives its nerve supply from the glossopharyngeal nerve.

Third degree burns is involving entire epidermis and dermis and all dermal appendages so there is no spontaneous healing of the wound, leaving an ulcer. Since the entire thickness of skin is burned with no tissue left for repair and regeneration, these will require skin grafting or will close by contractures wherein two raw surfaces fuse together.

Third molar see wisdom tooth.

Third pharyngeal pouch the ventral diverticulum endoderm proliferates and migrates from each side to form two elongated diverticulum that grow caudally into the surrounding mesenchyme to form the elements of thymus gland. The two thymic rudiments meet in the midline but do not fuse, being united by connective tissue. Lymphoid cells invade the thymus from hemopoietic tissue during the 3rd month of IU. The dorsal diverticulum endoderm differentiates and migrates caudally to form inferior parathyroid gland. The gland derived from the endodermal lining of the pouch loses their connection with the pharyngeal wall when the

pouches become obliterated during later development. The lateral glosso-epiglotic fold represents the third pharyngeal pouch.

Three – quarter crowns actually covers four – fifths of the tooth surface – mesial, distal, occlusal, lingual or palatal. They are always made up of cast metal and are used when the buccal surface of the tooth is intact. The advantage of these types of crowns is that they are more conservative of tooth tissue than complete crowns and the margin does not approach gingival margin buccally.

Thromboangitis obliterans is an inflammatory occlusive peripheral vascular disease of unknown etiology affecting arteries and veins especially of lower limbs. Smoking is the risk factor. Small and medium sized arteries are more involved. There is proliferation of intima and thrombosis. There develops digital ulceration or pain from ischemia. Arteriography and biopsy are confirmatory.

Thrombocythemia is an increased number megakaryocytes resulting in a raised level of circulating platelets that is mostly dysfunctional. Etiology is not known. Epistaxia and intestinal bleeding exists. Hemorrhage into skin is found. There may be spontaneous gingival bleeding. After dental extraction also excessive bleeding takes place. Radioactive phosphorus and blood transfusion helps.

Thrombocytopenia is very low quantity of platelets in circulatory system. These patients have tendency to bleed from small capillaries while in hemophilia bleeding is from larger vessels. As a result large punctate bleeding develops over skin. For bleeding count should fall below 50,000 per cu/mm. Level below 10,000 becomes lethal.

Thromboplastin – Substance is produced in blood. It plays a role in the coagulation process.

Throttling is a condition where the constriction is produced by pressure of fingers and palm. Finger marks may be found on either side of front of neck i.e. wind pipe. Marks are obliquely downwards and outwards one below the other.

Throwing power is a measure of the uniformity in plating thickness of irregular surface.

Thrush is known as psuedomembranous candidiasis. Actually it is a superficial infection of upper layers of mucosal epithelium. It forms a patchy white plaques or flecks on mucosal surface. Once you remove this area of erythema shallow ulceration is seen. Antifungal drugs are helpful. In infants lesions are soft, white or bluish. It is adherent to oral mucosa. Intraoral lesions are painless and being removed with difficulty. It leaves a raw bleeding surface. Any mucosal area of mouth may be involved. Constitutional symptoms are not present but in adults rapid onset of a bad taste may develop. Some may feel burning of mouth also. Causative organisms are yeast like fungus causing thrush. It occurs in both yeast and mycelia forms of oral cavity and infected tissue. Candida species are normal inhabitants of the oral flora. Concentration is 200-500 cells per ml of saliva. Carrier state is more in diabetics. The wearing of removal prosthetic appliances may also become asymptomatic carrier. Predisposing factors include – after administration of antibiotics, irritant dentures, long term consumption of cortisone, pregnancy, old age, AIDS and low immunity.

Thumb and digit sucking is defined as placement of the thumb or more fingers in varying depths into the mouth. Thumb and digit sucking is one of the commonest seen habit in children. Recent studies have shown that thumb sucking may be practiced even during intrauterine life. The presence of this habit until the age 31/2-4 years is considered normal. Persistence of the habit beyond this age can lead to various malocclusions.

Thymol is relatively a weak antiseptic. It is widely used as mouth washes. It has a good flavor.

Thymus is a primary lymphoid organ, bilobed structure located in the thorax anterior to the sternum. Histologically, each lobe contains lobules separated by connective tissue trabaculae. Each lobule is made up of an outer cortex with immature cells. Hassal Corpuscles in thymic medulla are containing degenerating suspected cells.

Thyroglossal tract cyst arises from remnants of thyroglossal duct and may develop anywhere along the embryonic thyroglossal tract between the foramen coecum of tongue and thyroid gland. It consists squamous and glandular epithelium. It generally develops in young person. It raises from a few mm to a few centimetres. It is asymptomatic and grows slowly. If large, it may cause dysphagia. Occasionally fistula may form.

Thyroid storm is a medical emergency. Fever may go up to 41° C with anxiety, tremor, weakness, heat intolerance, sweating and weight loss. Sinus tachycardia is always present. Atrial fibrillation develops. Reflexes become brisk.

Tic Doloreux where Tic is spasm and Dolor is the Latin word for pain. Because trigeminal neuralgia pain comes as electrical shock, each pain spasm is called tic doloreux.

Tics are a sudden rapid twitch like movement always of same nature and same type. These are generally common in childhood and disappear in adult life. All forms of tics can be suppressed clinically.

Tin oxide is a pure white powder that is used as a final polishing agent. Tine oxide is mixed with water alcohol or glycerine and is used as a paste. Finishing abrasives are coarse, hard particles and polishing abrasives are fine articles.

Tissue borne passive appliance are mostly located in the vestibule and have little or no contact with the dentition e.g. functional regulator or Frankel.

Tissue Health Index was developed by Sheiham A., Maizels J. and Maizels A., at the second alternative indices, which is a modification of the DMFT index. In the THI, selective weighting is given for Decayed, Filled and Sound teeth (i.e. '1' - Decayed, '2' - Filled and '4' - Sound).

Tissue repair is a process following inflammation white cells repair by filling the breach with a temporary repair called granulation tissue. New capillaries are formed, but repair cannot take place in presence of pus. Hence tooth requires extraction or root treatment to drain off pus.

Titanium is a material of choice because of its good biocompatibility, mechanical properties and in implantology, its proven ability to achieve osseointegration.

T-Lymphocytes precursor arise from bone marrow stem cell, the T-lymphocytes travel to the thymus where they mature. T-lymphocytes mediate cellular immunity and is important for defence against virus, fungi and bacteria. They play an important role in regulating immune system. Thymus is large in children and shrinks as an individual matures. Different types of T-cells have different functions. Some are memory cells. Some are T-helper cells increasing the function of B lymphocytes and increases the antibody response. Others are called T-suppress or cells decreasing the function of B lymphocytes. T-killer cells are active in vigilance against tumor or virally affected cells.

Tobacco chewer's white lesion develops where the tobacco is placed. Mucobuccal fold is the most common location. Epithelium gives a wrinkled appearance. There is a risk of malignancy with long exposure to tobacco.

Tobacco stains appear as light brown to dark brown or black. They may appear in various forms such as - Narrow crest following the gingival contour, Wide band extending from the cervical third to the middle third of the tooth and diffuse they are primarily present on the cervical third of the tooth but may involve any surface including pits and fissures and the lingual surface. These stains are generally formed from the smokeless tobacco and are mainly composed of tar and combustion products. The heavy deposits may penetrate the enamel and present as endogenous stains.

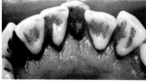

Tobacco stains

Tolerance occurs when the immune system is constantly exposed to self Ag (antigen) without inducing lymphocyte stimulation 'self tolerance'. It is a result of several mechanisms designed to distinguish between lymphocytes with potential to bind to self components and those with much higher binding specificity for antigenic determinants expressed by foreign Ag.

Tongue brushing is an act involving cleaning of tongue that should be combined with tooth brushing. Dorsum of the tongue is a primary source of infection. Tongue brushing can reduce the number of these organisms. It improves patient's taste perception also. Tongue should remain free of coating or debris. But tongue may not be scrubbed with tooth brush.

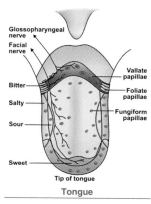

Tongue

Tongue papillae are the samll elevations present on dorsal surface of tongue. These are of variable size and represent different type of taste sensation. These can be classified into four types. (i) Filliform papillae – are numerous white hair like projection that covers the dorsal surface (ii) circumvallate papillae on tongue in a V formation on dorsal surface. It contains bitter taste buds. (iii) Foliate papillae are projection found on posterior lateral borders of tongue and consist of sour and acidic taste buds. (iv) Fungiform papillae among filliform papillae on the dorsal surface of tongue. These consists sweet, sour and salty buds.

Tongue thrust habit is defined as a condition in which the tongue makes contact with any teeth anterior to the molars during swallowing. Tongue thrust is a forward placement of the tongue between the anterior teeth and against the lower lip during swallowing (Schneider 1982) is an act of swallowing as the placement of the tongue tip forward between the incisors during swallowing (Profit 1990) or is an oral habit pattern related to the persistence of an infantile swallow pattern during childhood and adolescence and thereby produces an open bite and protrusion of the anterior tooth segments (Barber, 1975).

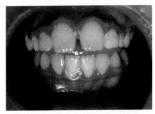

Tongue thrust

Tongue thrusting corrector appliance (Viazis, 1993) consists of a palatal wire that is inserted in the upper lingual molar sheaths, passes through the open-bite area, and carries over the lower incisors toward the labial vestibule, ending 1-2 mm above the labial surface. 'U'- shaped palatal loops are used to adjust the appliance in an anteroposterior or vertical direction with a three -prong plier. The TCA can also be expanded, like a palatal expansion appliance, to correct the posterior cross bites that often accompany open bites. It does not contact the teeth or the soft tissue. The TCA is designed to keep the

patient from inserting the thumb in the mouth, and it prevents tongue thrusting or abnormal tongue posturing during swallowing by blocking the tongue from the anterior teeth. This in turn helps close the open bite.

Tonic seizure there is a tonic contraction of muscle with altered consciousness but no clonic phase. These generally occur during NREM sleep with day drowsiness.

Tonsillitis is a common bacterial upper respiratory tract infection. Patients will complaint of sore throat with dysphagia. Child is not able to eat food. Pain and fever accompanies. There develops leucocytosis. Amoxicillin and analgesic anti-inflammatory drugs help.

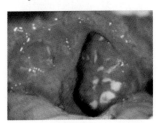

Tonsillitis-mononucleosis

Tooth ankylosis can be defined as fusion of tooth root to the underlying bone more often after an injury. Periapical inflammation is a well recognised cause of it by way of root absorption. If more of root surface is involved it may give a dull, muffed sound on percussion instead of normal sharp sound. It may be visible on radiograph there will be loss of normal thin radiolucent line with mild sclerosis of bone. There is no treatment. It serves well unless infected.

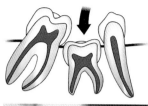

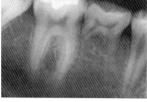

Submerged ankylosed teeth

Tooth banks are several banks to store tooth with different techniques such as chemical coagulation, vitrification, freeze drying and regular freezing.

Tooth borne active appliance includes modification of activator and bionator that include expansion screws or other active components like spring to provide intrinsic force to transverse or anteroposterior changes.

Tooth borne passive appliance are those appliances that have no intrinsic force generating components such as spring or screw. They depend on the soft tissues stretch and muscular activity to produce the desired treatment results. e.g. activator, bionator and herbst appliance.

Tooth brush filaments are the nylon filaments that are superior to natural bristles made of hog or boar hair. Nylon filaments flex 10 times more than breaking. These are more resistant to accumulation of bacteria and fungi. Soft nylon filaments are less traumatic to gingival tissues. Range of nylon filament diameter is 0.15 mm to 0.4 mm. Most bristles are 10 to 12 mm long. Thickness any from 0.007 to 0.12 mm are considered medium and 0.013 to 0.015 mm are classified as hard. End of the tooth brush filament can be cut bluntly or rounded. Round cut edges reduce gingival abrasion.

Tooth brushing is an act of cleaning done domestically after meals to removes plaque. Tooth brushes with a small head and multi tufted medium nylon bristles are most effective. Brushed in rinsed and pea size portion of fluoride tooth paste is added. Effective tooth brushing required time, knowledge and skill.

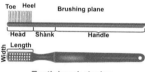

Tooth brush design

Tooth eruption is the process by which developing teeth emerge through the soft tissue of the jaws and the overlying mucosa to enter the oral cavity, contact the teeth of the opposing arch, and function in mastication (*see* **Figure** on page 454).

Tooth fracture is a common injury occuring due to trauma. It may occur at any age but children between the age of 2-3 yrs are most commonly affected. Minor chipping is common. Fracture has been classified in many ways. Prognosis depends whether pulp

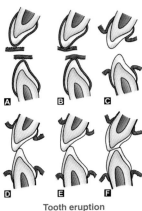

Tooth eruption

is involved, or crown/root is involved. If dentin over pulp is thin bacteria may penetrate producing pulpitis. Fractured crown is a more serious problem if the pulp is exposed.

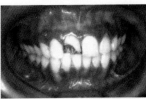

Ellis Class III dentoalvepoldar fracture

Tooth surface index of fluorosis (TSIF) is a index that was developed to measure the extent of fluorosis. TSIF was developed by Herschel S Horowitz, William S Driscoll, Rhea J Meyers, Stanley B Heifeta, and Albert Knigman in 1984. TSIF was developed in order to eliminate or reduce some of the short comings of 'Deans Index'. TSIF was applied in a survey to assess the prevalence of dental caries and dental fluorosis in communities having optimal and above optimal concentrations of naturally occurring fluoride in the drinking water.

Tooth wear is a mechanical process that occurs due to aging. It is an increasing problem in older adults due to long period of functioning. It has 3 causes abrasion, attrition and erosion. Reduction in lubricating effect of saliva may cause it.

Tooth zones are divided into imaginary third, named according to areas in which they are found. Root of tooth is divided into apical, middle and cervical third. Crown of the tooth is divided into cervico occlusal division, mesio distal division and buccolingual division.

Topical is application directly to an affected area for treatment.

Topical anesthesia is a medicament that eliminates sensation on surface tissues such as skin and mucosa. Oral mucosa can be anesthetized by wiping a topical anesthetic which will reduce the discomfort of dental injections, etc.

Topical fluoride is applied to the teeth but not ingested.

Topography is detailed description and analysis of features of an anatomic region.

Toronto automated probe is a diagnostic probe to measure clinical attachment levels. Here the sulcus is probed with the Ni-Ti wire that is extended under air pressure.

Torus mandibularis is an outgrowth of bone on the lingual surface of mandible opposite bicuspid tooth. These may be multiple and on both sides. It may be removed surgically.

Torus palatinus is slowly growing, flat base bone protuberance. It generally occurs in mid line of hard palate. Women are affected more. On trauma it becomes ulcerated. It never becomes malignant. It is not treated.

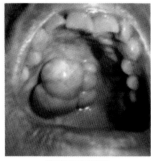

Toris palatinus

Toxic refer to Poisonous.

Toxic myocarditis occurs due to drugs that cause a direct toxic injury to the myocardial fibres. Response is cumulative and dose related. In this group drugs include arsenicals, catecholamines, lithium, cyclophosphamide emetine etc. Healing occurs by fibrosis.

Toxic shock syndrome is a multisystem illness caused by endotoxins produced by stains of staphylococcus aureus. Symptoms include fever, chills, diarrhea, dizziness, headache, myalgias and sore throat. Patient may develop hypotension with desquamation of skin.

Toxicology is the study of toxic and harmful effects of drugs and chemicals. It deals with the science of knowledge of sources, characters, properties and symptoms of poisons, their fatal effects, the lethal doses and remedies to be taken to counteract the effect.

Toxin is any poisonous substance of microbial, vegetable or animal origin that causes symptoms after a period of incubation. It can induce the elaboration of specific antitoxin in suitable animal.

Trabecular bone is similar to cortical bone but with spongy look. It is composed of rods and sheets of bone.

Tracheostomy is the term given to the surgical establishment of an opening in to the trachea. It is usually performed electively when the endotracheal intubation is likely to extend beyond 14 days. The opening is made in the anterior wall of trachea. It is done to have alternate pathway for breathing, improves alveolar ventilation, to give anesthesia.

Traction vertebral spurs projects horizontally and develops 1-2 mm above the vertebral edge. It is also known as Macnab spur. It is the small traction spur that is symptomatic.

Traditional alloy contain silver 66 to 72% by weight, tin 25-29%, copper 2 to 6%. Zinc 2% and mercury 3% by weight.

Tragus is the cartilaginous projection anterior to external opening of the ear.

Tramadol is an analgesic with both opioid as well as non opioid actions. It works like aspirin as well as like morphine. High doses of it should be avoided. It is used in the dose of 50-100 mg daily.

Tranquillizers are the drugs which decrease anxiety and tension without producing sedation.

T

Transient ischemic attack (TIA) also termed incipient stroke, transient cerebral ischemia is characterized by ischemic cerebral neurologic deficits that last for less than 24 hours. These attacks rarely last more than 8 hours and often resolve within 15-60 mins. Platelet, fibrin or other atherosclerotic embolic material from the neck or heart may lodge in a cerebral vessel and interfere transiently with blood flow causing the TIA.

Translocation is the change in position.

Translucency is the amount of incident light transmitted and scattered by that object. Translucency decreases with increasing scattered within materials. A high translucency gives a lighter color appearance. Translucency decreases with increasing scattering with in a material.

Translucent lesion are demonstrating translucent quality and are bullae or vesicle. Translucent pink lesions are due to accumulation of clear fluid such as serum, mucin or lymph. Blue translucent lesion indicates clear fluid or blood accumulation. Red or purple translucent lesion indicates blood accumulation.

Transmissible is the term which denotes a capacity of a lesion to maintain an infectious agent in successive passages through a susceptible host.

Transmission refers to the spread of disease from one person to another by various model such as saliva air, contact with contaminated instrument etc. of disease through saliva is low. Herpes virus may secrete into saliva. Coxsakie virus is also a latent infection and has a risk of transmission of virus through dental clinic.

Transosseous wiring is a type of intermaxillary fixation with osteosynthesis where direct wiring is done across the fracture line in order to achieve effective immobilization of the fracture of the body of the mandible including angle. The holes are drilled in the bone ends of both the sides of the fracture line and the soft stainless steel wire is passed through the holes across the fracture. After achieving the accurate reduction the free ends of the wires are twisted together and tucked in to a nearest hole. Achieving osteosynthesis by wiring has an advantage of requiring minimal equipment and can be used for many types of mandibular fractures.

Transplantation of organs refers to a removal of a viable and healthy organ and placing it into another body where the existing organ has become diseased or dysfunctional e.g. heart, kidney, brain and liver. The viability or transplantable organs falls sharply after somatic death such as liver must be taken out within 15 minutes, a kidney within 45 minutes and a heart within an hour. After molecular death it is not feasible.

Transseptal fibres are those fibres which extend interproximally over the alveolar bone crest and get embedded into the cementum of the adjacent tooth. These fibers can be considered as a part of gingival fibers as they lack osseous attachment.

Transverse ridge is a linear elevation that crosses a surface (usually the occlusal surface).

Trauma from occlusion (TFO) can be described as when occlusal forces exceed the adaptive capacity or margins of safety of the tissues, it results in tissue injury. This resultant injury is known as trauma from occlusion.

Traumatic cyst is not a true cyst not being lined by epithelium. Expansion ceases when cyst like lesion reaches the cortical layer of bone. When roots are involved cavity may become scalloped. A thin connective tissue lines the cavity. X-ray shows smoothly outlined radiolucent area of variable size with in sclerotic border.

Traumatic fibroma refers to fibroma.

Traumatic neuroma is not a true neoplasm but is an exuberant try to repair a damaged nerve trunk. It is a hyperplasia of nerve fibers and supporting tissue. Degeneration of distal nerve after injury begins with swelling, fragmentation and disintegration of myelin sheath and axis cylinder. Oral neuroma begins with small nodule or swelling of mucosa near mental foramen. Treatment includes surgical excision of nodule along with small proximal portion of nerve involved.

Traumatic occlusion is the term used when the injury is produced by the occlusion.

Traumatic ulcer results due to physical injury such as denture irritation, an ill fitting denture or biting of the mucosa. Traumatic ulcers are usually single of variable size and round in shape. The floor will be yellow with red margins and there will not be any induration. It is covered by a white or tan fibrin clot and generally located at lateral border. It can be painful. Recurrent trauma can make it firm and elevated with rolled borders. After removing the cause ulcer may heal within 1-2 days, occasionally ulcers persist for long. Traumatic ulcers may be accidental or deliberate biting or thermal burns from hot pasty foods.

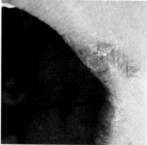

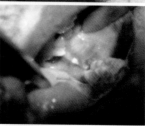

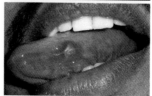

Traumatic ulcer of tongue

Treatment contract is the understanding between doctor and patient which includes frequency, number and duration of treatment.

Treatment index The 'F (filled) portion of the DMF Index best exemplifies a treatment index. In general, there are two types of dental indices. This type of dental index measures the 'number' of people affected and the 'severity' of the specific condition at a specific time or interval of time.

Treatment manual is a written material that identifies key concepts, procedure and tactic to treat a person.

Treatment plan is known as blue print for case management. It includes all the procedures required for the maintenance of oral health.

Tremor is the rhythmic oscillation of part of body around a fixed point. Tremors usually involve distal part of limb, head, tongue and rarely trunk. Tremors at rest even in lying supine are seen in parkinsonism. Essential tremors occur in anxiety, fatigue and due to alcohol while intentional tremors are seen in phenytoin toxicity, multiple sclerosis and in cerebellar disease.

Tremor of Parkinsonism consists of a rapid, rhythmic, alternating tremor. Pill rolling tremors are seen. It is usually unilateral.

Trench mouth refers acute necrotizing ulcerative gingivitis.

Trichloroethylene is a colorless volatile liquid with chloroform like smell. It is colored blue to avoid confusion with chloroform. It has a poor relaxation of skeletal muscles. It has good analgesic properties but induction and recovery are poor. Bradycardia and cardiac arrhythmias may occur.

Trichodento-osseous syndrome shows enamel defects in conjunction with morphologic dental anomalies. These patients have tightly curled kinky hair with osteosclerosis of bone cortices. The enamel is hypoplastic and hypocalcified, lacking mesiodistal contact with pitting.

Triclosan is a non-cationic antibacterial agent and has been added to several dentifrices to inhibit plaque and gingivitis. It has good antibacterial activity against Gram positive and Gram negative organisms and is compatible with anionic component of fluoride dentifrices. Two clinical studies over a 3-month period by Schiff et al (1990) and Lobene et al (1990) showed a statistically significant reduction of plaque formation.

Tricuspid regurgitation is common and most frequently occuring as a result of right ventricular dialatations. It may occur with right ventricular and inferior myocardial infarction. Symptoms and signs of tricuspid regurgitation are identical to those resulting from right ventricular failure of any cause. Symptoms are usually non specific and relate to reduced forward flow and venous congestion pansystolic murmur and systolic pulsation of liver.

Tricuspid stenosis is usually rheumatic in origin. It is suspected when right heart failure is marked with liver enlargement, ascites and dependent edema. Acquired

T

tricuspid stenosis needs valvotomy.

Trifurcation is forked or divided into three parts.

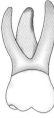

Trifurction

Trigeminal nerve is a fifth cranial nerve that contains both sensory and motor fibres. It is the largest and has 3 branches –(i) Ophthalmic nerve is purely sensory and is the smallest division. It divides into three branches lacrimal, frontal and nasociliary nerve. It supplies cornea, skin of forehead, scalp, eyelids, nose and also the mucus membrane of paranasal sinuses.(ii) Maxillary branch is purely sensory. It leaves the skull through foramen rotundum. It supplies skin over face over maxilla and the upper lip, teeth of upper jaw, mucus membrane of nose, maxillary air sinus and palate. (iii) Mandibular division is a mixed branch and is the largest branch. Motor part supplies muscles of mastication. Sensory supply is to skin of cheek, skin over mandible, lower lip and side of head, teeth of lower jaw, mucus membrane of mouth and anterior 2/3rd of tongue.

Trigeminal neuralgia is the most painful affliction of mankind. A single branch may be affected without affecting other branch. It is an intermittent brief, laminating pain in face. It is evoked by facial movement or by touching the skin. Pain is sudden, excruciating and brief like the stabbing. Peripheral receptors are not hyperalgesic. Pain does not extend outside area supplied by trigeminal nerve. The trigger may occur from light touch or movement of same receptor areas. Pain is usually unilateral and remains in the anatomical distribution of affected nerve. Typically individual pains are paroxysms of hot, shocking, burning or electric like lasting from a few seconds to several minutes. They may be repeated so frequently that pain becomes continuous. Paresthesia and motor symptoms are generally absent. No sensory loss is detected. No specific cause is known. Progressive degeneration and demyelination of trigeminal ganglion is seen. Secondary trigeminal neuralgia can result due to intracranial tumor, and vascular malformation, CNS lesions involving trigeminal

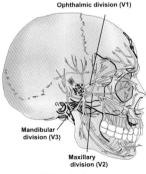

Ophthalmic division (V1)

Mandibular division (V3)

Maxillary division (V2)

Trigeminal nerve

pathways. Trigeminal neuralgia due to multiple sclerosis may have bilateral facial pain. There may be hypoesthesia too. In both cases carbamazpiene and GABA are used. Phenytoin in doses of 400 mg/day reduces the dose of carbamazepiene.

Trismus is a spasm of the muscles of mastication that results in difficulty in opening of mouth. Intraoral injections may result it.

Triturate is to mix together.

Trochlear nerve is a motor nerve, cranial nerve number four. It assists in turning eye ball downward and laterally. It emerges from posterior surface of mid brain. It enters the orbit through the superior orbital fissure (*see* Figure).

Tropic ulcer is found at anaesthetic sites. Injury may be mechanical and thermal. First and fifth metatarsals are commonly affected. There may be spontaneous blister or nodule. Ulcer may become infected. Deep tissues and bone may be involved. Floor of ulcer is covered by brownish tenacious and foul swelling slough. Surrounding skin is edematous regional lymph nodes may be enlarged and tender.

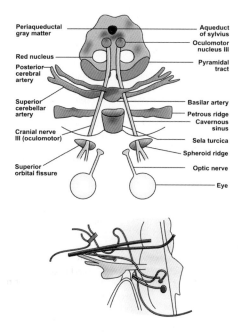

Trochlear nerve

True oral malodor Halitosis is most often a consequence of oral bacterial activity typically arising from anaerobes due to poor oral hygiene, gingivitis (ANUG), periodontal disease, infected extraction sockets, oral sepsis, residual blood postoperatively, debris under fixes or removable appliances, ulcers and dry mouth.

Tubercle is a small, rounded projection.

Tuberculin test was discovered by Von Pirquet in 1907. A positive reaction to test is accepted as evidence of past or present infection by M Tuberculosis. It is done to test in population.

Tuberculin type hypersentivity was originally, described by Koch in patients with TB who had fever and generalized sickness, following a spontaneous injection of tuberculin, a lipoprotein antigen from tubercle bacillus. 12 hrs after Intradermal tuberculosis challenge, T-lymphocytes are present at perivascular sites and this infiltrate, which extends outwards and disrupts the collagen bundles of the dermis increases to a peak at 48 hrs. Cells of the macrophage lineage are probably the main APCs in tuberculin hypersensitivity. As the lesion develops, it may become a granulomatous reaction.

Tuberculoid leprosy has well defined skin lesions with raised margins and healing centers are characteristic of tuberculoid leprosy. These lesions are anesthetic to touch and pin prick. The leprae are usually not detected on skin smear examination. Microscopically lesion shows collections of epitheloid cells and Langerhan's type giant cell. Caseation is usually absent. Temperature sensation is first to be affected followed by pressure, touch and pain. Margins of lesions are elevated and superficial. Larger nerves closer to skin are enlarged. Neuritic pain, muscle dystrophy, contracture and trauma from pressure and burns are common.

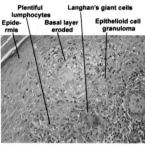

Tuberculoid leprosy

Tuberculosis is a granulomatous disease caused by acid fast bacillus. Patient may suffer from evening fever, fatigue, malaise and loss of weight. Spread is through blood or lymph TB of submaxillary and cervical lymph nodes may progress to the actual abscess. Glands are enlarged. Lesions of oral mucosa are seldom primary but secondary to pulmonary disease. Tongue is most commonly affected. Lesion is irregular, superficial or deep, painful ulcer which increases slowly. Mucosal lesions show swelling or fissuring. Tuberculous gingivitis is an unusual form of tuberculosis which produces hyperaemic, nodular or proliferative gingiva. Diffuse involvement of maxilla or mandible may occur (*see* Figure on page 462).

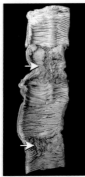

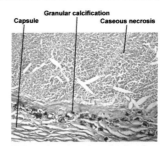

Capsule   Granular calcification   Caseous necrosis

Tuberculous lymph node showing
dystrophic calcification

Langhan's giant cells   Caseation necrosis
Lympho-   Intestinal   Epithelioid cell
cytes   mucosa   granuloma

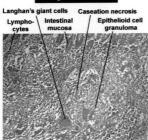

Tuberculosis of small intestine

Langhan's giant cell
Necrotic bone   Granulomatous
inflammation

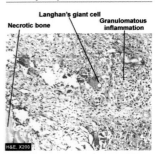

H&E, X200

Tuberculous osteomyelitis

Tuberculous lymphadenitis is a condition where cervical glands are commonly affected. Route may be via tonsils or oral mucosa. There will be a lump in neck. It is painful. In early stage swelling is firm and mobile. Later the mass becomes fixed. Lesion may be unilateral, bilateral single or multiple (*see* Figure).

Tuberculous meningitis may develop as a consequence of miliary TB. Human tubercular bacilli are responsible. Prodromal symptoms include lassitude, weight loss and anorexia. Diffuse headache and neck stiffness develops. Mild fever appears. Patient assumes a flexed position.

Caseation necrosis   Langhan's giant cells
Lymphoid   Epithelioid cell
tissue   granuloma

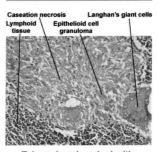

Tuberculous lymphadenitis

CSF pressure is raised. On long standing 'cob web' is formed. CSF sugar is low. Treatment is to begin with 3 anti TB drugs. Total duration of treatment is 6-9 month.

Tuberculous ulcer is caused by mycobacterium tuberculosis. It is an aerobic, slender, non motile, non spore forming, rod shaped organism. Most of people get infection in first year of life. Primary infection usually takes place in lungs. Hemoptysis, abundant sputum and pleuritic pain are very common. Tuberculous lesions of the oral cavity are secondary to pulmonary infections. Important oral lesions are tuberculous ulcers, tuberculous gingivitis, tuberculous osteomyelitis and tuberculosis of salivary gland. For tongue ulcers it is the most common site of occurrence. On lateral borders these appear either single or multiple lesions. On palate these may appear as small ulcer or granuloma. Lesions often produced small, granulating ulcers at the mucocutaneous junction. Gingival lesions of tuberculosis usually produce granulating ulcers or erosive lesions with gingival hyperplasia.

Tuberosity is a large, rounded projection.

Tuberous sclerosis is an autosomal dominant multisystem disorder of neuroectodermal origin. Presenting feature is mental deficiency with epilepsy. Seizures develop in first decade of life. Mental retardation may be noted. Radiograph shows intracranial calcification with generalized thickening and hyperostosis of cranial vault. Multiple cortical tubers are classical findings. Metacarpals and phalanges may show subperiosteal irregular new bone formation. Small well defined cysts are seen.

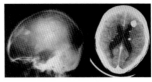

Tubercus sclerosis

Tumor necrosis factor alpha (TNF-α) shares many of its biological activities i.e. Pro-inflammatory properties, MMP stimulation, and bone resorption with IL-1. In addition, it's secretion by monocytes and fibroblast is stimulated by bacterial Lipopoly-saccharide.

Tumors of brain stem present with unilateral or bilateral paralysis of cranial nerves. Crossed hemiplegia, hemianesthesia and cerebellar symptoms develop.

Turkey tests include multiple comparison procedure.

Turku sugar studies were a series of collaborative studies carried out in Turku, Finland, by Scheinin, Makinen et al. They were investigated by a comprehensive program including clinical, radiographic, biochemical, and micro-bio-chemical determinants of health. In addition to the massive data indicating that xylitol would be an acceptable metabolite in humans, there was a dramatic reduction in the incidence of dental caries after two years of xylitol consumption. Subsequently a 1-year chewing gum study was conducted on 102 subjects who consumed the xylitol or sucrose chewing gum but otherwise pursued their usual dietary and oral hygiene habits.

T

Turner's spot is an enamel hypoplasia of permanent tooth as a result of local trauma or infection of a deciduous tooth. Infection restricts work of ameloblasts and results in poorly formed enamel.

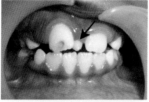

Turner's tooth

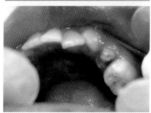

Turner's tooth involving premolar

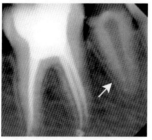

Turner's hypoplasia of premolars

Tweed's method is one of the method of performing serial extractions. It involves the extraction of the first molars around 8 years of age. This is followed by the extraction of the first premolars and the deciduous canine.

Twitch is the contraction of a muscle in response to a single action potential.

Type I hypersensitivity is characterized by an allergic reaction immediately following contact with an antigen referred to as an allergen. Allergy (coined by Von-Pirquet in 1906) is defined as the changed reactivity of the host when meeting an agent. In recent years allergy has become synonymous with Type I hypersensitivity. Dependent on the specific triggering of IgE sensitized mast cells by antigen, resulting in the release of pharmacological mediators of inflammation.

Typhoid is caused by *Salmonella Typhi*. The infection gets localized to small intestine. To start person may have headache, general body ache and malaise. Fever rises in step ladder fashion. Temperature increases every day especially in the evening. In morning fever comes down but never touches normal. It happens for 7-10 days. During the second stage patient usually looks very ill. Tongue is coated with clean tip. There will be relative bradycardia. During third week patient starts looking better. During acute stage, the organisms would be positive in first week and urine, stool culture becomes positive by second week. Widal test is positive during second week.

Tzanck cells are the epithelial cells which shows ballooning degeneration, consisting of acantholysis, nuclear clearing and nuclear enlargement. This is a histologic feature and can be appreciated only at a microscopic level.

Ulcer is a pathological condition in which there is a breakdown of epithelial tissue. There is a full thickness loss of surface epithelium with exposure to underlying connective tissue. In mouth ulcers are usually painful, except malignant one which may be initially painless. Biopsy is needed if ulcer is not responding for more than 3 weeks.

Ulceration colitis is a disease of young people between the age of 15-25 years. Symptoms range from small amount of rectal bleeding to prominent diarrhea and colonic hemorrhage with prostration. It may manifest as spondylitis, peripheral arthritis, iritis and skin disorders. Rectosigmoid colon is commonly involved.

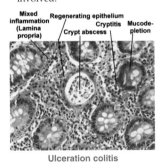

Mixed inflammation (Lamina propria) Regenerating epithelium Cryptitis Mucodepletion Crypt abscess

Ulceration colitis

Ultimate strength is the maximum stress a solid can support based on its original cross section area.

Ultrasonic cleaning is the loosening and removal of debris from instruments by sound waves travelling through a chemical solution. It has increased efficiency in cleaning and has reduced danger of aerosolization of infectious particles released during scrubbing. Injury to instrument is lesser and is an easy process.

Ultrasonic is the conversion of high frequency electrical current into mechanical vibrations. Ultrasonic is the use of sound waves for detection and this offers considerable potential as a diagnostic instrument. Ultrasonic imaging was introduced by Ng et al. (1988) as a method for detecting early caries in smooth surfaces. With the use of this instrumentation, sonic velocity and specific acoustic impedance can be determined for the dentin and enamel as well as for the soft tissue and bone.

Ultrasonic scaler is an electronically powered device that produces vibratory motions to dislodge deposits from teeth. Commonly used scalers operate in the 5000 to 7000 cycles/second range. Most magnetostrictive ultrasonic operate at 25000-30000 cycles per second while piezo electric ultrasonic operates at 40000 to 50000 cycles/second.

Ultrasonic scaling is a use of an ultrasonic scaler to remove mineralized deposits from tooth surface.

Ultrasound – Upper limit of hearing is 20 KHz (20,000 cycles per second). Ultrasound is very much above this therapeutic frequencies being in the region of 1 MHz to 3 MHz.

Uncontrolled diabetes – Oral manifestations include multiple periodontal abscesses, velvety red gingival and marginal proliferation of the periodontal tissues.

Undercut is the portion of tooth lying between the height and contour of gingiva.

Under cut cavity preparation We know that permanent filling canont be inserted directly into a cavity and preparation of cavity is required so that filling may not comeout.

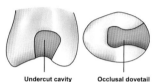

Undercut cavity   **Occlusal dovetail**

Cavity preparation for plastic fillings

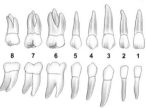

8   7   6   5   4   3   2   1

Upper and lower permanent teeth

Undermining resorption is the term used when the bone loss occurs from a healthy or viable periodontal ligament which is present adjacent to the necrotic areas.

Undifferentiated mesenchymal cells are the stem cells located in the cell-rich zone and the pulp proper which can differentiate into odontoblasts and / or fibroblasts.

Unfavorable fractures are the one where the vertical fracture or the horizontal fracture lines are opposed by the action of the muscle around them. However, these types of fractures are not so easy to reduce and stabilize.

Unicystic Ameloblastoma – There will be localized thinning and haziness of radiopaque rim. It generally occurs before the age of 30. Lesion slowly enlarges due to expansion of cortex. On palpation it is hard and bony.

Unilateral condylar neck fractures are the fractures involving the neck of the condyle and are of two types: low condylar neck fractures and high condylar neck fractures. If the fracture is undisplaced, no active treatment is required but in case of displaced fractures, dislocation will induce malocclusion. A low neck fracture can be treated by open reduction and a high condylar neck fracture with extensive displacement and malocclusion, intermaxillary fixation (IMF) is done for up to 3-4 weeks and maintained until bony union has occurred.

Unilateral extracapsular fractures refer unilateral condylar neck fractures.

Unilateral fracture usually ours on one side of the body but occasionally more than one fracture may be present. It is generally caused by direct violence.

Unilateral intracapsular fractures are the fractures occurring in the condyle. In these cases the occlusion is usually undisturbed and fracture should be treated conservatively. If malocclusion occurs the intermaxillary fixation (IMF) for 2-3 weeks is indicated.

U

Universal curettes are the one which can be used in most areas of the dentition by altering and adapting the finger rest and hand position of the operator. The blades of these curettes are curved in one direction.

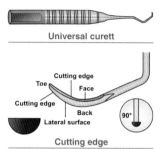

Universal curett

Cutting edge

Universal/National Numbering System is approved by the American Dental Association in 1968. Most commonly used throughout the United States. The permanent teeth are numbered from 1 to 32. Numbering begins with the upper right third molar, works around to the upper left third molar, drops to the lower left third molar, and works around to the lower right third molar. In the Universal Numbering System, the primary teeth are lettered with capital letters from A to T.

Upper lip prominence A line is drawn from subnasale (Sn) to soft-tissue pogonion (Pog'). The most prominent point of the upper lip (Ls) should be 3 ± 1mm anterior to this line.

Upper lip-lower lip-chin prominence is a vertical reference line drawn through subnasale (SnV) perpendicular to the true horizontal. The upper lip should be 1 to 2 mm ahead of this line. The lower lip should be on the line or 1 mm posterior to it. The chin (Pog') should fall within 1 to 4 mm posterior to SnV. Alternatively the distance from soft-tissue chin to a line perpendicular to FH through soft tissue nasion can be measured. This is also known as 0-degree meridian and Pog' is estimated to be 0 ± 2 mm from this line.

Uremic syndrome Early symptom of kidney failure is decreased creatinine clearance. As disease progresses glomerular filtration rate falls and blood urea nitrogen rises. Person may develop impaired ability to concentrate urine, nocturia and mild anemia. Advanced uremia is associated with pericarditis, pericardial effusion and neuropathies.

Ureter is a duct that transmits urine from kidney to bladder.

Urgency of urine is the sudden desire to void. It is seen in inflammatory conditions i.e. cystitis or neurogenic bladder.

Uric acid is the end product of purine metabolism.

Uricosuric drugs are those drugs that block tubular reabsorption of filtered urate and reduce the metabolic pool of urates, preventing the formation of new tophi. When given with colchicines these lessen the frequency of recurrence of gout.

Urinary tract obstruction – Severe obstruction can produce acute anuria, burning and pain on urination, overflow in continence or dribbling, voiding of small amount and flank pain. In secondary infection fever, chills malaise develop along with foul smelling urine.

Urine pregnancy test is a test that depends on the presence of human chorionic gonadotrophin in urine. Usually a concentration of about 2500 I.V. HCG per liter of urine is required to register a positive health. It usually occurs 12 days after the first missed period.

Urticaria results when antigen reaches specific skin areas causing localized anaphylactic reaction. Histamine on release results in red flare and increased permeability of capillaries resulting in swelling within a few minutes.

Useful habits include habits that are considered essential for normal function such as proper positioning of the tongue, respiration and normal deglutition.

Uterine fibroids – These are uterine leiomyoma. If large it produces a round, multinodular mass in suprapubic region. She may feel heaviness in abdomen and pressure on surrounding organs with frequency of urine. Menorrhagia develops. Edema and varicosities of lower extremities result.

Utilitarian ethics is an ethical theory based on the principle of the greatest good for the majority.

Uvula is a small muscular structure located on the free edge of soft palate. When you swallow the food it prevents your food from coming out of your nose. It directs the food down the throat into esophagus.

U

V

Vaccination is used to produce acquired immunity. Person can be vaccinated by injecting dead organisms which are no longer capable of causing disease but still have chemical antigen. These are used against typhoid, diphtheria, whooping cough and diphtheria. Secondly immunity can be achieved against toxins which have been treated with chemicals. These are used against tetanus and botulinism. Thirdly person can be vaccinated by infecting him with live organism that has been attenuated. These are used against polio, measles and other viral diseases.

Vagus nerve is a mixed tenth cranial nerve. Motor part supplies pharynx and larynx, bronchi and heart. Sensory fibres carry taste from epiglottis and vellecula.

Validity is the meaningfulness of test scores as they are used for specific tests.

Van Limborgh's Theory is a multifactorial theory put forward by Van Limborgh in 1970. According to van Limborgh, the three popular theories of growth were not satisfactory, yet each contains elements of significance that cannot be denied. Van Limborgh explains the process of growth and development in a view that combines all the three existing theories. He supports the functional matrix theory of Moss, acknowledged some aspects of Sicher's theory and at the same time does not rule out genetic involvement. Van Limborgh has suggested the following five factors that he believed controls growth: intrinsic genetic factors, local epigenetic factors, general epigenetic factors, local environmental factors, general environmental factors.

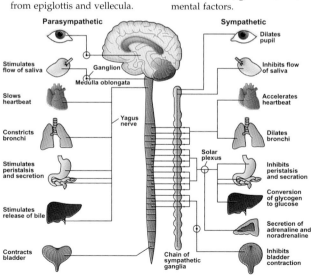

Vagus nerve

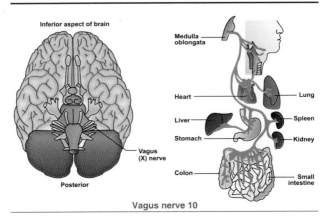

Vagus nerve 10

Veneer crown is a thin gold shell used in the construction of bridges. On back teeth it covers the entire crown known as full crown. On front it covers all but the labial surface and is called three quarter crown.

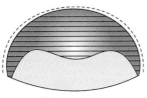

Veneer crown

Vapour pressure is a measure of liquid's tendency to evaporate. Materials with high vapor pressure at room temperature tend to evaporate readily.

Varicocele is a pampiniform plexus of veins of the spermatic cord. It is a consequence to venous stasis aided by gravity forces and prolonged standing. Intra-abdominal tumor also results increased pressure on the spermatic veins.

Varicose ulcer is a chronic ulcer of leg of insidious onset. Mostly ulcer is on medial side of leg. It is solitary. It is a shallow ulcer where floor is covered by bluish granulation tissue of pale slough. Edges are irregular and sloping. It is mobile on underlying bone. Surrounding skin is swollen and pigmented.

Varicose veins are an abnormal dilatation and tortousity of vein especially in leg. In legs these are abnormally dilated, elongated and tortuous. Incidence increases with age. It has familial tendency. Increased intraluminal pressure leads it. Affected veins are dilated, stretched, tortuous and nodular. There is irregular thinning and atrophy of vein. Thrombosis is common. Fibrosis results in tortuousity. Intima is thickened. Valvular defect causes an important defect. Long standing cases may develop fibrosis, chronic edema and skin pigmentation. Person feels dull, aching heaviness or a feeling of fatigue.

V

Varnishes are used as thin layers but don't provide thermal insulation. These serve to isolate the tubule contents from the cavity. Several applications are needed to prevent penetration of bacteria.

Vascular dementia is the single brain lesion which doesn't lead to dementia but affects mental function. The most common type of vascular dementia is caused by multiple supra tentorial infarcts. Hypertensive small vessel disease produces predominant deep white matter infarcts.

Vasculitis describes a diverse group of inflammatory disorder characterized by multi organ vessel involvement. There develops fever, malaise, weight loss and raised WBCs and ESR.

Vasoconstrictor drugs i.e. adrenaline and noradrenaline are useful when there is an access to the bleeding site. These are effective in controlling the oozing from capillaries. These are useful in controlling gingival bleeding. It is not useful in controlling heavy hemorrhage because these are diluted and washed out.

Vasodepressor syncope refers to sudden loss of consciousness that usually occurs secondary to a period of cerebral ischemia. Predisposing factors for vasodepressor syncope are psychogenic factors such as fright, anxiety, emotional stress, pain especially sudden and unexpected, sight of blood or surgical or other dental instruments. Non psychogenic factors include sitting in an upright position which permits blood to pool in the periphery decreasing cerebral blood flow; hunger from missed meal which decrease the glucose supply to brain, exhaustion, poor physical condition and hot, humid environment.

Vasomotor syncope may be due to excessive vagal tone or impaired reflex control of peripheral circulation. Common faint is initiated by a stressful, painful or claustrophobic experience.

Vehicle is a substance possessing little or no medicinal action used as a medium to confer a suitable consistency or form.

Vein – Blood vessel carrying blood from periphery to heart.

Veneer is a layer of tooth-colored material can be porcelain, composite, or ceramics attached to the front of the tooth to improve appearance. These are bonded to enamel by means of acid etch technique with the help of resin.

Venous hemorrhage – Wound bleeds with steady flow. The lost blood is dark red or bluish. The bleeding stops by elevating the part above the level of heart.

Ventral surface of the tongue is the underside of the tongue.

Vermilion means red.

Virgin teeth are those teeth that are free from decay or restorations.

Ventricular septal defect is the persistent opening in upper interventricular septum due to failure of fusion with aortic septum. It results in blood to pass from high pressure left ventricle into low pressure right ventricle. Large defects are associated with early left ventricular failure. Many VSD defects close spontaneously in early childhood.

Verrucal resembles like a wart.

V

Verrucous carcinoma is diffused; non metastasing well differentiated malignant neoplasm. It mostly develops in tobacco chewing patients. It is exophytic and papillary in nature. Commonest site involved is gingiva, alveolar mucosa and buccal mucosa. Surface of the lesion shows multiple deep clefts. Lesion may be single or multiple involving different parts of buccal mucosa. Pain may develop making chewing difficult. It becomes rapidly fixed to underlying bone. Regional lymph nodes are often enlarged. Malignant epithelial cells are usually well differentiated. Pain and difficulty in mastication are chief complaints. Anaplastic transformation occurs.

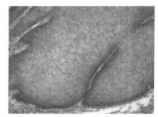
Verrucous carcinoma high power

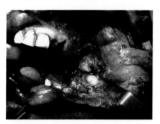
Operative photo of verrucous carcinoma of upper gingivo-buccal sulcus1

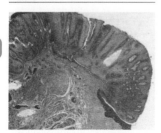
Verrucous carcinoma

Vertebral compression fracture it may result due to osteoporosis by bending, lifting, coughing or sneezing. There develops acute, severe pain at fracture site. Pain may radiate anteriorly to flank. Pain is typically worse in up right position. Signs include spinal tenderness over fractured spine along with paravertebral muscle spasm. Kyphosis and loss of height will develop. Weakness, sensory deficits incontinence or diminished deep reflexes develop.

Vertebral osteophytes occur due to repeated damage to the posterior joints especially lead to degenerative changes. It is a true osteo arthritic change and lipping of vertebra may take place.

Vertical bone loss is also known as angular bone loss. It does not occur in plane parallel to cementoenamel junction.

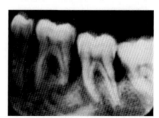
Verticle bone loss

V

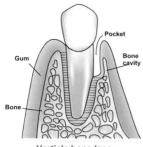

Verticle bone loss

Vertical defects are those bony defects of alveolar process which occur in an oblique direction, leaving a hollowed out trough in the bone alongside the root.

Vesibulocochlear nerve is the eighth cranial nerve consisting of two sets of sensory fibres vestibular and cochlear. Vestibular fibres are concerned with equilibrium. Cochlear fibres are concerned with hearing.

Vibration – Vibrations in the range of 10 to 500 Hz may be encountered in work of drills and hammer. After some months the fine blood vessels of fingers may become increasingly sensitive to spasm i.e. white fingers.

Vibrio cholerae is a microorganism that causes cholera. Their natural habitat is water. Watery diarrhea can be fatal. It is a gram negative slender bacilli, comma shaped with pointed ends. It is highly motile with single flagellum. It is seen under dark field microscopy.

Vimentin is the type of filament that is expressed in mesenchymal cells such as fibroblasts, and in endothelial cells. These fibres often end at the nuclear membrane and desmosomes. They are closely associated with micro-tubules, and they form cages around lipid droplets in adipose tissue.

Vincent's angina is an ulcerative infection of mouth and throat with enlarged lymph glands, pain and fever. Streptococcal sore throat also produces exudative membrane in throat. Throat becomes sore and extremely painful. Pharynx may show edema and reddening.

Vipeholm dental study was a 5-year investigation of 436 adult inmates in a mental institution at the Vipetional Hospital near Lund, Sweden. The dental caries rate in the inmates was relatively low. The experimental design divided the inmates into seven groups; sugar was introduced either at mealtime. The main conclusions of the study were as follows: An increase in carbo-hydrate definitely increases the caries activity. The risk of caries is greater if the sugar is consumed in a form that will be retained on the surfaces of teeth. The risk of sugar increasing caries activity is greatest if the sugar is consumed between meals and in a form that tends to be retained on the surfaces of the teeth. The increase in caries activity varies widely between individuals. Upon withdrawal of the sugar-rich foods, the increased caries activity rapidly disappears. Caries lesions may continue to appear despite the avoidance of refined sugar and maximum restrictions of natural sugars and dietary carbohydrate. A high concentra-tion of sugar in solution and its prolonged retention of tooth surfaces leads to increased caries activity. The clearance time of the sugar correlates closely with caries activity.

Viperine snake bite – local symptoms are persistent pain but salivation is rare. There is no paralysis of respiratory organs as in cobra bite. It produces extensive inflammation with cellulitis, discoloration and incessant oozing of hemolysed blood from the punctured point. Signs of collapse may be seen. Pupils are dilated and not reacting to light. There will be multiple hemorrhages, epistaxis, hematuria, hemoptysis and petechial hemorrhages. There may be complete unconsciousness. Death takes place due to cardiac failure within 1-2 days.

Viral fever is caused by influenza virus. Transmission is through inhalation of infected nasopharyngeal secretions.

Viral hepatitis viral hepatitis is an acute parenchymal necrotizing lesion where liver cell necrosis of hepatitis includes agents A, B, C, D, E, etc. During active disease one develops fever, nausea, vomiting fatigue, anorexia, headache and chills. There will be disturbance of taste. One can develop pruritic rash, arthritis and altered mental status. Urine will be dark and stools will be clay colored. Liver will be enlarged and tender.

Viral infection – Mumps is caused by a paramyxovirus. It may complicate gonads, CNS, pancreas and myocardium. Clinical features include sudden fever, malaise and anorexia. To start one sided parotid gland is involved then second is involved.

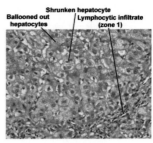

Viral hepatitis

Parotid gland enlarges for 2-3 days and return to normal within seven days. Submandibular gland may also be involved. Most of the causes are self limiting within a week. In some children meningitis or encephalitis may develop. Antibiotics and cortisone avoid complications.

Viral oral ulcer may be primary herpetic gingivostomatitis. Virus is transmitted by saliva and direct contact. Primary infection is subclinical. Multiple oral ulcers will result in painful gums, tongue and sore throat. Lips may be crushed with blood. Swallowing, eating, talking will be painful. Fever, nausea and vomiting may develop. Initially develop as vesicles which rupture later on. Ulcers are multiple and size is 2 to 3 mm.

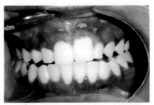

Herpetic gingivostomatitis

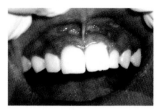
Herpetic gingivostomatitis

Virgin genitals – Question of virginity appears in case of marriage, divorce, defamation and rape. Labia majora are thick, elastic and will be rounded and will be in contact with each other to cover the vulva. Vagina is narrow and rugosed. Hymen a firm fold of mucous membrane may be intact. Hymen may be ruptured due to sports.

Virulence is the strength or disease producing capacity of a pathogen. The virulence of HIV is much less than that of hepatitis B virus. Needle prick involving blood from HBV carrier is 5 to 30% while from HIV positive is only 1%.

Virulent is capable of causing infection or disease.

Virus infections cause disease in mankind. Viruses are obligatory parasites. They cannot reproduce outside living cells. Disease caused by virus includes common cold, measles, chickenpox, mumps, AIDS, poliomyelitis and hepatitis.

Visceral pain is transmitted mainly in the fibres which may accompany sympathetic nerves, most visceral pain impulses travel with sympathetic nerves.

Viscosity is the ability of the material to flow. Thick or viscous liquids flow poorly while thin fluids flow easily. Impression materials have viscosities between 100,000 and 100,000 CP.

Visible luminescent spectroscopy The visible emission spectra and the fluorescent lifetimes for decayed and non-decayed regions of teeth differ. Quasi-monochromatic light from a tungsten source dispersed with a grating monochromator was focused on the teeth. Although, how exactly it works is unknown, this is a non-radiological, non-invasive clinical method to detect dental caries.

Visual agnosia is a failure to identify objects by sight alone even though visual acuity and cerebral functions are normal. Patient may be able to recognize shape and form but not the image or object as a whole. He can match two identical things but cannot recognize the object as a whole.

Vital capacity is the maximum volume of air that can be moved in or out of lungs.

Vital staining is the technique involving administration of certain dyes to the experimental animal, which get incorporated to bone. It is possible to study the manner in which one is laid down, site of growth, and the directions.

Vital statistics can be referred as a systematic approach to collect and compile in numerical form the information related to vital events. It is useful for maintaining records, to maintain control during execution of program or to create administrative standard of health.

Vital theory considered dental caries as originating within the tooth itself, analogous to the bone gangrene. At the end of eighteenth century this theory remained dominant until the middle of the nineteenth century. A clinically well known type of caries is characterized by extensive penetrations into the dentin, and even into the pulp, but with a barely detectable scratch or a fissure.

Vitamin A is a fat soluble vitamin, although vitamin A was not discovered until 1913, cod liver has been in use for centuries. It was chemically synthesized in 1930. Retinal is found only in foods of animal origin. Herbivorous obtain the vitamins from its precursor i.e. carotenoid pigment. Conversion of beta-carotene into retinal in small intestine is only 30 percent. Absorption of both retinal and carotene is facilitated by bile salts. Vitamin E prevents the destruction of vitamin A in the body. It plays a crucial role in normal vision and plays role in immunological defence mechanism. Liver, egg yolk, butter, milk and fish are good sources of vitamin A. yellow colored carrots 'pumpkin, papaya and mango are rich source of vitamin A. Its deficiency may cause night blindness, dry skin and scaly skins. Lack of vitamin A first causes night blindness or inability to see in dim light. Mother can easily detect in children. Conjuctival xerosis is the first clinical sign of vitamin A deficiency. Conjunctiva becomes dry and non wettable. Instead of looking smooth and swing it looks muddy and wrinkled. Bitot's spots are triangular, yellowish foamy spots on bulbar conjunctiva on either side of cornea.

Vitamin C is an ascorbic acid and it is a white crystalline colorless compound readily soluble in water. It is a strong reducing agent. It is comparatively stable in acid medium but is destroyed by heat and catalysts such as copper. Each cigarette smoked uses up to 25 mg of vitamin C equivalent of one orange. Being water soluble it cannot be stored in body. Vitamin C is a cementing material which holds the body cell in place. It helps in absorption of calcium and iron. Deficiency of it delays wound healing. Animal food is a poor source of it and amla is a richest source. Daily requirement is 50 mg and has to be consumed daily. Lemon and oranges are good source of it. Guava and drumsticks have high ascorbic acid content. Leafy vegetables such as cabbage contain lesser quantities. Sprouting converts part of carbohydrate and pulses into vitamin C.

Vitamin D a fat soluble vitamin is intimately connected with the metabolism of calcium and phosphorous. It promotes the absorption of calcium and phosphorous. It promotes the absorption of calcium from intestine and helps in mineralization of bones. It was synthesized in 1935. Exposing the skin to the sun enables the ultraviolet rays to react on the skin's surface oil to produce Vitamin D. The result is not achieved unless you "strip off" since an intervening layer of clothing or of glass impedes the production of Vitamin D. Vitamin D is found in small quantities and in a few animal foods. Foods of plant origin do not contain Vitamin D.

Vitamin E was isolated from wheat germ oil in 1936. It is also known as anti sterility vitamin. Chemically it is identified as tocoferol. This vitamin decreases oxygen requirement of body. Foods rich in poly unsaturated fatty acids are often rich in vitamin E. Vegetable oils, wheat germ oil and egg yolk are rich in vitamin. E. It minimizes wrinkles. It allows great storage of vit. A. It is destroyed by food refining.

Vitamin K was isolated in 1939 by Damin and his Colleagues. Coagulation or clotting of blood is a vitamin K's role function and in cases of deficiency hemorrhage occurs. Limited stores in liver are maintained. Green vegetables contain it well so deficiency does not occur. Soya bean, unrefined cereals, tomatoes, honey and wheat germ also supplies it. It is resistant to heat.

Vitamins are chemical compounds made of carbon, hydrogen and oxygen. Vitamins are soluble in either water or fat. Solubility affects their absorption, storage and excretion. Vitamins do not provide energy but are required for the metabolism of food. Vitamins cannot be synthesized by the body, if any then quantity is not sufficient, hence are to be supplied from outside. Body can make Vitamin D, Vitamin A and niacin if the required precursors are available. Microorganisms of G. I. Tract can synthesize Vitamin K and B_{12} but not to the requirement of body's need.

Vitiligo is a condition where there is partial or complete loss of pigment producing melanocytes within epidermis. Lesions are already seen in darkly pigmented individuals. Histologically there is loss of melanocytes.

Volatile anesthetic agents Basic properties of these agents are (i) liquid at room temperature, (ii) potent in low concentration and (iii) more soluble in blood, cell water and fat than anesthetic agents. Because of solubility of these, equilibration is retarded and induction is slow.

Volvulus is the rotation of a segment of intestine on an axis formed by its mesentery. Cecal volvulus causes colicky pain in right abdomen, obstruction and vomiting with abdominal distension. Plain X-ray will show hugely dilated ovoid cecum. To start single fluid level may be seen.

Von – Sallman Syndrome is a hereditary benign intra-epithelial dyskeratosis. It is rare autosomal dominant trait. Patient shows oral mucosal thickening with superficial gelatinous looking plaques on bulbar conjunctiva. Cytological scrapings show 'cells within cells'.

Von Willebrand's disease is a rare hemorrhage disorder inherited as a Mendelian dominant. There is an excessive capillary fragility. Postoperative dental hemorrhage is a potential hazard.

Vulcanite is a hard rubber prepared by vulcanizing India rubber with suffers. Previously it was used for making removable dentures.

Waddling gait is a gait of a duck. Body is tilted backwards with an increase in lumbar lordosis. Feet are planted widely apart and body sways side to side.

Walking/stepping reflex When the sole of the foot is pressed against the couch, the body tries to walk. It persists as a voluntary standing.

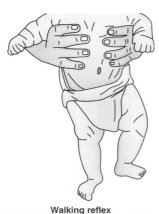

Walking reflex

Walking of the probe is probing technique where the probe should be inserted parallel to the vertical axis of the tooth and is 'walked' circumferentially around each surface of the tooth to detect areas of deepest penetration.

Wallace's "Rule of nine" is the most common technique for assessing the TBSA (total body surface area). This divides the body surface into eleven equal areas each of which is 9% of the total or in multiples of 9, e.g. each upper limb is 9% of the TBSA, each thigh is 9% of TBSA, each lower leg is 9% of TBSA, head and neck is 9%, front of chest is 9%, back of chest is 9%, front of abdomen is 9% and back of trunk is 9%. The perineal area is remaining 1% of TBSA. However, this technique cannot be applied for children because of the proportionately larger surface area of head and neck and smaller area of limbs. Hence modification is done for calculating BSA burned in children.

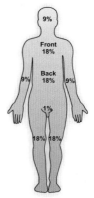

Rule of nine

Wallerian degeneration is the biochemical and morphological alterations following trauma which occur in a nerve due to loss of continuity of axon.

Warty Dyskeratoma involves Face, scalp and neck. Oral lesion are rare but do occur. These areas are small, whitish areas of mucosa with a central depression. Lesion is to be treated by surgical excision. There is no malignant transformation.

Warthin tumor is a common benign tumor of salivary gland. These arise from the lymph nodes with ectopic salivary tissue. Microscopically it shows an admixture of glandular and papillary epithelial structure.

Wasting is defined as any gradual loss of tooth substance which is characterized by the formation of smooth, polished surface. The various forms of wasting are erosion, abrasion and attrition.

Water 55 to 70% of total body weight is water. In old age water content decreases. Fat people contain less water. Urine contains 87% of water. Water is required for many chemical changes. Daily requirement is of 2 to 2.5 litres. Hypothalamus controls water balance. Any loss more than 10% of water is serious.

Water fluoridation is a procedure of adding fluoride to community water supply Grand Rapid's experiment in 1943 first showed conclusive evidence of the success of water fluoridation. 1ppm added, to the community water

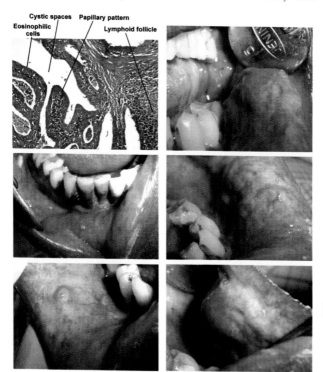

Warthin tumor of minor salivary gland

W

supply and used over 15 yrs. Reduced caries were experienced. By 50% the amount of fluoride varies with the temperature of the area and can be calculated using the formula: -Conc. Of F (PPM) = 0.34/E. Where E = 0.038 + 0.0062 Temperature of the area in F. In colder climates where water consumption is reducing, the concentration of F may be from 1 ppm whereas in hotter climates only up to 0.7 ppm is needed. In moderate temperature the optimum pH conc. is 1 PPM.

Water hammer pulse is having rapid upstroke and descent of pulse wave. It occurs in the case of aortic regurgitation, increased stroke volume results in abrupt upstroke.

Water soluble vitamins are those vitamins which are filtered through the kidneys and excreted in urine when consumed in excess. These are generally non toxic and to be supplied daily. Body reserve of these vitamins are minimal, hence toxicity does not develop. Water soluble vitamins include vitamin C and B complex including thiamine, niacin, riboflavin, pyridoxine, biotin, cynacobalamine and folate.

Water sorption means when some material absorb water. It is known as water sorption.

Water/powder ratio is the mixing proportion of plaster expressed as a decimal fraction. If 100 gm. of plaster is to be mixed with 50 gram of water the W/P ratio is 0.50.

Wave length is the distance between any two corresponding points in the wave. A measurement of physical size, which is important with respect to how the laser light is delivered to the surgical site and to how it reacts with tissue. Wavelength is measured in meters; microns ($10-6m$) and nanometers ($10-9m$).

Wedge fracture of vertebra results from a flexion force. Posterior elements are intact. Reduction is not required.

Wegener's granulomatosis was first described by Wegener in 1936. It is of unknown etiology involving vascular, renal and respiratory system. It may occur at any age. It may develop rhinitis, sinusitis and Otitis or ocular symptoms. Hemorrhage or vascular skin lesions are common. It is characterized by necrotizing granulomatous vasculitis of the respiratory tract and kidneys. Oral manifestations includes oral mucosal ulceration, abnormal tooth mobility, spontaneous exfoliation of teeth and delayed healing, Gingival enlargement may be localized to a single papilla or generalized, It appears as a florid, exospheric growth with a granular surface, Gingival is reddish purple in color and bleeds on provocation, Appearance is that of "over riped strawberry".

Weldability – Substance having the capability of being joined by the passage of a strong electric current.

Well circumscribed lesion is described when the borders of lesion are specifically not defined. Margins and extent of lesions are well seen.

Wernicke's Aphasia The speech is fluent and effortless but comprehension is impaired. Speech is without any meaning.

W

Reading is impaired and writing is full of spelling mistakes. In global aphasia all parameters of language are impaired due to lesion involving territory of middle cerebral artery. There is an extensive lesion of postero-superior temporal region.

Wernicke's encephalopathy is a cerebral form of thiamine deficiency. It presents acutely in thiamine deficiency. Patient is confused and bilateral symme-trical ophthalmoplegia, nystag-mus and ataxia may be present. There may develop permanent memory defect.

Wet gangrene develops when both arterial and venous supply are blocked suddenly. Wet gangrene is rare except in diabetes. Gangrene of internal organs is wet type strangulated hernia, torsions and intestinal adhesions may cause gangrene of bowel. Lesions of lung cause irregular greenish black cavities with foul smell.

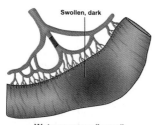

Wet gangrene (bowel)

Wetting is the spreading of a liquid drop on the surface of a solid.

Wheal – A red raised area over skin.

White gold alloy is an alloy containing gold and white metal e.g. silver or palladium that imparts a white appearance to entire mass.

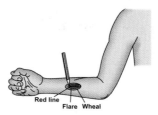

Wheal

White matter is made up of modulated nerve fibres and supporting glial cells. There are 3 types of fibres. Transverse fibers interconnect two cerebral hemis-pheres making up corpus collosum projection fibers con-nect the cerebral cortex with lower portions of brain and spinal cord. The short association fibres connect adjacent gyri.

White object is an object that reflects all incident color lights.

White sponge nevus is also known as cannon's disease. It is an autosomal dominant condition that affects only oral mucosa. Buccal mucosa is the site of lesions. Lesions are asympto-matic. Friction from mastication may strip off the keratotic layer. Cytological study will show empty epithelial cells. Centrally placed are pyknotic nuclei. There is no evidence of lesions being transformed into malignancy. White sponge nevus is an inherited anomaly. oral lesion may be wide spread involving cheeks, palate, gingiva and tongue. Mucus appears thick and folded with a spongy texture with white hue. Ragged white areas may be removed by gentle rubbing without bleeding. Numerous pedigrees of families may show it. There is no treat-ment for the condition.

W

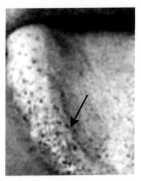

White spongy nevus

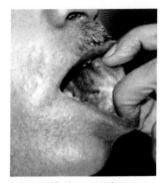

Wickhams straie

Whitlow is a purulent infection involving end of finger.

Whooping cough is caused by gram negative bacillus and principally affects younger person and children. Focal atelectasis, emphysema and peribronchial infiltration by lymphocytes are common. Incubation is 7-16 days. It has 3 stages. In catarrhal stage clinical picture resembles of respiratory catarrh. In paroxysmal stage the diurnal cough becomes paroxysm of 15-20 short coughs followed by deep inspiration with closed glottis producing whoop. Engorged conjunctiva and petechial hemorrhage in forehead and epistaxis are common. Erythromycin is a drug of choice.

Wickham's straie are white raised areas on the buccal, gingival and palatal soft tissues. Fungal infection, oral leukoplakia and lineal albicans are white but have different associations and not lacy in appearance.

Wine is produced by conversion of sugar present in fruits of different varieties into alcohol and CO_2.

Grapes contain 10 to 20% sugar. Fermentation is carried out in vats with the help of selected enzymes. Agreeable aroma and flavor are due to various aromatic principles present in fruits. The special bouquets develop only after wine has been aged for periods varying from four to five years to several decades. Alcoholic content varies from 10 to 20%.

Widening of sellaturcica takes place due to acromegaly or brain tumor. AP dimension ranges about 11 mm and vertical measure about 8 mm.

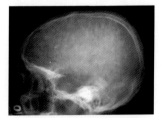

Widening of sellaturcica

Wisdom teeth means third molar. Several back molars appear later in life between 17-25 years of age.

At this age person becomes wise so are known as wisdom teeth. In many persons these may remain imbedded in jaw bone and are said to be impacted. These have to be removed otherwise remain the source of infection.

Working range of wire is the maximum deflection of a wire within the elastic range.

Working time is the duration from the start of mixing to the time when a test rod leaves a permanent identification in the material upon withdrawal.

Worm's theory is a theory explaining dental caries. According to the ancient Sumerian text, toothache was caused by a worm that drank the blood of the teeth and fed on the roots of the jaws. This legend of the worm was discovered on one of many clay tablets excavated. Niffer, Ur, and other cities within the Euphrates valley of the lower Mesopotamian area and estimated to date from about 5000 BC. The idea that caries is caused by a worm was almost universal at one time, as evidenced by the writing of Homer and popular lore of China, India, Finland and Scotland.

W

Xenograft refer Heterograft.

Xerophthalmia means where the sebaceous and hair follicles of skin and tear glands of eye become blocked with horny plugs of keratin so that their secretion diminishes. Lack of tears and heaping up of epithelium on the sclera and conjunctiva develops. In conjuctival xerosis conjunctiva looks muddy and wrinkled instead of transparent and clear. It becomes dry.

Xeroradiography is a technique that uses modified xerographic copying techniques to record images produced by diagnostic X-rays. They have an additional feature called "edge enhancement" effect. Due to these small structures and areas of subtle density differences are made more visible. They contain uniformly charged selenium plates. Advantages includes that half of X-ray radiation is required. 2. It produces real image. 3. Reflected light is used. 4. No need for chemical processing in dark room. 5. This technique is extensively used in the diagnosis of diseases of breast.6. It is economical.

Xerostomia is defined as the perception of oral dryness. There is a dryness of mouth and all degrees of dryness occur. It is often due to a reduction in salivary flow rates of the major and minor salivary glands. Humans suffering from decreased or lack of salivary secretions often experiences an increased rate of dental caries and rapid tooth destruction. Mucosa will appear dry and atrophic. It may be pale and translucent. Tongue may show fissuring and cracking. It may result in rampant dental caries.

X-ray absorptiometry is a diagnostic test where bone thickness is usually measured with bone density scan. Dual energy X-ray absorptiometry is a common test to measure bone thickness in spine, hips and wrists. This test gives two scores T score and X score. T score compares your bone thickness to the thickness of a healthy 30 years old. While X score compares your bone thickness to the bone thickness of other person of your age. T score lower than -2.5 means you have osteoporosis and T_1 score between -1 and -2.5 shows osteopenia.

Xylitol is the best nutritive sucrose substitute with respect to caries prevention. It is non-acidogenic, hence non-cariogenic. It is also non-cariogenic by inhibiting the growth of certain bacteria stimulating salivary flow and increasing salivary calcium concentration.

Yellow brown film is a processing error, where the film appears brown – yellow due to exhausted develop or fixer.

Yellow lesions give yellow color and are caused by carotene, accumulation of pus, exudation of serum and aggregation of lymphoid tissue. Yellow color is seen in ulcers or pustules. Serum is normally a yellow or straw colored fluid. Normal lipid containing structures such as Fordyce's granules usually appear yellow.

Yellow stains generally occur from the food pigments and are also associated with the presence of bacterial plaque; it has a dull, light yellow appearance due to bacterial plaque which is common to all ages and more prominent in patients where personal oral hygiene is neglected.

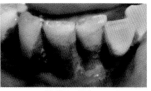

Yellow stains

Yield stress is the stress at which dislocation, motion and permanent deformation and plastic flow begin.

Young's frame is a U-shaped metal or plastic form used to hold a dental dam in place.

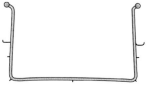

Youngs rubber dam frame

Z score is a deviation score divided by the standard deviation. It indicates how many standard deviations the raw score is above or below the mean.

Zimmerman – Lebarnd Syndrome patient develops gingival fibromatosis with defects of ear, nose, bones and terminal phalanges. Joints become hyperflexible. Spleen is enlarged.

Zinc is a mineral present in human body. Average human body contains 1.4 to 2.3 gram of zinc. Highest concentrations are found in liver, bone, prostate and eye. It is a constituent of insulin. Zinc plasma level is 96 micro grams per 100 ml in adults. Daily requirement is 5 to 10 mg. Deficiency of it results in anorexia, pernicious anemia, and thalassemia. It maintains normal taste.

Zinc oxide – Eugenol is suitable as a base under metallic restorations due to its sealing quality. Eugenol has bacteriostatic property. But if zinc oxide is placed close to pulp it may result in irritation. Within 8 weeks period an increasing amount of reparative dentin is noted. Although it causes only a slight pulp response and yet promotes reparative dentin formation in deep cavities. . It is a material of choice for use over injured pulps or as a base in deep cavity preparation.

Z-track technique is a method of giving injection that prevents mediation from leaking outside the muscle.

Zygote – The fertilized ovum.

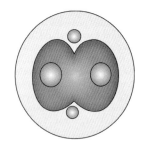

Zygote

Appendices

HISTORY OF DENTISTRY

Dentistry — Past and Present

Dental diseases have remained almost similar throughout history. Decay, toothaches, periodontal disease and premature tooth loss were documented in history. The exact time that dentistry has made its presence felt is not known but there are sufficient evidences of its existence among the various civilizations. Since Dental History is such a broad field, a few of the highlights of dentistry will be mentioned in order of importance and chronology.

Pre-historically

- Life consisted of simple creatures of the sea, which consisted of protoplasmic cells.
- They survived by engulfing themselves around a desired morsel, they were able to absorb food. Later a slit developed the forerunner of the oral cavity and great gut.
- Then there was development of tentacles and feelers developed around this slit, which helped them to carry the food to the slit, oral cavity and great gut.
- Then nature took the outer layer of skin and carried it inward to the oral cavity. This skin contained tentacles which were the forerunners of our teeth. These tentacles, also called shagreen, were calcified.
- Some of these sea creatures developed lungs and became amphibians.
- Some began to spend time on land. At first they crawled on their bellies, later they developed limbs and feet and arose from the ground. Faced with a new environment including a mixed diet, the creatures evolved into stronger animals made up of hard bone and tough muscle fiber. Originally three single tentacles fused and became tri-conodonts.
- These tri- conodonts later changed into teeth very similar to the Catarrine Apes. The descendants of these apes have the similar dental formula as humans.
- Fire and its benefits were discovered. Cooking made sea food more palatable. Fish and shell fish became the staple diet as well as nuts, fruits, and the flesh of animals, then the cultivated grains such as rice, wheat and barley were added to the diet.

- If we go back to the beginning of history at 4000 B.C., toothaches can be traced to the earliest records. In the Egyptian manuscripts known as Eber's Papyri, which dates back to 3700 B.C., where dental diseases such as toothaches and sore gums are mentioned.
- 3000 years ago, the Chinese manuscripts of that period, at least nine dental diseases were listed and also along with them were listed the prescriptions for their treatment. Ancient skulls showed the presence of decay. In the Giza Pyramids skulls were found with evidence of tooth decay.
- People of early ages had odd beliefs concerning teeth. The Egyptians believed that the mouse was under the direct protection of the sun therefore if one had a toothache, the split body of a warm mouse was applied to the affected side. In India the cuspid of Buddha was enshrined in a famous temple (at Kandi) and prayed to in fertility rites. Prayers were offered up to saints for the relief of pain. St. Apollonia of Alexandria, 249 A.D., was one such saint. She is now the Patron Saint of Dentistry.

Egyptians

- The first known dentist was an Egyptian named Hesi-Re (3000 B.C.). He was the chief dentist to the Pharaohs. He was also a physician, indicating an association between medicine and dentistry but in the 5th century B.C. Herodatus, a historian, described the medical art in Egypt: "The art of medicine is distributed thus: Each physician is a physician of one disease and no more; and the whole country is full of physicians, for some profess themselves to be physicians of the eyes, others of the head, teeth, stomach, and others of more obscure ailments". Dentistry today is somewhat specialized and is divided into eight specialities that are as follows:
    - 1901 Orthodontics
    - 1918 Oral surgery
    - 1918 Periodontics
    - 1918 Prosthodontics
    - 1927 Pedodontics
    - 1937 Public health
    - 1946 Oral pathology
    - 1963 Endodontics.
- The first evidence of a surgical operation was found in Egypt. A mandible with two perforations just below the root of the first molar indicated the establishment of drainage of an abscessed tooth.
- Egyptians practised the splinting of teeth which dates back to 2750 B.C where it shows two molars fastened with heavy gold wire.

Chinese

- The Chinese were known to have treated dental ills with knife, cautery, and acupuncture, a technique whereby they punctured different areas of the body with a needle. There is no evidence of mechanical dentistry at that time.

- Marco Polo in 2700 B.C. stated that the Chinese did cover teeth with thin gold leafs only for aesthetic purposes.
- The earliest practice of the prosthetic arts was among the ancient Phoenicians circa 500 B.C. Hammarabi, ruler of all lower Mesopotamia (1760 B.C.), established a state controlled economy in which fees charged by physicians were set.

Greeks

Greeks contributed mostly on the medical side. The ancient Greek physician,

- **Aesculapius (1250 B.C.)** gained great fame for medical knowledge and skill. Apollo was listed as his father. He originated the art of bandaging and use of purgatives. He also advocated cleaning of teeth and extractions.
- **Hippocrate (500 B.C.)** was supposed to be a descendant of Aesculapius. Hippocrates became famous both as practioner and writer on medical subjects. He did not believe in magic and stressed nature's role in healing. Hippocrates raised the art of medicine to a high level. Also in one of his texts (Peri-Arthron) he devoted 32 paragraphs to the dentition. He appreciated the importance of teeth. He accurately described the technique for reducing a fracture of the jaw and also for replacing a dislocated mandible. He was familiar with extraction forceps for this is mentioned in one of his writings.
- **Aristotle (384 B.C.)** who follows Hippocrates, accurately described extraction forceps and in his book De Partibus Animal Culum and also devoted a complete chapter to the teeth. He also stated that figs and soft sweets produce decay. He called it a putrefactive process instead of fermentative.

Etruscans

- **Etruscans (100 - 400 B.C.)** made their greatest contribution in restorative dentistry. In Italian museums there are numerous specimens of crowns and bridges. In 1870 the dental engine was invented. A very unusual specimen is a bridge that was constructed about 2500 years ago. This consists of several gold bands fastened to natural teeth and supporting three artificial teeth. Etruscan art, seen at its best in Florence, reflects some oriental influence but essentially it is their own. Conquered in 309 B.C., they were absorbed by the Roman Empire.

Romans

Famous Roman physicians are named below:

Celsus (25 BC-50 AD) Hippocrates did not believe in magic but Celsus believed that General Physical deterioration caused dental diseases. For toothaches he prescribed:

- Hot water fermentations
- Narcotics
- Mustard seed
- Counter irritants
- Use of the cautery
- Alum for soft tissue disease
- Extraction of badly broken down teeth. He recommended filling the cavity with lead prior to extraction as a means of lessening the chance of fracturing the crown.
- Introduced the technique for reducing fractures
- Introduced first technique for tooth straightening or positioning.

Archigenus (100 A.D.)
- Pulpitis was recognized by him
- Invented the dental drill to enter into pulp chamber

Galen (200 A.D.) was considered to be the greatest physician since Hippocrates, was the first to recognize that a toothache could be due to:
- Pulpitis (inflammation of the pulp)
- Pericementitis (inflammation of radicular portion of the tooth)
- He classified teeth into centrals, cuspids and molars.

Hebrews give first evidence of dentistry among the Jews:
- Relief of toothache and artificial restorations may be found in a collection of books known as the Talmud (352 A.D. - 407).
- The worm was blamed for decay. Also stated that gum disease started in the mouth but ended in the gut.
- As for extractions — all cultures expressed anxiety about removing a cuspid for fear of eye injury. This superstition continues today.

The Middle Ages

- 410 A.D. the clever and rational approaches of Hippocrates and Celsus had disappeared; magic and superstitious dominated. Then came the **Albucasis**, (1013 A.D.). He was considered the great exponent of dental surgery in the middle ages. In his book the first illustration of dental instruments was found which are as follows:
  - Surgical elevators
  - Surgical forceps
  - 14 scalers
  - Cautery
  - Dental saws and files for caries removal
  - Besides being a famous surgeon and competent writer, he was also a greater teacher and believed in the referred pain theory. He accurately described technique for extractions, with special emphasis on careful manipulation of soft tissue. He also described treatment for partially luxated teeth.

The Barber-Surgeons

- At the onset of the middle Ages, monks became physicians and dentists. Barbers had acted as assistants to the monks. When the pope in 1163 ruled that any operation involving the shedding of blood was incompatible with the priestly office, the barber took over the practice of Surgery. The barber surgeons were not the only ones doing extractions; another group made up of Vagabonds were known as tooth drawers. They plied their trade in public squares. For awhile then, dentistry was carried on by Barber-surgeons both in France and England. However, in France (1700) anyone desiring to practice oral surgery and restorative dentistry had to take a regular prescribed examination.

Founding of Universities and Introduction of Dental Texts

Chirurgia Magna was written by the famous French surgeon **Guy de Cahuliac** in 1386. In this text, he devoted some space to pathology and therapeutics of the teeth. Cahuliac was first to coin the term **dentator** and **dentists**. The English term dentist came from his original terms. Following Cahuliac came **Giovanni de Arcoli** in 1400. His opinions and instruments were somewhat modern. His pelican for extraction of teeth was used for years and his root forceps could be used today. He advised good oral cleaning habits and to avoid hot and cold substances as well as sweet stuff. He was first to mention filling teeth with gold.

Famous Scientists

Vesalius, 1500 of Belgium, became an anatomist at the University of Padua, Italy. In medical profession he laid the foundation for true scientific research which is the basis of our present day medical practice. He accurately described the teeth and pulp chambers.

Fallopius was another anatomist, a pupil of Vesalius. He is credited with the descriptions of the dental follicle, trigeminal nerve, auditory nerve, the glossopharyngeal, the hard and the soft palate. He stated that teeth were not true bone.

Eustachius (1500) gave the complete anatomical description of teeth and their development, the periodontal membrane and alveoli. He was credited with the first complete dental book, ninety five pages of anatomy, embryology, physiology, blood and nerve supply of the teeth. In this text, he completely describes the anatomy of the teeth, their development, the alveolus and the periodontal membrane.

Leonardo da Vinci (end of 15th Century) described the anatomy of the jaws, teeth and maxillary sinus. These drawings are the first to accurately describe the maxillary sinus. However, credit has been given to **Dr Nathaniel Highmore** of England (1650).

Ambrose Pare (16th Century) was a Barber - Surgeon at 16 years of age and became a member of the College of Surgeons at age 37. He was the first to describe Palatal Obturators, and transplant techniques, etc. His instruments though crude could be used today.

Malpighi (17th Century) a great anatomist and a founder of histology had made great use of the microscope for tissue studies.

Leeuwenhoek (17th Century) invented the microscope. He described the dental tubuli and was the first to see organisms of the mouth.

Purman of Breslau (middle 17th Century) is known for wax impressions.

Philip Pfaff (18th Century) introduced plaster for pouring up models.

Pierre Fauchard (18th Century - 1728) Father of Scientific Dentistry wrote a great text "Surgeon Dentist". He not only wrote a complete work on Odontology in two volumes but also recognized the intimate relationship between oral conditions and general health. He advocated the use of lead to fill cavities. He removed all decay and if the pulp was exposed, and used the cautery. He prescribed oil of cloves and cinnamon for pulpitis. He also described partial dentures and full dentures in his text and constructed dentures with springs and used human teeth. Gold dowels were used in root canals filled with lead. He was also known as Father of Orthodontics.

Robert Bunon (1743) printed the first dental therapeutics text, dentistry's first pharmacopeia.

Thomas Berdmore (1768) wrote "Disorders and Deformities of Teeth and Gums".

John Hunter (1771) wrote "Natural History of the Human Teeth".

Joseph Fox wrote Pupil of Hunter; wrote text, same title "Natural History of the Human Teeth".

John Greenwood (1789) dentures for George Washington were made by him.

Charles Goodyear (1840) discovered vulcanite rubber. It was used for denture bases. This discovery led to false teeth for the millions. Dentures were called vulcanite dentures.

EJ Dunning (1844) made plaster of Paris impressions, first shown in America.

M Bourdet (mid 18th Century) described use of gold for base plates.

FAMOUS SCIENTISTS

Vesalius

Fallopius

Eustachius

Leonardo da Vinci

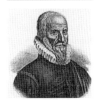
Ambrose Pare

Malpighi

Leeuwenhoek

Philip Pfaff

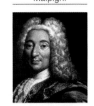
Pierre Fauchard

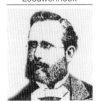
Robert Bunon

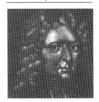
Thomas Berdmore

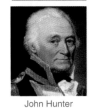
John Hunter

Charles Goodyear

EJ Dunning

M Bourdet

Role of Women in Dentistry

The first woman dentist in England was a widow of Dr Povey - 1719. When he died she took over his practice. The first woman dentist in the United States was Emeline Rupert Jones of Connecticut. She too, took over her husband's practice after he died. After his death, she took over and practiced for atleast 50 years. She was accepted in both the Connecticut State Dental Society in 1893 and National Dental Association in 1914. The honour of being the first woman graduate dentist goes to Dr Lucy Hobbs, 1865. She graduated from the Ohio Dental College.

HISTORICAL EVENTS OF DENTISTRY IN CHRONOLOGICAL ORDER

- 2750 B.C. Mandible of the ancient period shows evidence of having had a surgical operation to relieve an alveolar abscess.

- 2500 B.C. Egyptian, earliest evidence of simple retentive dental prosthesis as found in Tomb 984 at Gizeh, the linking together of the lower left second and third molar with gold wire woven around the gingival margins of the teeth.

- 1900 B.C. Code of **Hammurabi** established the civil and penal responsibility of the physician, dental penalties as to the extraction of teeth.

- 1700 B.C. **The Edwin Smith** Surgical Papyrus transcribed from an earlier manuscript contains methods for reducing fractures of the mandible.

- 700-510 B.C. Etruscan period of dentistry. i.e. Middle Italy, few examples of their fixed or removable bridgework has been preserved in various museums.

- 669-626 B.C. **King Ashurbanipal** has a Collection of Babylonian cuneiform tables and a library. Tooth worm theory. 5th Century Examples of Phoenician simple retentive dental prosthetics found at Sidon.

- Evidence of dental practice in India.

- 490-425 B.C. **Herodotus**, the Greek historian and traveller, describes Egypt as being the home of medical specialists. Confirmation of this was done by **Hermann Junker** in 1914.

- 480 B.C. Roman period begins. Dentistry was probably practiced before medicine.

- 460-370 B.C. **Hippocrates**, the founder of Medicine was first to recognize the teeth *in utero*, Humoral pathology, use of gold wire for fractures and instruction on how to handle instruments.

- 450 B.C. **Roman Laws** of the Twelve Tables and the permission to bury the dead with gold dental work with "which the teeth may be bound together. The use of Centuries B.C. gold shell crowns.

- 384-322 B.C. **Aristotle**, pupil of Plato was the first to make a study of comparative anatomy of the teeth. He also mentions the extraction of teeth with forceps.

- 30 A.D. Celsus wrote his De Medicina, is the earliest to mention the filling of teeth with lint or lead, however to extract the tooth more readily and not for its preservation. He suggested the binding of teeth in fractures of the jaw and orthodontic treatment.

- 48-117 A.D. Archigenes of Apameia , a roman physician recommended the use of the drill in filling teeth "right down to the center of the tooth, to give vent to the accumulated pus."

- 130-201 A.D. **Galen**, the Prince of Physicians, in 162 began to practice in Rome and in 168 was appointed as the imperial physician. His treatise (Venice 1490) was a standard textbook for centuries. He was also the earliest to mention the nerves of teeth. He recommended the use of file in removing the carious defect, he also mentioned about pulpitis and Pericementitis.

- 249 A.D. **St. Apollonia**, the Patron Saint of Dentistry, had her teeth extracted in Alexandria.

- 936-1013 A.D. **Albucasis a** physician born near Cordova, was one of the most learned physicians and surgeons of his time. His Dechirurgia, one of the great surgical treatises, contains illustrations of both surgical and dental instruments with detailed description of the use of them. He describes a method of transplanting teeth and the use of gold wire to ligate loose ones. Besides improving the type of extracting forceps he devised many elevators and scalers. He was also the one of the earliest to devise a method to correct deformities in the mouth and dental arches.

- 1308-1745 A.D. France, Guild of Barber-Surgeons founded and remained active until 1745.

- **Guy de Cahuliac** completes his celebrated work on surgery (published in 1478) and therein we obtain a clear and concise idea of the condition of dentistry during the fourteenth century. He coined the term dentators.

- 1452-1519 A.D. **Leonardo da Vinci**, who inspired the work of **Vesalius**, was an anatomist and original dissector of the human body. His manuscript presents the earliest accurate drawings of the skull, teeth, associated structures and maxillary sinus.1460 A.D. Earliest English medical manuscript Guy de Cahuliac's Surgery.

- 1468 A.D. **Barbers** in England obtain charter from King Edward IV.

- 1498 A.D. Invention of the modern toothbrush by the Chinese on June 24.

- 1514 A.D. Publication of **Giovanni's da Vigo's** work on surgery that passed through innumerable editions wherein we find the earliest printed record of the filling of teeth with gold foil after first excavation and shaping the cavity.

- 1538 A.D. **Andreas Vesalius**, the famous anatomist, was the first to use wood cuts to illustrate his writings; therein is to be found much relating to the tooth.

- 1542 A.D. **Ambrose Pare**, famous military surgeon, revived the old method of compression of nerve trunks to produce local anesthesia. He also mentions transplantation and filling of teeth and ligation of teeth with gold wire. He described palatal Obturators as well.

- 1543 A.D. **Andreas Vesalius** gave important observations on the development of teeth.

- 1561 A.D. **Gabriel Fallopius** writes about the dental follicle and development of teeth.

- 1651 A.D. **Nathaniel Highmore** describes maxillary sinus in the superior maxillary bone (1673) microorganisms (animalcules) in teeth and describes their tubular construction.

- 1683 A.D. **Anton van Leeuwenhoek** discovered the use of microscope

- 1728 A.D. First edition of **Pierre Fauchard** (founder of modern dentistry) textbook on "The Surgeon's Dentist."

- 1728 A.D. **Pierre Fauchard** great work "Le Chirurgien Dentiste"

- 1733-1735 A.D. **James Reading and James Mills** first tooth-drawers in New York and perhaps in America.

- 1756 A.D. **Philip Pfaff** made plaster models and describes taking the bite. He also practiced capping the pulp.

- 1759 A.D. The designation dentist first began to be used.

- 1763 A.D **John Baker,** M.D. Surgeon Dentist was the earliest qualified dentist to practice in Boston and in America.

- 1766 A.D. **Robert Woofendale**, pupil of Berdmore, arrives in America and locates in New York. Thomas Berdmore of London publishes the first English dental textbook in which he claims the use of sugar to be deleterious. He Became the Dentist to his Majesty.

- 1769 A.D. Title of Doctor began to be used.

- 1771 A.D. **John Hunter**, comparative anatomist and surgeon, publishes his classic description of the anatomy of the human teeth, he demanded the removal of the pulp before filling the teeth in the case of transplantation

- 1774 A.D. Introduction of porcelain into dentistry by French apothecary **Duchatenu**.

- 1778 A.D. Body of General Joseph Warren identified by dental work done in the mouth by **Paul Revere**.

- 1779 A.D. **Isaac Greenwood**, Sr., began to practice dentistry in Boston.

- 1784 A.D. **Isaac Greenwood**, Jr., begins his dental practice in New York.

- 1788 A.D. Improvement and development of porcelain dentures by **deChemant**.

- 1791 A.D. Establishment of the first dental clinic in the Dispensary of the City of New York.

- 1793 A.D. **Benjamin Bell's** interest in dental pathology and therapy led him to important observations on the pulp and pericementum.

- 1794 A.D. Earliest use of mineral paste teeth in America by **Le Breton**. **John Greenwood** began to swage gold bases for dentures. He made George Washington's dentures.

- 1801 A.D. First dental book to be published in America by **Richard Cortland Skinner**.

- 1806 A.D. Individual porcelain teeth with baked-in metal pins, invented by **Fonzi**.

- 1819 A.D. Mixing of coin silver fillings and mercury into a silver paste, by **Tavenu** in France.

- 1832 A.D. **Snell** - first dental chair.

- 1836 A.D. Arsenic introduced for the killing of pulps, by **Spooner**.

- 1839 A.D. First dental periodical, the American Journal of Dental Science.

- 1840 A.D. The American Society of Dental Surgeons, first national dental organization. The Baltimore College of Dental Surgery, the first school in the world for the training of dentists was founded by Harris and Harden.

- 1842 A.D. **Crawford W. Long** discovers anesthetic agent, but does not publicize it.

- 1844 A.D. Beginning of large scale manufacture of porcelain teeth by **S.S. White**. Discovery of nitrous oxide anesthesia by **H. Wells** and the use of plaster of Paris for impressions.

- 1851 A.D. **Patentt** for hard rubber (Vulcanite) granted to **Nelson Goodyear**.

- 1855 A.D. Cohesive gold foil for filling teeth, introduced by **Robert Arthur**.

- 1859 A.D. Organization of American Dental Association on a representative basis.

- 1863 A.D. Organization of National Association of Dental Examiners.

- 1864 A.D. Rubber dam suggested by **Sanford C. Barnum**.

- 1866 A.D. Organization of college faculties.

- 1866 Tiny multiple cysts of palate in fetus and neonates were first described by Heinrich Bohn and by Alois Epstein in 1880.

- 1868 A.D. Combination of nitrous oxide and oxygen for prolong anesthesia, by **Edmund Andrews**.

- 1872 A.D. First foot-engine, invented by **Morrison**.

- 1877 A.D. Hydraulic chair invented by **Wilkinson**.

- 1884 A.D. **Keller** suggests cocaine hydrochlorate for topical anesthesia. **W.S. Halstead** used conductive anesthesia in the mandible.

- 1885 **Malassez** named the term adamantinoma.

- 1887 A.D. Gutta percha root canal points.

- 1888 Mikulicz disease was described by **Mr Mikulicz**

- 1890 A.D **W.D. Miller** describes microorganism of the human mouth.

- 1891 A.D. Extension for prevention and scientific cavity preparation suggested by **G.V. Black**.

- 1892 A.D. The establishment of a three-year course in dental colleges.

- 1893 **Garre** described thickening of periosteum of long bones due to infection.

- 1893 A.D. System of dental nomenclature by **G.V. Black**

- 1895 A.D **Roentgen** discovers the X-ray. **G.V. Black** develops the balanced amalgam alloys.

- 1896 A.D. **C. Edward Kells** demonstrates use of Roentgen rays in dentistry.

- 1897 A.D. **B.F. Philbrook**, presents paper on "Cast Gold Fillings," the **Taggart** inlay method. American Dental Association and Southern Dental Association consolidate under the name of National Dental Association.

- 1899 A.D. One year of high school's a requirement for admission to dental school.

- 1901 A.D. **Weston A. Price** recommends the use of X-ray in root canal work.

- 1903 A.D. Four years course in dental colleges established.

- 1906 A.D. **Einhorn** recommends novacaine and adrenalin combination for local anesthesia.

- 1907 A.D. **William H. Taggart** demonstrates the cast gold inlay.

- 1909 A.D. Dental Educational Counsel of America organized.

- 1912 A.D. National Dental Association organized on a district basis.

- 1913 The term Tauriodontin was originated by **Sir Arthur Keith**. Body of tooth is enlarged at the cost of roots.

- 1914 A.D J. **Leon Williams** develops typical tooth forms.

- 1915 A.D. **McKay and Black** publishes results of investigation of fluoride in drinking water.

- 1916 Mottled enamel was described by **G.V. Black** and **F Mackay**.

- 1920 Dentin dysplasia was described by **Ballschmiede**.

- 1922 A.D. National Dental Association changed name to American Dental Association.

- Association publication changed from National to Journal of the American Dental Association.

- 1932 A.D. New type of denture materials introduced.

- 1933 The retrocuspid papilla was first described by **Hirshfeld** as a small, elevated nodule.

- 1936 Neonatal line in deciduous teeth was described by **Schour**.

- 1938 Dentinogenesis imperfect was diagnosed by **Finn, Hodge** and his **co-workers** confirmed in 1939.

- 1939 **Dodd** and her colleges isolated herpes simplex virus from gingivostomatitis.

- 1939 **Parker and Jackson** described Reticulum cell sarcoma.

- 1939-40 **Gall, Mallory, Jackson** and **Parker** developed classification for malignant lymphoma.

- 1940 The term eosinophilic granolona of bone was introduced by **Lichentenstrein** and **Jaffe** in 1940.

- 1942 Benign chondroblastoma of bone was named by **Jaffe** and **Lichtenstein**.

- 1942 **Stout** and **Murray** suggested the term heamangiopericytoma.

- 1945 Mucoepidermoid carcinoma was described by **Stewart Foote**.

- 1945 **Dublin** and **Johnson** described benign osteoblastoma.

- 1946 **Jaffe** and **Lichetenste**in described chondromyxoid fibroma.

- 1947 Adenoid squamous cell carcinoma was described by **Lever**.

- 1948 Verrucous carcinoma was defined **Ackerman**.

- 1949 **Macarthy** described pyostomatitis vegetans.

- 1952 **Christopherson** described Alveolar soft part sarcoma.

- 1953 A.D. **Dr. Nelson's** turbo-jet drill, 60,000 RPM.

- 1956 Clear cell carcinoma was described by **Coridan.**

- 1956 **Pindborg** was first to describe calcified epithelial odontogenic tumor.

- 1956 A.D. Air-rotor drill, 250,000 RPM **Dr Robert Borden**.

- 1957 Chronic granullomatour disease was identified.

- 1958 **Robinson** and his **co-workers** first described hand, foot and mouth disease.

- 1958-59 **Burkitt** reported African Jaw lymphoma.

- 1960 **Cooke** described recurrent herpetiform ulcer.

- 1962 **Steigman** foun out a strain of coxsackie virus causing acute lymphonodular pharyngitis.

- 1962 **Gorlin** and co-workers described calcified odontogenic cyst.

- 1963 Odontogenic Keratocyst was described calcified by **Philipsen.**
- 1967 Monomorphic adenoma was described by **Kleinasser.**
- 1971 Verruciform Xanthoma was first described by **Shafer.**
- 1975 **Pullon** reported squamous odontogenic tumor.
- 1988 **Sir William Osler** is 1888 first described hereditary form of angioneurotic oedemo.

INDIVIDUAL HISTORICAL BACKGROUND IN DENTISTRY

Gold Foil

- **Giovanni di Arcoli**, 15th Century described filling of cavity with gold leaf.
- **Pierre Fauchard**, 1728, used gold for restorations, and denture bases.
- In 1812, a manufacturer in **Hartford**, Connecticut specialized in beaten gold leaf for dental purposes.
- In 1855, **Dr Arthur** described a technique for using cohesive gold foil. the passing of gold foil through a flame would remove impurities and cause it to adhere to each other. One important condition for perfect cohesiveness was that the cavity had to be free of saliva. This wasn't overcome until **Dr Barnum** invented the rubber dam in 1864. The dam plus the dental engine helped gold foil achieve a high degree of perfection. In the early 1900s a leading authority on gold foil was **Dr Charles Woodbury** who taught for many years at Creighton.

Amalgam

- First used as a silver paste by **M. Taveau** of Paris in 1826, amalgam at first had its drawbacks. Some mixtures caused expansion resulting in fractured teeth. G.V. Black experimented with silver amalgam and developed a suitable formula which met all requirements. He found in his research that if alloy fillings are heated to a certain temperature they would remain stable for a long period.

Gutta Percha

- A rubber-like material which came into use in 1848. It is used as a temporary filling and also extensively used in Endodontics.

Zinc Oxyphosphate Cement

- Came into use in 1880.
- Used in cementing crowns, inlays, and as a protective base over nearly exposed pulps.

Porcelain

- Used since the 1800s for denture teeth.
- All porcelain crowns used since 1900, generally unacceptable.
- Porcelain fused to metal crowns developed in late 1950s.

Gold Inlay

- A new and accurate method of casting gold inlays was announced by **Dr William H. Taggart** in 1907.
- This technique was called the disappearing wax technique. He patented this technique but lost his patents when it was discovered that **Dr Philbrook** of Denison, Iowa had written an article concerning gold inlay castings 25 years earlier. A copy of this article was found in the dental library of the University of Iowa.

Composite

- In 1938 **Castan** invented epoxy resins formed the basis for composite resins.
- Acrylic **Resin** was used for anterior filling in the 1940s, but was unacceptable because of leakage.
- In 1948 an incremental layering technique involving an auto-cured acrylic resin was introduced. Later light-curing catalysis based an alpha-diketones amines were invented in Britain.
- Unfilled resins which were the predecessors of composite resins were introduced in late 1940s and early 1950s. They evolved as a restorative material because they are insoluble, aesthetic, insensitive to dehydration, inexpensive and relatively easy to manipulate but they were found to be only partially successful in meeting the requirements of a durable aesthetic restorative material for anterior teeth. High polymerization shrinkage, co-efficient of thermal expansion and Lack of abrasion resistance led to clinical deficiencies and permanent failure.
- In 1950 acrylic filling materials containing alumina silicate glass filler were formulated. Here silicate glass was precoated with polymer. Although this process improved the materials physical properties but it was still hard to manipulate.
- In an effort to improve the physical characteristics of unfilled acrylic resin, Development of Modern Dental Composite Restorative material started in the late 1950s early 1960s by **Dr. Raefel Bowen** to resolve the deficiencies caused by high polymerization shrinkage and high co-efficient of thermal expansion. Inert filler particles were added to reduce the volume of the resinous component but performance of composites were not too successful because the filler particles were not chemically bonded to the resin matrix. This resulted in fluid leakage, unacceptable surface appearance and poor wear resistance.
- A major advance occurred when **Bowen** developed a new type of composite material. His main innovations are Bis Phenal A. – glycidyl

methacrylate, (BISGMA) a dimethacrylate resin or Bowen's resin and use of a silane to coat filler particles that could bond chemically to resin.

- The improved matrix properties and Matrix bonding yielded a restorative material that was clearly superior to the unfilled resins. Since the early 1970's the composites have virtually replaced the unfilled acrylics for tooth restorations.
- The first commercial composites were introduced in early 1960s which includes TD71 (Dental Filling Ltd) and Addent (3M).

Bleaching

- Bleaching was unsuccessfully used in the middle ages.
- Modern bleaching technique began in 1918. **Abbot** used the combination of superoxol and heat.
- 1958 **Prarson** introduced intra pulpal bleach.
- 1967 **Nutting and Por** introduced walking bleach.
- 1978 Superoxol +heat + light.
- 1989 Haywood and Hayman gave night guard vital bleaching,10% carbimide peroxide.
- 1996 Laser tooth whitening officially started with the approval of ion laser technology, Argon and CO_2 lasers to be used with a potential system of chemicals.

Lasers

- The idea and concept of laser capability was first acknowledged in 1917. **Albert Einstein** first conceptualized the use of stimulated emission, which serves as the foundation of a laser. In the early to mid-1950's, Bell Labs' **Arthur L. Schawlow**, and **Charles H. Townes** invented the MASER (microwave amplification by stimulated emission of radiation), by means of ammonia gas and microwave radiation.
- The MASER was invented prior to the optical laser, yet the technology is very comparable.
- On May 16, 1960, **Theodore Maiman's** ruby laser became the first working laser in history.
- In the 1960's, **Dr Ali Javan** invented the first gas laser with Helium Neon.
- Four years later, the carbon dioxide laser was successfully shaped by **Kumar Patel** in 1964.
- A new realization of commercial and research opportunities through laser technology became widespread, and substrates and ions such as rare earths (Nd, Pr, Tm, Ho, Er, Yb, Gd, and Ur) were all eventually successfully "lased".
- Over the years, Goldman and Other researchers documented the ability of various types of lasers to cut, coagulate, ablate and vaporize biologic tissues.

- In 1968 L'Esperance was the first to report clinical use of an argon laser in ophthalmology.
- In 1972, Strong and Jako reported the first clinical use of a CO_2 laser in otolaryngology.
- Keifhaber et al documented the first clinical use of Nd: YAG laser in 1977 in gastro intestinal surgery.
- Historically, the first lasers to be marketed for intraoral use generally were CO_2 lasers with otorhinolaryngologic clearance authorized by FDA. In May 1990, the FDA cleared it for intraoral soft tissue surgery. A pulsed Nd: YAG laser developed by Myers and Myers, recognized as the first laser designed specifically for general dentistry.
- Other lasers and researches followed, and today lasers are used routinely across a broad spectrum of medical disciplines, including dentistry.

Caries Indices

- In 1931, **Bodecker, C.P** and **Bodecker H.W.C** described Caries Index. This Caries Index was found to be sensitive but too complex for use in epidemiological surveys.
- **Bodecker** modified this Caries Index later, where, in addition counting the surfaces decayed, an extra count was allotted for those surfaces that could experience multiple caries attacks. But this was also not used in major epidemiological studies.
- The approach to measuring caries by counting the numbers of teeth in the mouth visibly affected by caries was used in a systematic manner, by **Dean** and associated in their historical studies of the dental caries / fluoride relation.
- **Mellanby** M in 1934 described the carious lesions depending upon the degree of severity and numerical expressed it as follows:
  1 = Slight caries
  2 = Moderate caries
  3 = Advanced caries.
- However, the first systematic description of what is now known as the DMF index is usually attributed to **Henry Klein** and **Carole Paler** while carrying out their studies of dental caries in **Hagerstom**.

Retrograde Restorative Materials

- Mid 18th century- **Pfaff and Berdmore** performed root end resection and performed root end restorations with wax, lead or gold.
- 1880- **Brophy** provided a report on root end resection, root canal fill and management of the apical filling.
- 1884- **Farrar** first reports of placing a root end amalgam filling prior to resection.
- 1912- **Faulhaber and Neumann** used amalgam to fill root canals from resected root ends.

- 1913 –**Schuster** first reports of using gold foil.
- 1915-1920 Dental Literature carried articles with emphasis on sealing the gutta percha at the root apex with hot burnisher after resection.
- 1916-1919 - **Lucas** in a series of articles indicated that he first polished the resected root end, and then prepared a self retentive cavity with a small bur in the root end for placement of amalgam.
- 1917- **Ivy and Howe** recommended the sealing of the apical resected tubules with silver nitrate.
- In 1935- **Fernando Gracia** indicated an equal choice between amalgam and Zinc oxide eugenol, first indication of use of Zinc oxide eugenol.
- In 1939- **Castenfeldt** published an article on root end filling, a total seal with amalgam was recommended by removing all dentinal tubules at the resected root surface. A bevel was cut in the dentin from the canal orifice to the cemental junction.
- 1946- **Sommers** presented a technique for a root end fill with a silver cone. The cone was inserted into the canal at the resected root end, tapped to place with a chisel, and cut off and smoothed or burnished.
- Amalgam was the material of choice among Dentist all over in the next seven decades.
- However, reports in the 1960s, 1970s and 1980s continued to recommend the use of gold foils because of the ease of manipulation, marginal adaptation, surface smoothness and tissue biocompatibility.

Topical Fluorides

- Fluorine is an extremely reactive gas and is never found in its pure state, but always combined with other elements (fluorides). Before 1900, most water was consumed directly from the source, and had very little treatment. In some western cities, it was noted that people (especially children) who had grown up in these communities had teeth mottled with white or brown spots. Anecdotally, in the late 1800s it was noted that many of these people with mottled teeth had few cavities. Much later is was found that this mottling was caused by an excess of natural fluoride in the water.
- In 1901 **Dr Fredrick McKay** of Colorado (USA) accidentally discovered that many of his patients had an apparently permanent stain on their teeth that was often referred to as **'Colorado Stain'** by the local inhabitants.
- In the year 1908, as a first systemic endeavor, he presented a case at the annual meeting of state Dental Association in Boulder and found that the condition was not only confined to Colorado but extended to other towns as well.
- 1912 **McKay** came across an article written by **Dr. J.M. Eagar** (1902), a U.S. Marble hospital surgeon stationed in Italy, who reported that a high proportion of Italian residents in Naples, had ugly brown stains on their teeth known as 'denti di chiaie'.

- In 1916, **McKay** and **Black** examined 6,873 individuals in USA and reported that an unknown causative factor of mottled enamel was possibly present in domestic water during the period of teeth calcification.
- In 1930, **Kemp** and **McKay** observed that no mottling occurred in people who grew up in Bauxite prior to 1909, the year in which Bauxite had changed its supply from shallow wells to deep-drilled wells.
- In 1931, **Churchill H.V**, chief chemist of the aluminum company in New Kensington, Pennsylvania, after thorough spectrographic analysis of the rare element noted that fluoride was present in Bauxite water at a level of 13.7 ppm.
- In the same year, 1931, shoe leather survey by **Trendley H. Dean**, the most convincing evidence and direct proof was further established in depths.
- **Trendley H. Dean** was assigned the job to continue McKay's work and to find out the extent of geographical distribution of mottled enamel in the U.S by the U.S Public Health Service.
- Observations on 5,824 white Children in 22 cities of 10 states revealed that, where water concentration was 3 ppm or more, mottling was wide spread. Thus Dean established that concentration of fluoride in Drinking water was directly correlated with the severity of fluoride in enamel.
- In 1934, **Trendley H. Dean** introduced the mottling index, which is popularly known as Dean's index for Fluorosis.
- Simultaneously in 1940's, it was demonstrated that extracted teeth when exposed to dilute solutions of fluoride ion for a few seconds were found to have completely bound fluoride on the enamel surface, which subsequently was less soluble than the original enamel surface. These two facts brought forth the idea of topical application of fluoride solution for dental caries prevention.
- The classical study by **Dean** (1941) proved that individuals continuously living in a fluoride rich area had less caries as compared to the individuals who had lived in the same fluoride rich areas during calcification of teeth but had shifted to non-fluoride areas thereafter, which led to a stage of speculation that this effect after the completion of calcification of teeth may be because of repeated continuous contact of teeth with water containing fluoride.
- The year 1941 began the era of topical fluorides when the first clinical study of NAF was carried out by **Bibby**, using a 0.1% NAF solution.
- In 1942, the important milestone discovery was made by **Dean et al** that at 1 ppm Fluoride in drinking water, 60% reduction in caries experience was observed and only "sporadic instances of the mildest form of dental fluorosis of no practical or esthetic significance was observed".
- In 1945, world's first artificial fluoridation plant at Grant Rapids, USA.
- In 1946, **Klein** examined children of Japanese ancestry who had been transferred from a community containing 0.1 ppm fluoride or less to

Arizona, where water contained 3 ppm of fluoride. It was observed that teeth in process of eruption received maximum benefits from fluorides. Tooth exposed to fluoride shortly after eruption were protected but to a lesser degree.

- From all the above-mentioned studies and findings, fluoride was identified as the essential element for reducing dental caries and this led to introduction of various methods of topical application of fluoride.
- Subsequently over the years various other topical fluoride agents have been evolved in sequential order are SnF2 (1947), APF (1963), Sodium mono fluoro phosphate (NaMFP) (1963), Amine fluoride (1969) and Varnish containing fluoride (1964).

Systemic/Water Fluoridation

- **1901- Dr Frederick McKay**
  Permanent stains present on the teeth of the local inhabitant of Colorado Spring, U.S.A. known as 'Colorado Stains' noticed. Stains characterized by minute white flecks, yellow or brown spots scattered all over the surface of the tooth were termed as mottled enamel (most obviously and unmistakably defective enamel.
- **1902, Dr JM Eager**
  Described similar stains seen on the teeth of certain Italian emigrants embarking at Naples as 'denti di chiaie", denti scritti" – teeth with writing, "denti neri" – black teeth.
- **1925, Dr F McKay**
  Change of water supply from spring water of the Great salt lake of Oakley, Idaho city showed no brown stains in children who were born after changes of the water supply.
- **1933, Dr H Trendley**
  Shoe Leather Survey conducted in 97 localities with the help of questionnaire with the aim to find out minimal threshold of fluoride, the level at which it began to blemish the teeth.
- **Dean (1941)-21 cities study**
  Children of 12-14yrs, who were lifelong residents in 8 suburban areas of Chicago, where the water supplies were stable, but at various levels were examined. Moreover, data obtained from 13 other cities were included and showed a substantial difference in caries experience when the fluoride concentration in the water rose from 0.1-0.2 ppm F to 1-2 ppm F.
- **1944-1959 - Dean, Francies Arnold, Philip Jay and John Knutson (First artificial water fluoridation – 25th Jan, 1945)**
  Grand Rapids-muskegon Study (water fluoridation) - Grand Rapids as experimental town and sodium fluoride was added to water at 1 ppm and Muskegon as control. First crucial step proved caries reduction from 12.48 to 6.22DMF indicating that previously observed inverse relationship of fluoride in water and dental caries was a cause and effect relationship.

- **1945 – 1955-David et al**
  Newburgh-kingston (Control) Study - 10-year study. Newburgh children showed caries decline from 23.5 to 13.9% after water fluoridation.
- **1967(1946 - 1960)-Drs JR Blayney, TN Hill, SO Zilmmerman**
  Evanston-oak Park (Control) Study - 14-year study. Fluoridation in Evanston showed a 49% reduction of caries.
- **1951 - Hutton et al, 1965 - Brown and Poplove**
  Canadian study [Brantford (artificial fluoridation), Sarina (control) and Stratford]. Stratford with naturally present 1.3 ppm fluoride in water was auxillary control. After 17 year of fluoridation, Brantford showed a 50% reduction in caries than the control Sarina group.
- **1958- World Health Organization**
  Recommended for the first time 1 ppm fluoride in drinking water for a practicable and effective public health measure. This was reaffirmed in the report of the WHO director general in 1975:" fluoridation of communal water supplies where feasible should be cornerstone of any national programme of dental caries prevention.
- **1961- Backer Dirks et al**
  Dutch study (Tiel-Culemborg control). Tiel was fluoridated at the level of 1.1 ppm. Culemborg with 0.10 ppm served as a control. 13 years study showed 88% reduction in smooth surface caries and 31% in pit and fissure caries.
- **1965- Ludwig**
  New Zealand study. Study carried out in Hastings from 1954 to 1964-5 showed a DMF decline from 16.5 to 8.5 with reduction of approximal caries by 73% and occlusal caries by 39%.
- **Wideman et al. (1963)**
  Reported no radiographic evidence of skeletal abnormality in persons consuming water supply containing upto 4 ppm of fluoride throughout their lives.
- **Hodge (1963)**
  Observed no evidence of kidney or thyroid damage in persons who throughout their lives ingested water-containing 11ppm of fluoride.
- **Erricson (1978)**
  Compared the cancer mortality statistics in U.S.A. cities, with and without fluoridated water supplies and found no differences in the morbidity rates. Neither the United States Centre For Disease Control **(Rogot et al., 1978)** nor the National Heart Lung and Blood Institute **(Upton, A.C. 1977)** could find any evidence linking fluoride with cancer.

Pulp Therapy

- Pulp therapy for primary and young permanent teeth has for years been subject to change and controversy. The history of pulp therapy has been described to encompass four periods.

1. The **empirical era** that is prior to 1870.
2. The **antiseptic era** from 1870 to 1921.
3. The **aseptic era** ranging from 1921 to 1937.
4. The present **experimental era** or the **biologic era** from 1937 onwards.

- The reparative and the recuperative powers of dental pulp have long been recognized in dentistry. The young dental pulp particularly the pulp in primary teeth has a potential for repair because of high degree of cellularity and vascularity in this tissue prior to advanced physiological resorption of roots.

- In the mid eighteenth century, **Pierre Fauchard** advised that all caries in deeply carious sensitive teeth should not be removed because of danger of pulp exposure. As early as 1756, **Ptaff** reported placing a small piece of gold over a vital exposure in an attempt to promote healing. Principles of indirect pulp therapy was recognized by 1850 and published by **Foster**. Many medicaments have been tried since **Taft** (1860) and **Hunter** (1883). Hunter recommended covering an exposure with a mixture of Sorghum molasses and droppings of English sparrow.

- The first mention of a pulp treatment specifically for primary teeth was in 1872 in a column titled "Hints and Queri", the question, "What shall we do, with deciduous teeth in which pulps are exposed?" was answered by D.Cosmos in this manner - "They should be treated in somewhat the same manner as the permanent teeth. A Single application of the arsenical preparation in common use will so far destroy the vitality of the pulp in the crown so that it can be removed day after and then filled. Either Hill's stopping or osteoplastic may be used as filling, but no attempts should be made to fill the root".

- **Richardson** recorded the initial report on pulpotomy in 1860. The present day use of formocresol medicament has evolved from the use of formalin compounds in the past.

- **Hess** in 1929 reported pulp amputation as a method of treating exposed pulp and used this method most frequently on traumatic exposures and found it clinically successful to a certain extent.

- The formocresol technique used today is a modification of the original method reported by Sweet in 1930. The formocresol technique did not receive wide popularity as it mummified the pulp and was known as nonvital technique during the previous years. It was also overshadowed by the so-called vital pulpotomy using calcium hydroxide, which was introduced by **Teuscher** and **Zander** in 1938.

- With the Biological Era came a new concern for the histological evaluation of the injured and healthy pulp. The use of zinc oxide eugenol was emphasized during this era and has been considered one of the best pulpotomy dressings. **Glass** and **Zander** in 1949 reported that the so-called palliative zinc oxide eugenol preparation produced an acute inflammatory response with associated degeneration of odontoblasts.

- The search for more suitable medicament led investigations to test preparations containing antibiotics or corticosteroids.
- **Cook** and **Rowbotham** (1956) used zinc oxide eugenol only for pulpotomies in primary teeth, while **Seelig** in 1956 used dentin chips and other materials in pulpotomy procedure.
- After all these periods of using various compounds and medicaments in pulpotomy procedure a real study was taken up with Formocresol, which is one of the widely used medicament by **Massler** and **Mansukhani** in 1959.
- Doyle et al., 1962, introduced two-visit formocresol pulpotomy in human study. For a period of 10 years formocresol was completely dominating the other medicaments but as there is an unending quest for newer materials, investigators like **Hannah** in 1972 used glutaraldehyde. It is a dialdehyde known to be an excellent disinfectant, active against spores and bacteria and is generally used as 2% solution as quoted by s-Gravenmade in 1975. Shallow pulpotomy or partial pulpotomy was developed by **Granath L.E.** and **Hagman** (1971) and by **Cvek. M** (1978).
- Although **Laws A. J** reported electrocoagulation on the pulps of teeth in 1957, it was a decade later than Mack became the first U.S. dentist to perform electro surgical pulpotomy.
- In 1980 **Nevins et al** in a study demonstrated that cross-linked collagen phosphate gel could be used for regeneration and calcification of the pulp tissue within teeth that were partially pulpotomized. Electro surgical pulpotomy was supported histologically by **Ruemping** in 1983.
- **Shoji S et al.**, (1985) in a preliminary report on Laser pulpotomy, studied the histopathological changes in dental pulp irradiated by CO_2 laser. Freeze-dried bone **(Fadavi et al., 1988)** and demineralized dentin (Nakashima 1989) were tried.
- Bone morphogenetic protein was suggested by **Nakashima** in (1991). **Fei et al.** (1991) suggested ferric sulphate as a substitute for formocresol. **Seow WK** et al., (1993) evaluated anti-inflammatory agent – tetrandrine as a pulpotomy medicament and gave favorable results. Osteogenic protein was tried in animals by **Rutherford** et al., (1993)

Glass Ionomer Cements

- During the early and mid-1960s, science and technology of clinical dental materials were those materials that could be used directly by the dental surgeon. Silicate cement, the principal anterior restorative material of those days was recognized as flaw for use in the general dental practice. It had remained essentially the same for 50 years, even the nature of its setting and structure were imperfectly understood.
- This unsatisfactory state of affairs, however, produced a positive response, and the period of the late 1960s and early 1970s was a most creative one in the development of new materials. There was a general recognition that.

- Adequate physical properties are not enough by themselves.
- A restorative material should be more than just an inert stopping.
- Biocompatibility and adhesion are important.
- New materials and techniques should be developed with these characteristics.

- Scientific development of glass ionomer cement has been in two steps. First effort was devoted to improve properties to make it a fully practical material for anterior restorations. Second properties were modified in order to extend its range of application.
- Wilson collaboration with Kent and Lewis found that employing novel glass formulations, hydrolytically stable cements could be produced **(Wilson and Kent 1972)**.

Pit and Fissure Sealants

- The dental profession has known for some time that susceptibility to caries on tooth surfaces containing pit and fissure is related to the formation and depth of these pit and fissures. The fissure provides a protected reach for plaque accumulations. The rapidity with which dental caries occurs in pits and fissures is most likely related to the fact that the depth of the fissure is close to the DEJ and the underlying dentin, which is highly susceptible to caries.
- In 1803, **Hunter** noted that "caries is often observed on the hollow parts of the molars". In 1895, **Wilson** documented the use of current for blocking fissures in permanent molars.
- During the 1920s, two different clinical techniques were introduced in an attempt to reduce the extent and severity of pit and fissure caries in occlusal and smooth surfaces.
- In 1924, **Thaddeus Hyatt** advocated prophylactic restorations. This procedure consisted of preparing and conservative Class I cavity that included all pits and fissures at risk for caries development and then placing an amalgam restorations. The rationale for prophylactic restorations of an otherwise caries free surface was that the procedure prevented further insult to the pulp from caries, decreased loss of tooth structure and required less time for restorations when the tooth eventually succumbed to caries.
- A more conservative approach to prevention of pit and fissure caries was presented by **Bodecker** in 1929. Initially, he advocated cleaning the fissure with an explorer and flowing a thin mix of oxyphosphate current into the fissure – essentially an attempt to "Seal" the fissure. Later, he introduced an alternative method for caries prevention, the **prophylactic odontotomy**, which involved mechanical eradication of fissures into cleansable ones. These 2 techniques, prophylactic restoration and prophylactic odontotomy, were employed until the use of sealants became prevalent.
- The development of pit and fissure sealants was based on the discovery that etching enamel with phosphoric acid increased the retention of

resin restorative materials and improved marginal integrity considerably. The initial studies evaluating the effects of acid-etching on enamel were performed by **Buonocore** in 1955.

- The first sealant material that involved the acid - etch technique was introduced in the mid-1960s and was a cyanoacrylate substance; cyanoacrylates were not suitable as sealant materials owing to bacterial degradation of the material in the oral cavity over time.
- By the late in 1960s, a number of different resin materials had been tested, and a viscous resin was found to be resistant to degradation and produced a tenacious bond with etched enamel. This resin was formed by reacting Bisphenol A with glycidyl methacrylate, and this class of dimethacrylate resins has become known as BIS-GMA (Bowen 1982).
- Two methods of polymerization have been employed with BIS GMA sealants. Auto polymerization and photo activated polymerization.
- During the 1970s and early 1980s UV light with a wave length of 365 nm was used to initiate setting but was abandoned later. In its place, photo activation of sealant materials with a visible light source was introduced.
- Laser curing of visible light – activated sealant and resin materials has been advocated. In addition to BIS-GMA sealants, conventional glass Ionomer materials have also been used as pit and fissure sealants.
- Glass Ionomer bond to both enamel and dentin by physio - chemical mechanisms following polyacrylic acid conditioning. The primary advantage of glass ionomers over conventional BIS-GMA sealants is the ability of Glass ionomers to release fluoride.
- Hybrid materials composed of a variable mixture of glass ionomer and composite resin have been advocated as possible pit and fissure sealants because of the improved physical characteristics over glass ionomers, relative case of placement, adhesive compatibility with various dental substrates and fluoride releasing capability.

Dental Chairs

- The first dental chair by **James Snell** in 1832.
- The first hydraulic chair by **Wilkerson** in 1877.

Dental Drills

- Hand operated gear-driven by **John Lewis** in 1838.
- The air abrasive drill by **Dr Black** in **1945.**
- The first foot or threadle engine by Dr **Morrison** in 1872.
- The first electric dental engine by **Dr Green** in 1874.
- The water-turbine handpiece by **Dr Nelson** in 1954.
- The air-turbine handpiece by **Dr Borden** in 1957.
- Chemical methods, abrasives and lasers have been advocated for tooth removal, but as yet have not been sufficiently developed for widespread use.

George Washington's Dentures

- As there were no satisfactory filling materials or procedures at that time, decay usually proceeded until the patient had a toothache, the only remedy being. At the time of Washington's inauguration in 1790, he had only a lower premolar left, which was lost some time after. His diaries record many instances of prolonged toothaches, and his dental problems did not end with the loss of his teeth. Washington employed the best dentists of his day (John Greenwood was his favorite), many dentures made for him were unsatisfactory. Due to poor materials and procedures, the dentures made at that time fit the gingiva poorly. Although plaster was used to take impressions of the arches, the denture bases were carved or hammered to only approximate fit.
- The upper fit so poorly and had no retention; springs were attached to the upper and lower plates and pushed them against the tissue. It may be due to that there was little understanding of occlusion, so the uppers did not fit the lowers well. This type of denture could not have been comfortable. Although these dentures were mainly cosmetic, he still attempted to wear them for official occasions and dinners, although this did limit his speaking engagements.
- Even with these dentures, his mouth was badly sunken and the ivory used for the teeth stained quickly, common people of that time probably did not attempt to have dentures fitted, and even with their fame and affluence the washingtons did not have a very satisfactory prosthodontic result.
- Until the late 1800s, catalogues listed "masticators", which crushed food so that it could be consumed by those without teeth. Naturally retained upper dentures seem to have been discovered accidentally, as one of the case was documented by a **Dr Gardette of Philadelphia** in 1800. Gold was the preferred material for these bases, obviously at some cost. These were known as "suction dentures" and preceded Vulcanite dentures.

Vulcanite Dentures

- Before restorative dental care came into picture or became popular, the only treatment for dental pain was extraction which resulted in partial or complete edentulism. Unfortunately in those times there were neither materials nor techniques for the fabrication of satisfactory dentures and the lack of durable material added to the problem. It was **Nelson Goodyear** in 1851who discovered how to make hard rubber products. This hard rubber was named Vulcanite. This product found wide popularity in fabrication of denture bases, where it soon replaced all previously used materials, being far superior in cost and function The fit of these bases allowed self retaining dentures, making earlier spring type dentures obsolete. These Vulcanite dentures were the first functional, durable and affordable dentures, marking a great advance in dental treatment. After a lot of legal procedures, the Goodyear

Company obtained a patent for Vulcanite dentures in 1864. They proceeded to license dentists who used their material, and charged a royalty for all dentures made. Dentists who would not comply were sued. Although many dentists bought licenses, the dental profession as a whole opposed the patent and licensure of vulcanite denture.

- The struggle came to an end when Goodyear hired Josiah Bacon to prosecute noncompliant dentists, which he did across the country with almost malicious vigor. One he filed suit against was a well respected dentist named **Samuel Chalfant**. Chalfant was so distressed that he shot and killed Bacon in California in 1879. Chalfant served 10 years for second degree murder and resumed his practice upon his release. The Goodyear patents expired in 1881, and the company did not again seek to license dentists or dental products.

- Vulcanite dentures were very popular until the 1940s, when acrylic (pink plastic) denture bases replaced them.

Amalgam

- Despite of having great success stories, Mercury-silver amalgam material has always been a part of controversy since its earliest days. Many metallic powders (most commonly silver alloys), can be mixed with mercury to form amalgams, which are soft and then harden to metallic solids. Early attempts to use amalgam as a dental restoration were often failures, however. Silver was obtained from many sources, often shaved from coins. First, the ingredients and proportions were usually inconsistent, leading to early breakdown of the filling or tooth fracture from excessive expansion, and then the proportions and mixing procedure with mercury were also variable. The other problem was that the tooth preparation was usually haphazard, both from poor instrumentation and inadequate dental training. Because of these failures, in the middle to late 1800s the amalgam was subjected to many conflicts in the dental profession and was known as "amalgam wars".

- **G.V. Black's** greatest success was in the development of usable amalgams around 1900. After many studies and researches, he determined the correct proportions of silver, zinc, copper and tin and the proper processing of the powder. He also determined the right percentage of mercury and the proper mixing procedure.

- Along with the material he developed a systematic and scientific approach to cavity preparation, which was equally responsible for success. G.V.Black's amalgam and tooth preparation system, for the first time it was possible to successfully repair cavities quickly and inexpensively.

- While other restorative materials such were also in successful use during that period, they were not as widely used because of the time required and the cost. Throughout most of the 20th century, dental amalgam was the predominant material for the general repair of carious teeth. Although amalgam continues to develop and improve through the present time, it is not without problems. Perhaps the greatest disadvantage is the silvery or dark appearance, which is somewhat acceptable in posterior teeth but very unesthetic in the anterior teeth.

- The other concern is the mercury toxicity in amalgam. While some forms of mercury are very toxic and harmful, there has been no scientific evidence that the mercury in dental amalgams causes health problems in the general population. Nonetheless, many individuals and groups ascribe a wide variety of ills to the presence or release of mercury from amalgam restorations with the press often giving credence to these theories, so the controversy continues.

First Use of Inhalation Anesthesia

- Since prehistoric times, man has sought ways to lessen pain. With varying degrees of success he has utilized: mandrake, opium and other poppy extracts, fermented and distilled beverages, nerve compresses, cold, extreme fatigue from prohibiting sleep, bleeding to the point of fainting shock and hypnosis.
- One of these parties (ether frolics) in 1842, a young physician. **Crawford W. Long** of Georgia conceived the idea of administering to patient sufficient ether to inhale so that an operation could be performed without pain to the patient. After selecting his patient, Dr. Long removed a tumor from the neck while the patient was under the influence of ether. In that year, 1842, Dr. Long claimed three administrations of ether. Since that year, up to 1849, he had performed one or more surgical operations annually on patients under the influence of ether.
- **Dr Horace Wells** of Hartford, Connecticut. A young conscientious dentist. Being a very sensitive individual, the suffering he caused during the extraction of teeth troubled him greatly. These feelings prompted him to give considerable thought to the subject of pain relief during extractions. In 1838, he wrote, "An Essay on Teeth, Comprising a Brief Description of Their Formation, Diseases, and Proper Treatment".
- Horace Wells was constantly enlarging his knowledge and attended a lecture on chemical phenomena by **Gardner Q. Colton** in 1844. After manufacturing some nitrous oxide, known as "laughing gas", Mr. Colton invited spectators to come forward and inhale the fumes. Horace noticed that no sign was exhibited when the volunteers, under the influence of nitrous oxide, stumbled and scraped their shins on the heavy benches. Immediately, Wells conceived the idea of Inhalation Anesthesia. Though history notes that **Sir Humphrey Davy**, in 1799, published an account of his research and experiments with nitrous oxide, Horace Wells was not aware of it.
- Later Wells spoke with Colton and asked him to bring a bag of the gas to his office the next day. Wells had an aching tooth and felt that by inhaling sufficient nitrous oxide, the tooth could be extracted painlessly. Colton at first had objected as the gas might prove fatal.

- In 1844, Wells, sitting in his own dental chair, inhaled the gas until he lost consciousness. **Dr Riggs**, a friend and former pupil of Dr Wells stepped forward and extracted the arching third molar (wisdom tooth). On regaining consciousness, Wells exclaimed, "A new era in tooth pulling". After experimenting for weeks, he went to Boston, the medical center of the New England States. There, **William T.G. Morton** arranged the lecture and demonstrated nitrous oxide before the medical students of John C. Warren. However, this demonstration was a failure.
- Wells continued to use nitrous oxide and taught other dentists to use it. **William Thomas Green Morton** received the idea of inhalation anesthesia from Well's demonstration. He extracted a tooth for a patient under its influence. Morton saturated a handkerchief with it, giving it to the patient, he remarked that it was something better than mesmerization. The patient inhaled it and soon was unconscious. The tooth was removed painlessly. This took place in 1846.
- Morton then demonstrated ether as a practical anesthetic to the Harvard medical class. The surgeon in charge was **Dr John C Warren**. He is the man credited with giving both Morton and Wells their big opportunity to demonstrate publicly their anesthetic agents. Morton patented the ether under the name of Letheon and secretly promised to pay a percentage to Jackson.
- Morton, wealthiest of the three, gave up dentistry and became the first specialist in anesthesia. Wells, deranged by his self-experimentation with chloroform, committed suicide in 1848. In 1864, the American Dental Association gave full credit to Horace Wells for the discovery of practical anesthesia and its introduction to the United States of America.

Local Anesthesia

- Local anesthetics were first used in 1884. It was then that **Koller**, a young intern and house surgeon, first announced the use of cocaine to anesthetize the eye. That same year, William S. Halstead, surgeon at John Hopkins Hospital, demonstrated that the injection of a nerve trunk in any part of its course is followed by local anesthesia in its entire peripheral distribution. The nerve he first blocked was the mandibular branch of the trigeminal.
- Novocain (procaine hydrochloride) was introduced into by Professor **Braun** in 1905. Novocaine is a comparatively weak anesthetic agent possessing a low degree of toxicity. It is still potent enough to provide a safe, sure analgesia under practically all circumstances. When infiltrated around free nerve endings and fibers, onset of analgesia is almost immediate. At most, the onset is from 3 to 5 minutes. A two percent solution of novocaine is recommended for use in dental practice. This percentage will give approximately 12-15 minutes of analgesia. The addition of epinephrine 1:100,000 per milliliter prolong analgesis to 30-45 minutes. A 1:50,000 per milliliter produces

60-90 minutes of analgesia. Dental surgery performed under these conditions on a cardiac patient will present no special hazards. Novocaine is now seldom used. It has been replaced by stronger anesthetics such as: Primacaine, 1.5% solution, which is four times more potent than novocaine and slightly more toxic.

- Lidocaine (Xylocaine) Hydrochloride 2% solution was discovered in 1943 by two Swedish chemists, **Nils Lofgven** and **Bengt Lundquist**. After many experiments, Xylocaine was introduced to the medical and dental professions. Its acceptance by the dental profession of the United States in 1950 was rapid and dramatic. Soon afterwards, it was made available to hospitals. Xylocaine did not just happen, its recognition as one of the greatest contributions to the field of local anesthesia constitutes a success story but unlimited credit must be given to first, its discoverers, and the countless number of scientists and clinicians whose untiring efforts established the effectiveness and safety of Xylocaine. Lidocaine (Xylocaine) diffuses readily through the tissues, and nerve sheath giving a rapid onset of analgesia. It is detoxified in the liver and possesses slight vaso-constricting properties. Xylocaine has an early cortical depressant effect and it, thereby, potentiates the hypnotic effect of barbiturates. Therefore, in cases of pre-medication with barbiturates, the dosage should be decreased if Xylocaine is used. Xylocaine has been used effectively and safely in dentistry and in various specialties of medicine such as: Urology, Opthalmology, Otorhinolaryngology, Proctology, and Dermatology.
- Xylocaine is rapidly replacing novocain. It has been widely accepted by obstetricians who have become aware of its effectiveness and safety. The spread of Xylocaine has been phenomenal. It has even replaced novocaine in the field of intravenous anesthesia, the advantages being many, such as: a very low incidence of postoperative nausea, vomiting and chest complications. The idea of using anesthetic solutions or drugs in cartridges was developed by **Harvey Cook**. The idea was conceived from the cartridges used in rifles. Dr Cook fashioned his own syringes and cartridges. From this humble beginning, new agents and different types of syringes have sprung.

ANNEXURE - II

SYNDROMES

1. **Acanthosis Nigricans syndrome** can be manifested by development of gingival papillomatosis with periorofacial mucosal and skin lesions Gastric adenocarcinoma may develop.

2. **Acute coronary syndromes** comprise the spectrum of unstable cardiac ischemia from unstable angina to acute myocardial infarction. During many patients may show ST segment elevation, ST segment depression on T wave flattening or inversion. Chest pain is the commonest complaint

3. **AIDS** (Acquired Immuno Deficiency Syndrome) is a condition where acute infection occurs 3 to 6 weeks after initial contact with HIV (Human Immuno Virus). Initially non specific syndrome occurs during which joints pain, gastrointestinal symptoms and a macular rash predominate, and then these self limiting symptoms persist for 2-3 weeks. Eights to twelve weeks after infection, antibody to HIV can be detected in serum. After acute infection, person enters the symptomatic phase of the disease. The average time from infection to development of disease is 8 to 10 years. During this period T_4 lymphocytes comes down from 800 mm^3 to 50 mm^3.Oral manifestations in HIV infected patients are oral candidiasis that occurs in 30% to 90% cases. Persistent ulcers of mouth in AIDS should be biopsied for deep fungal infections. Hairy leukoplakia has been noted in HIV positive homosexuals. Recurrent herpes simplex virus progresses to large chronic oral lesions. Ulcers are surrounded by raised white border. Lesions may co-exist with genital and anal lesions. Painful oral ulcers caused by cytomegalovirus may be seen. Kaposi's sarcoma is the most common oral neoplasm in AIDS. Early lesions look like hemangiomas, flat or raised discolorations. Generalized gingivitis and periodontitis is also seen.

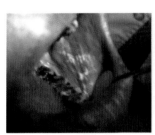

Oral candidiasis

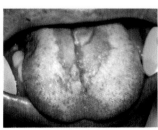

Hairy leukoplakia

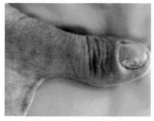

Recurrent herpes simplex

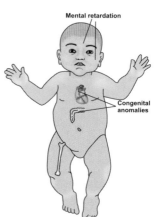

Mental retardation

Congenital anomalies

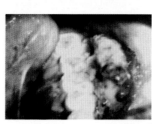

Kaposi's sarcoma

4. **Albright's syndrome** is like fibrous dysplasia of bone. There is replacement of spongy bone by a peculiar fibrous tissue. Radiographs will show radiopacity and radiolucency, some will appear like compact bone and other like cystic bone. The cause of endocrine manifestation in Albright's syndrome is not known. Transformation to malignancy occurs. Radiotherapy is not advised.

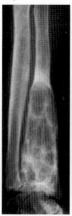 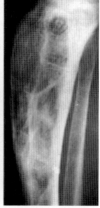

Albright's syndrome

5. **Aldrich syndrome** is rare hereditary disease transmitted as an x-linked recessive trait. It is characterized by thrombocytopenic purpura, eczema and increased susceptibility of disease. Spontaneous bleeding of gingiva is common. Palatal petechiae may be present.

6. **Amelo-onychohypohidrotic syndrome** can be manifested by defective nails with subungal hyperkeratosis is seen with hypofunction of sweat gland and severe hypoplastic-hypocalcified crowns.

7. **Amnesic syndrome** is said to have occurred where it becomes difficult to retaining new information. There may be polyneuritis.

8. **Auriculotemporal syndrome** develops due to damage of auriculotemporal nerve and subsequent reinnervation of sweat glands. There is flushing and sweating of involved side of face during eating. Sweating may increase with tart food. Also known as frey's syndrome.

9. **B.K. Mole syndrome** was described by Clark and co-workers. This autosomal dominant condition is characterized by large pigmented nevi. There is higher risk of development of melanoma.

10. **Behcet's disease** is an idiopathic disorder characterized by triad of symptoms i.e. recurrent oral ulcers, genital ulcers and eye lesions. Development of vasculitis of medium sized blood vessels is seen. Eye lesions consist of uveitis, retinal infiltrates, edema and vascular occlusion. Skin lesions are large papular lesions. Pustules may be formed in 24 hours. Ulcers may also be present on scrotum, penis or vulva. Cyclosporine with cortisone is useful.

11. **Bloch Sulzberger syndrome** is a disease that generally appears shortly after birth and is characterized by erythematous and vesico bullous lesion on trunk. There will be marked eosinophilia. Dental changes include delayed tooth eruption, peg or cone shaped crowns and congenitally missing teeth.

12. **Branchial arch syndrome** is clinically manifested by heterogeneous group of malformation including antimongloid palpebral fissures, deficiency of eyelashes, hypoplasia of facial bones, malformations of malar bones, facial clefts and skeletal deformities. Facies are characteristics.

13. **Burning mouth syndrome** is characterized by painful, burning sensation localized in the tongue or affecting other areas of the oral mucosa. The pain of burning tongue is rated similar to that of toothache. Tongue temperature is decreased. Some evidence suggests the existence of oral Somatosensory and special sensory deficits.

14. **Chediak – Higashi syndrome** is a congenital autosomal recessive defect. It is a fatal disease in early life. Defect is of granule containing cells as granulocytes and melanocytes. Clinical features include oculocutaneous albinism, photophobia, nystagmus and recurrent infections. Hypopigmentation will be seen in skin and hair. Some may develop neuropathy. Child dies before the age of 10 due to recurrent infection. Lymph nodes, spleen, liver and bone marrow

are infiltrated with lymphohistiocyte cell. Oral lesions include ulcerations of oral mucosa, severe gingivitis, glossitis and periodontal breakdown are common. Early loss of teeth is noted. There is no specific treatment.

15. **Cleidocranial dysplasia** is a hereditary disorder. There is an abnormal growth of bones of face, skull and clavicles. There is failure of tooth eruption. There is autosomal dominant trait. There is spontaneous mutations. Clinical features: There is hyper mobility of shoulder joint, frontal bossing is seen, underdevelopment of mid face, nose is wide, flat without bridge, multiple unerupted and impacted teeth, supernumerary teeth are seen and Clavicle is hypoplastic.

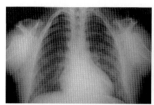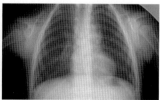

Cleidocranial dysplasia

16. **Complex regional pain syndrome** after an injury patient sometimes develop a variety of persistent unpleasant sensation in the previously injured area. Pain is severe and burning loss of hair may develop, complex regional pain syndrome typically occurs after nerve trauma, fractures and periods of immobilization pain may lead to reflex sympathetic dystrophy.

17. **Cowden's syndrome** There is hamartomas involvement of many organs with a potential of neoplastic transformation. It is inherited as autosomal dominant character. Multiple cysts over lips and gingiva are seen. Papilloma like lesions as well as pebbly lesion and fibromas at various sites in oral cavity are seen. Tongue is also fissured. Hemangiomas and neuromas are also seen.

18. **Cracked tooth syndrome** can be manifested by development or presence of a crack in a restored or an unrestored tooth due to excessive occlusal forces. There is sharp pain on biting. Pain is similar to that of trigeminal neuralgia. Radiographs are unable to show cracked tooth.

19. **CREST syndrome** is one of the forms of systemic sclerosis. Its findings include Reynaud's phenomenon, esophageal dysfunction, sclerodactaly and telangiectasia. Calcinosis cutis may also be there. Etiology is not known. Early mild edema of tongue, soft palate and larynx are seen. Tongue often becomes stiff and board like. Dysphagia and chocking sensations are seen. Bone resorption of angle of mandibular ramus in noted.

20. **Crouzon syndrome** is known as cranio facial dysostosis. Signs are due to early synostosis of the sutures. There is protuberant frontal region. There will be hypoplasia of maxillae with mandibular prognathism and a high arched palate.

21. **Cushing's syndrome** is seen due to adrenal hyperactivity. Patient may be hypertensive and hypoglycemic and may have moon face appearance. Gingiva, palate and buccal mucosa may appear blotchy due to melanin granules.

22. **de Quervain's syndrome** in 1985 Swiss doctor named Fritz de Quervain described pain syndrome involving tendons. Injury to nerve or repetitive wrist motions can cause swelling of tunnel through which tendon pass. Diabetes, thyroid disease, rheumatoid arthritis may also cause inflammation in this tunnel. Swelling irritates the tendon and causes pain. This syndrome causes pain at the base of thumb.

23. **Down syndrome/ Mongolism** /Trisomy 21 is a congenital disease caused by chromosomal abnormalities, it is characterised by mental deficiency and growth retardation. Oral manifestations present are periodontal disease with periodontal pockets, diastema, crowding and high freenal attachment.

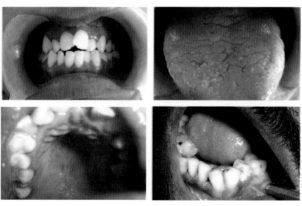

Down syndrome/Mongolism

24. **Dyskeratosis congenital (Zinsser – Engmann Cole Syndrome)** is a rare X-linked disorder characterized leading to atrophic, leukoplakic oral mucosa. Tongue and cheek are adversely affected. Oral lesions starting before the age of 10 presents as vesicles and white necrotic patches with Candida, ulcerations and erythroplakic changes.

25. **Ectodermal dysplasia** is an X – linked recessive disorder affecting essentially males. Defect is seen in all ectodermally derived structures.

Patient exhibit decreased sweating, sparse hair, many congenitally missing teeth. Hypodontia involves most stable teeth like maxillary central incisor and first molars.

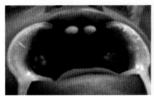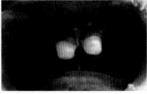

Ectodermal dysplasia

26. **Gardner's syndrome** consists of multiple polyposis of large intestine, osteoma's of bone, specially jaw and skull. There is occasional occurrence of desmoids tumors. Multiple epidermoid or sebaceous cysts of skin are noted.

27. **Godtfredsen's syndrome** consists of ophthalmoplegia and trigeminal neuralgia with paralysis of tongue. Tumor is located in cavernous and lateral sinus.

28. **Goltz-Gorlin syndrome** is a hereditary condition transmitted as an autosomal dominant trait. Cutaneous anomalies include plantar keratosis and dermal calcinosis. Dental and osseous abnormalities include odontogenic keratocysts, mandibular prognathism and rib anomalies. Ophthalmic abnormalities include wide nasal bridge, dystopia canthorum while sexual abnormalities include hypogonadism. Patient will develop gingival and other mucosal papillomatous lesions. Lips and teeth develop defects. Associated features include poikiloderma, syndactyly and adactyly.

29. **Gorham's syndrome** is a condition where spontaneous progressive resorption of bone is seen. Etiology is not known but there is an active hyperemia of bone. Osteolysis is most common in older children. Mandible and other bones may be involved. Patient may present with pain and facial asymmetry. There is a replacement of bone by connective tissue containing thin walled blood vessels.

30. **Gardner's syndrome** There is carcinomatous transformation of adenomatous intestinal polyps. There may be osteomas of jaw and accompanying cysts are indictors of Gardner's syndrome and bowel should be examined.

31. **Grinspan's syndrome** is a triad of lichen planus, diabetes mellitus and hypertension. It may predispose to squamous cell carcinoma.

32. **Guillain Barré syndrome** is caused by progressive demyelinating neuropathy. It is an autoimmune following a non specific disease. Impaired swallowing or parasthesia of mouth and face is the early sign. There may be ascending anesthesia and paralysis of legs and trunk. In severe case respiration is compromised.

33. **Hypohidrotic ectodermal dysplasia** has X-linked recessive inheritance. It present with hypodontia, hypotrichosis and hypoanhydrosis. There is marked frontal bossing, depressed nasal bridge, protuberant lips and lack of scalp hair. There will be hypodontia or Anodontia. There may be partial lack and dysplasia of minor salivary glands.

34. **Jacod's syndrome** is caused by intracranial lesion of middle cranial fossa. It has mandibular nerve pain and dental pain associated with maxilla.

35. **Jadassohn–Lewandowsky syndrome** causes congenital gross thickening of finger and toe nails. Along with it leukokeratosis is noted. Nail lesion is noted just after birth with a horny brownish material at nail bed. Oral leukokeratosis affects dorsum of tongue which becomes thickened and grayish white. Histologically these are similar to white sponge nevus. Frequent oral aphthous ulceration may develop.

36. **James Ramsay Hunt's Syndrome** is clinically manifested by facial paralysis as well as pain in external auditory meatus. In addition vascular eruption may occur in oral cavity. There may be hoarseness of voice.

37. **Jaw – Winking syndrome** may be hereditary. It may be seen after peripheral facial syndrome. On opening mouth, eye is closed. During chewing tears may flow.

38. **Klinefelter's syndrome** includes Taurodontism i.e. peculiar dental anomaly at the expense of roots. Such males have one more extra X-chromosome.

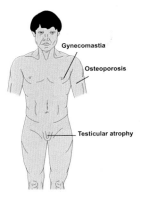

Klinefelter's syndrome

39. **Lysosomal storage syndrome** is manifested by formation of childhood gingival enlargement, widened alveolar ridges and widely spaced teeth. Certain viscera's are also enlarged.

40. **Maffucci's syndrome** is characterized by development of multiple hemangiomas of skin and oral mucosa. Multiple chondromas of jaw bone are seen. They represent calcification of organized blood clots in dilated vascular spaces.

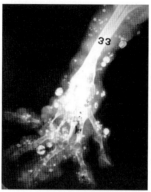

Maffucci's syndrome

41. **Marfan –Achard syndrome** is basically a disease of connective tissue and defective organization of collagen. There will be excessive length of tubular bones, shape of skull and face is long and narrow. There is hyper extensibility of joints and habitual dislocations. High arched palate vault is very common. Bifid uvula is very common. Temporomandibular dysarthrosis is noted.

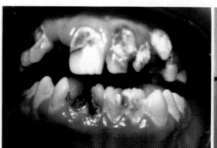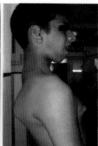

Marfan – Achard syndrome

42. **Meckel's syndrome** is characterized by midline clefting of tongue. Tongue is also thrown into multiple nodular or papillomatous projections.

43. **Median cleft face syndrome** includes hypertelorism, median cleft of premaxilla and palate. There will be bifidum occultum. It has no clinical manifestation.

44. **MEN syndrome** It is a group of syndromes characterized by tumors of various endocrine organs.

45. **Miescher's syndrome** is characterized by development of diffuse swelling of lip. Swelling may take place on vermillion border. Formation of scaling, fissuring, vesicle or pustule formation may take place.

46. **Mobius syndrome** is manifested by facial diplegia with bilateral paralysis of ocular muscles. Child is not able to close the eye during sleep. Lips are everted and mouth may remain open. There is difficulty in mastication and drooling of saliva may be seen. Mental defects and epilepsy may develop.

47. **Mucocutaneous lymph node syndrome** is a disease of unknown etiology. It is a self limiting febrile illness. Some think it is a collagen vascular disease. There may be dryness, redness and fissuring of lips. There may be acute, non purulent swelling of cervical lymph glands.

48. **Myofacial pain dysfunction syndrome (MPDS)** is characterized by pain and limited movements of TMJ. It may be caused by spasm of muscles of mastication and fatigue. Habitual grinding of teeth may also result in the condition. Clinical manifestations are generally seen as most of the females being the sufferer between the age group of 30-40 years, pain in temporomandibular joint, muscle tenderness, limitation of movements, sometimes clicking sound will be produced.

49. **Neck – Tongue syndrome** is characterized by unilateral upper nuchal or occipital pain with or without numbness in these areas. There is simultaneous numbness of tongue on the same side.

50. **Nevoid basal cell carcinoma syndrome** Individuals parent with jaw cysts, facies, calcification, bifid ribs and skin lesions. Multiple pink to brown papules appear on face. In 50% cases pitting of soles and palms is seen.

51. **Nursing bottle syndrome** occurs in babies who are on bottle feed that contain more of sugar. It results in multiple numbers of caries in many teeth mostly the lower one.

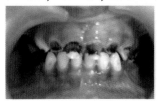 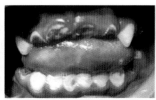

Nursing bottle syndrome

52. **Occulo-dento-osseous dysplasia** is characterized by micro-ophthalmus, iridal anomalies, bony anomalies of the digits and syndactyly, with enamel hypoplasia. The teeth show large multifocal hypoplastic defects and pitting yielding a moth-eaten pattern radiographically.

53. **Oral – facial digital syndrome** is characterized by cleft tongue as one of the part of this syndrome in association with thick fibrous bands in lower anterior mucobuccal fold. It is of little significance.

54. **Papillon - lefevre syndrome** is characterized by hyperkeratotic skin lesion, severe periodontal destruction, destruction of alveolar bone involving both deciduous and permanent dentitions. Inflammatory gingival enlargement, gingival ulceration, formation of deep pockets are frequently present and calcification of the dura, the cutaneous. The Dural changes generally occur before the age of 4 years. The syndrome is inherited and appears to follow an autosomal recessive pattern. Parents are not affected and may occur in siblings; males and females are equally affected.

55. **Paratrigeminal syndrome** is a disease with severe headache or pain in area of distribution of trigeminal nerve. Cause of disease is not known. Some of the signs may be of Horner's syndrome.

56. **Peutz – Jegher's syndrome** is characterized by an oral pigmentation. Multiple, focal, melanotic brown macules are concentrated on lips. Macules may go upto 3-5 cms in size. Anterior tongue may be involved. Histologically these show basilar melanogenesis without melanocytic proliferation.

57. **Pierre robin syndrome** consists of cleft palate, micrognathia and glossoptosis. There is hypoplasia of mandible. Patient may have congenital heart defects and ocular lesions.

58. **Plummer-vinson syndrome** develops chiefly in women of fourth and fifth decade of life. Clinically it may be manifested by the presence of anemia, cracks or fissures at corners of mouth, smooth red painful tongue with atrophy of filliform and later fungiform papillae. Mucus membrane and esophagus are atrophic and show loss of keratinization. Koilonychias develops. Blood will show hypochromic microcytic anemia.

59. **Pterygopalatine fossa syndrome** is caused by metastatic tumor to pterygopalatine fossa. It consists of maxillary dental pain, infraorbital and palatal anesthesia. There may also be associated blindness and paralysis of pterygoid muscle.

60. **Romon syndrome** can be clinically described where patient develops gingival and alveolar enlargement, microophthalmia. Cornea becomes cloudy. Hypopigmentation results with athetosis. Mental retardation is rare.

61. **Rubinstein-Taypi syndrome** is manifested by Talon cusp being the main feature along with development retardation, broad thumbs and great toes. Facial features are characteristic. Head circumference and bone age is below fifth percentile.

62. **Rutherford syndrome** is characterized by congenitally enlarged gingiva, delayed tooth eruption and superior corneal opacities. Patient may have mental retardation, aggressive behavior and dentigerous cysts.

63. **Scheuthauer–Marie sainton syndrome** is also known as cleidocranial dysplasia, patient may have high narrow arched palate. Maxilla is under developed. Mandible may be larger. There may be prolonged retention of deciduous tooth.

64. **Sinus of Morgagni syndrome** consists of mandibular nerve pain, palatal immobilization and trismus. There may be unilateral deafness. It is may be due to carcinoma.

65. **Sipple's syndrome** is characterized by parathyroid hyperplasia or adenoma but no tumors of pancreas. There is no peptic ulcer but may have pheochromocytomas of adrenal medulla.

66. **Sjögren's syndrome** is an multisystem autoimmune disorder of

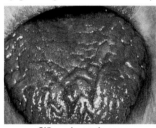
Sjögren's syndrome

exocrine glands which may be associated with neuropathy and lympho proliferative disorder with acinar destruction of glands. It is a condition originally described as triad consisting of Keratoconjunctivitis sicca, Xerostomia and rheumatoid arthritis i.e. Lacrimal and salivary glands are affected. In primary Sjögren's syndrome only salivary and lacrimal glands are involved. In this mouth and eyes becomes dry. In secondary Sjögren's syndrome along with above symptoms rheumatoid arthritis may also develop. Some may develop arthalgia. Person feels tired. Histological hallmark is focal lymphocytic infiltration of exocrine glands. Epstein – Barr or a type A retrovirus is the causative organism. Xerostomia is a major complaint in most patients as it results in difficulty in swallowing and talking. Taste sensations may also be distorted. Mucosa becomes red and parchment like look. Dorsum of tongue becomes red and atrophic. There may be fissuring. Parotid gland enlargement is seen along with enlargement of submandibular gland. There may be symptoms of rheumatoid arthritis. Kidney involvement is noted.

67. **Solitary median maxillary central incisor syndrome** presents with a single central incisor in the midline. This condition may be associated with other midline disturbances such as cleft lip and palate, imperforate anus, umbilical hernia, choanal stenosis.

68. **Stevens – Johnson syndrome** is also known as erythema multiforme when the vesicles and bulla involve skin, mouth, eyes and genitals. Generally young adults are involved. Discrete macula, papule or vesicles are distributed symmetrically over hands and arms, face and

neck. Oral mucus membrane lesions are very painful and mastication may not be possible. Mucosal vesicles rupture leaving surface covered with thick, white, yellow exudates. Erosions of pharynx are common. It may also occur secondary to a drug reaction. It can slough skin and mucosa. Electrolyte imbalance may develop.

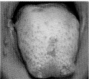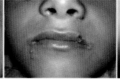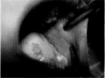

Stevens–Johnson syndrome

69. **Sturge–Weber syndrome** is described as where patients develops orofacial and meningeal angiomatosis with secondary mental deficiency. There may be seizures, hemiplegia and mild to severe enlargement of gingiva. Hyperplastic vascular gingival blanch on pressure. Bony hemangiomas and delayed tooth eruption may be noted.

70. **Sweat Retention syndrome** can be described as an extravasation of sweat in the tissue with subsequent inflammation, there is also keratin plug formation in sweat glands.

71. **Tietze syndrome** is a painful costochondral function syndrome. There is no palpable abnormality and pain is identified in medial quadrant of breast. It is generally unilateral and may develop at any age. Antiinflammatory drugs may give comfort.

72. **Trichodento-osseous syndrome** also shows enamel defects in conjunction with morphologic dental anomalies. These patients have tightly curled kinky hair with osteosclerosis of bone cortices. The enamel is hypoplastic and hypocalcified, lacking mesiodistal contact with pitting.

73. **Trisomy** – 13 develops due to multiple abnormalities of various organs. Child dies within a year. There may be bilateral cleft lip and palate, small or no eye at all. Superficial hemangioma of forehead, delayed growth, mental retardation, polydactyly of hands and fest are noted.

74. **Uremic syndrome** is a disease where signs and symptoms of kidney failure is seen, one of them is decreased creatinine clearance. As disease progresses, glomerular filtration rate falls and blood urea nitrogen rises. Person may develop impaired ability to concentrate urine, nocturia and mild anemia. Advanced uremia is associated with pericarditis, pericardial effusion and neuropathies.

75. **Von–Sallman syndrome** is a hereditary benign intra-epithelial Dyskeratosis. It is rare autosomal dominant trait. Patient shows oral mucosal thickening with superficial gelatinous looking plaques on bulbar conjunctiva. Cytological scrapings show 'cells within cells'.

76. **Zimmerman–Lebarnd syndrome** is characterized when patient develops gingival fibromatosis with defects of ear, nose, bones and terminal phalanges. Joints become hyperexible. Spleen is enlarged.

CAUSES OF DENTAL DISEASES

Causes of Pulpitis

- Fracture of crown/cusp
- Dental caries
- Thermal/chemical irritation.

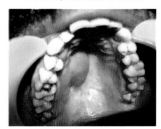

Causes of pulpitis

Causes of Resorption of Permanent teeth

- Impacted teeth putting pressure on adjacent teeth
- Periapical periodontitis
- Replanted teeth
- Neoplasm
- Idiopathic resorption.

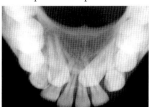

Causes of resorption of permanent teeth

Causes of Exacerbating Gingivitis

- Dental irregularities
- Restorations resulting in stagnation area

- Pregnancy
- Down's syndrome
- Uncontrolled diabetes.

Causes of Persistence of Plaque

- Overhanging restorations
- Calculus
- Mouth breathing
- Pocketing
- Irregular teeth.

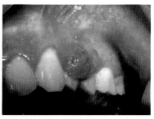

Causes of persistence of plaque

Causes of Premature Periodontal Tissue Destruction

- Severe uncontrolled diabetes
- Leukopenia
- HIV infections
- Hypophosphatasia.

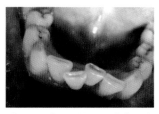

Causes of premature periodontal tissue destruction

Causes of Gingival Enlargement

- Genetic
- Drugs associated phenytoin
- Calcium channel blockers
- Pregnancy
- Inflammatory
  - Leukemia
  - Sarcoidosis
  - Scurvy.

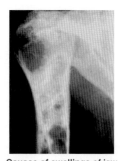
Causes of swellings of jaw

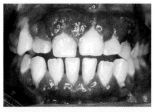
Causes of gingival enlargement

Causes of Cyst Like Areas of Jaw

- Ameloblastoma
- Hyperparathyroidism
- Pseudocysts
- Giant cell granuloma.

Drugs Causing Lichenoid Reactions

- Beta blockers
- Allopurinol
- Methyldopa
- Antimalarials
- Captopril
- Penicillamine.

Causes of Macroglossia

- Cretinism
- Amyloidosis
- Lingual thyroid
- Down's syndrome.

Causes of Xerostemia

- Functional causes
  - Dehydration
  - Hemorrhage
  - Anxiety/depression
  - Psychogenic
- Organic causes
  - Mumps
  - HIV infection
  - Sarcoidosis
  - Amyloidosis
- Drugs
  - Excessive diuretic
  - Atropine
  - Decongestants
  - Bronchodilators.

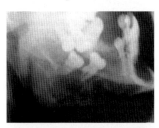
Causes of cyst like areas of jaw

Causes of Swellings of Jaw

- Odontogenic tumors
- Odontogenic cysts
- Giant cell lesion
- Metastatic neoplasm
- Fibrosseous lesions.

Causes of Ptyalism

- False ptyalism
  - Bell's palsy
  - Psychogenic
  - Stroke
  - Parkinsonism
- Local
  - Oral wounds
  - New dentures
  - Oral infections.

Causes of Sialodenosis

- Diabetes mellitus
- Drugs
- Idiopathic
- Alcoholism.

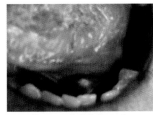

Causes of sialodenosis

Causes of Dental pain

- Dull throbbing pain
  - Pericoronitis
  - Late pulpitis
  - Dry socket
  - Herpes zoster
  - Atypical odontalgia
  - Atypical facial pain
- Burning pain
  - Post herpetic neuralgia
  - Burning mouth syndrome
- Sharp stapping pain
  - Exposed dentine
  - Early pulpitis
  - Trigeminal neuralgia
  - Fractured tooth.

Developmental Defects in Jaws

- Craniofacial anomalies
- Hereditary prognanthiasim

- Cleidocranial dysplasia
- Osteogenesis imperfecta
- Gardner's syndrome.

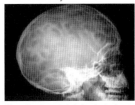

Developmental defects in jaws

Classification of Cysts of Jaw

- Inflammatory odontogenic cyst
  Radicular
  Paradental.
- Odontogenic developmental cysts
  Dentigerous cyst
  Eruption cyst
  Lateral peridontal cyst
  Gingival cyst.
- Non odontogenic developmental cysts
  Nasolabial cyst
  Nasopalantine duct cysts.

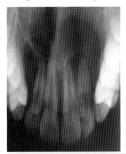

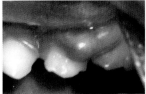

Classification of cysts of jaw

SYNONYMS/ALTERNATIVES

- **Perleche** — Angular cheilitis
- **Mucous retention cyst** — Mucocele
- **Dry socket** — Aleveolitis sicca dolorosa, Alveolar osteitis
- **Hand Schullar Christian disease** — Multifocal esonophilic granuloma
- **Histiocytosis** — Non lipid reticuloendotheliosis
- **Osteomalacia** — Adult rickets
- **Renal rickets** — Renal osteodystrophy
- **Marfan syndrome** — Arachnodactyly
- **Down's syndrome** — Trisomy 21 syndrome, Mongolism
- **Osteopetrosis** — Marble bone disease, Osteosclerosis
- **Achondroplasia** — Chondrodystrophia fetalis
- **Osteitis Deforman's** — Paget's disease
- **Van Buchem disease** — Generalized cortical hyperosteosis
- **Massive osteolysis** — Vanishing bone
- **Cherubism** — Familial fibrous dysplasia
- **Osteoarthritis** — Degenerative joint disease
- **Ankylosis** — Hypomobility
- **Pernicious anemia** — Addison's anemia
- **Sprue** — Coelic disease
- **Thalassemia** — Cooley's anemia
- **Polycythemia Vera** — Erythroblastic anemia
- **Agranulocytosis** — Granulocytopenia
- **Infectious mononucleosis** — Glandular fever
- **Thrombocythemia** — Thrombocytosis
- **Hemophilia** — Disease of King's
- **Acute necrotizing ulcerative gingivitis (ANUG)** — Vincent's infection, Ulcerative gingivitis, Trench mouth
- **Juvenile Periodontitis** — Periodontosis

- **Migraine headache** — Menstrual headache, Sunday headache, Monday morning headache, Sick headache
- **Acute septic osteitis** — Osteomyelitis
- **Dentinal sclerosis** — Transparent dentin
- **Secondary dentin** — Irregular dentin
- **Hypercementosis** — Cementum hyperplasia
- **Internal resorption** — Odontoclastoma, pink tooth of mummery
- **Scarlet fever** — Scarlatina
- **Sarcoidosis** — Boeck's Sarcoid
- **Uveoparotid fever** — Heerfordt's syndrome
- **Leprosy** — Hansen's disease
- **Botryomycosis** — Bacterial actinophytosis
- **Granuloma inguinale** — Granuloma venereum
- **Rhinoscleroma** — Scleroma
- **Midline lethal granuloma** — Malignant granuloma
- **NOMA** — Carcrum oris, Gangrenous stomatitis
- **Progenic granuloma** — Granuloma pyogenicum
- **Herpes Simplex** — Herpes Labialis
- **Recurrent Aphthous stomatitis** — Canker sorea
- **Herpangina** — Aphthous pharyngitis
- **Rubella** — German measles
- **Herpes zoster** — Shingles
- **Mumps** — Epidemic parotitis
- **Poliomyelitis** — Infantile paralysis
- **Coccidioidomycosis** — Valley fever
- **Candidiasis** — Moniliasis, Thrush
- **Periapical granuloma** — Atypical periodontia
- **Apical periodontal cyst** — Radicular cyst
- **Periapical abscess** — Alveolar abscess
- **Condensing osteitis** — Chronic focal sclerosing osteomyelitis
- **Traumatic ulcer** — Decubitus ulcer, Sore ulcers
- **Palatal papillomatosis** — Inflammatory papillary hyperplasia

- **Dental lamina cyst**   Gingival cyst,
                                                  Epstein's pearls,
                                                  Bohn's Nodules

- **Bifid rib syndrome**   Basal cell nevus syndrome,
                                                  Goltz syndrome

- **Calcifying odontogenic cyst**   Cystic keratinizing cyst

- **Enameloma**   Enamel Drop

- **Ameloblastoma**   Adamatinoma
                                                  Multilocular cyst

- **Primary intrasoseous   Primary intra alveolar epidermoid
  carcinoma**   carcinoma

- **Calcifying epithelial   Adenoameloblastma,
  odontogenic tumor (CEOT)**   Ameloblastic adenomatiod tumor

- **Squamous odontogenic tumor**   Benign epithelial odontogenic tumor

- **Peripheral odontogenic   Peripheral ossifying fibroma,
  fibroma**   calcifying fibrous eupilis

- **Odontogenic myxoma**   Cementoma,
                                                  Periapical osteofibroma,
                                                  Cementifying fibroma,
                                                  periapical fibrous dysplasia

- **Periapical cemental dysplasia**   Cementoma,
                                                  Periapical osteofibroma,
                                                  Cementifying fibroma,
                                                  Periapical fibrous dysplasia

- **Benign cementoblastoma**   True cementoma

- **Gigantiform cementoma**   Familial multiple cementoma

- **Ameloblastic fibroma**   Soft mixed odontogenic tumor,
                                                  Soft mixed odontoma

- **Ameloblastic fibroma**   Ameloblastic sarcoma

- **Ameloblastic odontoma**   Odontoameloblastoma calcified
                                                  odontoma

- **Terratoma**   Terotoblastoma

- **Primary lymphoma of bone**   Primary reticulum cell sarcoma

- **African Jaw lymphoma**   Burkitt's lymphoma

- **Multiple myeloma**   Plasma cell myeloma

- **Plasma cell myeloma**   Plasmacytoma

- **Angiomyoma**   Vascular leimyoma

- **Granular cell myoblastoma**   Granular cell tumor myoblastic
                                                  myoma

• **Traumatic neuroma**	Amputation neuroma
• **Alveolar soft part sarcoma**	Malignant granular cell myoblastoma
• **Multiple endocrine neoplasm**	Men syndrome
• **Neurofibroma**	Neurofibromatosis, Fibroma Molluscum
• **Neurolemma**	Schwannoma, Perineural fibroblastoma
• **Malignant schwannoma**	Neurofibrosarcoma
• **Olfactory neuro blastoma**	Esthesio neuroblastoma
• **Pleomorphic adenoma**	Mixed tumor
• **Papillary cystadenoma lymphomatosum**	Warthin's tumor Adeno lymphoma
• **Oxyphilic adenoma**	Oncocytoma, Acidophilic adenoma
• **Mikulicz's disease**	Benign lymphoepithelial lesion
• **Sjogren's syndrome**	Sicca syndrome
• **Malignant pleomorphic adenoma**	Malignant mixed tumor pleomorphic adenoma
• **Adenoid cystic carcinoma**	Cylindroma, Basaloid mixed tumor, Adenocystic basal cell carcinoma
• **Acinic cell carcinoma**	Seroud cell adenoma, Adenocarcinoma
• **Dentigerous cyst**	Follicular cyst
• **Apical periodontal cyst**	Radicular cyst, Periapical cyst, Dental root end cyst
• **Facial neuritis**	Bell's palsy
• **Ankylosed deciduous teeth**	Submerged teeth
• **Median anterior maxillary cyst**	Nasopalatine duct cyst, Incisive canal cyst
• **Nasoalveolar cyst**	Nasolabial cyst
• **Palatal cysts**	Epstein's pearls
• **Benign cervical lymphoepithelial cyst**	Branchial left cyst benign cystic lymph node
• **Keratoacanthoma**	Self healing carcinoma, Molluscum setaceum
• **Intraepithelial carcinoma**	Carcinoma in situ
• **Basal cell carcinoma**	Rodent ulcer

- **Epidermoid carcinoma** — Squamous cell carcinoma
- **Spindle cell carcinoma** — Carcinosarcoma, Lane tumor?
- **Adenoacanthoma** — Adenoid squamous cell carcinoma
- **Peripheral ossifying fibroma** — Peripheral odontogenic fibroma
- **Central ossifying fibroma** — Central fibro osteoma
- **Osteoclastoma giant cell Epulis** — Peripheral giant cell granuloma
- **Verruciform Xanthoma** — Histiocytosis 'Y'
- **Hemangioma** — Vascular nevus
- **Sturge Weber Syndrome** — Encephalotrigeminal angiomatosis
- **Rendu-Osler-Weber disease** — Hereditary hemorrhagic telangiectasia
- **Nasopharyngeal Angiofibroma** — Juvenile nasopharyngeal fibroma
- **Benign chondroblastoma** — Codman's tumor
- **Benign osteoblastoma** — Giant osteoid osteoma
- **Kaposi's sarcoma** — Angioreticuloendothelioma
- **Ewing's sarcoma** — Round cell sarcoma, Endothelial myeloma
- **Osteosarcoma** — Osteogenic sarcoma
- **Labial/oral melanotic macule** — Ephelis, Focal melanosis, Solitary labial lentigo
- **Focal epithelial hyperplasia** — Heck's disease
- **Fibromatosis gingiva** — Elephantiasis gingivae, Hereditary gingival fibromatosis,
- **Fissured tongue** — Scrotal tongue
- **Medium Rhomboid Glossitis** — Central papillary atrophy of tongue
- **Benign migratory glossitis** — Geographic tongue, Erythema migrans, Wandering rash of tongue
- **Lymphoid hamartoma** — Angiofollicular, Lymph node malformation
- **Angiolymphoid hyperplasia** — Kimuras disease, Eosinophilic folliculosis
- **Lymphoepithelial cyst** — Branchial cyst, Branchiogenic cyst
- **Aplasia** — Agenesis
- **Dens in dente** — Dens invaginatus, Dilated composite odontome, Occlusal enamel pearl

- **Amelogenesis Imperfecta** — Hereditary Brown opalescent teeth, Hereditary enamel dysplasia
- **Dentinogenesis Imperfecta** — Hereditary oplasescent dentin, Odonotogenic imperfecta
- **Regional odontodysplasia** — Ghost teeth
- **Plasma cells** — Effector cells
- **Rickett's E line** — E-line
- **Bell's palsy** — Facial neuritis
- **Accessory cusp** — Talon cusp
- **Supernumerary cusp** — Talon cusp
- **Gumma** — Tertiary syphilitic oral ulcer
- **Vitamin B$_1$** — Thiamine
- **Endogenous Malodor** — True oral malodor
- **Vasodepressor syncope** — Vasovagal syncope
- **Angular defects** — Vertical defects
- **Cannon's disease** — White spongy nervus
- **Sterlity** — Infertility
- **Nursing bottle caries** — Infancy caries
- **Soother caries** — Infancy caries
- **Kissing disease** — Infectious mononeucleosis
- **Infracrestal pocket** — Infrabony pocket
- **Infralveolar pocket** — Infrabony pocket
- **Centric occlusion** — Intecuspal position
- **Papillary gingival** — Inter dental gingiva
- **Supracontact** — Interference
- **Apoplexy** — Intracerebral hemorrhage
- **Chronic microcytic** — Iron deficiency anemia, Hypochromic anemia
- **Juvenile periodontitis** — Localized juvenile periodontis, Early onset periodontitis, Localized aggressive periodontitis
- **Warty dyskeratoma** — Keratosis foelleuleris
- **Kirkland knives** — Periodontal knives, Gingivectomy knives
- **Le-fort I** — Low level fracture
- **Le-fort II** — Pyramidal fracture, Subzygomatic fracture

• **Le-fort III**	High transverse fracture, Suprazygomatic fracture
• **Migratory glossitis**	Geographic tongue
• **Sulculur fluid**	Gingival fluid
• **Polyalkanoate cements**	Glass ionomer cements (GICS)
• **Meischer's syndrome**	Granulomatous cheilitis
• **Bicuspidization**	Hemiseptum
• **Witkop – von sallman syndrome**	Hereditary benign intraepithelial dyskeratosis
• **Thyrotoxicosis**	Hyperthyroidism
• **Mucoperiosteal flap**	Full thickness flap
• **German measles**	Rubella
• **Septic theory**	Parasitic theory
• **Partial thickness flap**	Mucosal flap, Split thickness flap
• **Servo system**	Pertrovic's hypothesis
• **Branchial arches**	Pharyngeal arches
• **Compomers**	Polyacid – modified composite resins
• **Orthostatic hypotension**	Postural hypotension
• **Dentinoid**	Predentin
• **Deciduous dentition**	Primary dentition
• **Unethical act**	Professional misconducts
• **Thrush**	Pseudomembranous candidiasis
• **Takayasu's disease**	Pulseless disease
• **Pyelonephritis**	Pyelitis
• **Progressive systemic sclerosis**	Scleroderma
• **Cartilaginous theory**	Scott's hypothesis
• **Fissured tongue**	Scrotal tongue
• **Diode lasers**	Semiconductor lasers
• **Steiner's line**	S-line
• **Incomplete fracture**	Split tooth
• **Contact stomatitis**	Stomatitis venenata
• **Suprabony pocket**	Supracrestal pocket, Supralveolar pocket
• **Neutrophilis**	Polymorphonuclear, Leukocytes, Microphage
• **Monocytes**	Macrophages
• **Unattached gingival**	Marginal gingiva
• **Transitional dentition**	Mixed dentition

ANNEXURE - V

TOOTH NUMBERING SYSTEM

I. AMERICAN NUMBERING SYSTEM OF PERMANENT TEETH

Upper Teeth

1. Maxillary right third molar
2. Maxillary right second molar
3. Maxillary right first molar
4. Maxillary right second premolar
5. Maxillary right first premolar
6. Maxillary right canine
7. Maxillary right lateral incisor
8. Maxillary right central incisor
9. Maxillary left central incisor
10. Maxillary left lateral incisor
11. Maxillary left canine
12. Maxillary left first premolar
13. Maxillary left second premolar
14. Maxillary left first molar
15. Maxillary left second molar
16. Maxillary left third molar

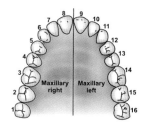

Lower Teeth

17. Mandibular left third molar
18. Mandibular left second molar
19. Mandibular left first molar
20. Mandibular left second premolar
21. Mandibular left first premolar
22. Mandibular left canine
23. Mandibular left lateral incisor
24. Mandibular left central incisor
25. Mandibular right central incisor
26. Mandibular right lateral incisor
27. Mandibular right canine
28. Mandibular right first premolar
29. Mandibular right first premolar
30. Mandibular right first molar
31. Mandibular right second molar
32. Mandibular right third molar

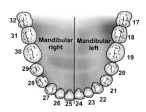

Upper Teeth

A. Maxillary right second molar
B. Maxillary right first molar
C. Maxillary right canine
D. Maxillary right lateral incisor
E. Maxillary right central incisor
F. Maxillary left central incisor
G. Maxillary left lateral incisor
H. Maxillary left canine
I. Maxillary left first molar
J. Maxillary left second molar

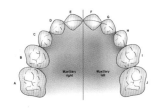

Lower Teeth

K. Mandibular left second molar
L. Mandibular left first molar
M. Mandibular left canine
N. Mandibular left lateral incisor
O. Mandibular left central incisor
P. Mandibular right central incisor
Q. Mandibular right lateral incisor
R. Mandibular right canine
S. Mandibular right first molar
T. Mandibular right second molar

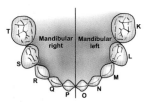

II. FEDERATION DENTAIRE INTERNATIONALE SYSTEM FOR PERMANENT TEETH

Quadrant number	Quadrant identification
1	Maxillary right
2	Maxillary left
3	Mandibular left
4	Mandibular right

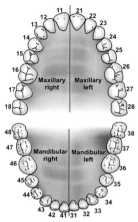

Federation Dentaire Internationale numbering system for
permanent dentition

FEDERATION DENTAIRE INTERNATIONALE SYSTEM FOR DECIDUOUS TEETH

Quadrant number	Quadrant identification
5	Maxillary right
6	Maxillary left
7	Mandibular left
8	Mandibular right

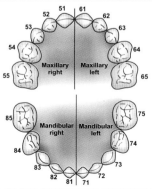

Federation Dentaire Internationale numbering system for
primary dentition

III. ZSIGMONDY-PALMER SYSTEM

It identifies specific teeth by using a grid system.

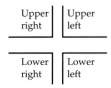

(A) ZSIGMONDY-PALMER SYSTEM FOR DECIDUOUS DENTITION

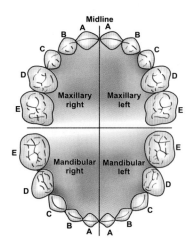

(B) ZSIGMONDY-PALMER SYSTEM FOR MIXED DENTITION

A

6	E	D	C	B	A	A	B	C	D	E	6
6	E	D	C	B	1	1	B	C	D	E	6

B

Symbol	Maxillary right	Symbol	Maxillary left
6	Maxillary right permanent first molar	A	Maxillar left deciduous central incisor
E	Maxillary right deciduous second molar	B	Maxillar left deciduous lateral incisor
D	Maxillar right deciduous first molar	C	Maxillar left deciduous cuspid
C	Maxillary right deciduous cuspid	D	Maxillar left deciduous first molar
B	Maxillary right deciduous lateral incisor	E	Maxillar left deciduous second molar
A	Maxillary right deciduous central incisor	6	Maxillar left deciduous first molar

Symbol	Mandibular right	Symbol	Mandibular left
6	Mandibular right deciduous first molar	1	Mandibular left deciduous central incisor
E	Mandibular right deciduous second molar	B	Mandibular left deciduous lateral incisor
D	Mandibular right deciduous first molar	C	Mandibular left deciduous cuspid
C	Mandibular right deciduous cuspid	D	Mandibular left deciduous first molar
B	Mandibular right deciduous lateral incisor	E	Mandibular left deciduous second molar
1	Mandibular right permanent central incisor	6	Mandibular left permanent first molar

A, **Schematic display of mixed dentition using Zsigmondy Palmer tooth identification system.** B, **Key to display shown in** A.

(C) ZSIGMONDY-PALMER SYSTEM FOR PERMANENT DENTITION

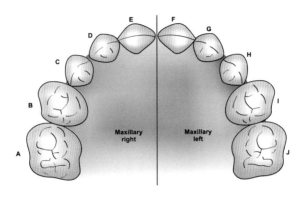

Number eight represents third molars
Number one represents central incisors

SITES FOR THE ADMINISTRATION OF ANESTHESIA

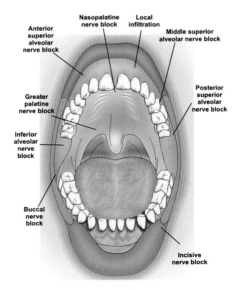

AREAS AFFECTED POST ADMINISTRATION OF LOCAL ANESTHESIA

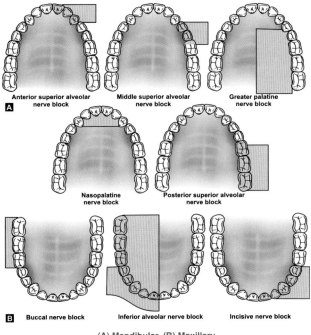

Anterior superior alveolar nerve block

Middle superior alveolar nerve block

Greater palatine nerve block

Nasopalatine nerve block

Posterior superior alveolar nerve block

A

Buccal nerve block

Inferior alveolar nerve block

Incisive nerve block

B

(A) Mandibular, (B) Maxillary

ANNEXURE - VI

TABLES

Lymph Nodes of the Head and Neck

Lymph nodes of the head	Drainage
Retroauricular nodes	Skin of ear and posterior parietal region of scalp.
Preauricular nodes	Auricle of ear and temporal region of scalp
Parotid nodes	Root of nose, eyelids, anterior temporal region, external auditory meatus, tympanic cavity, nasopharynx, and posterior portions of nasal cavity.
Facial nodes	
Infraorbital nodes	Eyelid and conjunctiva
Buccal nodes	Skin and mucous membrane of nose and cheek
Mandibular nodes	Skin and mucous membrane of nose and cheek
Submandibular nodes	Chin, lips, nose, nasal cavity, cheeks, gums, inferior surface of palate and anterior portion of tongue.
Submental nodes	Chin, lower, lip, cheeks, tip of tongue, and floor of mouth
Superficial cervical nodes	Inferior part of ear and parotid region
Deep cervical nodes	
Superior deep cervical node	Posterior head and neck, auricle, tongue, larynx, nodes esophagus, thyroid gland, nasopharynx, nasal cavity, palate and tonsils.
Inferior deep cervical node	Posterior scalp and neck, superficial pectoral region, and part of arm.

Muscles of the Face

Muscle	Origin	Action and comments
Orbicularis oris	Muscle fibers surrounding mouth	Closes lips, presses lips against teeth, protrudes lips and shapes lips in speech
Zygomaticus Minor	Zygomatic bone	Elevates upper lip
Major	Zygomatic bone	Draws angle of mouth upward and outward
Levator labii superioris	Maxilla and Zygomatic bone	Raises upper lip and turns it outward
Depressor labii inferioris	Mandible	Draws lower lip downward and a little laterally
Depressor anguli oris	Mandible	Draws angle of mouth downward and laterally
Buccinators	Mandible and maxilla in region near molars	Compresses cheeks against teeth, provides a stable lateral wall to oral cavity for pressure in speech, sucking and mastication
Levator anguli oris	Canine fossa of maxilla	Raises angle of mouth
Mentalis	Incisor fossa of mandible	Draws lower lip downward and a little laterally
Risorius	Facial of masseter muscle	Retracts angle of mouth

Muscles of Mastication

Muscle	Origin	Action and comments
Masseter	Maxilla, Zygomatic arch	Elevates mandible, closing jaw
Temporalis	Temporal fossa	Elevates mandible, closing jaw; draws mandible backward after protrusion, assists in lateral movements
Lateral pterygoid	Greater wing of the sphenoid bone and lateral pterygoid plate	Helps in opening mouth, protrusion of jaw, and grinding movements
Medial pterygoid	Pterygoid plate, palatine bone, and maxilla	Elevation and protrusion of mandible and side-to-side movements of jaw.

Muscles of the Neck

Muscle	Origin	Insertion	Action and comments
	Superficial lateral cervical muscles		
Platysma	Fascia covering pectoralis major and deltoid muscles skin and subcutaneous tissue of lower part of face	Body of mandible and	Wrinkles skin in neck, assists in lowering mandible, draws down lower lip and angle of mouth
Trapezius			
Sternocleidomastoid	Manubrium of sternum and clavicle cervical nerves	Mastoid process of temporal bone	Singly: tilts head toward shoulder of same side, rotates head to face opposite side; together ; draw head forward, flex cervical part of vertebral column; if head is fixed, they help raise the thorax in forced inspiration.
	Suprahyoid muscles		
Digastric	Mastoid portion of temporal bone, symphysis of mandible	Hyoid bone, occasionally mandible	Depresses mandible, can elevate hyoid bone

Contd...

Contd...

Muscle	Origin	Insertion	Action and comments
Stylohyoid	Styloid process of temporal bone	Hyoid bone	Elevates the hyoid bone and draws it back, elongating the floor of the mouth. Can stabilize hyoid bone for tongue muscle action
Mylohyoid	Mylohyoid line on mandible	Hyoid bone median raphe	Elevates floor of mouth in the first phase of swallowing elevates hyoid bone or depresses mandible.
Geniohyoid	Inferior mental spine on mandible	Body of hyoid bone	Elevates hyoid bone and draws it forward; depresses mandible when hyoid bone is fixed
Infrahyoid muscles			
Sternohyoid	Manubrium of the sternum	Bone of hyoid bone	Depresses hyoid bone after it has been raised as in swallowing
Sternothyroid	Manubrium of sternum and cartilage of first rib	Lamina of thyroid cartilage	Draws larynx downward after it has been elevated as in swallowing

Major Arteries of the Head and Neck

Artery	Major branches	Region supplied
External carotid artery	Superior thyroid artery	Thyroid gland and adjacent muscles
	Lingual artery	Tongue and floor of the mouth, oropharynx, sublingual gland, and neighboring muscles
	Facial artery	Muscles and tissues of the face below the level of the eyes, the submandibular gland, tonsil, and soft palate
	Occipital artery	Muscles, skin, and other tissue in the region behind the ear and the back part of the scalp
	Posterior auricular artery	Parotid gland, muscles, skin and other tissues of the ear and posterior scalp regions
	Superficial temporal artery	Parotid gland, temporo mandibular joint, outer, ear, forehead, temporal region of the scalp, adjacent muscles
	Maxillary artery	Upper and lower jaws, teeth, muscles of mastication, palate, nose, and dura mater
Internal carotid artery	Hypophyseal artery	Pituitary gland
	Ophthalmic artery	Eye, lacrimal gland, ocular muscles, nasal cavity, forehead
Right and left subclavicular arteries	Vertebral artery	Spinal cord, vertebrae and surrounding tissues, deep neck structures
	Thyrocervical trunk	Thyroid gland, neck muscles, trachea, esophagus
	Costocervical trunk	Muscles at the back of the neck, vertebral canal, first intercostals space

Major Branches from Various Segments of the Aorta

Artery	Major branches	Region supplied
Inferior mesenteric artery	Left colic artery	Transverse and descending colon
	Sigmoid arteries	Descending and sigmoid colon
	Superior rectal artery	Rectum
Lumbar arteries		Muscles and skin of the back, vertebral canal, and its contents intercostals
Median sacral artery		Sacral vertebrae, rectum
Common iliac arteries	External iliac	Pelvic region and legs
	Internal iliac	Leg
		Viscera and walls of the pelvis, perineum, and gluteal region

Cranial Nerves (Major Components)

No.	Name	Peripheral distribution	Functions
I	Olfactory	Mucous membrane of olfactory region of nose	Smell
II	Optic	Retina of eye	Vision
III	Occulomotor	Muscles (superior, inferior, and medial rectus; inferior oblique; and levator palpebrae	Eye movements, raise upper eyelid
		Pupillary constrictor and ciliary muscles of eye	Regulation of pupil size, accommodation of lens
IV	Trochlear	Superior oblique muscle	Eye movements
V	Trigeminal	Face, grater part of scalp, teeth, mouth, nasal cavity	Sensory from face, nose, and mouth
		Muscles (medial and lateral pterygoid, masseter, temporalis)	Chewing movements
VI	Abducent	Lateral rectus muscle	Eye movements
VII	Facial	Anterior part of tongue and soft palate	Taste
		Muscles of face, scalp, and outer ear	Facial expression
		Submandibular and sublingual salivary glands, lacrimal glands, glands of nasal and palatine mucosa	Secretions

contd...

contd...

No.	Name	Peripheral distribution	Functions
VIII	Acoustic	Hari cells of organ of corti, semi-circular canals, maculae, and saccule	Hearing, balance, change of rate of motion of head
IX	Glosso-pharyngeal	Back of tongue, pharynx, carotid sinus, and body Stylopharyngeus muscle Parotid salivary gland	Taste and other sensations of tongue, changes in levels of blood pressure and gases Swallowing movements Secretions
X	Vagus	Taste buds on epiglottis; larynx, trachea, pharynx, heart, lungs, esophagus, small intestine, part of colon Smooth muscle of bronchi, esophagus, stomach, and intestines; heart; striated muscles of pharyngeal constrictors and intrinsic muscles of larynx	Pain, stretching, changes in levels of blood pressure and gases, taste Movement and secretion by the organs supplied
XI	Accessory	Muscles of larynx, trapezius, sternocleidomastoid	Shoulder movements, turning head, voice production
XII	Hypoglossal	Muscles of tongue	Tongue movements

National Immunization Schedule

At birth	BCG and OPV
At 6 weeks	DPT-1, OPV-1 and Hepatitis B_1
At 10 weeks	DPT-2, OPV-2 and Hepatitis B_2
At 14 weeks	DPT-3, OPV-3 and Hepatitis B_3
At 9th month	Measles
16 and 24 months	DPT and OPV
At 10 and 16 years	Tetanus Toxoid second dose after 1 month
For pregnant women	$T_1 - TT_2$ after one month in first trimester

Mile Stone in Vaccination

Year	Vaccine
1798	Small pox vaccine
1885	Rabies vaccine
1892	Cholera vaccine
1913	Toxin/Diphtheria
1921	BCG
1923	Diphtheria Toxoid
1923	Pertusis vaccine
1937	Influenza vaccine
1949	Mumps vaccine
1954	Salk's Polio vaccine
1957	Sabin's live oral polio vaccine
1960	Measles vaccine
1962	Rubella vaccine
1968	Type C Meningococcal vaccine
1976	Hepatitis – B vaccine

Periods of Isolation

Disease	Duration of isolation
Measles	Catarrhal stage to 3rd day of stage
Chicken pox	Usually till 6 days
German measles	Women should not be exposed in first trimester
Cholera/Diphtheria	3 days after anti biotic
Shigellosis	Until stool becomes negative repeatively
Hepatitis A	3 weeks
Influenza	3 weeks after onset
Polio	2 weeks adult and six weeks children
T.B.	3 weeks of effective chemotherapy
Mumps	Until swelling subsides
Pharyngitis	6 hours of effective treatment

Methods for Sterilisations

Method	Used for	Advantages/Disadvantages
Hot air	2 hours, 160°C used for all instruments of root kits	It kills all micro-organisms/It is too long a procedure very limited use
Flaming autoclave	Immediate 3 minutes 134° C Most metal instruments swab, towels rubber, plastics hand pieces	Kills all organisms/ Equipment may be costlier

Impression Material

Material	Use	Advantage/Disadvantage
Alginate	Edentulous	Accuracy but dimension may change
Elastomers	For undercuts soft flabby ridges	Stronger than alginate but more extensive and takes longer to set
Impression compound	Edentulous impressions	Economical but dose not record the minute details
Impression paste	Lining base plates	Accuracy but sticks to lips/skin

Temporary Fillings

Fillings	Uses	Advantages	Disadvantages
Zinc oxide and eugenol cement	1. Temporary filling 2. Lining deep cavities 3. Sedative dressing for dry socket 4. Gingivectomy 5. Obturating material for primary teeth	1. Economical 2. Easily available 3. Can be used in deep cavities 4. Rate of resorption is closer to the primary tooth	1. Soft 2. Slow-setting 3. Irritant to soft tissue
Gutta-percha	1. Permanent filling for root canals 2. Vitality tests 3. Temporary obturator for cleft palates and cyst cavities 4. Lining for gunning splints	1. Inert 2. No mixing	1. Too soft 2. Periapically can act as a foreign body
Zinc phosphate cement	1. Thick mix: cavity lining; temporary filling 2. Thin mix: adhesive cement for inlays and crowns	1. Hard 2. Rapid set 3. Adhesive	1. Irritant in deep cavities
Polycarboxylate	1. Thick mix: cavity lining: temporary filling 2. Thin mix: adhesive cement for inlays, crowns and orthodontic bands	1. Less irritant 2. More adhesive	1. May be difficult to manipulate
Calcium hydroxide	1. Cavity lining 2. Endodontic treatment 3. Antibacterial 4. Pulp capping agent 5. Root induction procedures 6. Intracanal medicament	1. Non-irritant 2. Can be used in deepest cavities 3. Compatible with all materials 4. Restorable 5. Can be used in periapical areas	1. Sublining only, in deep cavities under metal fillings 2. Contraindicated in primary dentition as it causes internal resorption

Comparison of Permanent Filling

Filling	Uses	Advantage/Disadvantage
Glass Ionomer cement	• Permanent restoration for primary anterior teeth	It is cariostatic and non-irritant. It develops chemical bond to tooth. But it is too dark and opaque and is too soft for back teeth.
Amalgam	Permanent filling for posterior teeth	• It sets rapidly. Technique is simple but it requires lining.
Composite	• Permanent filling for front teeth	• Good strength suitable for large and complicated restorations.
	• Fissure sealents brackets	• It is good for undercut and • Bonding with teeth • But for back teeth it is not good.
Gold	• Crown for back teeth	It is much stronger but takes more time

Elastic Modulus of some Dental Material

Material	Pounds/inch^2
Human enamel	1,20,00,000
Dental amalgam	40,00,000
Gold alloy	1,40,00,000
Zinc phosphate cement	20,00,000
Glass ionomer cement	8,00,000
Human dentine	2,70,00,000

Tensile Strength of some Dental Material

Material	Tensile strength Pounds/inch^2
Human enamel	5000
Dental amalgam	7000
Gold alloy	60,000-120,000
Porcelain	5000
Nikel-chromium alloy	61000

Properties of Alloying Elements

	Platinum	Gold	Silver	Copper
	Pi	Au	Ag	Cu
Color	White	Yellow	White	Reddish
Tarnish resistence	Excellant	Excellant	Poor	Fair
Chemical activity	Inert	Inert	Active	Very active
Density	21.5	19.3	10.5	9

Different Alloys used for Orthodontic Wires

	Co-Cr	Stainless steel	B-T_1
Elastic limit	1100	1300	900
Stiffness	185 high	180 high	72 medium
Maximum flexibility	low	low	medium
Formability	medium	high	medium

Hardness Values

Material	Hardness
Cementum	40
Composite	30
Dentin	70
Amalgam	90
Gold alloy	100
Enamel	340
Porcelin	595
Tungsten	1900
Diamond	7000

Liners, Bases and Cements

Substance	Mixing time	Quality of proper mix	Setting time
Temporary cement luting agent	Mix all at one time 30 seconds	Uniform color	2 minutes
Calcium hydroxide cavity liner	Mix quickely 10 seconds	Uniform color	2-3 minutes
Zinc phosphate luting agent	Add divided increaments	Mix aril stretch 1"	5-6 minutes
As base	Add divided increaments	Thick putty like non sticking	5-6 minutes
Glass ionomer luting agent and base	Add powder to liquid	Glossy	7 minutes

Muscles of Tongue

Muscle	Nerve supply	Action
1. Intrinsic group		
• Inferior lingualis	Hypoglossal nerve	• Shortens tongue
• Transverase lingualis	Hypoglossal	• Narrous & stretches
• Vertical lingualis	Hypoglossal	• Flatterns tip of tongue
• Superior lingualis	Hypoglossal	• Contracts tongue and raises its tongue-tip and edges
2. Extrinsic group		
• Glossopharyngeus	Pharyngeal plexus	Contracts oropharynx
• Hypoglossus	Hypoglossal	Lipts and retracts tongue
• Geniohyglossus	Hypoglossal	Retracts, protrudes and depresses tongue
• Styloglossus	Hypoglossal	Raises and retracts the tongue

Tumors Associated with Trigeminal Nerve Pain

	Disease
Tumors	Trigeminal neurinoma Metastatic neoplasia Tuberculoma
Trauma	Traumatic neuroma
Infections disease	Leprosy Herpes zoster Sarcoidosis
Metabolic disease	Diabetes mellitus chronic alcoholism
Intoxications	Drug intoxications digitalis organic chemical intoxication

Tongue Deformities and Syndromes

Bald tongue	Familial dysautonomia Endocrine condidosis Epidermolysis bullosa
Fissured tongue	Cowden's syndrome Clefting syndrome Coffee-Lowry syndrome
Popillomatous tongue	Congenital lymphangioma Neurofibromatosis Meckel's syndrome
Bifurcated tongue	Fetal face syndrome Meckel's syndrome
Long narrow tongue	Tuberous sclerosis Ehlers-Danlo's syndrome
Ankyglossia	Cryptoph thalmos syndrome orofacial digetal syndrome
Macroglossia	Hyrler's syndrome Fetal face syndrome cretism Sturge-Weber syndrome Mucopolysaccharidosis

Cranial Nerves

Cranial Nerve	Function	Physical Findings
I (Olfactory)	Smell	No smell
II (Optic)	Vision	Decreased visual acuity
III (Oculomotor)	Eye movement Pupillary constriction	Failure to move eye in fild of motion of muscle Pupillary abnormalities
IV (Trochlear)	Eye movement	May be difficult to detect anything if 3rd nerve intact
V (Trigeminal)	Facial, nasal and oral sensation Jaw movement	Absent corneal reflex, weakness of masticatory muscles
VI (Abducens)	Eye movement	Failure of eye to abduct
VII (Facial)	Facial movement	Asymmetry of facial contraction
VIII (Auditory and vestibular	Hearing Balance	Decreased hearing Nystagmus, Ataxia
IX (Glossopharyngeal)	Palatal movement	Asymmetric palate
X (Vagus)	Palatal movement Vocal cords	Asymmetric palate Brassy voice
XI (Spinal accessory)	Turns neck	Paralysis of sterno-cleidomastoid muscle
XII (Hypoglossal)	Moves tongue	Wasting and fascicula-tion or deviation of tongue

The Muscles Acting on the Temporomandibular Joint

Muscle	Main actions
Temporalis	Elevates mandible, closing jaws; its posterior firbers retrude mandible after protrusion
Masseter	Elevates and protrudes mandible, thus closing jaws; deep fibers retrude it
Lateral pterygoid	*Acting together*, the protrude mandible and depress chain *Acting alone* and alternately, they produce side-to-side movements of mandible
Medial pterygoid	Helps to elevate mandible, closing jaws *Acting together*, the help to protrude mandible *Acting alone*, it protrudes side of jaw

NUTRITIONAL VALUES

Nutrition Ready Reckoner
These are average values for standard recipes found in most books and used in Indian kitchens

	Calories (Kcal)	Proteins (g)	Fats (g)	Carbo-hydrates (g)	Fibre (g)	Calcium (mg)	Iron (mg)	Caro-tene (mcg)	Retinol (mcg)	Vit B₁ (mg)	Vit B₂ (mg)	Niacin (mg)	Vit C (mg)	Serving Portion
BEVERAGES														
Hot Tea	34	0.6	1.0	5.7	0.0	31.0	0.0	0.0	7.00	0.01	0.01	0.0	0	1 Tea Cup
Instant Coffee	149	1.0	13.3	6.3	0.0	31.0	0.0	0.0	7.00	0.01	0.01	0.0	0	1 Tea Cup
Cold Coffee (with Cream)	279	3.9	17.0	27.7	0.0	144.0	0.3	487.0	183.00	0.06	0.23	0.1	2	1 Tall Glass
Banana Milk Shake	228	6.2	7.5	33.8	0.0	223.0	0.5	40.0	101.00	0.11	0.37	0.4	7	1 Tall Glass
Mango Milk Shake	237	6.2	7.7	35.6	0.8	227.0	1.3	2067.0	608.00	0.15	0.41	9.0	16	1 Tall Glass
Lemonade	107	0.3	0.3	25.7	0.5	21.0	0.1	0.0	0.00	0.01	0.00	0.0	12	1 Glass
BREAKFAST CEREALS														
Cracked Wheat Porridge	292	10.0	10.4	39.7	2.5	296.0	1.5	152.0	39.00	1.29	0.49	1.3	5	1 Bowl
Semonlina Porridge	293	9.8	10.2	40.4	0.0	291.0	0.8	139.0	36.00	1.24	0.47	0.6	5	1 Bowl
Vermicelli Porridge	294	9.4	10.2	41.1	2.5	292.0	0.9	139.0	36.00	1.24	0.47	0.6	5	1 Bowl
Oat Meal Porridge	217	6.6	6.6	32.8	2.0	154.0	1.0	70.0	18.00	0.80	0.26	0.3	2	1 Bowl
Cornflakes with Milk	291	9.8	10.8	38.7	1.2	290.0	0.9	157.0	41.00	1.28	0.48	0.6	5	1 Bowl

Contd...

Contd...

	Calories (Kcal)	Proteins (g)	Fats (g)	Carbo-hydrates (g)	Fibre (g)	Calcium (mg)	Iron (mg)	Caro-tene (mcg)	Retinol (mcg)	Vit B_1 (mg)	Vit B_2 (mg)	Niacin (mg)	Vit C (mg)	Serving Portion
Semolina Upma	147	2.3	7.7	17.1	9.9	11.0	0.5	1.0	0.00	0.04	0.01	0.4	2	1 Bowl
Vermicilli Upma	296	4.0	15.2	35.7	5.4	24.0	1.2	2.0	1.00	0.10	0.03	0.9	5	1 Bowl
Vegetable Upma	192	4.4	9.7	21.7	1.5	22.0	0.9	107.0	27.00	0.20	0.02	1.6	4	1 Bowl
Poha	158	2.8	7.3	20.2	1.5	10.0	4.2	6.0	1.00	0.10	0.02	2.0	3	1 Bowl
Vegetable with Poha	202	4.9	9.3	24.7	2.1	21.0	4.6	111.0	28.00	0.18	0.03	3.1	5	1 Bowl
EGGS														
Boiled Egg	87	6.7	6.7	0.0	0.0	25.0	0.7	300.0	180.00	0.05	0.20	0.1	0	1 Egg
Poached Egg	87	6.7	6.7	0.0	0.0	25.0	0.7	300.0	180.00	0.05	0.20	0.1	0	1 Egg
Fried Egg	160	6.7	14.8	0.0	0.0	25.0	0.7	620.0	260.00	0.05	0.20	0.1	0	1 Egg
Scrambled Egg	172	6.7	15.8	0.8	0.0	57.0	0.7	620.0	267.00	0.06	0.22	0.1	0	1 Egg
Baked Egg	124	6.7	10.8	0.0	0.0	25.0	0.7	460.0	220.0	0.05	0.20	0.1	0	1 Egg
Fluffy Omelette	160	6.7	14.8	0.0	0.0	25.0	0.7	620.0	260.00	0.05	0.20	0.1	0	1 Egg
Cheese and Mushroom Omelette	308	12.9	27.1	3.0	0.0	182.0	1.3	780.0	373.00	0.09	0.42	1.5	1	1 Egg
SOUPS														
Minestrone Soup	90	1.4	5.2	9.4	1.2	43.0	0.7	491.0	123.00	0.07	0.03	0.5	17	1 Bowl
Chicken Soup Corn Soup	322	25.5	13.5	24.6	6.0	23.0	2.6	10.7	93.00	0.21	0.34	8.6	6	1 Bowl
French Onion Soup	208	4.8	11.6	21.1	2.4	102.0	0.8	321.0	110.00	0.08	0.05	0.6	8	1 Bowl

Contd...

Contd...

	Calories (Kcal)	Proteins (g)	Fats (g)	Carbohydrates (g)	Fibre (g)	Calcium (mg)	Iron (mg)	Carotene (mcg)	Retinol (mcg)	Vit B_1 (mg)	Vit B_2 (mg)	Niacin (mg)	Vit C (mg)	Serving Portion
Tomato Soup	82	2.1	4.5	8.3	2.3	101.0	1.3	862.0	216.00	0.25	0.21	0.8	55	1 Bowl
Green Pea Soup	186	9.0	6.4	23.1	2.2	70.0	1.9	375.0	109.00	0.28	0.08	1.1	11	1 Bowl
Spinach Soup	561	3.9	8.9	116.2	5.9	81.0	1.5	5902.0	1475.00	0.06	0.27	0.08	29	1 Bowl
Mixed Vegetable Soup	146	3.3	9.2	12.5	1.4	124.0	0.9	779.0	225.0	0.11	0.16	0.6	23	1 Bowl
Cream with Tomato Soup	245	5.4	16.6	18.5	2.3	180.0	1.5	984.0	287.00	0.32	0.25	1.0	45	1 Bowl
Cream with Spinach Soup	307	8.5	23.2	16.0	5.1	200.0	2.2	6214.0	1644.00	0.20	0.52	0.9	32	1 Bowl
Cream with Carrot Soup	250	4.6	16.2	21.5	2.0	172.0	1.4	1935.0	531.00	0.17	0.17	0.9	6	1 Bowl
Cream of Pea Soup	342	12.4	18.2	32.2	2.6	132.0	2.4	590.0	188.00	0.44	0.17	1.4	15	1 Bowl
Cream with Potato Soup	282	5.4	13.1	35.7	3.1	118.0	1.1	415.0	144.00	0.24	0.17	1.6	21	1 Bowl
Cream with Mixed Vegetable Soup	263	7.5	13.4	28.0	3.2	179.0	2.0	1160.0	331.00	0.33	0.24	1.5	45	1 Bowl
Cream with Mushroom Soup	308	6.6	22.4	19.9	0.7	136.0	1.5	554.0	189.00	0.13	0.41	2.9	6	1 Bowl
Hot and Sour Soup	181	11.2	9.3	13.2	1.6	65.0	2.8	86.0	22.00	0.22	0.25	23	6	1 Bowl

Contd...

Contd...

Contd...

	Calories (Kcal)	Proteins (g)	Fats (g)	Carbo-hydrates (g)	Fibre (g)	Calcium (mg)	Iron (mg)	Caro-tene (mcg)	Retinol (mcg)	Vit B₁ (mg)	Vit B₂ (mg)	Niacin (mg)	Vit C (mg)	Serving Portion
CEREALS														
Chapati	273	9.7	1.4	55.5	5.6	38.0	3.9	23.0	5.00	0.39	0.14	3.40	0	3 or 4
Plain Parantha	363	9.7	11.4	55.5	5.6	38.0	3.9	23.0	6.00	0.39	0.14	3.40	0	3 Medium
Potato Stuffed Parantha	632	11.2	31.5	75.8	7.9	56.0	4.4	42.0	10.00	0.49	0.15	4.50	16	3 Medium
Pea Parantha	693	20.7	31.5	75.8	7.9	78.0	6.3	148.0	37.00	0.78	0.15	4.70	16	3 Medium
Cauliflower Parantha	577	12.0	31.7	60.9	7.1	74.0	5.0	47.0	12.00	0.44	0.22	4.30	47	3 Medium
Radish Parantha	574	10.8	31.5	61.8	8.2	90.0	4.5	27.0	7.00	0.48	0.16	4.10	20	3 Medium
Daal Parantha	665	16.2	33.1	75.6	9.0	65.0	5.6	62.0	15.00	0.55	0.19	4.20	3	3 Medium
Sprouted Dal Parantha	727	22.1	32.0	87.6	10.2	85.0	6.0	48.0	12.00	0.64	0.24	4.70	2	3 Medium
Paneer Parantha	713	20.9	43.9	58.5	5.9	173.0	4.0	243.0	61.00	0.45	0.15	3.50	4	3 Medium
Onion-Green Chilli Parantha	594	10.9	31.5	66.6	7.1	85.0	4.5	23.0	6.00	0.57	0.15	3.80	11	3 Medium
Keema Parantha	712	24.8	42.1	58.4	5.9	169.0	6.2	25.0	13.00	0.55	0.25	9.00	3	3 Medium
Methi Parantha	652	14.2	32.4	75.8	8.1	293.0	7.2	1230.0	303.00	0.52	0.32	4.50	0	3 Medium
Pooris (10 g oil absorbed)	375	9.2	12.1	57.4	4.0	28.0	3.0	42.0	11.00	0.24	0.10	2.70	0	3 Medium
Daal Stuffed Pooris	427	12.8	12.3	66.3	51.5	5.0	3.6	47.0	12.00	0.31	0.13	3.00	0	4 or 5
Palak Pooris	388	10.2	12.4	58.8	64.9	6.0	3.6	2832.0	708.00	0.26	0.23	2.9	14	4 or 5

Contd...

	Calories (Kcal)	Proteins (g)	Fats (g)	Carbo-hydrates (g)	Fibre (g)	Calcium (mg)	Iron (mg)	Caro-tene (mcg)	Retinol (mcg)	Vit B₁ (mg)	Vit B₂ (mg)	Niacin (mg)	Vit C (mg)	Serving Portion
Besan Pooris	380	11.2	13.0	54.6	5.5	35.0	3.6	62.0	16.00	0.32	0.12	2.7	0	4 or 5
Pea Pooris	431	13.6	12.1	66.9	5.0	40.0	3.9	91.0	23.00	0.39	0.10	3.2	5	4 or 5
Pea Kachori (10 g oil absorbed)	215	6.9	7.4	30.2	1.8	17.0	1.6	49.0	13.00	0.16	0.03	1.1	5	2
Khasta Kachori (10 g oil absorbed)	441	11.4	18.9	56.3	3.2	45.0	2.4	163.0	41.00	0.16	0.8	1.8	0	2
Naan	200	6.7	2.1	38.5	1.5	60.0	1.4	31.0	9.00	0.19	0.10	1.2	1	1
Bhatura	176	5.6	3.8	29.9	1.2	28.0	1.2	51.0	27.00	0.06	0.07	0.1	0	2 or 3
Boiled Rice	277	6.0	0.8	61.4	3.6	8.00	2.6	2.0	0.40	0.17	0.13	3.1	0	1 Full plate
Curd Rice	484	15.1	12.5	77.8	5.3	253.00	3.8	66.0	26.00	0.33	0.41	3.7	2	1 Full plate
Zeera Pulao	400	8.2	10.5	68.1	4.4	25.00	2.9	78.0	45.00	0.22	0.18	3.5	6	1 Full plate
Mixed Vegetable Pulao	523	17.6	9.0	92.9	7.2	71.0	5.2	126.0	32.00	0.60	0.15	4.6	21	1 Full plate
Pea Pulao	510	12.1	9.1	94.8	8.1	108.0	4.6	1033.0	258.00	0.44	0.17	4.8	28	1 Full plate
Channa Daal & Vegetable Pulao	529	15.1	10.1	94.3	8.5	102.0	5.3	1014.0	254.00	0.47	0.19	4.6	14	1 Full plate
Black Channa Pulao	464	10.9	10.2	82.1	7.5	82.00	4.0	49.0	11.00	0.28	0.17	4.1	6	1 Full plate
Mushroom Pulao	411	9.7	9.7	71.2	4.3	38.00	4.4	2.0	0.40	0.31	0.55	8.1	9	1 Full plate
Paneer Pulao	520	13.3	20.4	70.9	4.3	272.0	4.9	2.0	0.40	0.21	0.13	3.3	6	1 Full plate
Mutton Pulao	622	22.6	28.5	68.7	4.3	216.0	5.1	13.0	12.00	0.37	0.29	8.8	6	1 Full plate
Chicken Pulao	661	27.9	30.5	68.7	4.3	110.0	4.6	88.0	90.00	0.33	0.34	11.4	6	1 Full plate

Contd...

Contd...

	Calories (Kcal)	Proteins (g)	Fats (g)	Carbo-hydrates (g)	Fibre (g)	Calcium (mg)	Iron (mg)	Caro-tene (mcg)	Retinol (mcg)	Vit B₁ (mg)	Vit B₂ (mg)	Niacin (mg)	Vit C (mg)	Serving Portion
Idli	157	6.7	0.5	31.5	2.5	33.00	1.6	8.00	2.00	0.14	0.08	1.4	0	3 or 4
Plain Dosa	261	7.1	4.6	47.8	3.2	28.00	1.6	166.0	41.00	0.17	0.08	2.2	0	2
Masala Dosa	208	3.0	4.2	39.5	4.5	39.00	1.1	36.0	9.00	0.19	0.02	2.0	31	1
Mixed Vegetable Dosa	184	4.8	4.4	31.2	4.2	79.00	1.8	624.0	156.00	0.20	0.10	1.8	43	1
Paneer Filling	130	3.8	8.8	8.9	1.3	144.0	0.6	176.0	44.00	0.10	0.00	0.4	19	1
Uttapam	316	7.8	8.7	51.6	3.9	55.0	2.1	465.0	116.00	0.20	0.10	2.5	23	2
Beans and Macaroni	352	12.1	16.8	38.0	3.7	243.0	2.2	673.0	242.00	0.20	0.20	1.5	40	1 Plate
Spaghetti Bolognese	346	14.6	14.9	38.3	33.0	174.0	3.2	867.0	236.00	0.28	0.21	4.8	30	1 Shallow dish
Chicken Chowmein	542	31.4	24.2	49.6	3.9	104.0	5.6	9.8	333.00	0.39	0.36	8.1	59	1 Shallow dish
PULSES														
Dal Moong	104	7.3	0.4	17.9	2.6	23.0	1.2	15.0	4.00	0.14	0.06	0.7	0	1 Curry Bowl
Cumin Seed Baghar	47	0.0	5.0	0.5	0.0	0.0	0.0	100.0	25.00	0.00	0.00	0.0	0	Contd...
Onion Tomato Baghar	59	0.4	5.1	2.8	0.5	17.0	0.2	153.0	38.00	0.03	0.01	0.1	6	
Mustard Seed Baghar	45	0.0	5.0	0.0	0.0	0.0	0.0	100.0	25.00	0.00	0.00	0.0	0	
Urad Sp.	94	7.9	5.5	3.3	3.1	78.0	1.5	82.0	21.00	0.19	0.08	0.9	11	1 Curry Bowl

Contd...

Contd...

	Calories (Kcal)	Proteins (g)	Fats (g)	Carbo-hydrates (g)	Fibre (g)	Calcium (mg)	Iron (mg)	Caro-tene (mcg)	Retinol (mcg)	Vit B₁ (mg)	Vit B₂ (mg)	Niacin (mg)	Vit C (mg)	Serving Portion
Dehusked Dry Arhar Daal with Spinach	159	7.7	5.9	18.7	4.4	58.0	1.4	2830.0	707.00	0.50	0.19	1.1	14	1 Curry Bowl
Channa Daal with Ghia	117	6.3	1.7	19.1	3.4	27.0	1.8	39.0	10.00	0.16	0.06	0.8	0	1 Curry Bowl
Sambar	119	5.6	2.5	18.4	3.2	45.0	1.7	88.0	22.00	0.13	0.08	0.9	19	1 Curry Bowl
Green Gram Whole	100	7.2	0.4	17.0	1.2	37.0	1.3	28.0	7.00	0.14	0.08	0.6	0	1 Bowl
Dry Khatta Channa	232	6.0	11.7	25.6	4.8	83.0	1.9	369.0	91.00	0.16	0.07	1.3	14	1 Bowl
Rajma Curry	268	10.5	11.0	31.8	3.7	162.0	2.6	193.0	49.00	0.29	0.12	1.2	20	1 Bowl
Lobia Curry	259	10.9	10.9	29.3	2.8	89.0	4.1	182.0	46.00	0.31	0.12	0.9	19	1 Bowl
Besan Gatte Curry	497	21.3	30.6	34.0	5.5	255.0	2.9	367.0	96.00	0.34	0.22	1.4	14	1 Bowl
Besan Kadhi with Pakoris	408	9.9	30.2	24.1	3.7	140.0	2.2	73.0	23.00	0.21	0.19	1.0	1	1 Bowl
MEATS														
Keema Matar	411	26.9	23.7	22.6	2.8	215.0	4.9	298.0	84.00	0.53	0.19	8.0	29	1 Bowl
Roganjosh	404	25.0	30.6	7.2	0.8	276.0	4.0	114.0	45.00	0.31	0.27	8.0	12	1 Bowl
Mutton Korma	439	24.0	34.7	7.7	0.8	259.0	3.7	149.0	54	0.30	0.22	8.50	6.0	1 Bowl
Palak Meat	374	19.1	28.4	10.6	5.2	290.0	3.8	5600.0	1410	0.24	0.46	620	34.0	1 Bowl
Shahi Keema Kofta Curry	508	23.8	41.3	10.2	1.5	238.0	4.3	217.0	65	0.34	0.21	8.70	23.0	1 Bowl

Contd...

Contd...

Contd...

	Calories (Kcal)	Proteins (g)	Fats (g)	Carbohydrates (g)	Fibre (g)	Calcium (mg)	Iron (mg)	Carotene (mcg)	Retinol (mcg)	Vit B₁ (mg)	Vit B₂ (mg)	Niacin (mg)	Vit C (mg)	Serving Portion
Boti Kabab	365	23.6	27.8	5.0	0.5	232.0	3.6	8.0	19	0.24	0.22	8.30	9.0	1 Bowl
Shammi Kabab	435	25.0	25.8	25.8	3.6	180.0	3.4	890.0	58.00	0.29	0.21	7.4	3.7	1 Bowl
Shepherd's Pie	486	23.8	34.5	20.0	2.2	206.0	3.5	339.0	98.00	0.31	0.18	9.2	15	1 Bowl
Roast Chicken	297	25.3	21.8	0.0	0.0	18.0	2.0	334.0	166.0	0.13	0.20	10.0	0	1 Bowl
Chilli Chicken	464	27.3	35.5	8.8	1.9	46.0	3.1	222.0	135.0	0.35	0.31	10.9	50	1 Bowl
Chicken Sweet and Sour	420	27.0	33.3	3.1	0.8	39.0	2.7	270.0	181.0	0.28	0.35	10.6	30	1 Bowl
Chicken Korma	493	28.1	36.4	13.2	2.1	188.0	3.2	94.0	127.0	0.23	0.32	10.2	11	1 Bowl
Bengal Fish Curry	296	18.4	17.5	16.3	1.6	731.0	1.7	22.4	7.00	0.14	0.11	1.1	35	1 Bowl
Tandoori Fish	174	25.7	6.8	2.4	0.0	7.0	3.1	10.0	11.00	0.01	0.02	0.0	0	1 Bowl
Fried Fish with Chips	443	26.3	26.2	25.4	2.3	307.0	3.3	165.0	94.00	0.09	0.11	0.9	9	1 Bowl
Fish in Coconut Milk	371	27.0	17.1	27.2	3.2	150.0	3.2	4.0	1.00	0.06	0.03	0.5	7	1 Bowl
Prawn Curry	342	30.1	19.9	10.5	2.7	509.0	9.3	3.0	0.80	0.05	0.18	7.5	4	1 Bowl
Crispy Baked Fish	390	32.3	15.1	31.2	4.1	461.0	4.1	496.0	153.00	0.13	0.13	1.3	16	1 Bowl
VEGETABLES AND PANEER														
Nutri Nugget Sweet and Sour	252	12.8	18.3	9.1	8.0	22.0	1.0	180.0	79.00	0.16	0.16	1.0	30	1 Bowl
Nutri Nugget Korma	347	14.2	23.4	20.0	2.1	217.0	1.4	28.0	12.00	0.11	0.13	0.6	11	1 Bowl

Contd...

	Calories (Kcal)	Proteins (g)	Fats (g)	Carbo-hydrates (g)	Fibre (g)	Calcium (mg)	Iron (mg)	Caro-tene (mcg)	Retinol (mcg)	Vit B_1 (mg)	Vit B_2 (mg)	Niacin (mg)	Vit C (mg)	Serving Portion
Mashroom Matar	239	10.3	10.8	25.2	2.8	68.5	3.3	298.0	75.00	0.41	0.30	4.1	31	1 Bowl
Nutri Nugget Matar	283	18.4	10.5	28.6	2.8	68.5	2.4	298.0	75.00	0.35	0.05	1.0	29	1 Bowl
Palak Mushroom	161	5.2	10.6	11.3	7.7	149.0	2.9	708.0	2177.00	0.17	0.59	3.0	60	1 Bowl
Vegetable Nargisi Kofta	394	17.1	33.1	6.8	6.7	188.0	2.0	146.0	103.0	0.30	0.06	2.6	43	1 Bowl
Paneer Makhani Curry	659	9.5	61.3	17.4	3.0	305.0	2.9	2046.0	580.0	0.36	0.19	1.3	64	1 Bowl
Pea Potato Curry	267	8.9	10.3	34.6	4.1	62.8	2.2	165.0	41.00	0.37	0.03	1.7	30	1 Bowl
Pea Paneer Curry	351	17.3	20.8	23.6	2.8	162.0	2.0	153.0	94.00	0.36	0.04	1.1	23	1 Bowl
Pea Curry	311	15.3	10.3	39.2	4.5	78.0	3.5	236.0	60.00	0.60	0.04	2.0	30	1 Bowl
Pea/Cholia Vadi Curry	309	11.7	15.3	31.0	3.7	68.0	2.8	195.0	49.00	0.50	0.03	1.5	26	1 Bowl
Potato Curry	221	2.5	10.2	29.9	3.6	47.7	1.0	94.0	23.60	0.17	0.03	1.5	29	1 Bowl
Egg Curry	314	15.5	17.6	23.3	2.8	85.0	2.8	483.0	237.00	0.38	0.25	1.2	21	1 Bowl
Dahi Aloo	260	4.2	12.2	33.4	3.9	119.0	1.0	169.0	58.00	0.22	0.12	1.8	35	1 Bowl
Dum Aloo	291	2.1	21.1	23.2	2.5	41.5	0.5	29.0	8.00	0.11	0.03	1.2	17	1 Bowl
Ghia Kofta Curry	273	3.6	20.9	17.5	2.9	70.0	1.9	122.0	31.00	0.17	0.05	0.9	15	1 Bowl
Potato Kofta Curry	290	2.9	15.3	35.1	4.1	51.0	1.3	101.0	25.00	0.19	0.03	1.80	33	1 Bowl

Contd...

Contd...

	Calories (Kcal)	Proteins (g)	Fats (g)	Carbo-hydrates (g)	Fibre (g)	Calcium (mg)	Iron (mg)	Caro-tene (mcg)	Retinol (mcg)	Vit B_1 (mg)	Vit B_2 (mg)	Niacin (mg)	Vit C (mg)	Serving Portion
Cabbage Kofta Curry	297	5.9	21.0	21.0	4.0	85.0	2.1	210.0	52.00	0.20	0.14	1.1	136	1 Bowl
Paneer Kofta Curry	383	11.2	30.7	15.5	1.5	149.0	0.9	74.0	74.00	0.13	0.04	0.6	15	1 Bowl
Aloo Methi	221	5.8	11.0	24.7	4.1	404.0	2.5	2361.0	590.00	0.12	0.32	1.8	66	1 Bowl
Gajar Methi	180	5.2	11.0	15.0	3.5	460.0	2.8	3854.0	963.00	0.08	0.33	1.3	55	1 Bowl
Sarson Ka Saag	157	8.5	6.7	15.7	3.2	200.0	25.0	6734.0	1682.00	0.22	0.14	0.5	66	1 Bowl
Palak Paneer	240	11.2	17.5	9.4	7.7	228.0	2.1	8545.0	2180.00	0.16	0.43	1.1	59	1 Bowl
Palak Aloo	230	5.1	11.3	27.0	9.7	153.0	2.5	8564.0	2141.00	0.20	0.40	2.0	72	1 Bowl
Mooli Bhujia	144	4.6	10.6	7.6	2.3	294.0	0.8	5300.0	2.00	0.23	0.49	1.2	91	1 Bowl
Bathua Bhujia	152	6.0	10.7	7.8	0.3	236.0	6.8	2614.0	1.00	0.04	0.22	1.0	55	1 Bowl
Peas and Cabbage Subzi	122	5.5	5.2	13.2	2.2	50.0	1.7	164.0	41.00	0.19	0.10	0.8	129	1 Bowl
Dry Arbi (Fried)	254	3.6	15.2	25.6	1.6	62.0	0.9	79.0	14.00	0.14	0.04	0.6	8	1 Bowl
Masala Arbi	187	3.0	10.1	21.1	1.0	40.0	0.4	24.0	0.00	0.09	0.03	0.4	0	1 Bowl
Bingan Bhartha	192	2.8	15.5	10.4	4.5	55.0	0.9	216.0	54.00	0.12	0.19	1.6	29	1 Small Bowl
Stuffed Tomatoes	233	6.0	15.6	17.1	2.8	138.0	1.5	829.0	228.00	0.27	0.08	1.1	41	2 Tomatoes
Bhindi Subzi	189	2.6	15.0	11.0	6.3	93.0	0.7	62.0	16.00	0.11	0.12	0.8	19	1 Bowl
Stuffed Bhindi	132	2.3	10.2	7.7	5.9	79.0	0.5	62.0	16.00	0.08	0.12	0.7	16	1 Bowl
Stuffed Karela (Wet)	225	1.9	20.2	8.9	2.6	39.0	1.0	101.0	25.00	0.10	0.08	0.6	76	1 Bowl
Stuffed Karela (Dry)	156	1.3	15.2	3.4	1.8	16.0	0.5	100.0	25.00	0.06	0.07	0.4	70	3 Pcs
Kathal (Dry)	300	2.2	20.3	27.0	7.1	89.5	1.3	201.0	51.00	0.15	0.02	1.1	12	1 Bowl

Contd...

Contd...

	Calories (Kcal)	Proteins (g)	Fats (g)	Carbo-hydrates (g)	Fibre (g)	Calcium (mg)	Iron (mg)	Caro-tene (mcg)	Retinol (mcg)	Vit B$_1$ (mg)	Vit B$_2$ (mg)	Niacin (mg)	Vit C (mg)	Serving Portion
Cauliflower, Peas and Potato Subzi	196	5.1	10.3	20.7	2.9	49.0	1.6	143.0	36.00	0.21	0.07	1.4	42	1 Bowl
Stuffed Ghia	456	21.3	31.8	21.1	2.5	323.0	2.9	632.0	304.00	0.22	0.34	4.1	3	1/2 Marrow
Rost Potatoes	191	2.4	5.0	34.0	3.8	15.0	0.8	228.0	57.00	0.15	0.01	1.8	26	1-2 Potatoes
Stuffed Baked Potato	334	7.1	18.8	34.0	3.8	33.0	1.3	698.0	248.00	0.19	0.16	1.8	26	1-2 Potatoes
Creamed Spinach	429	21.4	29.8	18.8	9.3	458.0	3.5	11812.0	3195.00	0.25	1.00	1.4	58	1 Small Bowl
Creamed Spinach and Mushrooms	363	13.4	25.8	19.2	7.1	366.0	2.9	8692.0	2284.00	0.23	0.90	3.5	45	1 Bowl
SALADS														
Russian Salad	959	19.7	85.6	27.5	3.3	100.0	3.8	879.0	333.00	0.38	0.33	5.4	39	1 Small Bowl
Beetroot and Egg Salad	366	8.9	30.8	13.4	3.6	62.0	2.1	300.0	180.00	0.12	0.29	0.6	15	1 Small Bowl
Tossed Green Salad	153	1.5	12.2	9.2	2.0	50.0	0.9	225.0	57.00	0.18	0.04	0.5	43	1 Small Bowl
Cucumber and Yogurt Salad	29	1.3	1.3	2.9	1.0	53.0	0.5	10.0	4.00	0.04	0.05	0.2	6	1 Small Bowl
French Dressing	722	0.0	80.0	0.4	0.0	1.0	0.0	0.0	0.00	0.00	0.00	0.01	1	3/4 Cup
Mayonnaise	1220	7.1	131.8	1.3	0.0	56.0	1.4	380.0	229.00	0.08	0.26	0.0	4	1 Cup
Mayonnaise without Eggs	886	7.7	90.1	11.0	0.0	288.0	0.5	139.0	36.00	1.20	0.46	0.3	6	1 Cup

Contd...

Contd...

	Calories (Kcal)	Proteins (g)	Fats (g)	Carbo-hydrates (g)	Fibre (g)	Calcium (mg)	Iron (mg)	Caro-tene (mcg)	Retinol (mcg)	Vit B$_1$ (mg)	Vit B$_2$ (mg)	Niacin (mg)	Vit C (mg)	Serving Portion
RAITAS														
Tomato Onion Raita	79	3.7	4.1	6.7	0.6	173.0	0.5	120.0	36.00	0.10	0.18	0.3	11	1 Bowl
Cucumber Raita	68	3.3	4.1	4.5	0.8	155.0	0.6	32.0	14.00	0.07	0.16	0.2	5	1 Bowl
Carrot Raita	85	3.6	4.1	8.3	0.9	189.0	0.7	977.0	250.00	0.07	0.17	0.4	3	1 Bowl
Ghia Raita	67	3.2	4.1	4.3	0.3	159.0	0.4	32.0	14.00	0.06	0.17	0.2	1	1 Bowl
Potato Raita	110	3.9	4.1	14.3	1.3	154.0	0.5	44.0	17.00	0.10	0.17	0.7	10	1 Bowl
Spinach Raita	143	7.7	8.7	8.5	4.9	231.0	1.6	5616.0	1410.00	0.17	0.43	2.6	29	1 Bowl
Bathua Raita	147	9.3	8.4	8.5	0.4	308.0	4.7	1776.0	15.00	0.15	0.31	2.7	36	1 Bowl
Sprouted Green Gram Raita	105	5.8	4.1	11.2	1.2	166.0	0.7	37.0	15.00	0.11	0.18	0.4	3	1 Bowl
Boondi Raita	224	7.3	15.0	15.0	2.1	160.0	1.3	58.0	21.00	0.15	0.20	0.6	1	1 Bowl
Pineapple Raita	84	3.3	4.1	8.4	0.0	159.0	1.4	41.0	16.00	0.15	0.22	0.2	21	1 Bowl
Banana Raita	118	3.7	4.1	16.6	0.4	158.0	0.4	71.0	24.00	0.08	0.20	0.4	5	1 Bowl
Mango Raita	97	3.4	4.2	11.5	0.5	156.0	0.9	1404.0	357.00	0.09	0.20	0.6	9	1 Bowl
Grape Raita	91	3.4	4.2	10.0	1.4	159.0	0.5	33.0	14.00	0.06	0.17	0.2	2	1 Bowl
DESSERTS														
Rice Kheer	257	7.2	8.3	38.3	0.4	241.0	0.7	12.0	104.00	0.12	0.40	0.6	4	1 Bowl
Sevian Kheer	271	7.9	9.2	39.2	1.2	273.0	0.6	12.0	111.00	0.12	0.40	0.4	4	1 Bowl
Carrot Kheer	218	6.9	8.3	29.0	0.9	280.0	0.9	957.0	340.00	0.12	0.38	0.5	6	1 Bowl
Apple Kheer	244	6.5	8.5	35.4	0.6	245.0	0.8	12.0	104.00	0.10	0.38	0.2	5	1 Bowl
Phirni	258	7.1	8.3	38.8	0.4	241.0	0.5	12.0	104.00	0.11	0.39	0.4	4	1 Bowl
Carrot Halva	472	8.3	24.5	54.5	2.7	443.0	1.6	3137.0	844.00	0.14	0.30	1.0	7	1 Small Bowl

Contd...

variable duration. Distended arteries are extremely tender on palpation. Headache, scalp hyperalgesias and painful mastication are present. It is a type of immunologic vasculitis and is a self limiting disease of many days.

Temporal lobe tumor produces expressive aphasia and impaired performance of hearing. Auditory illusions, hallucination psychomotor seizure or visual hallucination develop.

joint and pain during chewing and swallowing.

Temporomandibular dysfunction involves both muscle and joint derangements. Physical therapy and relaxation techniques are beneficial. Intraoral splints provide relief.

Temporomandibular joint (TMJ) is a synovial joint where temporo (temporal bone), mandibular (lower jaw) is the connecting hinge between the lower jaw and base of the skull.

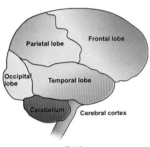

Brain

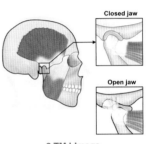

2.TMJ-Image

Temporary bridges are those intermitent restorations that are necessary between visits to prevent pain and space closure.

Temporary fillings are a first aid measure to relieve pain. Zinc oxide, Zinc phosphate and gutta percha are used. These are soft and soluble and will not remain for long hence are not to be used for permanent filling.

Temporomandibular disorder is a deviation from normal function which includes restricted movement of mandible, 2 mm deviation of mandible on opening, pain on palpation of masticatory muscles. There may be sound in temporomandibular

Temporomandibular joint arthritis occurs during periods of severe psychic stress, clenching and bruxism may become exaggerated and lead to severe mandibular joint and muscle pain. Marital problems, menopause and fatigue all may result the condition. X-ray may show evidence of bone resorption or irregularity of head of condyle or anterior slope of glenoid fossa.

TENS stands for Transcutaneous electrical nerve stimulation which has been used in the treatment of phantom limb pain; peripheral nerve injury joint pain, etc. Electrical stimulus is typically generated from a portable battery operated device. Mode of action is not very well understood. It blocks pain signals carried over to small unmyelinated 'C' fibres.

Tension headache is bilateral and diffuse. It is felt as a sense of tightness, pressure in head and band like constriction. Onset is gradual and may persist for a few days. During worry and anxiety headache is worst. These responses best to anxiolytics and antidepressants.

Teratogenesis is the development of organic defects due to certain drug used in pregnancy.

Teratoma is the neoplasm composed of multiple tissues including those which are normally not found in the organ in which it arises. It is a heterotopic collection of various forms. Benign tumors are cystic lesions. Walls of lesion are thickened. These contain hair, sebaceous material and teeth. Teeth are uncommon in malignant form of teratoma. Teeth resemble bicuspid.

Tertian fever refers to the type of fever that comes on alternate day.

Tertiary health care offers super specialized care. It is proved by regional and central level of institutions.

Tertiary prevention is a post pathogenic prevention. It includes techniques designed to replace lost tissues and rehabilitate a normal like function. It is done to prevent any further damage and maintain homeostasis.

Tertiary syphilis develops after 5-10 years of primary lesion affecting every organ of the body. It mainly affects CNS and CVS. Typical lesion is 'gumma'. It is a localized chronic granulomatous lesion having either nodular or ulcerated surface. Ulcer is a punched out ulcer having vertical walls. Base is dull, red granulomatous with irregular outline. Skin lesions leave tissue paper like scars.

Tertiary syphilitic oral ulcer is a very rarely seen after the invent of penicillin. It is known as gumma, a destructive granulomatous process. It is painless. Usually palate, tongue and tonsils are affected. Shape is round with punched out areas. Floor is depressed with a pale appearance. Edges are punched out.

Testes are located in scrotum. Testosterone is a steroid secreted on the stimulation of luteinizing hormone. It helps in maturation of sperm and is responsible for

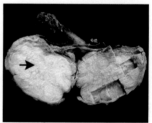

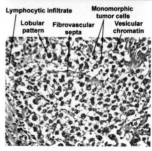

Lymphocytic infiltrate   Monomorphic tumor cells

Lobular pattern   Fibrovascular septa   Vesicular chromatin

Seminoma testis

sex characteristics. It helps in growth and development of male reproductive organs, musculo-skeletal growth, growth and distribution of hair and enlargement of larynx accompanied by voice changes.

Tetanus is a disease that is caused by a gram positive, actively motile, anerobic spore bearing rod called clostridium tetani. It is found in soil and horse dung. Organism may enter through injury. Clinical features develop within 14 days. Symptoms appear once toxins fix to cell bodies of motor nerves. Incubation period is 5 to 15 weeks. Short duration indicates of serious disease. Titanic spasm follows within 24-72 hours of lock jaw. Diagnosis is clinical and does not require clinical confirmation. Convulsion becomes less frequent after 10 days and survivors recover completely by 4 weeks. There develops pain and stiffness in jaws and neck muscle. It results in dysphagia. After stimuli reflex spasm develops. Cranial tetanus paralyses 7th nerve.

Tetany is a condition that occurs due to low extracellular calcium condition developing with marked muscle cramps, twitching and convulsions.

Tetracycline is a broad spectrum antibiotic drug which forms complex with calcium and deposit on tooth. Tetracycline has a wider range of activity. Spectrum includes most species of gram positive and gram negative bacteria and spirochetes. These are absorbed slowly from GIT. Larger the dose, less of proportion is absorbed. Peak levels in blood occur after 3 hours hence 6 hour interval between two doses is sufficient. All tetracyclines are chelating agents. In fetus or growing child permanent staining of teeth may occur. The degree and color of staining varies with different tetracycline in different doses. Retardation of fetal growth is noted down when given during pregnancy.

Tetracycline pigmentation fluoresces bright yellow under ultraviolet light. Tetracycline can cross the placenta to stain the developing teeth and fetus. It is deposited along the incremental lines of dentine. Long treatment produces broader band of stain and deeper discoloration. Stain is permanent and incisors become ugly.

Tetracycline stains are endogenous stains that occured due to the use of tetracycline drug at the time of prenatal or postnatal dental development. The drug was widely used once upon a time to fight variety of infections. At that point little was known about the side effects of the drug. The antibiotic has an affinity towards the mineralized tissue and gets absorbed by the hard tissues of the body. Since the drug also has a capability to pass across the placenta and enters the fetal circulation, so when the expecting mother is administered this drug during the third trimester, the drug gets deposited in the forming bones and teeth of the fetus. Discoloration can also occur when the drug is administered to the child in infancy and early childhood.

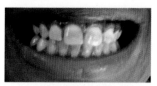
Tetracycline stains

Thalamic pain can occur due to spinal cord lesions that affects spinothalamic tracts resulting in painful limbs. Similarly a lesion of thalamus itself may cause severe pain in the contralateral face and arm/leg. Thalamic pain is intense, burning and continuous. It is felt around angle of mouth and cheek.

Thalassemia is a group of chronic hemolytic anemia. The disease is inherited as autosomal dominant trait. It produces thin, fragile erythrocytes. In this condition, there is insufficient synthesis of alpha and beta chains of hemoglobin. It is detected in first two years of life. There may be jaundice, fever with chills. Marked anemia is of microchronic microcytic type. WBC count is high with malaise. Bone marrow shows cellular hyperplasia with large number of immature primitive and stem form of red cells. Spleen is enlarged. Mongoloid face is due to prominence of premaxilla. Death often occurs during puberty. Oral manifestations include spacing of anterior maxillary teeth. Pallor of oral mucosa, bimaxillary protrusion and Prominent molar bones with delayed pneumatization of sinuses develop discoloration of teeth is due to iron. Skull bones will show "hair on end"

appearance. Jaw bones may show "salt and pepper effect".

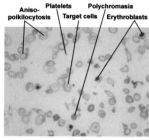
Thalassemia

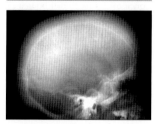
Sun ray appearance

Thelarche is faster breast development in absence of additional signs of sexual maturation. Exact cause is not known.

Theory is a paper about relationship specially defined concepts that describe, explain or predict some phenomenon in professional discipline/action.

Therapeutic Inhalation Menthol and eucalyptus form an aromatic inhalation and this when mixed with hot water gives rise to vapors. These when inhaled sooths the inflamed mucous membrane. Steam serves the purpose of humidifying the dry mucosal secretions and facilitate their removal.

Therapeutic occlusion is said to be present where the specific interventions are designed to treat the disease.

Therapy refers to the treatment of a disease.

Thermal conductivity is a measure of speed at which heat travels per second through a given thickness of 1 cm when one side of material is maintained at a constant temperature i.e. 1° C higher than the other side. Thermal conductivity depends on the distance heat travels, area through which heat travels and the difference of temperature between source and destination.

Thermal diffusivity is a measure of heat transfer of a material in the time dependant state.

Thermogenic is a process that creates heat.

Thermometer is the device used to measure temperature.

Thermoplastic is the property of softening on heating and hardening on cooling.

Thermoset is a polymer which is not able to undergo softening upon heating.

Thiamine (Vitamin B$_1$) was the first of the Vitamin B complex discovered. Thiamine B$_1$ vitamin is water soluble and is destroyed by refining, exposure to alkalies such as baking powder. Up to 50% is lost in cooking water and 15% during baking. Toasting of bread destroys further 15% for thick slice or up to 30% for thin slice. Recommended daily intake is 0.4 mg/ 1000 Kcal or about 1.2 mg in adult man. Limited amount is synthesized by microorganisms in GIT. Normally, about 25-35 mg is stored in the body. Deficiency of it leads to accumulation of pyruvic and lactic acid in tissues and body fluids. Severe deficiency may lead to neurological and mental deficiency.

Thiazides are derivatives of sulphonamides and are used as weaker diuretics. These exert their diuretic effect by inhibiting the Na$^+$ CL$^-$ transport in early distal convoluted tubules. These cause increased loss of K$^+$ and Mg but reduce calcium excretion. These are indicated in hypertension, mild heart failure, and idiopathic hypercalciuria.

Thiopentone has largely been superseded in outpatient dental practice by short acting methohexitone. Thiopentone is freshly prepared to produce 2.5% solution by dissolving powder in sterile distilled water. Dose is 4 to 7 mg/kg body weight. It is a powerful myocardial depressant.

Third branchial arch Branchial arches are formed in the pharangeal wall due to the prolyeratring ateral plate mesoderm and migrating neural crest cell. The arches are clearly seen as bulges on the lateral aspect of the embryo and are externally separated by small cleft called branhial grooves and internally small depression called pharyngeal pouches. The cartilage of this small arch produces the greater horn and caudal part of the body of the hyoid bone. The remainder of the cartilage disappears. The mesoderm forms the stylopharyngeal muscle, inerveted by the IXth nerve glossopharyngeal supplying the arch. The mucosa of the posterior third of the tongue is derived from this arch, which accounts for its sensory innervations by the glossopharyngeal nerve. The artery of this arch contributes to the common carotid and part of the internal carotid arteries. Neural crest tissue in the third arch forms the carotid body which first appears as a mesenchymal condensation around the third aortic arch artery. This chemoreceptor body thus derives its nerve supply from the glossopharyngeal nerve.

Third degree burns is involving entire epidermis and dermis and all dermal appendages so there is no spontaneous healing of the wound, leaving an ulcer. Since the entire thickness of skin is burned with no tissue left for repair and regeneration, these will require skin grafting or will close by contractures wherein two raw surfaces fuse together.

Third molar see wisdom tooth.

Third pharyngeal pouch the ventral diverticulum endoderm proliferates and migrates from each side to form two elongated diverticulum that grow caudally into the surrounding mesenchyme to form the elements of thymus gland. The two thymic rudiments meet in the midline but do not fuse, being united by connective tissue. Lymphoid cells invade the thymus from hemopoietic tissue during the 3rd month of IU. The dorsal diverticulum endoderm differentiates and migrates caudally to form inferior parathyroid gland. The gland derived from the endodermal lining of the pouch loses their connection with the pharyngeal wall when the

pouches become obliterated during later development. The lateral glosso-epiglotic fold represents the third pharyngeal pouch.

Three – quarter crowns actually covers four – fifths of the tooth surface – mesial, distal, occlusal, lingual or palatal. They are always made up of cast metal and are used when the buccal surface of the tooth is intact. The advantage of these types of crowns is that they are more conservative of tooth tissue than complete crowns and the margin does not approach gingival margin buccally.

Thromboangitis obliterans is an inflammatory occlusive peripheral vascular disease of unknown etiology affecting arteries and veins especially of lower limbs. Smoking is the risk factor. Small and medium sized arteries are more involved. There is proliferation of intima and thrombosis. There develops digital ulceration or pain from ischemia. Arteriography and biopsy are confirmatory.

Thrombocythemia is an increased number megakaryocytes resulting in a raised level of circulating platelets that is mostly dysfunctional. Etiology is not known. Epistaxia and intestinal bleeding exists. Hemorrhage into skin is found. There may be spontaneous gingival bleeding. After dental extraction also excessive bleeding takes place. Radioactive phosphorus and blood transfusion helps.

Thrombocytopenia is very low quantity of platelets in circulatory system. These patients have tendency to bleed from small capillaries while in hemophilia bleeding is from larger vessels. As a result large punctate bleeding develops over skin. For bleeding count should fall below 50,000 per cu/mm. Level below 10,000 becomes lethal.

Thromboplastin – Substance is produced in blood. It plays a role in the coagulation process.

Throttling is a condition where the constriction is produced by pressure of fingers and palm. Finger marks may be found on either side of front of neck i.e. wind pipe. Marks are obliquely downwards and outwards one below the other.

Throwing power is a measure of the uniformity in plating thickness of irregular surface.

Thrush is known as psuedomembranous candidiasis. Actually it is a superficial infection of upper layers of mucosal epithelium. It forms a patchy white plaques or flecks on mucosal surface. Once you remove this area of erythema shallow ulceration is seen. Antifungal drugs are helpful. In infants lesions are soft, white or bluish. It is adherent to oral mucosa. Intraoral lesions are painless and being removed with difficulty. It leaves a raw bleeding surface. Any mucosal area of mouth may be involved. Constitutional symptoms are not present but in adults rapid onset of a bad taste may develop. Some may feel burning of mouth also. Causative organisms are yeast like fungus causing thrush. It occurs in both yeast and mycelia forms of oral cavity and infected tissue. Candida species are normal inhabitants of the oral flora. Concentration is 200-500 cells per ml of saliva. Carrier state is more in diabetics. The wearing of removal prosthetic appliances may also become asymptomatic carrier. Predisposing factors include – after administration of antibiotics, irritant dentures, long term consumption of cortisone, pregnancy, old age, AIDS and low immunity.

Thumb and digit sucking is defined as placement of the thumb or more fingers in varying depths into the mouth. Thumb and digit sucking is one of the commonest seen habit in children. Recent studies have shown that thumb sucking may be practiced even during intrauterine life. The presence of this habit until the age 31/2-4 years is considered normal. Persistence of the habit beyond this age can lead to various malocclusions.

Thymol is relatively a weak antiseptic. It is widely used as mouth washes. It has a good flavor.

Thymus is a primary lymphoid organ, bilobed structure located in the thorax anterior to the sternum. Histologically, each lobe contains lobules separated by connective tissue trabaculae. Each lobe is made up of an outer cortex with immature cells. Hassal Corpuscles in thymic medulla are containing degenerating suspected cells.

Thyroglossal tract cyst arises from remnants of thyroglossal duct and may develop anywhere along the embryonic thyroglossal tract between the foramen coecum of tongue and thyroid gland. It consists squamous and glandular epithelium. It generally develops in young person. It raises from a few mm to a few centimetres. It is asymptomatic and grows slowly. If large, it may cause dysphagia. Occasionally fistula may form.

Thyroid storm is a medical emergency. Fever may go up to 41° C with anxiety, tremor, weakness, heat intolerance, sweating and weight loss. Sinus tachycardia is always present. Atrial fibrillation develops. Reflexes become brisk.

Tic Doloreux where Tic is spasm and Dolor is the Latin word for pain. Because trigeminal neuralgia pain comes as electrical shock, each pain spasm is called tic doloreux.

Tics are a sudden rapid twitch like movement always of same nature and same type. These are generally common in childhood and disappear in adult life. All forms of tics can be suppressed clinically.

Tin oxide is a pure white powder that is used as a final polishing agent. Tine oxide is mixed with water alcohol or glycerine and is used as a paste. Finishing abrasives are coarse, hard particles and polishing abrasives are fine articles.

Tissue borne passive appliance are mostly located in the vestibule and have little or no contact with the dentition e.g. functional regulator or Frankel.

Tissue Health Index was developed by Sheiham A., Maizels J. and Maizels A., at the second alternative indices, which is a modification of the DMFT index. In the THI, selective weighting is given for Decayed, Filled and Sound teeth (i.e. '1' - Decayed, '2' - Filled and '4' - Sound).

Tissue repair is a process following inflammation white cells repair by filling the breach with a temporary repair called granulation tissue. New capillaries are formed, but repair cannot take place in presence of pus. Hence tooth requires extraction or root treatment to drain off pus.

Titanium is a material of choice because of its good biocompatibility, mechanical properties and in implantology, its proven ability to achieve osseointegration.

T-Lymphocytes precursor arise from bone marrow stem cell, the T-lymphocytes travel to the thymus where they mature. T-lymphocytes mediate cellular immunity and is important for defence against virus, fungi and bacteria. They play an important role in regulating immune system. Thymus is large in children and shrinks as an individual matures. Different types of T-cells have different functions. Some are memory cells. Some are T-helper cells increasing the function of B lymphocytes and increases the antibody response. Others are called T-suppress or cells decreasing the function of B lymphocytes. T-killer cells are active in vigilance against tumor or virally affected cells.

Tobacco chewer's white lesion develops where the tobacco is placed. Mucobuccal fold is the most common location. Epithelium gives a wrinkled appearance. There is a risk of malignancy with long exposure to tobacco.

Tobacco stains appear as light brown to dark brown or black. They may appear in various forms such as - Narrow crest following the gingival contour, Wide band extending from the cervical third to the middle third of the tooth and diffuse they are primarily present on the cervical third of the tooth but may involve any surface including pits and fissures and the lingual surface. These stains are generally formed from the smokeless tobacco and are mainly composed of tar and combustion products. The heavy deposits may penetrate the enamel and present as endogenous stains.

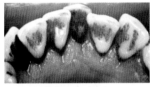

Tobacco stains

Tolerance occurs when the immune system is constantly exposed to self Ag (antigen) without inducing lymphocyte stimulation 'self tolerance'. It is a result of several mechanisms designed to distinguish between lymphocytes with potential to bind to self components and those with much higher binding specificity for antigenic determinants expressed by foreign Ag.

Tongue brushing is an act involving cleaning of tongue that should be combined with tooth brushing. Dorsum of the tongue is a primary source of infection. Tongue brushing can reduce the number of these organisms. It improves patient's taste perception also. Tongue should remain free of coating or debris. But tongue may not be scrubbed with tooth brush.

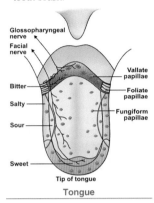

Tongue

Tongue papillae are the samll elevations present on dorsal surface of tongue. These are of variable size and represent different type of taste sensation. These can be classified into four types. (i) Filliform papillae – are numerous white hair like projection that covers the dorsal surface (ii) circumvallate papillae on tongue in a V formation on dorsal surface. It contains bitter taste buds. (iii) Foliate papillae are projection found on posterior lateral borders of tongue and consist of sour and acidic taste buds. (iv) Fungiform papillae among filliform papillae on the dorsal surface of tongue. These consists sweet, sour and salty buds.

Tongue thrust habit is defined as a condition in which the tongue makes contact with any teeth anterior to the molars during swallowing. Tongue thrust is a forward placement of the tongue between the anterior teeth and against the lower lip during swallowing (Schneider 1982) is an act of swallowing as the placement of the tongue tip forward between the incisors during swallowing (Profit 1990) or is an oral habit pattern related to the persistence of an infantile swallow pattern during childhood and adolescence and thereby produces an open bite and protrusion of the anterior tooth segments (Barber, 1975).

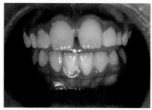

Tongue thrust

Tongue thrusting corrector appliance (Viazis, 1993) consists of a palatal wire that is inserted in the upper lingual molar sheaths, passes through the open-bite area, and carries over the lower incisors toward the labial vestibule, ending 1-2 mm above the labial surface. 'U'- shaped palatal loops are used to adjust the appliance in an anteroposterior or vertical direction with a three -prong plier. The TCA can also be expanded, like a palatal expansion appliance, to correct the posterior cross bites that often accompany open bites. It does not contact the teeth or the soft tissue. The TCA is designed to keep the

patient from inserting the thumb in the mouth, and it prevents tongue thrusting or abnormal tongue posturing during swallowing by blocking the tongue from the anterior teeth. This in turn helps close the open bite.

Tonic seizure there is a tonic contraction of muscle with altered consciousness but no clonic phase. These generally occur during NREM sleep with day drowsiness.

Tonsillitis is a common bacterial upper respiratory tract infection. Patients will complaint of sore throat with dysphagia. Child is not able to eat food. Pain and fever accompanies. There develops leucocytosis. Amoxicillin and analgesic anti-inflammatory drugs help.

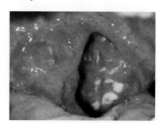

Tonsillitis-mononucleosis

Tooth ankylosis can be defined as fusion of tooth root to the underlying bone more often after an injury. Periapical inflammation is a well recognised cause of it by way of root absorption. If more of root surface is involved it may give a dull, muffed sound on percussion instead of normal sharp sound. It may be visible on radiograph there will be loss of normal thin radiolucent line with mild sclerosis of bone. There is no treatment. It serves well unless infected.

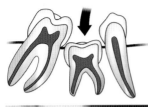

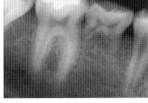

Submerged ankylosed teeth

Tooth banks are several banks to store tooth with different techniques such as chemical coagulation, vitrification, freeze drying and regular freezing.

Tooth borne active appliance includes modification of activator and bionator that include expansion screws or other active components like spring to provide intrinsic force to transverse or anteroposterior changes.

Tooth borne passive appliance are those appliances that have no intrinsic force generating components such as spring or screw. They depend on the soft tissues stretch and muscular activity to produce the desired treatment results. e.g. activator, bionator and herbst appliance.

Tooth brush filaments are the nylon filaments that are superior to natural bristles made of hog or boar hair. Nylon filaments flex 10 times more than breaking. These are more resistant to accumulation of bacteria and fungi. Soft nylon filaments are less traumatic to gingival tissues. Range of nylon filament diameter is 0.15 mm to 0.4 mm. Most bristles are 10 to 12 mm long. Thickness any from 0.007 to 0.12 mm are considered medium and 0.013 to 0.015 mm are classified as hard. End of the tooth brush filament can be cut bluntly or rounded. Round cut edges reduce gingival abrasion.

Tooth brushing is an act of cleaning done domestically after meals to removes plaque. Tooth brushes with a small head and multi tufted medium nylon bristles are most effective. Brushed in rinsed and pea size portion of fluoride tooth paste is added. Effective tooth brushing required time, knowledge and skill.

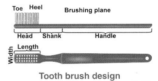

Tooth brush design

Tooth eruption is the process by which developing teeth emerge through the soft tissue of the jaws and the overlying mucosa to enter the oral cavity, contact the teeth of the opposing arch, and function in mastication (*see* Figure on page 454).

Tooth fracture is a common injury occuring due to trauma. It may occur at any age but children between the age of 2-3 yrs are most commonly affected. Minor chipping is common. Fracture has been classified in many ways. Prognosis depends whether pulp

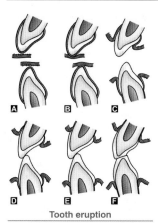

Tooth eruption

is involved, or crown/root is involved. If dentin over pulp is thin bacteria may penetrate producing pulpitis. Fractured crown is a more serious problem if the pulp is exposed.

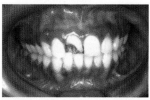

Ellis Class III dentoalvepoldar fracture

Tooth surface index of fluorosis (TSIF) is a index that was developed to measure the extent of fluorosis. TSIF was developed by Herschel S Horowitz, William S Driscoll, Rhea J Meyers, Stanley B Heifeta, and Albert Knigman in 1984. TSIF was developed in order to eliminate or reduce some of the short comings of 'Deans Index'. TSIF was applied in a survey to assess the prevalence of dental caries and dental fluorosis in communities having optimal and above optimal concentrations of naturally occurring fluoride in the drinking water.

Tooth wear is a mechanical process that occurs due to aging. It is an increasing problem in older adults due to long period of functioning. It has 3 causes abrasion, attrition and erosion. Reduction in lubricating effect of saliva may cause it.

Tooth zones are divided into imaginary third, named according to areas in which they are found. Root of tooth is divided into apical, middle and cervical third. Crown of the tooth is divided into cervico occlusal division, mesio distal division and buccolingual division.

Topical is application directly to an affected area for treatment.

Topical anesthesia is a medicament that eliminates sensation on surface tissues such as skin and mucosa. Oral mucosa can be anesthetized by wiping a topical anesthetic which will reduce the discomfort of dental injections, etc.

Topical fluoride is applied to the teeth but not ingested.

Topography is detailed description and analysis of features of an anatomic region.

Toronto automated probe is a diagnostic probe to measure clinical attachment levels. Here the sulcus is probed with the Ni-Ti wire that is extended under air pressure.

Torus mandibularis is an outgrowth of bone on the lingual surface of mandible opposite bicuspid tooth. These may be multiple and on both sides. It may be removed surgically.

Torus palatinus is slowly growing, flat base bone protuberance. It generally occurs in mid line of hard palate. Women are affected more. On trauma it becomes ulcerated. It never becomes malignant. It is not treated.

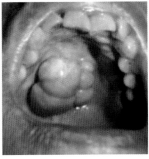

Toris palatinus

Toxic refer to Poisonous.

Toxic myocarditis occurs due to drugs that cause a direct toxic injury to the myocardial fibres. Response is cumulative and dose related. In this group drugs include arsenicals, catecholamines, lithium, cyclophosphamide emetine etc. Healing occurs by fibrosis.

Toxic shock syndrome is a multisystem illness caused by endotoxins produced by stains of staphylococcus aureus. Symptoms include fever, chills, diarrhea, dizziness, headache, myalgias and sore throat. Patient may develop hypotension with desquamation of skin.

Toxicology is the study of toxic and harmful effects of drugs and chemicals. It deals with the science of knowledge of sources, characters, properties and symptoms of poisons, their fatal effects, the lethal doses and remedies to be taken to counteract the effect.

Toxin is any poisonous substance of microbial, vegetable or animal origin that causes symptoms after a period of incubation. It can induce the elaboration of specific antitoxin in suitable animal.

Trabecular bone is similar to cortical bone but with spongy look. It is composed of rods and sheets of bone.

Tracheostomy is the term given to the surgical establishment of an opening in to the trachea. It is usually performed electively when the endotracheal intubation is likely to extend beyond 14 days. The opening is made in the anterior wall of trachea. It is done to have alternate pathway for breathing, improves alveolar ventilation, to give anesthesia.

Traction vertebral spurs projects horizontally and develops 1-2 mm above the vertebral edge. It is also known as Macnab spur. It is the small traction spur that is symptomatic.

Traditional alloy contain silver 66 to 72% by weight, tin 25-29%, copper 2 to 6%. Zinc 2% and mercury 3% by weight.

Tragus is the cartilaginous projection anterior to external opening of the ear.

Tramadol is an analgesic with both opioid as well as non opioid actions. It works like aspirin as well as like morphine. High doses of it should be avoided. It is used in the dose of 50-100 mg daily.

Tranquillizers are the drugs which decrease anxiety and tension without producing sedation.

Transient ischemic attack (TIA) also termed incipient stroke, transient cerebral ischemia is characterized by ischemic cerebral neurologic deficits that last for less than 24 hours. These attacks rarely last more than 8 hours and often resolve within 15-60 mins. Platelet, fibrin or other atherosclerotic embolic material from the neck or heart may lodge in a cerebral vessel and interfere transiently with blood flow causing the TIA.

Translocation is the change in position.

Translucency is the amount of incident light transmitted and scattered by that object. Translucency decreases with increasing scattered within materials. A high translucency gives a lighter color appearance. Translucency decreases with increasing scattering with in a material.

Translucent lesion are demonstrating translucent quality and are bullae or vesicle. Translucent pink lesions are due to accumulation of clear fluid such as serum, mucin or lymph. Blue translucent lesion indicates clear fluid or blood accumulation. Red or purple translucent lesion indicates blood accumulation.

Transmissible is the term which denotes a capacity of a lesion to maintain an infectious agent in successive passages through a susceptible host.

Transmission refers to the spread of disease from one person to another by various model such as saliva air, contact with contaminated instrument etc. of disease through saliva is low. Herpes virus may secrete into saliva. Coxsakie virus is also a latent infection and has a risk of transmission of virus through dental clinic.

Transosseous wiring is a type of intermaxillary fixation with osteosynthesis where direct wiring is done across the fracture line in order to achieve effective immobilization of the fracture of the body of the mandible including angle. The holes are drilled in the bone ends of both the sides of the fracture line and the soft stainless steel wire is passed through the holes across the fracture. After achieving the accurate reduction the free ends of the wires are twisted together and tucked in to a nearest hole. Achieving osteosynthesis by wiring has an advantage of requiring minimal equipment and can be used for many types of mandibular fractures.

Transplantation of organs refers to a removal of a viable and healthy organ and placing it into another body where the existing organ has become diseased or dysfunctional e.g. heart, kidney, brain and liver. The viability or transplantable organs falls sharply after somatic death such as liver must be taken out within 15 minutes, a kidney within 45 minutes and a heart within an hour. After molecular death it is not feasible.

Transseptal fibres are those fibres which extend interproximally over the alveolar bone crest and get embedded into the cementum of the adjacent tooth. These fibers can be considered as a part of gingival fibers as they lack osseous attachment.

Transverse ridge is a linear elevation that crosses a surface (usually the occlusal surface).

Trauma from occlusion (TFO) can be described as when occlusal forces exceed the adaptive capacity or margins of safety of the tissues, it results in tissue injury. This resultant injury is known as trauma from occlusion.

Traumatic cyst is not a true cyst not being lined by epithelium. Expansion ceases when cyst like lesion reaches the cortical layer of bone. When roots are involved cavity may become scalloped. A thin connective tissue lines the cavity. X-ray shows smoothly outlined radiolucent area of variable size with in sclerotic border.

Traumatic fibroma refers to fibroma.

Traumatic neuroma is not a true neoplasm but is an exuberant try to repair a damaged nerve trunk. It is a hyperplasia of nerve fibers and supporting tissue. Degeneration of distal nerve after injury begins with swelling, fragmentation and disintegration of myelin sheath and axis cylinder. Oral neuroma begins with small nodule or swelling of mucosa near mental foramen. Treatment includes surgical excision of nodule along with small proximal portion of nerve involved.

Traumatic occlusion is the term used when the injury is produced by the occlusion.

Traumatic ulcer results due to physical injury such as denture irritation, an ill fitting denture or biting of the mucosa. Traumatic ulcers are usually single of variable size and round in shape. The floor will be yellow with red margins and there will not be any induration. It is covered by a white or tan fibrin clot and generally located at lateral border. It can be painful. Recurrent trauma can make it firm and elevated with rolled borders. After removing the cause ulcer may heal within 1-2 days, occasionally ulcers persist for long. Traumatic ulcers may be accidental or deliberate biting or thermal burns from hot pasty foods.

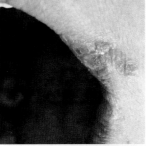

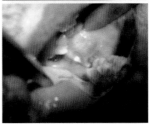

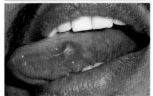

Traumatic ulcer of tongue

Treatment contract is the understanding between doctor and patient which includes frequency, number and duration of treatment.

Treatment index The 'F (filled) portion of the DMF Index best exemplifies a treatment index. In general, there are two types of dental indices. This type of dental index measures the 'number' of people affected and the 'severity' of the specific condition at a specific time or interval of time.

Treatment manual is a written material that identifies key concepts, procedure and tactic to treat a person.

Treatment plan is known as blue print for case management. It includes all the procedures required for the maintenance of oral health.

Tremor is the rhythmic oscillation of part of body around a fixed point. Tremors usually involve distal part of limb, head, tongue and rarely trunk. Tremors at rest even in lying supine are seen in parkinsonism. Essential tremors occur in anxiety, fatigue and due to alcohol while intentional tremors are seen in phenytoin toxicity, multiple sclerosis and in cerebellar disease.

Tremor of Parkinsonism consists of a rapid, rhythmic, alternating tremor. Pill rolling tremors are seen. It is usually unilateral.

Trench mouth refers acute necrotizing ulcerative gingivitis.

Trichloroethylene is a colorless volatile liquid with chloroform like smell. It is colored blue to avoid confusion with chloroform. It has a poor relaxation of skeletal muscles. It has good analgesic properties but induction and recovery are poor. Bradycardia and cardiac arrhythmias may occur.

Trichodento-osseous syndrome shows enamel defects in conjunction with morphologic dental anomalies. These patients have tightly curled kinky hair with osteosclerosis of bone cortices. The enamel is hypoplastic and hypocalcified, lacking mesiodistal contact with pitting.

Triclosan is a non-cationic antibacterial agent and has been added to several dentifrices to inhibit plaque and gingivitis. It has good antibacterial activity against Gram positive and Gram negative organisms and is compatible with anionic component of fluoride dentifrices. Two clinical studies over a 3-month period by Schiff et al (1990) and Lobene et al (1990) showed a statistically significant reduction of plaque formation.

Tricuspid regurgitation is common and most frequently occuring as a result of right ventricular dialatations. It may occur with right ventricular and inferior myocardial infarction. Symptoms and signs of tricuspid regurgitation are identical to those resulting from right ventricular failure of any cause. Symptoms are usually non specific and relate to reduced forward flow and venous congestion pansystolic murmur and systolic pulsation of liver.

Tricuspid stenosis is usually rheumatic in origin. It is suspected when right heart failure is marked with liver enlargement, ascites and dependent edema. Acquired tricuspid stenosis needs valvotomy.

Trifurcation is forked or divided into three parts.

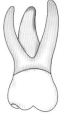

Trifurction

Trigeminal nerve is a fifth cranial nerve that contains both sensory and motor fibres. It is the largest and has 3 branches –(i) Ophthalmic nerve is purely sensory and is the smallest division. It divides into three branches lacrimal, frontal and nasociliary nerve. It supplies cornea, skin of forehead, scalp, eyelids, nose and also the mucus membrane of paranasal sinuses.(ii) Maxillary branch is purely sensory. It leaves the skull through foramen rotundum. It supplies skin over face over maxilla and the upper lip, teeth of upper jaw, mucus membrane of nose, maxillary air sinus and palate. (iii) Mandibular division is a mixed branch and is the largest branch. Motor part supplies muscles of mastication. Sensory supply is to skin of cheek, skin over mandible, lower lip and side of head, teeth of lower jaw, mucus membrane of mouth and anterior 2/3rd of tongue.

Trigeminal neuralgia is the most painful affliction of mankind. A single branch may be affected without affecting other branch. It is an intermittent brief, laminating pain in face. It is evoked by facial movement or by touching the skin. Pain is sudden, excruciating and brief like the stabbing. Peripheral receptors are not hyperalgesic. Pain does not extend outside area supplied by trigeminal nerve. The trigger may occur from light touch or movement of same receptor areas. Pain is usually unilateral and remains in the anatomical distribution of affected nerve. Typically individual pains are paroxysms of hot, shocking, burning or electric like lasting from a few seconds to several minutes. They may be repeated so frequently that pain becomes continuous. Paresthesia and motor symptoms are generally absent. No sensory loss is detected. No specific cause is known. Progressive degeneration and demyelination of trigeminal ganglion is seen. Secondary trigeminal neuralgia can result due to intracranial tumor, and vascular malformation, CNS lesions involving trigeminal

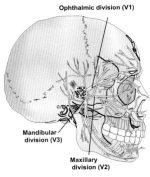

Ophthalmic division (V1)

Mandibular
division (V3)

Maxillary
division (V2)

Trigeminal nerve

pathways. Trigeminal neuralgia due to multiple sclerosis may have bilateral facial pain. There may be hypoesthesia too. In both cases carbamazpiene and GABA are used. Phenytoin in doses of 400 mg/day reduces the dose of carbamazepiene.

Trismus is a spasm of the muscles of mastication that results in difficulty in opening of mouth. Intraoral injections may result it.

Triturate is to mix together.

Trochlear nerve is a motor nerve, cranial nerve number four. It assists in turning eye ball downward and laterally. It emerges from posterior surface of mid brain. It enters the orbit through the superior orbital fissure (*see* Figure).

Tropic ulcer is found at anaesthetic sites. Injury may be mechanical and thermal. First and fifth metatarsals are commonly affected. There may be spontaneous blister or nodule. Ulcer may become infected. Deep tissues and bone may be involved. Floor of ulcer is covered by brownish tenacious and foul swelling slough. Surrounding skin is edematous regional lymph nodes may be enlarged and tender.

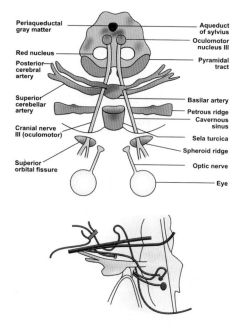

Trochlear nerve

True oral malodor Halitosis is most often a consequence of oral bacterial activity typically arising from anaerobes due to poor oral hygiene, gingivitis (ANUG), periodontal disease, infected extraction sockets, oral sepsis, residual blood postoperatively, debris under fixes or removable appliances, ulcers and dry mouth.

Tubercle is a small, rounded projection.

Tuberculin test was discovered by Von Pirquet in 1907. A positive reaction to test is accepted as evidence of past or present infection by M Tuberculosis. It is done to test in population.

Tuberculin type hypersentivity was originally, described by Koch in patients with TB who had fever and generalized sickness, following a spontaneous injection of tuberculin, a lipoprotein antigen from tubercle bacillus. 12 hrs after Intradermal tuberculosis challenge, T-lymphocytes are present at perivascular sites and this infiltrate, which extends outwards and disrupts the collagen bundles of the dermis increases to a peak at 48 hrs. Cells of the macrophage lineage are probably the main APCs in tuberculin hypersensitivity. As the lesion develops, it may become a granulomatous reaction.

Tuberculoid leprosy has well defined skin lesions with raised margins and healing centers are characteristic of tuberculoid leprosy. These lesions are anesthetic to touch and pin prick. The leprae are usually not detected on skin smear examination. Microscopically lesion shows collections of epithelioid cells and Langerhan's type giant cell. Caseation is usually absent. Temperature sensation is first to be affected followed by pressure, touch and pain. Margins of lesions are elevated and superficial. Larger nerves closer to skin are enlarged. Neuritic pain, muscle dystrophy, contracture and trauma from pressure and burns are common.

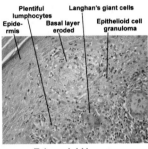

Tuberculoid leprosy

Tuberculosis is a granulomatous disease caused by acid fast bacillus. Patient may suffer from evening fever, fatigue, malaise and loss of weight. Spread is through blood or lymph TB of submaxillary and cervical lymph nodes may progress to the actual abscess. Glands are enlarged. Lesions of oral mucosa are seldom primary but secondary to pulmonary disease. Tongue is most commonly affected. Lesion is irregular, superficial or deep, painful ulcer which increases slowly. Mucosal lesions show swelling or fissuring. Tuberculous gingivitis is an unusual form of tuberculosis which produces hyperaemic, nodular or proliferative gingiva. Diffuse involvement of maxilla or mandible may occur (*see* Figure on page 462).

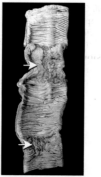

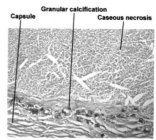

Tuberculous lymph node showing dystrophic calcification

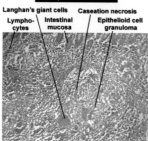

Tuberculosis of small intestine

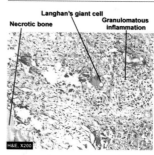

Tuberculous osteomyelitis

Tuberculous lymphadenitis is a condition where cervical glands are commonly affected. Route may be via tonsils or oral mucosa. There will be a lump in neck. It is painful. In early stage swelling is firm and mobile. Later the mass becomes fixed. Lesion may be unilateral, bilateral single or multiple (*see* Figure).

Tuberculous meningitis may develop as a consequence of miliary TB. Human tubercular bacilli are responsible. Prodromal symptoms include lassitude, weight loss and anorexia. Diffuse headache and neck stiffness develops. Mild fever appears. Patient assumes a flexed position.

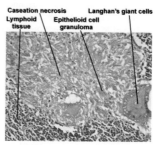

Tuberculous lymphadenitis

CSF pressure is raised. On long standing 'cob web' is formed. CSF sugar is low. Treatment is to begin with 3 anti TB drugs. Total duration of treatment is 6-9 month.

Tuberculous ulcer is caused by mycobacterium tuberculosis. It is an aerobic, slender, non motile, non spore forming, rod shaped organism. Most of people get infection in first year of life. Primary infection usually takes place in lungs. Hemoptysis, abundant sputum and pleuritic pain are very common. Tuberculous lesions of the oral cavity are secondary to pulmonary infections. Important oral lesions are tuberculous ulcers, tuberculous gingivitis, tuberculous osteomyelitis and tuberculosis of salivary gland. For tongue ulcers it is the most common site of occurrence. On lateral borders these appear either single or multiple lesions. On palate these may appear as small ulcer or granuloma. Lesions often produced are small, granulating ulcers at the mucocutaneous junction. Gingival lesions of tuberculosis usually produce granulating ulcers or erosive lesions with gingival hyperplasia.

Tuberosity is a large, rounded projection.

Tuberous sclerosis is an autosomal dominant multisystem disorder of neuroectodermal origin. Presenting feature is mental deficiency with epilepsy. Seizures develop in first decade of life. Mental retardation may be noted. Radiograph shows intracranial calcification with generalized thickening and hyperostosis of cranial vault. Multiple cortical tubers are classical findings. Metacarpals and phalanges may show subperiosteal irregular new bone formation. Small well defined cysts are seen.

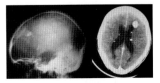

Tubercus sclerosis

Tumor necrosis factor alpha (TNF-α) shares many of its biological activities i.e. Pro-inflammatory properties, MMP stimulation, and bone resorption with IL-1. In addition, it's secretion by monocytes and fibroblast is stimulated by bacterial Lipopolysaccharide.

Tumors of brain stem present with unilateral or bilateral paralysis of cranial nerves. Crossed hemiplegia, hemianesthesia and cerebellar symptoms develop.

Turkey tests include multiple comparison procedure.

Turku sugar studies were a series of collaborative studies carried out in Turku, Finland, by Scheinin, Makinen et al. They were investigated by a comprehensive program including clinical, radiographic, biochemical, and micro-biochemical determinants of health. In addition to the massive data indicating that xylitol would be an acceptable metabolite in humans, there was a dramatic reduction in the incidence of dental caries after two years of xylitol consumption. Subsequently a 1-year chewing gum study was conducted on 102 subjects who consumed the xylitol or sucrose chewing gum but otherwise pursued their usual dietary and oral hygiene habits.

Turner's spot is an enamel hypoplasia of permanent tooth as a result of local trauma or infection of a deciduous tooth. Infection restricts work of ameloblasts and results in poorly formed enamel.

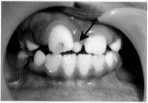

Turner's tooth

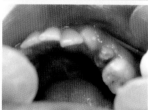

Turner's tooth involving premolar

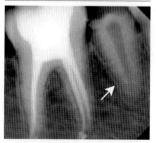

Turner's hypoplasia of premolars

Tweed's method is one of the method of performing serial extractions. It involves the extraction of the first molars around 8 years of age. This is followed by the extraction of the first premolars and the deciduous canine.

Twitch is the contraction of a muscle in response to a single action potential.

Type I hypersensitivity is characterized by an allergic reaction immediately following contact with an antigen referred to as an allergen. Allergy (coined by Von-Pirquet in 1906) is defined as the changed reactivity of the host when meeting an agent. In recent years allergy has become synonymous with Type I hypersensitivity. Dependent on the specific triggering of IgE sensitized mast cells by antigen, resulting in the release of pharmacological mediators of inflammation.

Typhoid is caused by *Salmonella Typhi*. The infection gets localized to small intestine. To start person may have headache, general body ache and malaise. Fever rises in step ladder fashion. Temperature increases every day especially in the evening. In morning fever comes down but never touches normal. It happens for 7-10 days. During the second stage patient usually looks very ill. Tongue is coated with clean tip. There will be relative bradycardia. During third week patient starts looking better. During acute stage, the organisms would be positive in first week and urine, stool culture becomes positive by second week. Widal test is positive during second week.

Tzanck cells are the epithelial cells which shows ballooning degeneration, consisting of acantholysis, nuclear clearing and nuclear enlargement. This is a histologic feature and can be appreciated only at a microscopic level.

Ulcer is a pathological condition in which there is a breakdown of epithelial tissue. There is a full thickness loss of surface epithelium with exposure to underlying connective tissue. In mouth ulcers are usually painful, except malignant one which may be initially painless. Biopsy is needed if ulcer is not responding for more than 3 weeks.

Ulceration colitis is a disease of young people between the age of 15-25 years. Symptoms range from small amount of rectal bleeding to prominent diarrhea and colonic hemorrhage with prostration. It may manifest as spondylitis, peripheral arthritis, iritis and skin disorders. Rectosigmoid colon is commonly involved.

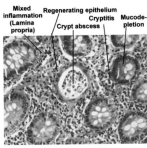

Mixed inflammation (Lamina propria) Regenerating epithelium Cryptitis Crypt abscess Mucode-pletion

Ulceration colitis

Ultimate strength is the maximum stress a solid can support based on its original cross section area.

Ultrasonic cleaning is the loosening and removal of debris from instruments by sound waves travelling through a chemical solution. It has increased efficiency in cleaning and has reduced danger of aerosolization of infectious particles released during scrubbing. Injury to instrument is lesser and is an easy process.

Ultrasonic is the conversion of high frequency electrical current into mechanical vibrations. Ultrasonic is the use of sound waves for detection and this offers considerable potential as a diagnostic instrument. Ultrasonic imaging was introduced by Ng et al. (1988) as a method for detecting early caries in smooth surfaces. With the use of this instrumentation, sonic velocity and specific acoustic impedance can be determined for the dentin and enamel as well as for the soft tissue and bone.

Ultrasonic scaler is an electronically powered device that produces vibratory motions to dislodge deposits from teeth. Commonly used scalers operate in the 5000 to 7000 cycles/second range. Most magnetostrictive ultrasonic operate at 25000-30000 cycles per second while piezo electric ultrasonic operates at 40000 to 50000 cycles/second.

Ultrasonic scaling is a use of an ultrasonic scaler to remove mineralized deposits from tooth surface.

Ultrasound – Upper limit of hearing is 20 KHz (20,000 cycles per second). Ultrasound is very much above this therapeutic frequencies being in the region of 1 MHz to 3 MHz.

Uncontrolled diabetes – Oral manifestations include multiple periodontal abscesses, velvety red gingival and marginal

U

proliferation of the periodontal tissues.

Undercut is the portion of tooth lying between the height and contour of gingiva.

Under cut cavity preparation We know that permanent filling canont be inserted directly into a cavity and preparation of cavity is required so that filling may not comeout.

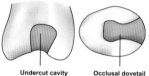

Undercut cavity   **Occlusal dovetail**

Cavity preparation for plastic fillings

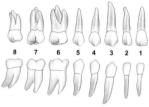

8   7   6   5   4   3   2   1

Upper and lower permanent teeth

Undermining resorption is the term used when the bone loss occurs from a healthy or viable periodontal ligament which is present adjacent to the necrotic areas.

Undifferentiated mesenchymal cells are the stem cells located in the cell-rich zone and the pulp proper which can differentiate into odontoblasts and / or fibroblasts.

Unfavorable fractures are the one where the vertical fracture or the horizontal fracture lines are opposed by the action of the muscle around them. However, these types of fractures are not so easy to reduce and stabilize.

Unicystic Ameloblastoma – There will be localized thinning and haziness of radiopaque rim. It generally occurs before the age of 30. Lesion slowly enlarges due to expansion of cortex. On palpation it is hard and bony.

Unilateral condylar neck fractures are the fractures involving the neck of the condyle and are of two types: low condylar neck fractures and high condylar neck fractures. If the fracture is undisplaced, no active treatment is required but in case of displaced fractures, dislocation will induce malocclusion. A low neck fracture can be treated by open reduction and a high condylar neck fracture with extensive displacement and malocclusion, intermaxillary fixation (IMF) is done for up to 3-4 weeks and maintained until bony union has occurred.

Unilateral extracapsular fractures refer unilateral condylar neck fractures.

Unilateral fracture usually ours on one side of the body but occasionally more than one fracture may be present. It is generally caused by direct violence.

Unilateral intracapsular fractures are the fractures occurring in the condyle. In these cases the occlusion is usually undisturbed and fracture should be treated conservatively. If malocclusion occurs the intermaxillary fixation (IMF) for 2-3 weeks is indicated.

Universal curettes are the one which can be used in most areas of the dentition by altering and adapting the finger rest and hand position of the operator. The blades of these curettes are curved in one direction.

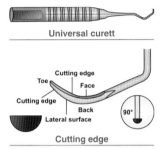

Universal curett

Cutting edge

Universal/National Numbering System is approved by the American Dental Association in 1968. Most commonly used throughout the United States. The permanent teeth are numbered from 1 to 32. Numbering begins with the upper right third molar, works around to the upper left third molar, drops to the lower left third molar, and works around to the lower right third molar. In the Universal Numbering System, the primary teeth are lettered with capital letters from A to T.

Upper lip prominence A line is drawn from subnasale (Sn) to soft-tissue pogonion (Pog'). The most prominent point of the upper lip (Ls) should be 3 ± 1mm anterior to this line.

Upper lip-lower lip-chin prominence is a vertical reference line drawn through subnasale (SnV) perpendicular to the true horizontal. The upper lip should be 1 to 2 mm ahead of this line. The lower lip should be on the line or 1 mm posterior to it. The chin (Pog') should fall within 1 to 4 mm posterior to SnV. Alternatively the distance from soft-tissue chin to a line perpendicular to FH through soft tissue nasion can be measured. This is also known as 0-degree meridian and Pog' is estimated to be 0 ± 2 mm from this line.

Uremic syndrome Early symptom of kidney failure is decreased creatinine clearance. As disease progresses glomerular filtration rate falls and blood urea nitrogen rises. Person may develop impaired ability to concentrate urine, nocturia and mild anemia. Advanced uremia is associated with pericarditis, pericardial effusion and neuropathies.

Ureter is a duct that transmits urine from kidney to bladder.

Urgency of urine is the sudden desire to void. It is seen in inflammatory conditions i.e. cystitis or neurogenic bladder.

Uric acid is the end product of purine metabolism.

Uricosuric drugs are those drugs that block tubular reabsorption of filtered urate and reduce the metabolic pool of urates, preventing the formation of new tophi. When given with colchicines these lessen the frequency of recurrence of gout.

Urinary tract obstruction – Severe obstruction can produce acute anuria, burning and pain on urination, overflow in continence or dribbling, voiding of small amount and flank pain. In secondary infection fever, chills malaise develop along with foul smelling urine.

U

Urine pregnancy test is a test that depends on the presence of human chorionic gonadotrophin in urine. Usually a concentration of about 2500 I.V. HCG per liter of urine is required to register a positive health. It usually occurs 12 days after the first missed period.

Urticaria results when antigen reaches specific skin areas causing localized anaphylactic reaction. Histamine on release results in red flare and increased permeability of capillaries resulting in swelling within a few minutes.

Useful habits include habits that are considered essential for normal function such as proper positioning of the tongue, respiration and normal deglutition.

Uterine fibroids – These are uterine leiomyoma. If large it produces a round, multinodular mass in suprapubic region. She may feel heaviness in abdomen and pressure on surrounding organs with frequency of urine. Menorrhagia develops. Edema and varicosities of lower extremities result.

Utilitarian ethics is an ethical theory based in the principle of the greatest good for the majority.

Uvula is a small muscular structure located on the free edge of soft palate. When you swallow the food it prevents your food from coming out of your nose. It directs the food down the throat into esophagus.

U

Vaccination is used to produce acquired immunity. Person can be vaccinated by injecting dead organisms which are no longer capable of causing disease but still have chemical antigen. These are used against typhoid, diphtheria, whooping cough and diphtheria. Secondly immunity can be achieved against toxins which have been treated with chemicals. These are used against tetanus and botulinism. Thirdly person can be vaccinated by infecting him with live organism that has been attenuated. These are used against polio, measles and other viral diseases.

Vagus nerve is a mixed tenth cranial nerve. Motor part supplies pharynx and larynx, bronchi and heart. Sensory fibres carry taste from epiglottis and vellecula.

Validity is the meaningfulness of test scores as they are used for specific tests.

Van Limborgh's Theory is a multifactorial theory put forward by Van Limborgh in 1970. According to van Limborgh, the three popular theories of growth were not satisfactory, yet each contains elements of significance that cannot be denied. Van Limborgh explains the process of growth and development in a view that combines all the three existing theories. He supports the functional matrix theory of Moss, acknowledged some aspects of Sicher's theory and at the same time does not rule out genetic involvement. Van Limborgh has suggested the following five factors that he believed controls growth: intrinsic genetic factors, local epigenetic factors, general epigenetic factors, local environmental factors, general environmental factors.

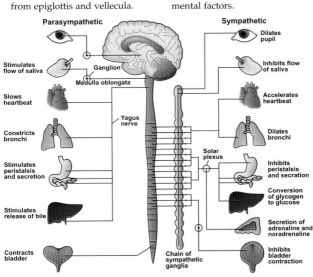

Vagus nerve

V

Inferior aspect of brain

Posterior

Vagus (X) nerve

Medulla oblongata

Heart — Lung

Liver — Spleen

Stomach — Kidney

Colon — Small intestine

Vagus nerve 10

Veneer crown is a thin gold shell used in the construction of bridges. On back teeth it covers the entire crown known as full crown. On front it covers all but the labial surface and is called three quarter crown.

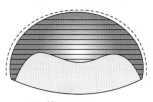

Veneer crown

Vapour pressure is a measure of liquid's tendency to evaporate. Materials with high vapor pressure at room temperature tend to evaporate readily.

Varicocele is a pampiniform plexus of veins of the spermatic cord. It is a consequence to venous stasis aided by gravity forces and prolonged standing. Intra-abdominal tumor also results increased pressure on the spermatic veins.

Varicose ulcer is a chronic ulcer of leg of insidious onset. Mostly ulcer is on medial side of leg. It is solitary. It is a shallow ulcer where floor is covered by bluish granulation tissue of pale slough. Edges are irregular and sloping. It is mobile on underlying bone. Surrounding skin is swollen and pigmented.

Varicose veins are an abnormal dilatation and tortuosity of vein especially in leg. In legs these are abnormally dilated, elongated and tortuous. Incidence increases with age. It has familial tendency. Increased intraluminal pressure leads it. Affected veins are dilated, stretched, tortuous and nodular. There is irregular thinning and atrophy of vein. Thrombosis is common. Fibrosis results in tortuousity. Intima is thickened. Valvular defect causes an important defect. Long standing cases may develop fibrosis, chronic edema and skin pigmentation. Person feels dull, aching heaviness or a feeling of fatigue.

V

Varnishes are used as thin layers but don't provide thermal insulation. These serve to isolate the tubule contents from the cavity. Several applications are needed to prevent penetration of bacteria.

Vascular dementia is the single brain lesion which doesn't lead to dementia but affects mental function. The most common type of vascular dementia is caused by multiple supra tentorial infarcts. Hypertensive small vessel disease produces predominant deep white matter infarcts.

Vasculitis describes a diverse group of inflammatory disorder characterized by multi organ vessel involvement. There develops fever, malaise, weight loss and raised WBCs and ESR.

Vasoconstrictor drugs i.e. adrenaline and noradrenaline are useful when there is an access to the bleeding site. These are effective in controlling the oozing from capillaries. These are useful in controlling gingival bleeding. It is not useful in controlling heavy hemorrhage because these are diluted and washed out.

Vasodepressor syncope refers to sudden loss of consciousness that usually occurs secondary to a period of cerebral ischemia. Predisposing factors for vasodepressor syncope are psychogenic factors such as fright, anxiety, emotional stress, pain especially sudden and unexpected, sight of blood or surgical or other dental instruments. Non psychogenic factors include sitting in an upright position which permits blood to pool in the periphery decreasing cerebral blood flow; hunger from missed meal which decrease the glucose supply to brain, exhaustion, poor physical condition and hot, humid environment.

Vasomotor syncope may be due to excessive vagal tone or impaired reflex control of peripheral circulation. Common faint is initiated by a stressful, painful or claustrophobic experience.

Vehicle is a substance possessing little or no medicinal action used as a medium to confer a suitable consistency or form.

Vein – Blood vessel carrying blood from periphery to heart.

Veneer is a layer of tooth-colored material can be porcelain, composite, or ceramics attached to the front of the tooth to improve appearance. These are bonded to enamel by means of acid etch technique with the help of resin.

Venous hemorrhage – Wound bleeds with steady flow. The lost blood is dark red or bluish. The bleeding stops by elevating the part above the level of heart.

Ventral surface of the tongue is the underside of the tongue.

Vermilion means red.

Virgin teeth are those teeth that are free from decay or restorations.

Ventricular septal defect is the persistent opening in upper interventricular septum due to failure of fusion with aortic septum. It results in blood to pass from high pressure left ventricle into low pressure right ventricle. Large defects are associated with early left ventricular failure. Many VSD defects close spontaneously in early childhood.

Verrucal resembles like a wart.

Verrucous carcinoma is diffused; non metastasing well differentiated malignant neoplasm. It mostly develops in tobacco chewing patients. It is exophytic and papillary in nature. Commonest site involved is gingiva, alveolar mucosa and buccal mucosa. Surface of the lesion shows multiple deep clefts. Lesion may be single or multiple involving different parts of buccal mucosa. Pain may develop making chewing difficult. It becomes rapidly fixed to underlying bone. Regional lymph nodes are often enlarged. Malignant epithelial cells are usually well differentiated. Pain and difficulty in mastication are chief complaints. Anaplastic transformation occurs.

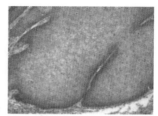
Verrucous carcinoma high power

Vertebral compression fracture it may result due to osteoporosis by bending, lifting, coughing or sneezing. There develops acute, severe pain at fracture site. Pain may radiate anteriorly to flank. Pain is typically worse in up right position. Signs include spinal tenderness over fractured spine along with paravertebral muscle spasm. Kyphosis and loss of height will develop. Weakness, sensory deficits incontinence or diminished deep reflexes develop.

Vertebral osteophytes occur due to repeated damage to the posterior joints especially lead to degenerative changes. It is a true osteo arthritic change and lipping of vertebra may take place.

Vertical bone loss is also known as angular bone loss. It does not occur in plane parallel to cementoenamel junction.

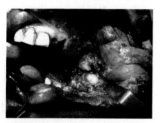
Operative photo of verrucous carcinoma of upper gingivo-buccal sulcus1

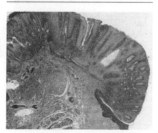
Verrucous carcinoma

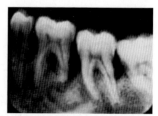
Verticle bone loss

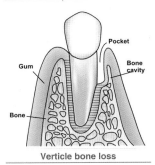

Verticle bone loss

Vertical defects are those bony defects of alveolar process which occur in an oblique direction, leaving a hollowed out trough in the bone alongside the root.

Vesibulocochlear nerve is the eighth cranial nerve consisting of two sets of sensory fibres vestibular and cochlear. Vestibular fibres are concerned with equilibrium. Cochlear fibres are concerned with hearing.

Vibration – Vibrations in the range of 10 to 500 Hz may be encountered in work of drills and hammer. After some months the fine blood vessels of fingers may become increasingly sensitive to spasm i.e. white fingers.

Vibrio cholerae is a microorganism that causes cholera. Their natural habitat is water. Watery diarrhea can be fatal. It is a gram negative slender bacilli, comma shaped with pointed ends. It is highly motile with single flagellum. It is seen under dark field microscopy.

Vimentin is the type of filament that is expressed in mesenchymal cells such as fibroblasts, and in endothelial cells. These fibres often end at the nuclear membrane and desmosomes. They are closely associated with micro-tubules, and they form cages around lipid droplets in adipose tissue.

Vincent's angina is an ulcerative infection of mouth and throat with enlarged lymph glands, pain and fever. Streptococcal sore throat also produces exudative membrane in throat. Throat becomes sore and extremely painful. Pharynx may show edema and reddening.

Vipeholm dental study was a 5-year investigation of 436 adult inmates in a mental institution at the Vipetional Hospital near Lund, Sweden. The dental caries rate in the inmates was relatively low. The experimental design divided the inmates into seven groups; sugar was introduced either at mealtime. The main conclusions of the study were as follows: An increase in carbohydrate definitely increases the caries activity. The risk of caries is greater if the sugar is consumed in a form that will be retained on the surfaces of teeth.The risk of sugar increasing caries activity is greatest if the sugar is consumed between meals and in a form that tends to be retained on the surfaces of the teeth. The increase in caries activity varies widely between individuals. Upon withdrawal of the sugar-rich foods, the increased caries activity rapidly disappears. Caries lesions may continue to appear despite the avoidance of refined sugar and maximum restrictions of natural sugars and dietary carbohydrate.A high concentration of sugar in solution and its prolonged retention of tooth surfaces leads to increased caries activity. The clearance time of the sugar correlates closely with caries activity.

Viperine snake bite – local symptoms are persistent pain but salivation is rare. There is no paralysis of respiratory organs as in cobra bite. It produces extensive inflammation with cellulitis, discoloration and incessant oozing of hemolysed blood from the punctured point. Signs of collapse may be seen. Pupils are dilated and not reacting to light. There will be multiple hemorrhages, epistaxis, hematuria, hemoptysis and petechial hemorrhages. There may be complete unconsciousness. Death takes place due to cardiac failure within 1-2 days.

Viral fever is caused by influenza virus. Transmission is through inhalation of infected nasopharyngeal secretions.

Viral hepatitis viral hepatitis is an acute parenchymal necrotizing lesion where liver cell necrosis of hepatitis includes agents A, B, C, D, E, etc. During active disease one develops fever, nausea, vomiting fatigue, anorexia, headache and chills. There will be disturbance of taste. One can develop pruritic rash, arthritis and altered mental status. Urine will be dark and stools will be clay colored. Liver will be enlarged and tender.

Viral infection – Mumps is caused by a paramyxovirus. It may complicate gonads, CNS, pancreas and myocardium. Clinical features include sudden fever, malaise and anorexia. To start one sided parotid gland is involved then second is involved.

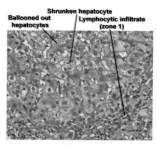
Viral hepatitis

Parotid gland enlarges for 2-3 days and return to normal within seven days. Submandibular gland may also be involved. Most of the causes are self limiting within a week. In some children meningitis or encephalitis may develop. Antibiotics and cortisone avoid complications.

Viral oral ulcer may be primary herpetic gingivostomatitis. Virus is transmitted by saliva and direct contact. Primary infection is subclinical. Multiple oral ulcers will result in painful gums, tongue and sore throat. Lips may be crushed with blood. Swallowing, eating, talking will be painful. Fever, nausea and vomiting may develop. Initially develop as vesicles which rupture later on. Ulcers are multiple and size is 2 to 3 mm.

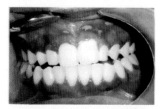
Herpetic gingivostomatitis

V

Causes of Malformed Permanent Teeth

- Infective   Congenital syphilis
- Metabolic   Rickets
                      Hypothyroidism
- Drugs   Tetracycline
- Fluorosis genetic   Dentigenesis imperfecta
                      Dental dysplasia
                      Odontodysplasia

Quality of Carcinogenic Bacteria

- It is to be acidogenic and can produce pH <5
- It should be able to decalcify tooth substance
- It should be able to adhere to smooth surface
- It should be able to produce adhesive isoluble plaque polysaccharides.

Stages of forMation of Plaque

- Deposition of salivary glycoprotein
- Bacterial action precipitating salivary proteins
- Colonization of S. sanguis and S mutans in 24 hours
- Progressive build up of plaque by bacterial polysaccharides.

Important Biopsy Principles

- Choose red area when premalignancy is suspected
- Avoid necrotic, slough area
- Dont give local anesthesia in lesion/mass
- Always include normal tissue margin
- For large areas many samples may be collected.
- Suture and control any bleeding.

Different Oral Pigmentations

i. Brown/black pigmentation
    Malignant melanoma
    Pigmented naevi
    Addision's disease
ii. Purple or red pigmentation
    Hemangioma
    Purpura
    Lingual varices
    Giant cell euplis

Oral Diseases in HIV Cases

- Viral
  Herpes simplex
  Leukoplakia

- Bacterial
  HIV associated gingivitis
  Necrotising gingivitis
- Fungal
  Thrush
- Tumor
  Kaposis sarcoma
- Enlarged glands.

Sweetness/Cariogenicity

Sweetness	Cariogenicity
• Sucrose	Highly cariogenic
• Glucose/fructose	Less cariogenic
• Lactose/galactose	Less cariogenic
• Glucose syrups	Less cariogenic than sugar
• Sorbitol/manitol	Non cariogenic
• Saccharin	Non sugar sweetness
Aspartame	Non cariogenic
Cyclamate	